A History of
Transplantation Immunology

A History of
Transplantation Immunology

Leslie Brent BSc PhD FInst Biol Hon MRCP
Emeritus Professor of Immunology
St Mary's Hospital Transplant Unit
Paddington, London, UK

ACADEMIC PRESS

San Diego   London   Boston
New York   Sydney   Tokyo   Toronto

Academic Press, Inc.
525 B Street, Suite 1900, San Diego, California 92101–4495, USA

Academic Press Limited
24–28 Oval Road, London NW1 7DX, UK

ISBN 0–12–131770–6

Library of Congress Cataloging-in-Publication Data
A history of transplantation immunology / by Leslie Brent.
p. cm.
Includes index.
ISBN 0–12–131770–6 (alk. paper)
1. Transplantation immunology – History.   I. Title.
[DNLM. 1. Transplantation Immunology.   2. Allergy and Immunology –
history.   3. Transplantation – history.   4. Allergy and Immunology –
biography.   WO 11.1 B839h 1996]
QR188.8.B74 1996
617.9'5 – dc20
DNLM/DLC
for Library of Congress   96-36685
                                                              CIP

A catalogue record for this book is available from the British Library

Typeset by Florencetype Ltd, Stoodleigh, Devon
Printed and bound in Great Britain by
Biddles Ltd, Guildford and King's Lynn

97 98 98 99 00 01 02 EB 9 8 7 6 5 4 3 2 1

Cover
The author and the publishers would like to thank the following for
use of the images on the cover:

Front cover:
Diagrammatic representation of IgG antibody molecule (left). Structure of
the human histocompatibility molecule HLA–A2 (centre) (courtesy of
Dr P.J. Bjorkman and Macmillan Magazines Ltd for the use of figure 2a in
Nature 329, p. 509). Kidney undergoing acute cellular rejection (right)
(courtesy of Professor K.A. Porter). Tolerant mouse carrying
a healthy allogenic skin graft
(main picture).

Back cover:
Small blood lymphocyte (top). Scanning electronmicrograph
of B lymphocyte (bottom)

Contents

Preface

"I should have liked to produce a good book. This has not come about, but the time is past in which I could improve it."

L.J.J. Wittgenstein

Preface to *Philosophical Investigations*, 1953

"Writing a good book about it is a good way to learn immunology, but I cannot recommend it to anyone as a pleasant way to pass the afternoons."

J. Klein

Preface to *Immunology: The Science of Self–Nonself Discrimination*, 1982

Like other academics I have read and examined numerous PhD and MD theses. Regardless of their quality I have often been struck by the candidates' ignorance of the historical background to their studies. This has always concerned me, for I believe that a full understanding of the present requires a knowledge of past ideas and discoveries. If scientists knew the history of their science perhaps there would be fewer instances of rediscovering the wheel. That apart, historical developments – in immunology as in any other branch of learning – are bound to be of interest and a source of insight and often of wonder to the modern practitioner.

This thinking led me to my decision to write a history of transplantation immunology six years ago, and I was delighted to find an encouraging response from Academic Press. I was well aware that for someone like myself who has been an active participant during the second half of the twentieth century there are drawbacks and pitfalls in such a venture, and I became even more acutely aware of this as I proceeded. Compared with a professional historian it is probably more difficult to maintain objectivity and to discard any prejudices or preconceived notions. If my account has deficiencies – and I know that it has – it will at least enable a professional historian to write a more definitive account, if indeed there can be such a thing. However, I would at the same time like to think that my close involvement over the last four to five decades enables me to provide an extra dimension.

I decided from the outset that I would want to make this history as up to date as possible. This has unquestionably complicated my task, and it leaves me open to the more than plausible charge that I have at times misjudged the importance of recent discoveries. Nonetheless it is my hope that by bringing the story (or the many stories) right up to the present time this book will prove to be especially useful and of interest to those for whom it is primarily intended. Had I ignored the last two decades or so a variety of exciting new developments would have been left in limbo – for example, the structure and function of the histocompatibility antigens, the sophisticated analysis of graft rejection mechanisms with monoclonal antibodies, and some interesting ideas on immunoregulation in adult life.

During the preparation of this book I have come to realize that there are several approaches I could have followed. For example, I could have focused primarily on only the giants in the field. Although this would have simplified my task and made the book more digestible it would be comparable to writing a history of England based entirely on the actions and thoughts of the kings and queens, without considering the aspirations and interventions of their subjects and the social milieu prevailing at the time. Similarly, although Hitler and Stalin were the dominant personalities of the twentieth century – both it so happens to the detriment of the world – they would not have succeeded (or nearly succeeded) to realize their ambitions without countless and diverse allies, and they themselves were products of the social, economic and political milieu of their time. Likewise, I was persuaded during the course of my research that remarkably few discoveries in transplantation immunology failed to have some sort of antecedent. Those that did not include Gorer's discovery of the first histocompatibility antigens of the mouse (though the human blood groups had already been well described) and Owen's demonstration of a naturally occurring form of tolerance in cattle dizygotic twins. Most other important findings arose from the scientific climate of their time. Furthermore, most would probably have been made sooner or later by someone other than the persons whose names are associated with them, and quite a few were made more or less simultaneously in more than one laboratory. I therefore decided to write not only about the generals but also about the foot soldiers who made the whole thing possible.

Another approach would have been to dwell only on ideas, to the detriment of the step-by-step progress made by experimental studies. That would clearly have been M. Cohn's preference, for he is impatient with the trials and errors that "are coupled to the lingering and unheralded death of that which is no longer heuristic or correct" (Cohn, M. 1994 *Annu. Rev. Immunol* **12**, 3). He went on to say that "The leading contributors of ideas in immunology have been empiricists in theoreticians' clothing." This is illustrated by Mitchison who wrote: "Cohn makes an eloquent case for large theories. Personally I prefer small ones, perhaps mostly from habit. They may not be the currency of Nobel prizes, but they are the familiar coinage of everyday science, and they provide the excitement that keeps us going on dull afternoons... An unattractive feature of large theories is that they force us to discard a great deal of perfectly respectable benchwork... In contrast, small theories invite us to confess our ignorance, by focusing attention on the gaps which they leave unexplained," (Mitchison, N.A. 1990 In *Cell to Cell Interactions*, ed. M.M. Burger, B. Sordat and R.M. Zinkernagel, pp. 232–234, Karger, Basel)." My history will make it clear that I tend to side with Mitchison.

A point of interest is the dichotomy between how individuals perceive their roles in the historical process and how the historian comes to assess them. I sent part of a chapter to one early worker who had made a large contribution to the development of the topic in question, hoping for some constructive comments. The gist of the reply was that he felt that I had done him "scant justice", an accusation that I found both upsetting and hard to credit. This anecdote illustrates that the contribution of many scientists seen in its historic context is not always commensurate with the towering achievement it may have seemed at the time it was made, or even when viewed in retrospect by the individual him- or herself. Even P.B. Medawar, who was one of the most dominant intellectual and experimental figures in transplantation immunology from the mid-1940s, often had indications (however tenuous) from the work of others before him that he was ploughing a worthwhile furrow. Indeed, it is fascinating that someone like the American tumor biologist J.B. Murphy, working in the first three decades of the twentieth century, came astonishingly close to realizing that small lymphocytes play a role in graft rejection.

Who, then, do I expect to want to read this book or to use it selectively for reference? It is definitely not written for the layperson, but it should be of interest to anyone working in the wider field of transplantation such as surgeons, physicians, pathologists, geneticists, immunologists, and biologists. This includes those studying tumor immunology as tumor biologists have certainly contributed to the development of transplantation. I would go so far as to say that I believe it should be required reading for any young person entering the field and this would ensure that future PhD theses would be historically less benighted than in the past. Furthermore, any clinician with a reasonable background in immunology should be able to derive some benefit from dipping into its pages.

Having researched and written the book entirely on my own I cannot blame others for its imperfections. Any errors or omissions have been made in good faith and I plead for the reader's indulgence. I have no hesitation in associating myself with the two quotations at the head of this Preface! Perhaps I should add that I enjoyed writing the biographical sketches interspersed in the book because they gave me the opportunity to learn a great deal about a diverse group of people. However, I went through much heart-searching in deciding upon which 20 individuals (all, alas, men) to include, and there are others I would like to have included. My choice can be defended in that all of them have made major original contributions to the development of transplantation.

Finally, I wish to acknowledge how immensely grateful I am to Ray Owen, who made such a seminal contribution to the discovery of immunologic tolerance half a century ago, for having so readily agreed to peruse the manuscript and for writing the Foreword.

Leslie Brent
London, May 1996

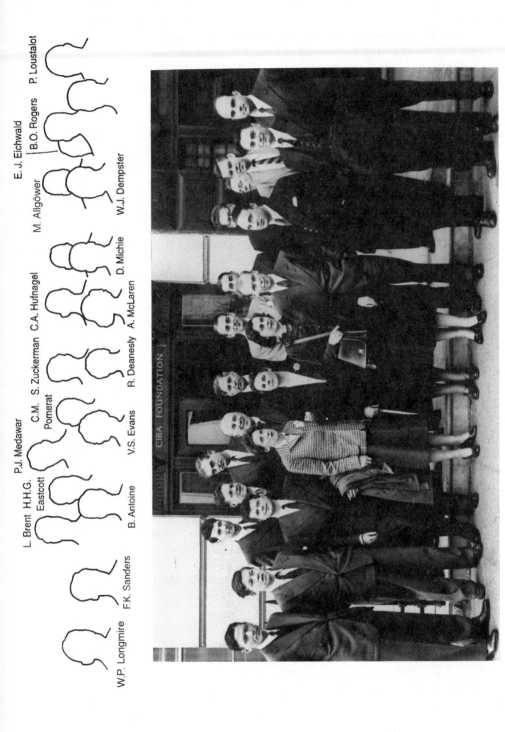

L. Brent H.H.G. P.J. Medawar   E. J. Eichwald
          Eastcott C.M. S. Zuckerman C.A. Hufnagel M. Allgöwer B.O. Rogers P. Loustalot
                    Pomerat   W.J. Dempster

W.P. Longmire F.K. Sanders B. Antoine V.S. Evans R. Deanesly A. McLaren D. Michie

Some participants at the Ciba Foundation on the Preservation of Normal Tissues for Transplantation, London, March 1953. (Not all have been identified or with certainty. Courtesy of the Ciba foundation).

Foreword

Immunology has its roots in concern for infectious disease: protection, recovery, and immunity. To understand the specificity of recognition and response in the immune system and its quality of memory has been a primary challenge for basic studies, and to control responses for useful effect has been an objective for adaptive research. It early became evident that a system capable of generating responses to external threats needed to evolve ways of avoiding or subduing the dangers of reaction to "self" potential immunogens. Transplantation research took the lead in defining that concept.

Approaches to understanding the immune system have been undertaken at all levels, at first the organismal and interactions among organisms at the population level, later the physiological, cellular and molecular levels. Vocabularies developed to suit accurate and concise communication among specialists within each of the various levels. Intercommunication among areas became difficult, and new associations developed outside the historic field as immunology came to illuminate other intellectual territories – genetics, molecular recognition, cell signalling pathways, cell–cell interactions, programmed cell death, somatic cell commitment and differentiation and other riddles of developmental biology, phylogeny and evolution.

At intervals, thoughtful people are impelled to take stock of science or of one of its branches, to ask where we are, how we got here, and where we are going. For some the future has seemed uninviting; compare, for example, the *Golden Age* perceived in 1969, when "the field has now lost its appeal for the kind of person who is driven to explore uncharted territory. Scholars and technologists replace the knights-errant and work out the details,"[1] with *The End of Science*, as foreseen in 1996.[2] Immunology has had its share of such philosophy. In 1967 we were told that we were on the brink of the final solution, *Waiting for the End*[3]; in 1969, ". . . what scientists will be doing during the following thousand years. In fact, they will be doing nothing, because all scientific knowledge worth knowing will be known."[4] And in a 1996 review, "Having solved the problem of the molecular basis of specificity immunology reached the end of its history . . . a state of such maturity that the time has come to seek out its intellectual roots."[5] At the end, it seems, little remains but history.

So far, none of the apocalyptic predictions has turned out to be true, either for science in general or particularly for immunology. Our science flourishes as we gain an ability to ask new and more searching questions, to seek and achieve new insights, to set new goals. Our students, and their students in turn for unforeseeable generations will be confronted with a world, not where everything worth knowing is known, but where they will continue to enjoy exploring frontiers to which we see no end.

Among the territories within our immunology frontiers none is more fertile, more inviting for the future, than transplantation. Recognized only within our lifetime as a legitimate aspect of immunology, it has both contributed to and profited from advances in other components of our science. Its prehistory is long and provocative; its development is a succession of primary discoveries, each usually followed by streams, waves, floods, avalanches, and explosions (to borrow a few of the terms used by the author of this history) of papers, by advances and retreats, discoveries forgotten and rediscovered, confirmations and denials. Our author's aim, "to be objective in matters of controversy", is on the whole admirably realized. One can count almost 3000 citations in his manuscript. Some of these are listed for more than one chapter, but obviously he has provided a fine resource, bringing together critically so large and select a collection. And the references are much more useful than a series of simple citations; they include selected direct quotations conveying the essence of contributions, many conference summaries, recollections and reviews. Through all the detail, the threads of the fabric remain intact, to repay study not only by the transplantaters to come, but for anyone approaching from another part of the field of immunology as well. And scholars outside our science can learn from this work much of how our field began, developed right up to the present day, and holds promise for the future.

A more subjective, human aspect of objective science is outlined in the twenty biographical sketches included with the successive chapters. They often reflect personal acquaintances of the author, an experienced participant in the history, and require little comment here except to note an important omission. The author himself deserves a place among twenty-one. A sketch of his life and contributions would be among the most valuable of the collection. As to his contributions, the reader can glean from the text and citations that he has been a leader in transplantation research and immunology over the whole of its modern history. As to his life, an account of it would be as inspiring as any in his collection. Happily, like our science, it isn't over yet.

And as to our science, as we learn more about our complex system with its many checks and balances our perceptions tend to become increasingly complicated, comprehensible only to the initiate, often only to those in the sub-field in which they are absorbed. Can we hope that beneath the complexity there is a set of principles subject to simple statement that almost everyone has a chance of understanding? If and when immunology reaches that point we might be willing to grant that it has "matured." Meanwhile, and even then, there will be much to be learned, and in the learning a guarantee of continuing wonder.

RD Owen

Emeritus Professor of Biology
California Institute of
Technology
July 1996

References

1. Stent, Gunther (1969). *The Coming of the Golden Age. A View of the End of Progress.* New York: The Natural History Press.
2. Hogan, John (1996). *The End of Science. Facing the Limits of Knowledge* in *The Twilight of the Scientific Age.* Reading, Massachusetts: Addison-Wesley.
3. Jerne, Niels (1967). "Summary: Waiting for the End." *Cold Spring Harbor Symposia on Quantitative Biology* v. XXXII, pp. 591-603.
4. Jerne, Niels (1969). "The Complete Solution of Immunology." *Australian Annals of Medicine* 4: 345-348.
5. Rosen, Fred S. (1996). "The End of History." *Nature* 379: 36.

Dedication

I dedicate this book to all those, whether or not they appear in its pages, who have furthered the cause of tissue and organ transplantation, making it an intellectually challenging and exciting science and a highly successful life-saving art; and to Milo.

Acknowledgements

I would like to express my grateful thanks to the many who have helped me in one way or another in the preparation of this book. Their help has varied from reading and commenting on chapters to advice on specific issues, familiarizing me with the Word Processor or sending and receiving numerous FAX messages. For fear that some of my fellow immunologists might be blamed for errors and omissions I will refrain from identifying those who have looked at specific chapters!

First and foremost I wish to thank three groups associated with St Mary's Hospital or its Medical School, without whom I could not have contemplated such an audacious enterprise. With great foresight members of my former Department of Immunology, in particular Dr Anthony Pinching, Mr Alan Bain and Mrs Jill Bridges, provided me with the electronic equipment and some other resources without which I would certainly have failed in my task. Dr David Taube most generously made available an office in his Transplant Unit despite an acute shortage of space and I warmly thank him and his colleagues for putting up with me for rather longer than they or I had anticipated. I also wish to acknowledge the sustained and excellent assistance I have had from the School Library staff – Mr Nigel Palmer, Ms Sally Smith, Ms Rachel Shipton, Ms Dinah Akan and Ms Sue Stoter – and to thank them for permitting me to use the library out of hours whenever necessary.

Librarians are a special breed – knowledgeable, devoted to their profession and unfailingly courteous – and those working in other London libraries, especially at the Royal Society of Medicine, University College and the British Library Science Reference and Information Service have also been a great help, as have Ms Elizabeth Allan, the Qvist Curator of the Hunterian Museum and Ms Josephine Marshall, librarian of the Walter and Eliza Hall Research Institute in Melbourne.

Others whose help it is a pleasure to acknowledge are: Ms Jessica Allwood, Dr Barbara Bain, Prof. Clyde Barker, Prof. Richard Batchelor, Prof. Ruth Bellairs, Ms Deborah Birrell, Dr Tom Cairns, Dr Philip Chandler, Dr Frank Billett, Prof. Rupert Billingham, Dr David Billington, Ms Mieke van Dam, Dr Douglas Darcy, Mr Julian Dye, Dr David Evans, Prof. John Fabre, Prof. Frank Fenner, members of the Finance Department of the Medical School, Dr Lawrence Goldberg, Mrs Elizabeth Gorer, Prof. Claus Hammer, Mr John Handford, Dr Vera Hašková, Dr Marta Hašková, Dr Vladimir Holáň, Prof. N. Hughes Jones, Mrs Joyce Johnson, Dr Nathan Kaliss, Prof. S. Kennaway, Dr Gerry Klaus, Prof. Robert Lechler, Prof. David Linch, London Borough of Islington, Dr Ian Mackay, Dr Keith Nye, Dr Steven Mackinnon, Ms Anne-Marie Meyer, Prof. P.L. Mollison, Prof. P.J. Morris, Prof. James Mowbray, Mrs Pauline Murfet, Prof. Ray Owen, Dr Mike Owen, Mr N.R. Parrott, Prof. F.T. Rapaport, Dr M. Rauscherová, Dr Ken Reid, Ms Greta Riley, Dr Ian Sargent, Dr Arthur Silverstein, Prof. Morten Simonsen, Prof. Elizabeth Simpson, Dr Fiona Smith, Dr George Snell, St Mary's Hospital and Medical School, Prof. Tom Starzl,

Dr David Steinmuller, Prof. Rainer Storb, Prof. Wayne Streilein, Mrs Dorothy Thomas, Prof. Erik Thorsby, Prof. John Turk, Dr Jenny Underwood, Dr Håkan Widmer, Dr Arthur Wild and Prof. Michael Woodruff.

My special thanks go to my editor, Dr Tessa Picknett, without whose patience and faith in me I would have abandoned this project long ago, and to the Academic Press production team, particularly Ms Manjula Goonawardena, for processing the book so quickly.

Finally, I wish to thank my wife Carol for her constant encouragement and support and her steadfast willingness to forego my company on many an evening and weekend.

A Note on Nomenclature

Grafts transplanted from one individual to another of the same species were called, until the early 1960s, homografts or homologous grafts, or even homoiografts. Those transplanted between species were described as heterografts or heterologous grafts. Grafts transplanted to another part of the same individual were autografts and, within the same inbred strain, isografts, first used by G.D. Snell (1).

In 1960 P.A. Gorer (2) published a wittily written critique of these terms, in his article entitled "Transplantese". He pointed out that immunologists used the terms homologous and heterologous in quite different senses and made some suggestions as to how matters could be improved. A year later, together with J.F. Loutit (who clearly had had a classical education!) and H.S. Micklem (3), he fleshed out his proposals. In 1964 G.D. Snell (4) proposed a modified terminology, having felt that despite the previous attempts to introduce sanity into the nomenclature of transplantation "the confusion has not been ablated", with investigators using a variety of terms. Snell's proposals, which he framed following a ballot of leading workers and which were quickly accepted by transplanters, were as follows:

- Homografts would become allografts, or allogeneic grafts, and the term "homologous" was to be abandoned.
- Autograft (or autogeneic or autogenous graft) would stay.
- Isogeneic would replace isologous or isogenic, with syngeneic as an alternative.
- Xenograft (or xenogeneic graft) would replace heterograft and heterologous.
- The term histocompatibility would relate to "the growth or failure to grow of tissue or tumor transplants".
- Histocompatible would denote "a relationship between the genotype of donor and host such that a graft cannot be resisted".

I have adhered to the old terminology whenever quoting directly from the older literature but, apart from this I have consistently used the new terms.

References

1. Snell, G.D. (1953) In *The Physiopathology of Cancer*, p. 338, P.B. Hoeber Inc., New York.
2. Gorer, P.A. (1960) *Ann. N.Y. Acad. Sci.* 87, 604.
3. Gorer, P.A., Loutit, J.F. & Micklem, H.S. (1961) *Nature* 189, 1024.
4. Snell, G.D. (1964) *Transplantation* 2, 655.

1 Landmarks in Immunology

*"I have given reasons for believing that the only possible
type of approach is by a 'selective' theory of immunity which must be
developed on a cellular, and probably a clonal, basis."*

F.M. Burnet, 1961

As emphasized in the preface, this book is not a history of immunology, which is a topic of immensely greater scope than transplantation immunology. That has been admirably told and analyzed by A.M. Silverstein (1) in *A History of Immunology*, published in 1989. Silverstein, a developmental and ocular immunologist who became a full-time historian, has written with special felicity and insight about seminal theories and experimental observations up to the seventh decade of the twentieth century and the scientists who initiated them. A complementary historical text that uses a very different approach, singling out many pioneers and presenting their most influential publications in detail is *Milestones in Immunology. A Historical Exploration* by D.J. Bibel (2). Another history is that of A.M. Moulin, *Le Dernier Langage de la Médicine. Histoire de l'Immunologie de Pasteur au Sida* (3), though there is not as yet an English translation. Multi-author texts include those edited by P.M.H. Mazumdar (4) and by R.B. Gallagher, J. Gilder, G.J.V. Nossal and G. Salvatore (5); the former is largely based on papers presented at the Sixth International Congress of Immunology held in Berlin in 1986, and the latter on contributions to the eighth course of the International School of Biological Sciences organized in 1992 by the Stazione Zoologica "Anton Dohrn" in Naples. Preceding all these by several decades is the succinctly written historical introduction to the textbook *Immunology for Medical Students*, first published in 1963 by J.H. Humphrey and R.G. White (6), while many historic aspects are explored in J. Klein's (7) vast tome entitled *Immunology. The Science of Self–Nonself Discrimination*.

Nonetheless it is important for the reader of this volume to be reminded of the events heralding the dawn of immunology and of the immunologic milieu in which transplantation and transplantation immunology have flourished during the twentieth century. I have therefore highlighted in this introductory chapter some of the landmarks in immunology that have profoundly influenced the development of transplantation immunology, even though many of them are also referred to in other chapters. Here, no attempt has been made to trace the development of any one topic; instead, the aim has been to identify the seminal papers that opened up a field in terms of either theoretic development or experimental investigation.

The Great Early Pioneers

Vaccination

The momentous activities of the great pioneers working in the two decades on either side of the beginning of the twentieth century have been well described in the above-mentioned historical texts (1–7). L. Pasteur, the giant of early bacteriology and immunotherapy, is often described as the father of immunology (8), but vaccination was practised long before his lifetime, at a time when nothing was known of the disease-causing organisms. According to J. Needham, the eminent British biochemist who immersed himself in the study of Chinese culture and science, a primitive form of smallpox vaccination was used in China from the tenth century (9). It was also used in the thirteenth century in Egypt, according to Fenner *et al.* (10) in their definitive and exhaustive tome on *Smallpox and its Eradication*. Voltaire (11), in his engaging letters, credits Lady Mary Wortley Montagu, the wife of the English Ambassador in Constantinople and who had been left pockmarked from smallpox in 1715 (12), with having encountered smallpox vaccination in Circassia; here children of the wealthy were frequently protected against the disease by inoculation of material taken from "a pustule taken from the most regular, and at the same time the most favorable, sort of smallpox that could be procured". Indeed, so impressed was this lady that on her return to London in 1718 she had her six-year-old son inoculated in likewise fashion (13). Silverstein (14) relates how medical men had reported these Chinese and Turkish vaccination practices to the Royal Society in London early in the seventeenth century, but that despite some publicity only one American physician, Z. Boylston, was persuaded to take up the cause of smallpox vaccination during an epidemic in Boston (15).

As Silverstein (1) points out, by the time the English physician E. Jenner (16) had published his important memoir in 1798 on the use of cowpox material to protect human beings from smallpox, the use of material from relatively non-virulent human smallpox pustules was already tolerably well known. Even so, Jenner's evidence was greeted with skepticism and generated widespread opposition in England until formally approved by a body of prominent physicians and surgeons in London. *En passant*, it should be noted that smallpox vaccination remained a controversial topic for many years (1, 10) and that the modern vaccine was based on the vaccinia virus rather than on the viruses responsible for cowpox or smallpox. In one respect Jenner proved to be wholly wrong, for vaccination was later shown not to give the life-long protection that he had claimed.

These were the seeds from which immunization in a far wider context began to flourish with the work of L. Pasteur, R. Koch, and others, and the identification of the micro-organisms responsible for many infections was, of course, to play a vital role. Pasteur's extraordinary contributions through the development of attenuated chicken cholera and veterinary anthrax organisms are well known, as is his dramatic discovery and application of a rabies vaccine. However, the mechanisms responsible for the protective effects remained obscure and in 1880 (17) Pasteur, Chamberland and Roux proposed a somewhat vague concept – the "exhaustion hypothesis" – according to which protection was brought about by the utilization by microbes of host nutrients essential to microbial growth, thus leading to the disappearance of these nutrients and their unavailability to subsequently introduced organisms. This notion soon had to give way to hypotheses involving an active response on the part of the host though, strangely, it was briefly resuscitated by P. Ehrlich (18) in 1906 to explain why second tumor transplants sometimes failed to grow (the "athrepsia" hypothesis). This is discussed in Chapter 2 (p. 66), as is Ehrlich's far more perceptive acknowledgement in the same paper of another phenomenon described by him as "an actively acquired immunity". I would like to argue that it was, on the one hand, Ehrlich, von Behring and other chemists and pathologists and, on the other, the Russian zoologist E. Metchnikoff, who are to be regarded as the fathers of immunology, in so far as that term has any meaning, rather than those pioneers who founded the science of bacteriology so successfully in the closing decades of the nineteenth century.

The cellular hypothesis

It was Metchnikoff (19, 20) who proposed that phagocytic cells form the natural defense of the body against foreign intruders. This theory was based on careful microscopic examination of starfish larvae into which tiny foreign bodies had been inserted and on yeast-infected water fleas (*Daphnia*). He later developed an all-embracing theory that these cells were the vital and beneficial ingredient in many if not all inflammatory conditions and in the pathogenesis of many diseases (21). For him, the phagocytic system was the most primitive and at the same time the most important defense mechanism of the body. His theory was strongly opposed by the "humoralists" (i.e. those who believed that chemical substances found in the blood – antitoxins and alexin, which was later called complement – were primarily responsible for the body's defense against microbial infection). The controversy between these two schools was often acrimonious and it was to continue for some time until the Englishmen A.E. Wright and S.R. Douglas (22), working at St Mary's Hospital, London, proposed an acceptable compromise, when they found in 1903 that phagocytic cells ingested bacteria far more efficiently when the latter had first been coated with fresh serum factors (opsonization). (In Chapter 2 (p. 74) I refer to a similar controversy, though one pursued in more gentlemanly fashion, half a century later between Medawar's "cellular" school of allograft rejection and those, foremost among them P.A. Gorer, who favored antibody-mediated rejection mechanisms. Like its predecessor it died a natural death when it became apparent that both played a role, depending on the tissues involved and the immunologic status of the host.) Metchnikoff was way ahead of his time, for it was many decades later that the role of macrophages and other cells of the reticuloendothelial system such as dendritic cells in the induction and, in some cases, the execution of immune responses became known.

The "humoral" school

Bibel (2) has claimed that although the first description of protective antitoxins is commonly attributed to Von Behring and Kitasato, their work "stems from experiments on snake venom by Henry Sewall", an American physiologist working at Johns Hopkins University. Although it is true that in his 1887 paper (23), which preceded Von Behring and Kitasato's by three years, Sewall described how the repeated inoculation of subtoxic and continually increasing doses of snake venom protected pigeons against a normally fatal dose and he used the terms "immunity" as well as "resistance", it is not at all clear that this was intended to imply an immunologic cause. Indeed, Sewall had no explanation for the protective effect he described. Furthermore, it is doubtful that Von Behring and Kitasato were aware of his experiments, for they do not refer to them and their profoundly influential studies were carried out with bacterial toxins. Arguably more relevant was the study by two other Americans, D.E. Salmon and T. Smith (24), published in 1886. These workers had shown that organisms thought to be the cause of swine plague induced immunity in pigeons that had been inoculated with the organisms together with their culture fluid after heat-inactivation. (Bibel (2) relates that Salmon had not been in any way involved in these experiments and that the inclusion of his name had been forced on Smith as a purely political move – an issue that led to great recriminations and that will find resonance with many modern scientists!) Be that as it may, the German Von Behring and the Japanese Kitasato (25), working in Koch's laboratory in Berlin, were able to show that it was possible to immunize rabbits against tetanus bacilli, that the blood or cell-free serum of such rabbits neutralized or destroyed the tetanus toxin, and that the protective effect could be transferred to normal mice by the transfer of blood or serum from immune donors. Neutralization of the toxin was demonstrated by mixing toxin with immune serum for 24 hours and then inoculating the mixture into mice, with the calculated dose of toxin exceeding the fatal dose more than 300-fold. This procedure proved to be harmless to the experimental subjects. Although the vital serum component was unknown at the time, these experiments clearly established serum-borne immunity as a powerful protective mechanism and these authors fully deserve the credit for having been the first to demonstrate the efficacy of serum factors (antibodies) as therapeutic agents.

Paul Ehrlich was an extraordinary man whose influence, as the first proponent of a selective theory of antibody formation, is still felt eight decades after his death in 1915. As an organic chemist he made many other important contributions outside the field of immunology, such as the development of diazo dyes, the discovery of Salvarsan – the drug that was used in the treatment of syphilis until antibiotics became available towards the middle of the century – and a variety of discoveries in the fields of histopathology, oncology and hematology. However, today he is known mainly as the founder of immunochemistry with a paper published in 1897 (26) and as the proponent of the side-chain theory of antibody formation. In this paper he studied the interaction of diphtheria toxin and antitoxin as in a chemical reaction and he determined the point of equivalence, when the antitoxin had neutralized a given amount of toxin. He postulated that at this point the mixture should be non-lethal when inoculated into guinea pigs, but soon found that the process of neutralization was highly complicated and he speculated that there were a number of toxoids differing in their affinity for the antitoxin. He interpreted the ability of toxin and antitoxin to enter into a chemical reaction as indicating that the toxin possessed a specific group of atoms with a particular affinity for another group of atoms in the antitoxin, and he used the lock and key analogy. He also recounted experiments with tetanus showing that the ability of the toxin to combine with the antitoxin was independent of its toxicity for animals, for toxin that had been rendered non-toxic (the "toxoid") with carbon sulfide nonetheless evoked immunity in guinea pigs. He believed that because the specific combining capacity of the different toxoids was intact, there must have been chemical changes "in the remainder of the atom complex" to account for the loss of toxicity at equivalence. In this paper Ehrlich also tentatively introduced the concept of the side-chain theory of antibody formation, which he was to develop more fully and with vivid illustrations in his Croonian Lecture to the Royal Society in 1900 (see below).

The last decade of the nineteenth century saw a succession of remarkable discoveries from the German school (Behring, Ehrlich, Buchner, Pfeiffer and Kraus foremost among them) and the French school led by Bordet. Silverstein (1) has discussed these in detail, together with the controversies they generated and the underlying national chauvinism that gave the debates a special and rather disagreeable edge. The published papers were often written in a dense and opaque style that makes their reading in German or French extremely arduous; summaries were rarely included and detailed references to the work of others were often scanty. What is more, some of the journals in which they were published, like the *Centralblatt für Bakteriologie* (note the C rather than the usual Z, a cause of confusion in the literature) had fuller names and sometimes underwent changes. It is therefore hardly surprising that references to these early papers are not always correct in modern texts. At a conceptual level, the conclusions drawn are sometimes complicated by confusion between specific antibodies (natural or acquired) and the naturally occurring agent that was first given the name alexin and later described as complement.

Among the most important contributions on the protective role of antitoxins, in addition to those already mentioned, are the following. Ehrlich described how he induced immunity in mice to the toxins ricin (27) and abrin (28) by feeding mice with minute amounts of the toxins incorporated in their diet, and he described how immunity appeared suddenly on day six and persisted for the duration of his observations. The blood of immune animals possessed antitoxins that *specifically* neutralized the toxin and which could be transferred passively to normal animals. The passively transferred antibodies persisted in the recipients for "a relatively long time" though the protective effect had more or less disappeared by the thirty-fifth day. Because of the specificity he observed Ehrlich concluded that other toxins that could incite the production of antibodies were chemically quite distinct.

R. Pfeiffer's (29) great contribution was to show that serum from animals immune to cholera not only killed the relevant bacteria but brought about their demise within minutes of exposure by a bactericidal process leading to their fragmentation into small granules. By sampling the peritoneal fluid of immune and reinfected guinea pigs he was able to describe the process kinetically – first immobility of the organisms, followed by degeneration and the formation of granular clumps and, in strongly immunized individuals, their total dissolution "under my eyes". Though sympathetic to Metchnikoff's phagocytic theory he was able to rule out the participation of phagocytes except as an epiphenomenon. He felt that the body cavity acted not merely as a receptacle, but played an active role under the influence of the immune serum in activating bactericidal function. He thus erroneously believed that the bactericidal substances were not preformed, but produced in response to the combined action of the pathogens and the antitoxin in the peritoneal cavity. He was, however, perfectly clear that they acted specifically and that their action was chemical rather than physical.

The observation that bacterial toxins and antibodies can react through a process of flocculation and precipitation we owe to R. Kraus (*30*), working in Vienna towards the end of the last century. He studied cell-free filtrates of cholera, typhus and plague and their reaction with the homologous immune serum. He concluded that precipitation was specific, that the substances interacting with the sera were bacterial components, and – rather curiously – that precipitation was not observed when he used diphtheria toxin and antitoxin. As Bibel (*2*) has pointed out, this was possibly due to the use of these agents in the wrong proportions. It was the Frenchman J. Bordet (*31*) working in, of all places, Metchnikoff's laboratory at the Institut Pasteur, who demonstrated convincingly that antibody could bring about the agglutination as well as the lysis of red blood cells. However, he did rather more than that.

Alexine, the forerunner of the complement system

Before Bordet's studies, others had already found evidence that more than one serum component was involved in the bactericidal action of normal sera. G.H.F. Nuttall (*32*), an American working at that time in Germany, was probably the first to show that normal sera, too, could be bactericidal, though less strongly than immune sera. He carried out *in vitro* experiments with hanging drop cultures using blood from rabbits, sheep, dogs and humans and observed the death of several kinds of bacteria, followed by their ingestion by phagocytes. An important observation was that the bactericidal potency of blood waned with time and thereafter the blood became a "good nutritive medium". He thought that the instability of the agent involved might have been caused by decomposition by other blood elements or by a process of fermentation. Nuttall favored the latter explanation because heating the blood to about 55° C for 10–45 minutes abolished the bactericidal effect. He concluded that the death of the organisms was quite independent of blood leukocytes and in stating that "Metchnikoff is wrong by claiming that the destruction of the bacilli in the living body is caused only by phagocytic activity" he struck a doughty blow against Metchnikoff's cellular hypothesis.

Nuttall's observations were taken up enthusiastically, but not uncritically, by H. Buchner, working in Munich. In a paper on the bactericidal action of cell-free blood serum (*33*), published in 1889, he drew attention to Nuttall's failure to remove cells from the plasma and he therefore regarded Nuttall's experiments as indecisive. By rectifying this deficiency using some primitive centrifugation methods or defibrination followed by natural sedimentation, Buchner proceeded to prove that the bactericidal properties of normal blood resided in the cell-free plasma. He confirmed Nuttall's observation that heating at 55° C for one hour destroyed the effect, but found that function was maintained for 7–8 days, and even up to 20 days, if the plasma was stored at 6–8° C. Buchner believed that some contradictory results obtained by him were caused by the presence of two opposing variables – a bactericidal factor and a nutritional factor, and he thought that the latter could mask the former. In another paper in the same year (*34*) he attempted to dialyze the serum against water, only to find that the activity disappeared totally. Believing that this had been caused by the removal of salts he repeated dialysis against a salt solution, this time successfully. Buchner concluded correctly that salts were needed for the normal action of the serum factors. He attempted to explain the loss of activity at room temperature in terms of either chemical changes or a physical rearrangement within the "albumen" molecule.

In his massive 1893 paper Buchner (35) continued to explore the properties of the active component of normal serum, "the so-called alexine", which he believed to share certain characteristics with enzymes (e.g. heat lability). Because he believed that instability was not due to heat *per se* but to the action of water molecules he dried plasma and found it to be stable in this form. Further, he demonstrated, following in Von Behring and Kitasato's footsteps, that mice could be protected against lethal doses of tetanus by small amounts of serum from immunized rabbits, regardless of whether the serum was mixed with the tetanus organisms before inoculation or given just before: ". . . and so we are in the pleasant position to experiment conveniently and reliably with these interesting substances, possibly the most interesting that medical science has so far had at its disposal."

This is where Bordet came in when he showed in 1895 (36) in a lengthy paper that the bacteriolytic and bactericidal action of immune sera against cholera *Vibrio* organisms had two quite separate components – a thermolabile factor that was also present in normal serum (i.e. it resembled alexine) and a thermostable and highly specific factor present in immune sera (i.e. antibody). Conclusive proof was obtained when he demonstrated that the bactericidal power of heated serum could be restored by the addition of fresh, but not pre-heated, serum from normal donors, and he showed that unlike immune serum, the heat-labile component acted nonspecifically. He followed Buchner's lead by calling the heat-labile factor alexine. Four years later Bordet (31) followed up these studies with his decisive demonstration that rabbit red blood cells were destroyed by immune guine pig sera. Such sera pre-heated to 55° C merely agglutinated the cells, but when fresh normal serum (either rabbit or guinea pig) was added the cells were lysed in a specific manner. *In vivo* experiments confirmed his conclusions and, in pointing to the similarity of the data obtained previously with cholera *Vibrio*, he expressed his conviction that the alexine active in the two systems was probably the same and that it therefore served a basic function that went beyond the need to counter infectious organisms.

Thus it can be seen that the basic principles of immunology were established in two extraordinary decades before the turn of the century and that modern immunology is based on the work of pioneers who had to conduct their studies without precedents and with the most primitive laboratory tools. With the avalanche of evidence favoring antibodies as the principal mediators of immunity it is hardly surprising that Metchnikoff's phagocytic theory went into decline, and it was only later incorporated into a more comprehensive framework of immunity. It is a fascinating and momentous story and I make no apologies for dwelling on it. From these early years are derived, in rapid succession, the subsequent discoveries of anaphylaxis by P. Portier and C. Richet (37), the Arthus reaction by M. Arthus (38) and serum sickness by Von Pirquet and Schick (39), all paradoxically harmful manifestations of antibody formation, which opened up the field of hypersensitivity.

The Discovery of Blood Group Antigens

The identification of the human blood group antigens by another great pioneer, K. Landsteiner (40), at the turn of the century was one of the most critically important discoveries in hematology and in medicine in general, but it also marked the beginning of the study of immunogenetics. It predated the discovery of histocompatibility antigens by several decades (see Chapter 4) and made it possible to establish that the ABO antigens were important in the transplantation of certain organs such as the kidney. Landsteiner put the blood group antigens and antisera against them to good use in the study of antibody specificity. Because blood group antigens are central to the story of blood transfusion their discovery has been considered in Chapter 3.

P.B. Medawar and the Immunologic Basis of Allograft Rejection

The science of modern transplantation had profoundly important antecedents through the work of the early surgeons who attempted skin and kidney transplantation, and the pathologists and biologists who were interested in the experimental transplantation of tumors. These antecedents are described in some detail in Chapter 2. However, by providing wholly convincing evidence for the immunologic basis of skin allograft rejection in a patient (41) in 1943 and in rabbits a year or two later (42, 43) Medawar laid the foundation for the modern study of alloreactivity. Again, Medawar's early work is fully considered in Chapter 2. Although in his classic studies he described the infiltration of skin allografts undergoing rejection by large numbers of small mononuclear cells, his interpretation was at that time in terms of specific antibodies rather than cell-mediated phenomena. The creation of the field of cellular immunology, to which he and his colleagues were to make substantial contributions, came about from the study of certain forms of hypersensitivity involving other kinds of antigens (see below). However, by giving the study of tissue transplantation a solid immunologic basis he not only made tissue transplantation credible and respectable but also opened up new vistas for immunology, giving the field a great boost.

Tolerance and Autoimmunity

The discovery of the phenomenon of acquired immunologic tolerance – a state of specific unresponsiveness that can be established by the introduction of allogeneic cells into immunologically immature animals such as murine fetuses or neonates – proved to be of critical importance in immunology. It provided a counterpart to the state of immunity, had to be taken into account in the development of theories of antibody formation, threw a new light on the origins of autoimmune manifestations, and provided the opportunity for the study of cellular events such as negative selection in the thymus. In the field of transplantation it provided the gold standard for tolerance induction in adults, and although it was not directly applicable clinically, it encouraged both experimentalists and clinicians to look for and deliberately further the induction of tolerance in adults.

The steps leading to the discovery of neonatal tolerance are described in detail in Chapter 5 and the development of immunoregulatory mechanisms in adult animals in Chapter 6. Here I wish to draw attention to a few of the most important publications responsible for the recognition that tolerance to foreign antigens can be acquired either naturally or experimentally and that it constitutes the chief safeguard against autoimmune diseases.

Despite the unexplored evidence from some of the early embryologists that allogeneic and even xenogeneic embryonic chick grafts can grow unhindered in other chick embryos (see Chapter 5), the real tolerance story must start with R.D. Owen's (44) remarkable observations in 1945 that cattle dizygotic twins normally possessed not only their own red blood cells, but also red cells that were demonstrably derived from their twin partners. In other words, cattle dizygotic twins were shown to be cellular chimeras. Owen was working at the time in the Department of Genetics at the University of Wisconsin, Madison, and living as he did in a state in which cattle outnumbered its human inhabitants, he soon became interested in the serology and genetics of cattle blood groups. He was surprised to find that each twin was chimeric in its repertoire of red blood corpuscles, a discovery that made sense to him only when he realized that F.R. Lillie had shown, many years earlier, that cattle dizygotic twins shared the same placenta and that their blood streams were therefore naturally anastomosed. Owen realized that such anastomoses must lead to a free exchange of blood, and because he found foreign (twin) red cells in the circulation many years later he rightly assumed that the exchange must have involved not only blood cells, but also precursor cells. These were assumed to have established themselves in their hosts and to have continued to produce red cells true to their genetic lineage.

Immunologists, whose sights at that time were fixed on more humdrum matters, did not become aware of Owen's findings, or if they did, failed to appreciate their great importance. The exception was provided by F.M. Burnet and F. Fenner (45), two Australian virologists who wrote a wide-ranging, speculative and brilliant monograph on the production of antibodies, which included the formulation of the self-marker hypothesis to explain why autoimmunity was the exception rather than the rule. They had read Owen's paper and proceeded to weave his findings into a theory that presupposed tolerance induction to be a normal event (i.e. that tolerance developed in fetal life to self-markers, but not to foreign antigens, leaving the immune system free to recognize the latter and to respond to them). Apart from quoting Owen's paper they also referred to some observations by E. Traub (see Chapter 5), who had demonstrated in the 1930s that non-fatal infections of embryos with choriomeningitis virus left the mice healthy carriers of the virus in adult life and resistant to intracerebral challenge later in life without the production of neutralizing antiviral antibodies. Burnet's subsequent attempt to demonstrate the induction of tolerance to influenza virus had met with failure.

The next milestone was the demonstration by Billingham, Brent and Medawar (46, 47), working in London, that tolerance to skin allografts could be induced in mouse or chicken embryos by the direct inoculation of viable cells from the skin graft donor or donor strain. The ensuing tolerance, which was frequently permanent, was highly specific and it was invariably accompanied by the presence of donor cells in the tissues of the tolerant hosts. Of particular relevance to Owen's observations in cattle was their finding that the embryos of fertile double-yolked eggs displayed anastomosis of their chorioallantoic circulation and that such twins were not only red cell chimeras but were also mutually tolerant to each other's skin. It is, however, of historical interest that Medawar's group had approached the question of tolerance not so much through knowledge of Owen's previous work or even the speculations of Burnet and Fenner, but as a result of studying skin graft survival in dizygotic cattle twins in the hope of solving the agricultural conundrum of distinguishing between mono- and dizygotic twins! These and other matters, such as the independent contribution of M. Hašek and his colleagues in Prague, are fully discussed in Chapter 5.

The discovery of tolerance is especially important because it was soon found that tolerance could be induced to a wide variety of molecules other than histocompatibility antigens, and the phenomenon therefore became central to an understanding of the immune system in all its diversity and complexity. In their 1956 monograph Billingham, Brent and Medawar (47) drew attention to its relevance to autoimmunity; were it not for tolerance, it was argued, autoantibodies would be the rule rather than the exception, and where such antibodies *could* be demonstrated there were usually special dispensations, such as the production of the antigens at a developmental stage when the immune system had already reached some degree of maturity (e.g. casein in milk and spermatozoal antigens). In other cases the tissues carrying the antigens might be sequestered from the developing immune system, such as the antigens of the lens. This theme was developed at greater length by Brent and Medawar (48) in 1959.

So far as autoimmunity is concerned, the first half of the twentieth century was adversely dominated by the concept of "horror autotoxicus" as enunciated by Ehrlich and Morgenroth (49), according to which autoantibodies are either not produced or, if they are, somehow prevented from acting to the detriment of the organism. Nonetheless, as early as 1904 it became apparent from the work of J. Donath and K. Landsteiner (50) that in certain circumstances autoantibodies capable of destroying red blood corpuscles could indeed be formed. Such was the case in a disease that came to be known as paroxysmal cold hemoglobinuria, in which the autoantibody bound to the red cells only at low temperature and lysed the cells in the presence of complement on warming.

The topic of autoimmunity and the ups and downs of its recognition have been well discussed by Silverstein (1), Bibel (2) and others such as Mackay (51). It received full recognition by the publication of papers in 1957 on both sides of the Atlantic. Thus E. Witebsky, N.R. Rose and K. Terplan (52), working at the University of Buffalo, set out to test the validity of the concept of horror autotoxicus by injecting rabbit thyroid extracts containing thyroglobulin incorporated in Freund's adjuvant into rabbits and testing the sera from such animals for specific antibodies using several highly sensitive techniques. One of these techniques revealed specific antibodies in the great majority of experimental subjects. They went on to demonstrate that antibodies were produced by rabbits inoculated with their own thyroid extract. Removal of an animal's thyroid, followed by the inoculation of thyroid extract from other rabbits, led to the formation of antithyroid antibodies reactive with the animal's own organ. Purified thyroglobulin was effective as the immunogen and the response to it led to histopathologic changes in the thyroid. Similar observations were made in dogs and guinea pigs. The sera of patients with chronic thyroiditis proved to have antithyroid antibodies and it was therefore postulated that the human condition was caused by the same mechanism as the thyroiditis in experimental animals (i.e. by the formation of autoantibodies against thyroglobulin). The authors thought that the slow release of thyroglobulin in patients mimicked the effect of adjuvant-incorporated thyroglobulin in animals. They proposed four criteria that they thought needed to be met to establish a role for an autoantibody in the pathogenesis of a disease and believed that the antibodies described by them had fulfilled these criteria. Interestingly, and unlike D. Doniach and I.M. Roitt in another publication that year (53), they did not attempt to place their data within the conceptual framework of tolerance.

Doniach and Roitt (53), having demonstrated thyroid-specific precipitating auto-antibodies in the sera of patients with Hashimoto's disease and identified thyro-globulin as the antigen, related their findings to the phenomenon of tolerance. "The concept of immunologic tolerance provides a rational basis for the phenomenon of auto-antibody formation, since animals may fail to acquire this tolerance for constituents which do not gain access to the sites of antibody formation during the critical developing period and may therefore produce antibodies in response to any subsequent release of these constituents. ... The failure to detect antibodies under normal conditions suggests that human beings may not be immunologically tolerant to this protein", they wrote. By being taken into the mainstream of immunology autoimmunity had at last achieved credibility and respectability.

The Development of Cellular Immunology

Apart from Metchnikoff and his band of followers, who held that it was the phago-cytic cell that was primarily responsible for the body's defense against infectious organisms, the champions of protective and therapeutic antibodies held centerstage for the first four decades of the twentieth century. This came about despite some straws in the wind pointing quite strongly, though not conclusively, to the involve-ment of mononuclear cells in immune reactions. Thus in Chapter 2 (p. 67) I refer to the histologic and experimental observations of J.B. Murphy at the Rockefeller Research Institute and some of the other tumor research workers who came very close to implicating small lymphocytes in the destruction of tumor allografts. Likewise, the work in 1921 of H. Zinsser (54) on "bacterial allergy" and that of L. Dienes and E.W. Schoenheit (55) on delayed-type hypersensivity to simple protein antigens injected together with tubercle bacilli paved the way for the realization that mononuclear cells were vitally important in the pathogenesis of these immunologic manifestations.

The passive (adoptive) transfer of sensitivity

However, a telling if not entirely decisive blow was struck by Landsteiner and Chase (56) in 1942. (Landsteiner had long left his native Germany and settled in the United States, and this was to be one of his last papers before his death in the following year.) They sensitized guinea pigs with simple chemical compounds such as picryl chloride together with tubercle bacilli as adjuvant. Having established a strong tuber-culin hypersensitivity demonstrable by skin tests, they transferred peritoneal exudate cells to naive animals and found that most of these developed cutaneous sensitivity to picryl chloride. The effect was not mediated by the peritoneal fluid but by the cells found in it; when the cells were killed by heat treatment, sensitivity was not transferred. They more or less ruled out active sensitization with antigen carried over with the cells, partly by following the kinetics of passive sensitization, which was evident within two days and then faded away rapidly. They concluded that "Consequently one would be inclined to assume that the sensitivity is produced by an activity in the recipient of the surviving cells, if not by antibodies carried by these." No attempt was made to identify the cells transferring sensitivity by separation of the different cell populations present in the exudate. It was later shown by Mitchison (see below) that the short-lived transfer effect was due to the fact that Landsteiner and Chase had used outbred animals, so that the transferred allogeneic cells were soon eliminated.

Chase, who later became the scourge of anyone illustrating his or her oral presentation at meetings with overhead slides that had been poorly devised and/or contained too much material, continued with these studies at the Rockefeller Institute. In 1945 he published data (57) demonstrating very clearly the cellular transfer of delayed hypersensitivity to tuberculin. As in his previous paper with Landsteiner, the hypersensivity could be shown to be present within two days, with maximal reactivity between three and four days. Transfer was not achieved with cells that had been killed by heating or by freezing and thawing, and he showed that not only peritoneal exudate cells but also splenic or lymph node cells from actively sensitized donors were capable of transferring sensitivity.

It was N.A. Mitchison (58) who in the course of his Ph.D. studies at Oxford found almost a decade later that the passive cellular transfer of sensitivity – this time to allogeneic tumors – was far more easily accomplished when the cell donors and recipients belonged to the same inbred strain. Thus, lymph node fragments, but not peritoneal exudate cells, transferred the sensitivity so that tumors transplanted to the cell recipients were rejected in accelerated fashion. Serum was ineffective, and Mitchison ruled out the possibility that active sensitization might have been responsible. The duration of the passive sensitivity was longer than in the experiments of Chase and came to an end after about 20 days (but see below). Mitchison concluded that his investigation "shows that transplantation immunity shares with immunity to simple chemical compounds and immunity to tuberculin the property of being transferred with greater facility by cells than by serum".

Billingham, Brent and Medawar (59), one year later, confirmed these findings for skin allografts. They showed that the cells from the lymph nodes draining the site of the allograft soon after rejection were especially effective compared with splenic cells and that cells obtained from the contralateral nodes or from the blood, like serum, were inactive. The duration of what they called "adoptively" transferred immunity (to distinguish it from passive transfer with antiserum) was at least 30 days, and they expressed the view that transplantation immunity was similar to delayed-type hypersensitivity. The adoptive transfer test, which was later made semiquantitative, became established in the wider field of immunology, helped to identify the cells responsible, and was commonly used to identify cellular chimerism in tolerant animals before the introduction of technologically more sophisticated methods.

Cellular immunology therefore became an accepted and rapidly developing field of study, complementing the study of antibodies as mediators of the multifarious responses of the immune system. It also marked the beginning of the "cellular school" in transplantation immunology, opposed by the "humoralists". The stage was now set for the remarkable discoveries of B. Glick, J.F.A.P. Miller, J.L. Gowans and others, which at last explained at a cellular level the basis of cell-mediated immune reactions and led to the recognition that lymphocytes are far from homogeneous.

The mysterious lymphocyte

Although workers like Murphy (see above and Chapter 2) came close to appreciating the participation of lymphocytes in graft rejection, and despite substantial studies by numerous workers, the function of lymphocytes remained a mystery until the beginning of the 1960s. Even as late as 1961 the British Bristol-based anatomist J.M. Yoffey (60), who had spent much of his life puzzling over the distribution, kinetics and function of lymphocytes, still thought it possible that lymphocytes were hemopoietic stem cells. Ironically, Yoffey's 1961 paper was published in the same *Ciba Foundation Monograph* – the proceedings of a meeting held earlier that year – as a paper by Gowans, Gesner and McGregor (61). This Oxford group, working not so many miles from Yoffey's laboratory, discussed their evidence for believing that thoracic duct lymphocytes have a clear and incontrovertible immunologic function (see below). For historians the discussions of these two contributions are well worth perusing.

Lymphocytes had certainly been regarded as the "Cinderella" of the immune system – generally neglected and an object of the most profound ignorance and even disdain. The general consensus was that they were in all probability short-lived cells, and that this, together with a lamentable scarcity of cytoplasm, meant that they were hardly equipped to fulfill any function of note. It should, however, be remembered that apart from the non-immunologic functions considered by workers like Yoffey, others such as Ehrich and Harris (62), Dougherty, Chase and White (63) amd Harris *et al.* (64) had thought it likely in the mid-1940s that lymphocytes were intimately involved in antibody formation, though Dougherty, Chase and White added the caution that "The actual production of antibodies by lymphocytes has not been established".

Lymphocytes as recirculating cells

One of the defining moments in the history of the lymphocyte came with the suggestion by J.L.Gowans (65), based mainly on his own observations on the kinetics of thoracic duct lymphocytes, that small lymphocytes, which enter the lymphatics from the blood, are part of a large pool of cells that circulate from the blood into the lymph and back again into the blood. A few years later he and Knight (66), in one of a classic series of papers using radiolabeled thoracic duct lymphocytes, provided a solid basis for this hypothesis, for they showed that the output of small lymphocytes from the thoracic duct is normally maintained by large-scale recirculation of cells from blood to lymph. The main channel for this flow lay within the lymph nodes, and small lymphocytes entered the nodes by crossing the walls of specialized blood vessels known as the post-capillary venules. In an accompanying paper Marchesi and Gowans (67) provided electron microscopic evidence for this migration and they showed that lymphocytes crossed the wall of the venules by entering the endothelial cells rather than passing through the intercellular junctions. So much for the "inert" small lymphocyte!

Small lymphocytes are immunologically active

Meanwhile considerable efforts had been made to ascertain whether lymphocytes are "immunologically competent" – an expression coined by Medawar in his 1958 Croonian Lecture (68) and the subject of his introduction (69) to the 1963 Ciba Foundation Monograph on "*The Immunologically Competent Cell*." The American P.I. Terasaki (70), working as a post-doctoral fellow in Medawar's department at the time, was the first to show that purified chicken blood white cells with a 99% content of small lymphocytes could bring about graft-versus-host reactions (GVHR) in newly hatched chicks. He was closely followed by the discoverer of GVHR in the chicken, M. Simonsen (71) in Copenhagen and by M.F.A. Woodruff's group in Edinburgh (72) and R.E. Billingham's team in Philadelphia (73). (Billingham had emigrated from the United Kingdom to the United States several years earlier.) The latter two groups reported that cells of the thoracic duct lymph (TDL) were capable of inducing GVHR in rats, and in view of the earlier demonstration by Gowans (74) that 95% of the cells in rat lymph were small lymphocytes (the remainder being medium or large lymphocytes), there was a strong presumption that the reactions had been caused by small lymphocytes. It should, however, be noted that Anderson, Delorme and Woodruff (72) thought it likely that the minority of large lymphocytes were the immunologically active cells because they were known to divide in culture.

It was at this point that Gowans, Gesner and McGregor in Oxford (61) provided fresh evidence for the induction of graft-versus-host disease (GVHD) in young adult F1 hybrid rats by the inoculation of parental TDL. Further, tolerance induced in neonatal animals could be broken by such cells, regardless of whether they were "naive" or presensitized, thus repeating the abolition of skin graft tolerance achieved in the mid-1950s by Billingham, Brent and Medawar (47) using unpurified spleen and lymph node cells. They ruled out the large lymphocyte as the culprit and concluded that "It is probably the small lymphocyte which initiates the graft-against-host reaction and, in doing so, it may change into a new type of cell" – the large pyroninophilic cell that was capable of cell division to form more small lymphocytes. This theme was developed further with new experimental data by Gowans *et al.* in their 1962 *Nature* paper (75). Here they offered "strong evidence" that small lymphocytes are involved in the inductive phase of antibody formation, probably because "they interact with antigen (or with antigen that has been "processed" by reticuloendothelial phagocytes), become fixed in lymphoid tissues and give rise to a dividing cell-line of the kind identified by Nossal and Mäkela" (76). (See also the account by Gowans (77) in the 1962 volume of the *Annals of the New York Academy of Sciences*, with its exquisite radiographic and histologic evidence for this cellular transformation.) Both Gowans' laboratory and many others were soon to confirm and extend these data: the small lymphocyte had come of age and cellular immunology was firmly established as a major branch of immunology. Several years later McGregor, McCullagh and Gowans (78) went on to show that small lymphocytes were the precursors of cells capable of producing antibodies to sheep red blood cells.

For the biographic sketch of Gowans see p. 116. He has recently written a vivid account (79) of the discoveries establishing the small lymphocyte as a dominant force in immunology.

The bursa of Fabricius and the thymus: immunologic finishing schools

The bursa

While these important discoveries were being made there were stirrings of an equally momentous nature in other quarters. Indeed, the discovery that the bursa of Fabricius of birds (exemplified by the chicken) had an immunologic function was made several years earlier. However, because B. Glick, T.S. Chang and R.G. Jaap (80) chose to publish their data in the journal *Poultry Science* – a journal which immunologists would normally have little cause to read over breakfast – their studies remained virtually unknown until A.P. Mueller, H.R. Wolfe and R.K. Meyer (81) repeated and extended them and published their own work in a mainstream immunologic journal in 1960.

The discovery of the immunologic function of the bursa – a blind sac connected to the cloaca by a duct and thought to have the same mysterious function as the mammalian thymus – was almost inevitably made by serendipity. Glick, Chang and Jaap (80) relate how, in the course of studying antibody formation to *Salmonella typhimurium*, a group of chickens that had been bursectomized six months earlier had been accidentally included. Most of these birds died 12 days after inoculation of the organisms, but the three survivors failed to generate any antibodies, in contrast to birds with an intact bursa. Antibody formation in chickens deliberately bursectomized two weeks after hatching was then studied and it was again found that there was a shortfall in antibody production in the majority of bursectomized birds, even when the immunization protocols were extremely rigorous. "These results demonstrate that the bursa of Fabricius plays a vital role in the production of antibodies to *S. typhimurium*," they wrote in their 1956 paper. Because the bursa was known to atrophy gradually 7–13 weeks after hatching the authors thought it unlikely that bursectomy after the thirteenth week could "have a direct influence on antibody production". Several more papers were published in the same specialist journal over the next two years, but the immunologic world continued to live in blissful ignorance until Mueller, Wolfe and Meyer (81) published their confirmation in the *Journal of Immunology*. (According to Bibel (2) the brief manuscript by Glick, Chang and Jaap had originally been sent to *Science*, in whose pages it would certainly have created a stir, but the editors declined it on the grounds that it was "of no general interest"!) It was left for Ackerman and Knouff (82) to describe the development of bursa lymphocytes from undifferentiated endodermal epithelial cells.

Mueller, Wolfe and Meyer (81) had bursectomized chicks both chemically by inoculating fertile eggs with the hormone 19-nortestosterone and surgically 1–2 weeks after hatching. Such birds were later unable to form precipitating antibodies to bovine serum albumin, and it was shown that bursectomy as late as ten weeks after hatching had little or no effect. These authors opined that "the bursa of Fabricius is thought to be similar to that of the thymus". The full implications of these observations were not appreciated until the function of the mammalian thymus had been uncovered.

The thymus

Claims for the discovery of the immunologic function of the thymus seem to be somewhat controversial, as will be apparent to anyone who has followed the articles on the thymus in the "Immunology Yesterday" series of the journal *Immunology Today* (83–85). I have taken special care to study all the relevant early papers on the subject, and am therefore reasonably confident that my assessment of this important chapter in the history of immunology is objective. More than one laboratory appears to have taken an interest in the thymus at roughly the same time. One of these was that of J.F.A.P. Miller, in whose biographic sketch (p. 54) I have described how he came to work at the Chester Beatty Research Institute in London in the late 1950s and how he came to be interested in the role of the thymus in leukemogenesis. All this is well described in a recently published historic monograph (86). Having completed his Ph.D. on the etiology and pathogenesis of mouse leukemia, he had formulated the hypothesis that the Gross leukemia was tumorogenic only when inoculated into newborn mice because the young thymus offered it a particularly fertile environment. Hence he decided to find out whether the virus grew in mice that had been thymectomized either neonatally or at the age of 6–8 weeks. His hypothesis proved to be mistaken in 1959 (87) but he noticed that those mice that after early thymectomy, had not been cannibalized by their mothers wasted away and died, regardless of whether they had been given the virus. This led him to formulate and explore a new hypothesis (i.e. that the thymus in the neonatal mouse "may be essential to life") and the result was a preliminary account of his renewed studies published in the *Lancet* in September 1961 (88).

The upshot was that mice thymectomized within 16 hours of birth had a higher mortality than the sham-operated controls, mainly due to common laboratory infections. Maintaining the mice under "near pathogen-free" conditions reduced this mortality. The mice had a much lowered blood lymphocyte/polymorph ratio six weeks after birth and their lymph nodes and spleens displayed a great deficiency of germinal centers and a shortfall of plasma cells. Of critical importance was the finding that the majority of thymectomized mice that were given skin allografts six weeks after birth failed to reject them, the grafts growing "luxuriant crops of hair." Some of the grafts survived beyond two months, when they were destroyed by a chronic form of rejection. Of the greatest importance was the demonstration that thymectomized mice grafted subsequently with syngeneic fetal thymuses destroyed skin allografts transplanted three weeks later within 15 days – almost normally. Miller wrote: "The above results indicate that thymectomy in the immediate neonatal period is associated with severe depletion in the lymphocyte population and serious immunological defects in the mature animal. Several hypotheses might account for these results. One is that the thymus, particularly in early life, regulates lymphocyte production, not only by being the main producer of such cells, but also by secreting a factor, such as Metcalf's lymphocytosis-stimulating factor. . . In mice thymectomized at birth, the deficiency of lymphocytes would simply weaken the host's immunological defense as a whole. Another hypothesis attributes to the thymus a more direct role in the development of immunologic response. During embryogenesis the thymus would produce the originators of immunologically competent cells many of which would have migrated to other sites at about the time of birth. This would suggest that lymphocytes leaving the thymus are specially selected cells, and this might possibly be correlated with their epithelial ... origin during embryogenesis ... In accordance with elective theories of antibody formation, genetically distinct clones of cells might differentiate at various stages during thymic morphogenesis."

This pioneering study, which provided the foundation for "thymology", was the only one published in 1961 showing conclusively that the thymus of mice plays a pivotal role in the development of immune responses. O. Archer and J.C. Pierce (89) from Good's department had, it is true, a brief abstract in *Federation Proceedings* in the same year reporting some experiments on thymectomy in young rabbits (see below), but the data were scanty and unrefereed. Fichtelius, Laurall and Philipsson (90), a Swedish group, had thymectomized young guinea pigs immediately after the administration of *Salmonella typhi* H antigen and had found that antibody production was reduced, though not in the secondary response. These workers concluded that "...the thymus very probably plays a role in antibody formation".

The American embryologist R.F. Ruth (91), in reviewing the ontogeny of blood cells, was aware of the effects of bursectomy in chickens, realized that the thymus involuted with the attainment of sexual maturity, and speculated on the origin of cells from the endoderm and mesoderm. One of his speculations entailed that "endodermal lymphocytes may migrate to other sites before or during the involution of the organs in which they first appear. In embryological terms, the two types of lymphocytes have different prospective fates. ....". Further, the American zoologist R. Auerbach (92) published a paper in 1961 on the genetic control of thymus lymphoid differentiation, in which he described the fate of mouse thymus rudiments from 12-day-old fetuses after culture in the anterior chamber of the eye. His unified view of events in the thymus included the suggestion that "Cells selected and/or directed toward lymphoid differentation then develop into thymic lymphoid cells which migrate from the thymus into specific areas of the developing spleen. Here, in a new environment, they directly or indirectly become foci for production of antibody-forming cells." The concept of cell migration from the thymus is clearly enunciated here. Auerbach went on to state that "the hypothesis, though speculation, is attractive in being readily amenable to testing. One would predict that embryonic thymectomy would lead to a reduction of the antibody-forming capacity; this experiment can be performed in lower vertebrates." As it happens, Miller had performed exactly that kind of experiment though in neonatal mice before Auerbach's perceptive paper had been submitted for publication. Finally, it should be noted that the tumor biologist W.H. Woglom (93) mentioned in a massive 1929 review on "Immunity to transplantable tumors" that several workers had reported the effects of removing the adult rabbit, rat and mouse thymus on the growth of tumors, but with widely conflicting results.

Miller's next three notable contributions, in which he published the bulk of his data, came in 1962. First, the manuscript of a paper read at the Ciba Foundation Symposium on "Transplantation" in 1961 was published in the following year (94); second, his *magnum opus*, submitted to the Royal Society, appeared in the *Proceedings of the Royal Society* (95) in September after a lengthy gestation period, and third, a paper read by him at the *Fifth Homotransplantation Conference* in New York in February 1962 appeared later that year (96). (At this meeting Good's group chose to present data on the passive transfer of allograft sensitivity and delayed allergy.) Neonatal thymectomy had been performed in several mouse strains, the depletion of lymphocytes had been fully documented, severe impairment of antibody production to *Salmonella typhi* H antigen and to allo- and xenogeneic skin grafts was described, the wasting syndrome and the mortality were discussed in relation to runt disease (97), and the effects of restoring the mice with syngeneic thymic tissue were given in detail. Of great importance was the finding that mice whose immune function had been restored with thymus grafts had normal lymphoid tissue that had been repopulated with cells from the thymus donors, and that such mice rejected skin allografts and became immune. Miller concluded (95): ". . . during very early life, the thymus produces the progenitors of immunologically competent cells which mature and migrate to other sites. Present evidence does not, however, exclude the production by the young thymus of a humoral factor necessary to the maturation or proliferation of lymphocytes elsewhere in the body."

In his 1991 account of the contribution he and his colleagues made to the discovery of thymic function, Good (85) recalled that his interest in the thymus stemmed from clinical observations concerning a patient who had agammaglobulinemia as well as a benign thymoma. In 1956 he reported, together with L.D. Maclean *et al.* (98), that excision of the thymoma had no effect on the enhanced susceptibility the patient had displayed to infections, and the group expressed the view that there was likely to be "an essential relationship" between the two conditions because ". . . it seems unlikely that two such rare diseases have occurred together by mere fortuity". They quoted T.N. Harris, J. Rhoods and J. Stokes (99) as having failed to show consistent differences in antibody production when adult rabbits had been thymectomized. The same group's attempt to improve on the results of Harris, Rhoods and Stokes by thymectomizing young adult rabbits were equally unsuccessful (100).

The only indication from Good's stable that thymectomy carried out early in life had led to immunoincompetence was the abstract by Archer and Pierce (89), published in 1961. Five- to seven-day-old rabbits were used, and subsequent attempts to immunize the animals with bovine serum albumin (BSA) apparently failed to generate antibody responses. The authors concluded that "the thymus is necessary for the normal development of the immune response in the rabbit". These data were published in *Nature* in the middle of the following year (101) in a letter that contradicted the abstract, in that thymectomy before the fifth day led to a substantial (though not complete) reduction in anti-BSA responses whereas removal of the thymus between days five and seven merely resulted in a difference that was not statistically significant. The authors wrote: "Our present hypothesis is that the thymus in newborn mammals and the bursa of Fabricius in newly hatched fowl represent important centres of centrifugal distribution of immunologically competent cells to other lymphatic organs."

There followed a number of brief papers, each with a limited objective, from Good's laboratory, all published in 1962. Neonatal thymectomy in mice:

(1) Led to prolonged survival of H-2 compatible, but not H-2 incompatible, skin allografts and reduced numbers of blood lymphocytes (102).
(2) Made the mice highly susceptible to common infections and, now, allowed skin allografts in all strain combinations tested, including H-2 incompatible grafts, to survive (103).
(3) Permitted an allogeneic mammary carcinoma to grow (104).

(4) Almost abolished the capacity to make antibody against T2 bacteriophage (*105*).

These data were consolidated in an article in the *Journal of Experimental Medicine* (*106*) received by the journal in July 1962, in which they confirmed that complete thymectomy of rabbits before the fifth day led to a reduction in antibody formation although it left the response to skin grafts intact. The authors drew attention to the wasting phenomenon in mice and showed that spleen and lymph node cells from thymectomized mice did not respond in a GVHR assay. The mice showed an "inordinate susceptibility to runt disease" when they were given allogeneic spleen cells some weeks after thymectomy on the fourteenth day after birth. Neonatal thymectomy led to a wasting syndrome and a short lifespan, and the mice "do not develop a mature lymphoid structure" in their spleens and lymph nodes. They concluded, as they had in their other articles, that "It is our current hypothesis that the thymus makes a major contribution toward the centrifugal distribution of lymphoid cells which, in turn, is essential to the full expression of immunological capacity."

In a further paper Papermaster and Good (*107*) compared the relative contribution of the bursa and the thymus of the chicken. Chemical bursectomy was achieved using 19-nortestosterone, and spleen cells from such 14-day-old birds were unable to initiate splenomegaly (i.e. GVHR). Others had already indicated that bursectomy led to a reduced, but by no means absent thymus, and histologic examination of various lymphoid organs was carried out. They suggested that "any immunological potential . . . might be related to the presence of small amounts of thymus tissue," and they went on to say that "In mammals, the thymus may be the most important organ supplying lymphoid cells to other organs in the reticuloendothelial system, as originally postulated by Ruth (see *91*). It may also influence the *de novo* development of lymphoid cells in such organs as the spleen and intestine through humoral factors influencing lymphopoiesis. . . . cells from the thymus and bursa could enter the spleen, gut tract, and other areas of lymphoid cell accumulation, and continue to proliferate and/or differentiate into immunologically competent cells." Finally, Papermaster and Good concluded that "The lymphoid development of the thymus and the bursa in the chick are similar, and the function of these two organs . . . may also prove to be similar". The distinction between T and B lymphocytes and their different "education" had yet to be made.

A third group that made an important early contribution to "thymology" was that of B.H. Waksman. According to B.D. Janković (*84*), they began their studies at Harvard quite independently of Miller in the spring of 1961 and a brief manuscript outlining their preliminary results was sent to *Nature* in August. Janković claims that the journal, having accepted the manuscript, then unaccountably lost it, so that a second copy had to be sent eventually. (All this happened before John Maddox had become editor and modernized the editorial structure.) The paper by Arnason, Janković and Waksman (*108*) was published by *Nature* in the following year. It seems surprising that the editors did not add a note acknowledging their negligence, which may have added several months to the date of publication, and that the authors failed to insist on it. In any event, Arnason, Janković and Waksman reported on two types of delayed-type hypersensitivity reaction after neonatal thymectomy in rats: the cutaneous delayed reaction that can be revealed following footpad sensitization with BSA in Freund's complete adjuvant, and the clinical manifestations of experimental allergic encephalomyelitis in rats sensitized with spinal cord tissue in Freund's complete adjuvant. Both were substantially, but not entirely depressed. Further, skin allografts enjoyed better survival as judged on the tenth day after transplantation, and circulating lymphocyte counts were reduced. The authors concluded that "these experiments emphasize the importance of the thymus in the initiation of delayed hypersensitivity reactivity". A note was added in proof referring to Miller's paper, which had meanwhile been published.

This group published three other articles in 1962 (109–111), all received by the *Journal of Experimental Medicine* on the same day in April of that year. They considerably extended the data that had been published in *Nature* and in one paper (*110*) they made the point that the inhibition of the Arthus reaction correlated with a drop in the titer of precipitating and hemagglutinating antibodies although natural antibodies were unaffected. Further, no serum protein abnormalities, including gamma-globulin, were detected. In another paper (*109*) they stated: "It is concluded that small lymphocytes of the spleen and lymph nodes may come, in large part, directly from the thymus and are not derived from the medium or large lymphocytes of the germinal centers. It is suggested that there is a second population of small lymphocytes whose function is unrelated to the thymus lymphocytes." This might well have foreshadowed the distinction between B and T lymphocytes. It was Waksman's group that was to make the astonishing and neglected discovery a few years later that antigens inoculated intrathymically induced systemic tolerance (see Chapter 6, p. 284).

Two other papers published in 1962 deserve mention because they were the first to point to a clear dissociation of function between the bursa and the thymus. The Australians N.L. Warner and A. Szenberg (*112, 113*), by demonstrating that early thymectomy in chicks, but not bursectomy, largely abolished the ability of the animals to reject skin allografts, established that the bursa and the thymus of birds have quite different functions, the former involving the production of antibodies and the latter of cell-mediated responses like allograft rejection. This paved the way for the distinction between T and B lymphocytes.

These are the bare bones relating to the discovery of the immunologic function of the thymus. It is likely that the three groups – Miller, Good's and Waksman's – approached the problem of the thymus quite independently, but there can be little doubt that it was Miller who first published the results of a detailed and convincing investigation in a refereed journal.

T and B lymphocytes and their interactions

Once it was appreciated that small lymphocytes had diverse functions, and that their development into mature cells was regulated by the two primary lymphoid organs, the bursa in birds and the thymus in mammals, cellular immunology developed fast and furiously in the 1960s and 1970s. Rather as in the golden period of the discovery of antitoxins towards the end of the last century, important discoveries were made with almost bewildering rapidity on the nature of the cells involved and their great heterogeneity, diverse functions and complex interactions. These developments were largely facilitated by technologic advances that made it possible to identify cell surface markers and to separate subpopulations. Here I wish to draw attention to only a few of the more seminal developments.

One of these was the publication of a report by an American group working at the University of Colorado. In 1966 H.N. Claman, E.A. Chaperon and R.F. Triplett (*114*) published the results of experiments intended to show that there are immunologically competent, antibody-forming cells in the thymus. To do this, they transferred thymus and/or bone marrow cells from normal mice into irradiated syngeneic recipients, which were then stimulated with sheep red blood cells. Hemolytic antibody production was measured in cultures of spleen fragments in the presence of guinea pig complement. A mixture of thymus and bone marrow cells was far more effective than either cell type on its own and they carefully studied the kinetics of antibody formation. Because thymus cells from normal or presensitized donors did not produce antibodies on their own, Claman, Chaperton and Triplett concluded that the amount of antibody generated from a mixture of cells was not simply an additive effect but one that involved synergy. They concluded that only one of the cell populations (the effector cells) was capable of producing antibodies, but that they required the presence of the other (auxiliary cells). They were cautious about identifying the cell populations, but felt "that it is most likely that the effector cell . . . is bone marrow-derived, and that the thymus provides the auxiliary cells".

J.F.A.P. Miller and G.F. Mitchell published a pair of papers in 1968 which took matters a big step further. The inoculation of syngeneic or even allogeneic thymus or thoracic duct lymphocytes was found to be "absolutely essential" in the generation of normal 19S anti-sheep red cell hemolysins by spleen cells obtained from neonatally thymectomized mice (*115*) – a result not achieved by injecting bone marrow cells. They concluded that the antibody-forming cells were of host origin and that thymus and TDL possessed cells that could react specifically with antigen and induce the formation of antibody-forming cells in the hosts. In the accompanying paper (*116*) Mitchell and Miller went on to show that there was synergy between syngeneic thymus and bone marrow cells when both cell types were inoculated together into heavily irradiated animals and that thoracic duct cells were even more effective than thymus cells in this respect. A similar observation was made in thymectomized and irradiated mice that had been protected with syngeneic bone marrow. Using anti-histocompatibility antigen (H-2) sera they were able to show that the antibody-forming cells in the spleens of these animals were bone marrow-derived. Mitchell and Miller concluded that thoracic duct lymphocytes comprised two lymphocyte populations – one acting as hemolysin-forming cell precursors and the other capable of reacting with antigen and of initiating the differentiation of the precursors of antibody-forming cells. In contrast, bone marrow possessed only antibody-forming cell precursors and the thymus only antigen-reactive cells, though in lower numbers compared with TDL. These conclusions were confirmed in a further study analyzing single antibody-forming cells (*117*).

It should be noted that the inability of thymus cells to produce antibody had already been highlighted by the work of A.J.S. Davies and his colleagues at the Chester Beatty Research Institute. This group (*118*) had used the mouse CBA strain T6T6 chromosomal marker in the study of radiation chimeras and had shown in 1967 that following transplantation of a single neonatal thymus lobe under the kidney capsule of thymectomized radiation chimeras, immunologic competence of host spleen and lymph nodes was restored by cells demonstrably derived from the thymus graft. A year later they showed that these thymus-derived cells, though responding to antigenic stimulation, were incapable of antibody production, whereas host bone marrow-derived cells produced limited amounts. However, when both kinds of cells were exposed to antigen together far more antibody was generated (*119*).

Of great importance was the demonstration by Mitchison, Rajewsky and Taylor (*120*) of the hapten–protein carrier effect, involving "help" from thymus-derived lymphocytes in the generation of antibody. These and many other studies underlined the dichotomy between thymus-derived and bone marrow-derived cells and the ability of these two cell types to cooperate in the production of antibodies to certain antigens and in other immunologic responses. By 1969 progress had been sufficient to enable I.M. Roitt *et al.* (*121*) to propose a unified hypothesis according to which thymus-dependent lymphocytes were designated as T cells and the thymus-independent (bursa-equivalent) lymphocytes as B cells. Although strenuous efforts were made, for example by Good's group, to identify in mammals an organ analogous to the avian bursa, and gut-associated lymphoid tissue was considered to be a candidate, these all came to nought and it was eventually concluded that in mammals the B cells were those bone-marrow derived cells that had not entered the thymus and come under its educative influence.

It was M.C. Raff (*122*) who in 1969 identified a cell surface marker (θ) on T lymphocytes and thereafter it became possible to distinguish between T and B cells on morphologic as well as functional grounds. (The θ marker had first been described by Reif and Allen (*123*) in the thymus and brain of inbred mouse strains.) A year later Raff provided evidence for the existence of two distinct populations of peripheral lymphocytes – T cells with the θ marker and B cells carrying naturally occurring immunoglobulin determinants on their membranes. The distribution of these two subpopulations was characteristic of various organs, with almost 100% T cells in the thymus and 30–50% in the spleen.

The full recognition of T cell subclasses came in the mid-1970s. Following some earlier leads indicating that there were three genetic loci (Ly-1, 2 and 3) coding for cell surface antigens on cells undergoing thymus-dependent differentiation, H. Cantor and E.A. Boyse (*124*) were able to group peripheral T cells into two distinct subclasses on the basis of their differential expression of the three antigens. Ly-1 enriched populations were capable of providing "help", but could not generate cytotoxic activity, whereas the reverse was true for cells enriched for Ly-2,3. This was the beginning of the dichotomy between T helper and T cytotoxic lymphocytes and foreshadowed the modern CD4 and CD8 terminology (see Chapter 2). In a companion paper Cantor and Boyse (*125*) described how Ly-1-positive cells assisted in the maturation of Ly-2,3-positive killer cells without themselves contributing to the cytotoxicity, and that this effect was brought about by recognition of the cell marker "Ia" coded for by the immune response (I) region of the major histocompatibility system (see Chapter 4). In the same year Simpson and Cantor (*126*), in an Anglo-American collaboration, described how thymectomy in adult mice affected humoral and cellular responses. They concluded that the adult thymus "maintains a regulatory population of T cells in peripheral tissues which suppress early T cell proliferation to cytotoxic effector cells and potentiates the development of immune memory".

This section has been given some prominence because the events described here have been fundamental to subsequent developments in the fields of immunology and transplantation. It can also be said that transplantation immunology, by contributing a variety of experimental approaches such as skin allotransplantation, adoptive transfer of sensitivity and graft-versus-host assays, and knowledge of the histocompatibility antigens – not to mention immunologic tolerance – made a considerable contribution.

Concurrent Developments on the Antibody Front

Although cellular immunology was to become *the* area of growth in the three post-war decades, exciting developments also occurred in the realm of immunochemistry, for great leaps were made in understanding the structure and function of antibodies, and a few of the highlights will now be mentioned.

The Swedish chemist S. Arrhenius (*127*) believed that antigen–antibody reactions obeyed the laws of mass action and that, in contradiction to Ehrlich, the union between the two was relatively easily reversible. He therefore made the study of antigen–antibody reactions amenable to quantitative and biochemical study. K. Landsteiner who, as the discoverer of the human ABO blood groups, is the hero of Chapter 3, explored the specificity of antigens and the antisera raised against them and demonstrated that the introduction of alkyl radicals into protein molecules created a new structural specificity (*128*). He demonstrated with the utmost clarity how molecular structure affected antigenicity and how small molecular entities of a large antigen (determinants), though not themselves immunogenic, could react with antibodies made against the whole antigen. The concepts of "hapten" and "carrier" thus became established. His numerous investigations were embodied in a classic monograph, *The Specificity of Serological Reactions*, which was first published in 1936 and republished in revised form in 1947 (*129*), a few years after his death. In it he exhaustively analyzed serologic specificity, the nature of cellular antigens, the properties of artificial conjugated antigens, serologic reactions with simple chemical compounds, the antigenic and immunogenic qualities of non-protein antigens such as polysaccharides, and the kinetics of antigen–antibody reactions. His was a towering contribution to the flowering of immunochemistry.

The investigations in the 1930s of two groups of workers paved the way for the unraveling of the structure of antibodies two decades later. J.R. Marrack (*130*) in London formulated a hypothesis concerning hydrogen bonding in antigen–antibody interactions and the formation of aggregates and lattices, and he postulated that precipitating antibodies would have to have at least two binding sites. At a time when nothing whatever was known of the structure of antibodies this was a remarkable prediction which turned out to be correct. The other contribution came from Uppsala, Sweden. A. Tiselius had already discovered electrophoresis, the technique that permitted the separation of molecules of different molecular weights by differential migration in an electric field, when he was joined by the American immunologist E.A. Kabat to help him apply his technique to the separation of antibodies. Tiselius and Kabat (*131*) described the results of their studies in 1939. Using a new electrophoretic apparatus designed by Tiselius they succeeded in separating the serum components into albumin and α, β and γ fractions and showed that antibodies were associated with the γ fraction. They wrote that "The method should be most useful for obtaining purified antibodies to protein antigens . . ." and the subsequent isolation and purification of antibodies was indeed largely based on their technique and observations.

The crowning glory of the antibody story – the elucidation of their structure – came about once again as a result of work independently carried out on both sides of the Atlantic. R.R. Porter was a biochemist at the National Institute for Medical Research in north London (later, in 1960 he became the first Professor of Immunology in the United Kingdom at St Mary's Hospital Medical School) when he turned his attention to antibodies. Using carboxymethylcellulose chromatography and the proteolytic enzyme papain he was able to recognize three fractions – I, II and III – in gammaglobulin isolated from rabbit antisera against several protein antigens such as BSA as well as against pneumococcal polysaccharide type 3. Although none of the fractions precipitated the corresponding antigen, fractions I and II inhibited precipitation of the antigen by the homologous antiserum (132). This inhibition was antigen-specific, but it could not be observed for any fractions from antipolysaccharide antisera unless much higher concentrations of fractions were used. This pointed to a quantitative rather than a qualitative difference. In contrast, fraction III seemed to be totally inert. To cut a long story short, strong evidence was provided that fractions I and II were virtually the same in terms of amino acid content, molecular weight, antigenic specificity and antigen-binding capacity. The apparently inert fraction III could be crystallized and possessed most of the antigenic sites of the original molecule. The molecular weights suggested for the fractions were 50 000 (I), 53 000 (II) and 80 000 (III), with the whole molecule having a value of 188 000. Among the different possible structures envisaged by Porter, all based on the assumption of a single polypeptide chain for the whole antibody molecule, was one in which fractions I and II, carrying the combining sites, came from the same portion of the molecule and fraction III from the remainder. Although he pointed out that this structure was "reminiscent of Pauling's theory of antibody formation" (see below) he wrote: "Nor is there any evidence on the essential feature of Pauling's theory, that the amino acid sequence of all antibodies is identical and that the different antibody-combining sites are formed only by refolding of the same polypeptide chain." Fractions I and II were later designated as "Fab" (fragment antigen-binding) and fragment III as "Fc" (fragment crystalline).

The other vital contribution to the elucidation of antibody structure came from the American biochemist G.M. Edelman, who was to share the 1972 Nobel Prize with Porter. He published a brief and densely written letter in 1959 (133) describing the dissociation of human gammaglobulin and a pathologic macroglobulin with sulfhydryl compounds, the dialysis of the products and the determination of their molecular weight (48 000). He concluded that "human gammaglobulin contains subunits linked at least in part by bisulfide bonds". This was to have a profound influence on the interpretation of Porter's proposed model. Together with M.D. Poulik (and now working at the Rockefeller Institute) he made some further critical observations that appeared two years later (134). Spurred by Edelman's earlier observation, they used a number of procedures, including papain and peptide digestion, in the expectation of breaking the postulated disulfide bonds of human and rabbit 7S gammaglobulins. The molecular weight of the products fell to about one-third of the original value, and the partial separation of these products, using chromatography and starch gel electrophoresis, enabled them to determine their amino acid composition. Similar treatment of a pathological macroglobulin yielded a fragment with a molecular weight of 41 000, and human myeloma proteins behaved in much the same way and led to the appearance of sulfhydryl groups. They concluded that 7S gammaglobulin is made up of "several discrete subunits or polypeptide chains linked by disulfhydryl bonds". They proposed a "unifying hypothesis" based on their own studies and those of Porter and of Nisonoff, Wissler and Lipman (135), who in 1960 had identified a univalent antibody fragment with a molecular weight of 56 000, which they were able to recombine by what they assumed to be reoxidation of the sulfhydryl groups. According to this unifying hypothesis, 7S antibodies were bivalent and composed of two chains of similar or identical structure, and 19S gammaglobulin was multivalent and made up of 5–6 multichain units of the size of 7S molecules.

Thus were laid the foundations of modern immunochemistry, and a four-chain structure (two light and two heavy) for immunoglobulins was soon arrived at. Disulfide bonds link the two light chains (at the N-terminal end) to the heavy chains, and the same kind of bond links the carboxyl terminal ends of the heavy chains. Both the structure and function of the Fab and Fc fragments of antibodies could now be established in fine detail. The univalent Fab polypeptide chains, possessing sites of variable amino acid composition, were shown to harbor the molecule's antigen-binding receptor sites. The Fc fragment, comprising the C-terminal portions of the two heavy chains, was found to have a variety of biologic functions including complement activation via complement receptors. It was now possible to study questions such as specificity, affinity, diversity and heterogeneity and the interaction of antibodies with various cell types at a new level of sophistication. This level was raised still further with the advent of monoclonal antibodies in the 1970s (see below).

Theories of Antibody Formation

These can be broadly divided into instructive and selective theories. Before World War II little was known of the structure of antibodies except that they were proteins made up of amino acids. The sequence of events in the synthesis of proteins – with the "flow" of information going from the nuclear deoxyribonucleic acid (DNA) to the cytoplasmic ribonucleic acid (RNA), followed by assembly of the proteins from amino acids – was at that time totally unknown and it is therefore not surprising that the theory that first held sway, in one form or another, was of an instructional kind. The history of various kinds of instructive theory have been well discussed by Silverstein (1) and here I shall focus mainly on the direct template theory of F. Breinl and F. Haurowitz and others, especially that of L. Pauling.

The direct template hypothesis

Because it seemed inconceivable that information about the vast array of possible antigens to which the body is exposed could be stored in the nucleus, Breinl and Haurowitz (136), at that time working in Prague, proposed that one way of explaining the extraordinary diversity of antibodies, including antibodies formed to molecules that do not exist in nature, was to regard the antigen as a template. Once inside the antibody-producing cell, antibody would be synthesized in close conjunction with the antigenic molecule, the shape of which would determine the precise sequence and spatial arrangement in which the amino acids were assembled. Such a mechanism could account for the specificity of antibodies as well as for the ability of an organism to respond to a wide variety of antigens. The theory also seemed to explain why minute amounts of antigen could elicit the formation of a huge number of antibody molecules, though inherent in it was the assumption that antigen persisted within cells for as long as antibody production was in progress. Breinl and Haurowitz listed the possible objections to their proposal, including the fact that antigen mixed with normal serum did not result in the formation of antibodies, but they dismissed Ehrlich's suggestion of preformed antibodies (see below) because, on the face of it, it could not explain the induction of antibodies to synthetic antigens.

Ten years later the American chemist Linus Pauling, a multiple Nobel Laureate, came up with an extension of the template theory, which seemed more plausible than the notion of Breinl and Haurowitz because it circumvented the need to synthesize antibodies directly from amino acids, a point that nobody had been able to explain satisfactorily. Working at the California Institute of Technology he published a paper in 1930 in *Science* together with M. Delbrück (*137*) – Delbrück was at the time at Vanderbilt University – in which they considered the stereochemical interactions between molecules. Having rejected P. Jordan's notion of a "quantum-mechanical resonance phenomenon" they proposed that ". . . the process of synthesis and folding of highly complex molecules in the living cell involves, in addition to covalent-bond formation, only the intermolecular interactions of van der Waal's attraction and repulsion, electrostatic interactions, hydrogen-bond formation etc. . . ." They envisaged that antibodies were formed by the folding of normal globulin molecules, and basic to this was the notion of complementariness, with one molecule influencing the shape of the other.

This hypothesis was further developed by Pauling (*138*) in the same year in relation to specific antibody formation. It entailed:

(1) First, synthesis of a normal globulin chain consisting of several hundred amino acid residues, with the middle of the chain having a much more stable configuration than the two ends.
(2) Second, the chain ends would coil up into the most stable of the accessible configurations by the formation of hydrogen bonds and other weak bonds and be "liberated" to lie outside the cell membrane.
(3) Third, the central portion of the chain would be liberated.
(4) Fourth, the central portion would assume a stable folded configuration to yield the completed globin molecule.

If at stage one an antigen molecule found itself held by the polypeptide chain, the coiling of the two ends of the molecule would be moulded to the surface configuration of the antigen and the two ends would adopt a complementary structure based on electrostatic attraction and repulsion. In the presence of the antigen the chain ends would become stable. The configuration of the chain ends could be "any one of a large number, depending upon which part of the surface of the antigen happens to exert its influence . . . and how large a region of the surface happens to be covered by it." What happened after complete liberation of the antibody molecule would depend on the strength of the bonds holding it to the antigen: in the presence of strong bonds "nothing further of interest will happen". If the bonds were weak, however, the antibody molecule would dissociate from the antigen, the central portion would coil up to achieve its normal configuration and the completed antibody molecule would "float away". The antigenic molecule could serve as a pattern for another globin molecule until it is degraded or "escapes from the region of globin formation. . .".

The template theory held sway until it became apparent in the 1950s that it was no longer tenable in the light of new knowledge of information flow from DNA to protein, and it was superseded by selective theories.

Selective theories

J.D. Watson and F.H.C. Crick (*139*) dropped their bombshell in 1953 when they published their two-chain helical model of the structure of DNA, and by 1958 the "central dogma" of molecular biology had been established, namely that there was a residue-by-residue sequential transfer of information from DNA to RNA to protein assembly (see *140, 141*). R.S. Schweet and R.D. Owen (*142*) at the California Institute of Technology made a valiant attempt to take this into account by proposing a modification of the template hypothesis. Thus antigen would in the first instance interact with the DNA of the globulin gene to provide a new RNA template, thereby setting up the cell to make a specific antibody, and subsequently the antigen acted as a template for the productive phase of antibody formation. However, this hypothesis too was swept away by the tide favoring a selective approach.

Such an approach had been followed by P. Ehrlich (*26, 143*) near the end of the nineteenth century, when he described his side chain theory of antibody formation. This was based on the notion that in order to incorporate nutrients into the cell there would have to be special receptors on the cell surface with which the nutrients reacted chemically. Similarly, to cope with toxic substances the same receptors had specificity for toxins. For example, the ganglion cells of the nervous system were thought to possess groups of atoms or side chains capable of binding tetanus toxin. The number of side chains of different kinds present in an organism would be "many hundreds", all capable of binding a specific toxin. To explain the relationship between side chain and its toxin Ehrlich used the male and female screw analogy, and the lock and key analogy, attributed to L. Pasteur and E. Fischer, respectively. Cells without side chains for a particular toxin could not be harmed by that substance. Because a cell whose side chains were occupied by toxins could not survive for lack of nutrients, regeneration of side chains was postulated. During the course of immunization with an antigen the specific side chains would be produced in ever increasing quantities, so that eventually there would be too many "for the cell to carry, and (they) are, after the manner of a secretion, handed over, as superfluous ballast, to the blood". Antibody production was thus seen as an overproduction of side chains in response to an antigen such as a bacterial toxin. The side chains (receptors) were present naturally on the cell surface and all the antigen did was to select the appropriate cell, which would in due course shed free antibodies into the circulation. Though wrong in detail and though the diagrammatic illustrations of the side chains were fanciful, Ehrlich's theory was clearly the forerunner of modern selective theories.

We owe the development of the natural selection theory of antibody formation largely to the work of N. Jerne and F.M. Burnet in the mid-1950s, by which time immunologic tolerance had been discovered and the basis of cellular immunology had been laid. Jerne, working at the Danish State Serum Institute in Copenhagen, published his wide-ranging speculations in 1955 (*144*) after having spent some months in M. Delbrück's laboratory at the California Institute of Technology. (It was Delbrück who encouraged Jerne to publish his ideas and it was he who communicated the paper to the *Proceedings of the National Academy of Sciences*.) What Jerne proposed was that the antigen acts neither as a template (as the instructive theories would have it) nor as an enzyme modifier (as Burnet and Fenner (*45*) had suggested), but that it is "solely a selective carrier of spontaneously circulating antibodies to a system of cells which can reproduce this antibody". The spontaneously circulating antibodies would be the natural antibodies, which Jerne assumed to be continuously "synthesized in an enormous variety of different configurations" though how this had come about was not specified. "The introduction of an antigen ... leads to the selective attachment to the antigen surface of those globulin molecules which happen to have a complementary configuration." This would result in internalization of the antigen by phagocytes, the dissociation of the globulin from the antigen and the elimination of the antigen, which had now "accomplished its role." The presence of the dissociated globulin within the cell would provide a signal for the synthesis of identical molecules, which would then be released into the circulation. Further antigen of the same specificity introduced into the body would select the "better-fitting" globulins and thus bring about a more rapid production of "an improved assortment of antibody molecules". The spontaneous production of antibodies was thought to have occurred early in the life of the animal, and the natural antibodies needed to be present in only very small numbers. "Those among them that will attach themselves to structures in the body of the animal itself will be removed and will therefore not be available for reproduction."

Jerne thought that his theory thus accounted for the booster effect (i.e. the secondary response), changes in avidity of antibody on repeated stimulation, the exponential rise in antibody, the continued production of antibody after elimination of the antigen, and the fact that the surface of particulate antigens played a dominant role in determining specificity. He believed that there was an "amply sufficient number of natural globulin molecules in the serum of animals to take care of the many different antigens that might be encountered", and he noted that cross-reactivity was not a rare event. He considered the plasma cell as the probable source of antibody production, but was undecided about the role of lymphocytes in this respect. His theory was an extension of that of Burnet and Fenner (*45*), who had postulated self-markers to explain how the body distinguished between self and not-self, in that the disappearance of antibodies with specificity for the organism would be removed and "lead to the permament disappearance of this type of specificity" and remove the danger of autoimmunity. It therefore took full account of immunologic tolerance. Strangely, there was no mention of Ehrlich's earlier speculations. The theory's weak point was that it ran counter to the "central dogma" of molecular biology (see above) and this was pointed out in 1957 by D.W. Talmage (*145*). Two years later both Talmage (*146*) and J. Lederberg (*147*) in the United States extended Jerne's theory into the cellular domain.

Meanwhile F.M. Burnet had been grappling with the same theoretic problems, which in his case arose from investigations of GVHRs of lymphoid cells transplanted to the chorioallantoic membrane of chick embryos. Because proliferating cells tended to appear in groups or plaques the idea came to him that it was not the antibody but the antigen that selected – not antibodies, but cells of the appropriate specificity. Thus was born the germ of the clonal selection hypothesis, a preliminary version of which was published in an Australian science journal (*148*), with a full account given two years later in his famous monograph *The Clonal Selection Theory of Acquired Immunity* (*149*), which was to provide the theoretic basis for modern immunology.

In this book, which was every bit as wide-ranging as his 1949 monograph, he considered virtually all aspects of immunology, including allograft immunity and tolerance. He felt that Jerne's theory "appears to be out of line with any of the current ideas on protein synthesis" and it was this objection that led him to formulate a clonal selection theory. "My own view is that any tenable form of Jerne's theory must involve the *existence of multiple clones of globulin-forming cells*, each responsible for one genetically determined type of antibody globulin." To allow for this he postulated that antibody-producing cells possess natural antibodies on their surface and that once an antigen engaged with such antibodies it would set in motion the process of antibody production by that cell. Each cell would carry cell-bound antibodies (receptors) of one particular specificity. "When an antigen is introduced it will make contact with a cell of the corresponding clone, presumably a lymphocyte, and by so doing stimulate it to produce in one way or another more globulin molecules of the cell's characteristic type." Jerne's natural antibody notion was therefore given a clear-cut cellular and clonal orientation while preserving the selective element. "Changing views on the life-history of the lymphocyte have made it admissible to postulate that a lymphocyte appropriately stimulated could give rise to a clone of descendant cells. In particular, work from Florey's laboratory (Gowens, 1957) (*sic*!) shows that lymphocytes can undergo more than one cycle between tissue and circulation." He had little doubt that following the work of Astrid Fagraeus (*150, 151*), in which she had demonstrated antibodies within mature plasma cells, that the antibody-producing cell *par excellence* was the plasma cell. He kept an open mind on small lymphocytes, in which he saw no sign of immunologic activity; but using his speculative powers to the full Burnet went on to say that "The position might, however, take on an entirely different aspect if small lymphocytes can be converted into other functional forms," as indeed proved to be the case with B lymphocytes. He concluded that his theory represented "a Darwinian approach which, pressed to its logical conclusion, demands that immunologic specificity is based on a special type of differentiation occurring in embryonic life plus a high subsequent potential for somatic mutation in that region of the genome concerned with immunologically significant pattern."

In his development of the clonal selection hypothesis Burnet was strongly underpinned by G.J. Nossal and J. Lederberg's (*152*) demonstration in 1958 that rat cells stimulated in microdroplets with two *Salmonella* serotypes produced antibody against one or the other, but not both. Their experiments had been "provoked by current hypotheses on the role of clonal individuation in antibody formation, with which they are consistent so far as they go", and they quoted Burnet's (*148*) and Talmage's

(*145*) 1957 papers. Nossal was later to confirm this powerful evidence in favor of clonal selection (see *153*). Following publication of Burnet's 1959 monograph (*149*) clonal deletion became the most attractive hypothesis for the induction of neonatally induced tolerance (see Chapter 5).

A very readable account of the origins of cell selection theories has recently been published by D.W. Talmage (*154*). For Burnet's biographic sketch, see p. 53.

Some 15 years after these important developments, Jerne published yet another highly influential theory – the network theory of the immune system (*155, 156*) in which he postulated an idiotype–antiidiotype network of interacting molecules on cells either stimulating or inhibiting each other, depending on the circumstances. In the same year this remarkable theoretician became a Nobel Laureate.

A further theory, proposed by P. Bretscher and M. Cohn in 1970 (*157*), provided an additional explanation for self–nonself discrimination in that it postulated the need for two signals, 1 and 2, for the induction of antibody formation. Whereas J. Lederberg (*147*) had proposed that a cell capable of antibody production first passed through a phase in which it could be paralyzed (tolerized) by antigen, Bretscher and Cohn suggested that cells retained the potential for both paralysis and antibody formation. Whether paralysis or induction came about depended on whether the cell received only one signal or two: a single antigenic determinant recognized by the cell's specific receptors would result in paralysis, whereas the second signal (provided by antibody against the protein carrier and bound to the antigen) would result in induction. This hypothesis was controversial and not universally accepted, but although ideas about the nature of the two signals have changed with the years, especially once the structure of the T cell receptor had been elucidated, it proved to be essentially correct. In modern terms, signal 1 is transmitted by the specific antigen to the B or T cell receptor of the resting B or T lymphocyte, while signal 2 in the form of interleukin-1 (IL-1) is provided by antigen-presenting cells (APC). Thus, antigenic peptides associated with class II histocompatibility antigens on the surface of an APC fulfill both these requirements, and the absense of signal 2 is more likely to lead to tolerance (see Chapters 5 and 6).

Cohn (*158*) has recently surveyed the evolution of the two signal concept. So far as its application to the transplantation of tissues is concerned, it is to the credit of Lafferty and Cunningham (*159*) (see also the review of Lafferty's group, *160*) that they were the first to appreciate its significance in 1975 in order to explain the activation of lymphocytes in response to allogeneic histocompatibility antigens, though many transplantation immunologists were skeptical at the time.

Some Other Important Developments

The 1970s and 1980s saw the most extraordinary upsurge in immunology, largely fueled by the application of technology derived from molecular biology. Nothing could have been further removed from the unfortunate statement made in the 1960s by one eminent elderly scientist (who shall remain anonymous) that there was nothing of importance left to be discovered in immunology – that it was now a question of dotting the is and crossing the ts! Among the most exciting developments from the point of view of transplantation were:

(1) The realization that immune responses were major histocompatibility complex (MHC)-restricted.
(2) The unraveling of the structure of the T cell receptor (TcR).
(3) X-ray crystallography of the human leukocyte antigen HLA-A2 molecule with the revelation of its peptide-binding groove.
(4) The role of accessory cells in the induction of immune responses.
(5) The participation of a battery of intercellular signals in the shape of the cytokines.
(6) The production of monoclonal antibodies.
(7) The isolation of T cell clones and the creation of T–T cell hybrids.

All these were of the most profound importance for the growth of transplantation immunology and some will be discussed in other chapters. Indeed, transplantation immunology played an honorable part in some of these discoveries. Here I will restrict myself to indicating the beginnings of these developments, leaving it to the reader to consult immunology reviews and textbooks for up-to-date and detailed information.

Major histocompatibility complex restriction

The role played by MHC molecules in the incitement of alloreactivity will be dealt with in Chapters 2 and 4. However, ever since the discovery of these molecules in the mouse and in humans (see Chapter 4) it had been clear that the main action of the transplantation antigens, as they were then called, must have served a more basic purpose than to frustrate the ambitions of twentieth-century transplant surgeons. Such a purpose was brilliantly revealed by the experiments of R.M. Zinkernagel and P.C. Doherty (*161, 162*), and of G.M. Shearer, in 1974 (*163*), long before the structure of the TcR had been elucidated.

Zinkernagel (a Swiss) and Doherty (*161, 162*), working at the time in Canberra, Australia, examined the possibility that the *in vitro* killing of virus-infected fibroblasts (L cells) by cytotoxic T lymphocytes might be MHC-restricted. Their inspiration came from data by two American groups (164–166) showing that in the mouse *in vivo* cooperation between T cells and antibody-forming cell precursors (B cells) in the production of antibody was controlled by the H-2 complex: helper activity by the T cells came about only when the two cell types shared at least one H-2 antigen with the B cells. Zinkernagel and Doherty proceeded to show that this was especially true for *in vivo* cytotoxic activity of T cells that had previously been sensitized *in vivo* with the lymphocytic choriomeningitis virus (LCM). When such cells were placed on monolayers of LCM-infected L cells, high level killing took place only when the T and L cells shared at least one H-2 haplotype (H-2K). The same was found to be true when infected macrophages from a number of allogeneic mouse strains were tested: again, specific lysis was restricted to the syngeneic system. Because lysis could be abrogated with an anti-θ (i.e. anti-T cell) antiserum the authors believed that they were dealing with MHC-restricted cytotoxicity by T lymphocytes. They pointed out that when the lymphocytes were specifically sensitized against alloantigens present on the targets such restriction was not required, as Cerottini, Nordin and Brunner (*167*; see also Chapter 2) had demonstrated when they first established the assay for cellular cytotoxicity. Indeed, it was later shown that MHC restriction is a phenomenon that applies to the so-called minor antigens, whether viral or histocompatibility (see Chapter 4). Zinkernagel and Doherty considered the possibility that what the cytotoxic lymphocytes were recognizing was "altered self", (i.e. a self-MHC molecule subtly altered by the incorporation of a viral moiety). They considered other possibilities in further articles published in the same (168) and in the following (169) year.

G.M. Shearer (163) made a related observation, likewise in 1974, but with a totally different antigenic system. Mouse spleen cells were exposed *in vitro* to trinitrophenyl (TNP)-modified syngeneic spleen cells, and the resultant effector cells were shown to be cytotoxic to TNP-modified target cells, but not to unmodified targets. This activity was shown to be a property of T cell effectors. Shearer concluded that his results were "compatible with the hypothesis that cell surface components (probably proteins) can be modified by TNP so as to be immunogenic to syngeneic lymphocytes, and that these structures are controlled by genes within distinct regions of the major histocompatibility complex." Shearer's interpretation did not postulate MHC restriction in the same graphic way as Zinkernagel and Doherty, but he felt that his evidence suggested that "these proteins are conformationally changed so as to be immunogenic to syngeneic thymus-derived lymphocytes".

The concept of MHC restriction provided the first clear indication that histocompatibility antigens serve a profoundly important biologic function, both in the induction and execution of certain immunologic responses. It was foreshadowed by the previous findings of two groups of transplantation immunologists that the ability of females to reject syngeneic male skin grafts (carrying the "minor" H-Y antigen) was largely determined by the H-2 genotype of the female (see Chapter 4, p. 164 – a point that was subsequently further illuminated by the work of Gordon *et al.* (see Chapter 4, p. 165). Other workers soon confirmed the data of Zinkernagel and Doherty that the sharing of class I antigens between virus-infected cells and effector cells was a necessity and this has been reviewed by Zinkernagel and Doherty (170), Swain and Dutton (171), and Dialynas *et al.* (172). In 1986 the British group of Townsend *et al.* (173) showed conclusively that short synthetic peptides derived from the nucleoprotein of the influenza A virus were recognized by mouse and human cytotoxic T lymphocytes (CTL) and that recognition was in association with class I histocompatibility antigens. In the same year Maryanski *et al.* (174) published their data demonstrating that the phenomenon extends beyond viral and minor antigens, in that a class I-restricted mouse CTL clone recognizing HLA class I products lysed HLA-negative syngeneic mouse targets in the presence of a synthetic HLA peptide. Both these studies supported the notion that class I-restricted T cells, like those restricted by class II molecules (see reviews, 175–177), recognize degraded or denatured antigenic fragments expressed on the cell surface in association with MHC molecules rather than the entire antigen.

B cell hybridomas: the advent of monoclonal antibodies

Rarely has a technologic innovation affected the course of immunology as dramatically as the fusion of myeloma cells with antibody-producing cells, resulting in the establishment of cell lines in continuous culture and able to secrete specific antibodies. Until 1975 immune sera, usually with a wide range of epitope specificities, had to be used as immunologic tools, whether to identify cellular antigens (e.g. those characterizing the cells of the immune system or the histocompatibility antigens) or to suppress the immune response, which antilymphocyte globulin had done very effectively though without defined specificity (see Chapter 6).

The circumstances that led to this discovery and, incidentally, to the award of the Nobel Prize in 1984 (together with Niels Jerne) to both scientists involved, have been described in the summary of a recent Wellcome Trust "*Witness Seminar*" on monoclonal antibodies (*178*). Cesar Milstein, an Argentinian established at the Medical Research Council Laboratory of Molecular Biology in Cambridge, was joined by a young German postdoctoral worker, Georges Köhler, in 1974. Köhler had thought about the possibility of fusing antibody-producing cells with tumor cells to confer longevity on the former and, having discussed the idea with Milstein, it was decided that he should carry out his project in Milstein's laboratory. Milstein had expressed considerable enthusiasm for it, particularly because he too had thought of making such an attempt. Most of the techniques required were readily available in Cambridge, and the experiments were carried out with mouse myeloma cells and cells from the spleens of mice that had been sensitized against sheep red blood cells.

I will spare the reader the technical details of cell fusion, which can be found in Köhler and Milstein's first publication in 1975 (*179*). Although myeloma cells had previously been used as a source of antibodies, they were "not a satisfactory source of monoclonal antibodies of predefined specificity". The critical experiments were preceded by fusion experiments between two known myeloma lines in order to investigate "the expression and interactions of the Ig chains from the parental lines". They concluded that "Ig molecules are produced as a result of mixed association between heavy and light chains from the two parents following an intracellular process" and the precise consequences of this were determined. Köhler and Milstein then went on to fuse mouse myeloma and spleen cells from mice presensitized to sheep red blood cells. They established a number of lines secreting anti-sheep red blood cell antibody after the elimination of unfused cells, and the cell clones (which were visible to the naked eye) could be observed to grow in distinct plaques and to secrete immunoglobulin IgM antibody into the surrounding medium, causing sheep red cells to be lysed. Köhler and Milstein concluded that ". . . cell fusion techniques are a useful tool to produce specific antibody directed against a predetermined antigen. It further shows that it is possible to isolate hybrid lines producing different antibodies directed against the same antigen and carrying different effector functions (direct and indirect plaque)."

Having produced a large number of antibody-producing cells from three fusion experiments, 3% were positive for IgM (i.e. forming direct plaques) three weeks after the initial fusion. "It remains to be seen whether similar results can be obtained with using other antigens."

These results were confirmed a year later (*180*), the subclasses of Ig were determined, and the principle was extended to a wholly different kind of antigen, 2,4,6-TNP. Different lines expressed different combinations of the four possible chains in each hybrid line (the myeloma γ and κ chains and the specific antibody heavy and light chains) – an issue that was further analyzed by Köhler, Hengartner and Shulman (*181*) after Köhler's move to the Basel Institute for Immunology. In none of these publications, which were mainly concerned with the technology and the nature of the antibodies secreted, was there any intimation of the revolutionary effect their experiments were to have on immunologic (and other) research, although Milstein was well aware of their importance.

Once the immunologic community had taken on board the almost unlimited possible applications of the cell fusion technique, monoclonal antibodies were produced against a wide range of antigens, and such antibodies were used to identify the presence of antigens on cells of all kinds and on bacteria and parasites. For example, as early as 1979 Brodsky *et al.* (*182*) published a massive review entitled "*Monoclonal antibodies for analysis of the HLA system,*" for the fine specificity of these antibodies permitted a much more precise identification, and in many cases the splitting, of previously identified HLA antigens. In the same year Kung *et al.* (*183*) and Reinherz *et al.* (*184*), a large group working with S.F. Schlossman in Boston, used monoclonal antibodies to identify the CD3 proteins that are intimately associated with the TcR. Gillis and Henney (*185*) identified the important cytokine IL-2, and monoclonal technology subsequently facilitated recognition of a very large family of cytokines with a variety of functions (see below). The analysis of the TcR (see below) could not have been achieved without it. Of great importance for transplantation was the fact that monoclonal antibodies, whether directed against T lymphocytes or other cells of the immune system, or against cytokines or their cell receptors, were to replace to a great extent the cruder polyvalent antisera such as antilymphocyte globulin as immunosuppressive agents in the reversal of clinical rejection crises (see Chapters 6 and 7).

A historic account of hybridoma technology, published recently, is that of Cambrioso and Keating (*186*). Sadly, Georges Köhler, who in 1985 had become director of the Max Planck Institute for Immunobiology in Freiburg, died in 1995 at the age of 48 (see obituary by F. Melchers, *187*).

One further important spin-off proved to be the production of T cell hybridomas, which have been used extensively in the dissection of immune T cell mechanisms. Thus Goldsby *et al.* (*188*) succeeded in 1977 in fusing mouse spleen cells with a mouse T lymphocyte lymphoma line, the hybridoma cells expressing T cell markers. The spleen donors were either normal or had been sensitized to DNP-KLH, and the hybridomas yielded continuous cell populations with T cell surface markers. Shortly afterwards Fathman and Hengartner (*189*) blazed the trail by the creation of T cell clones from cells that had been in long-term mixed lymphocyte culture (MLC) and whose specificity they studied. Their continuous culture became possible by the discovery and application of T cell growth factors. All clones displayed specificity for the priming stimulator cells used in MLC and some recognized unique F1 hybrid MLC determinants. T cell clones have since been used to great effect in the study of immune mechanisms and in the analysis of TcRs.

Lymphocyte receptors – early speculations

As explained above, the distinction between T and B lymphocytes became possible in 1969, when Raff (*122*) showed that murine B but not T lymphocytes possessed surface Ig, and that T cells carry a specific cell surface marker, θ. A number of groups subsequently demonstrated a similar dichotomy in human lymphocyte populations. Thus human T cells formed rosettes with sheep red blood cells and could be labeled or killed with certain xenogeneic antisera such as antilymphocyte serum.

B lymphocytes were shown to have Fc receptors that bound aggregated Ig, formed rosettes with sheep red blood cells only when the latter had bound IgM and complement (i.e. via the complement receptors) and, most importantly, had cell surface Ig (see *188*). Brown and Greaves (*190*) added to the markers characterizing human lymphocyte subpopulations by showing that absorbed antibrain antisera were T lymphocyte-specific. It soon became clear that whereas B lymphocytes were involved in antibody production, T lymphocyte played a role in the induction of immune responses and as effectors in viral and allograft sensitivity (see above and Chapter 2).

It was therefore assumed that surface Ig – probably different from serum Igs in only minor respects – was the antigen receptor for B lymphocytes. Although nothing was known of the structure of the antigen receptor of T lymphocytes in the early 1970s it was thought by some that it bore a close resemblance to that of B lymphocytes. The B cell receptor (BcR) was later shown to be a membrane-bound IgM monomer, specific for each B lymphocyte clone. Although some workers claimed that T lymphocytes were capable of antibody synthesis, others refuted this (see Binz, Kimura and Wigzell, *191*). Indeed, there was a strong current of opinion, led mainly by H. Binz and H. Wigzell and their colleagues in Stockholm, that T and B cells possessed closely similar idiotypic determinants, with the implication that the antigen receptors were identical or very similar. (Idiotypes are unique antigenic molecules in the variable regions of serum antibodies and they are likewise present on B lymphocyte surface Ig. They may thus act as autoantigens and lead to the formation of anti-idiotypic antibodies against an individual's own antibodies. This fact was the starting point of Jerne's network theory (*155, 156*). It is thus possible for the immune system to make anti-idiotypic antibodies, either spontaneously or assisted by the presentation of antibodies with suitable adjuvants.)

The evidence for BcR and TcR similarity or identity was largely derived from a number of papers from the Swedish team in the mid- to late-1970s. However, the first indication that this might be the case came from Ramseier and Lindenmann's findings using a rather crude assay (PAR) measuring the "product of antigen recognition" in one-way MLC reactions (for review, see *192*). Ramseier (*193*) argued that PAR was a function of TcR activation, and his 1975 data appeared to show that these receptors or recognition sites (RS) for alloantigen were shed spontaneously and could be used for the production of anti-RS antibodies in appropriate F1 hybrid mice (*194*). Ramseier and Lindenmann (*195*) believed that the cellular receptors for alloantigens had similar antigenic determinants to those on the combining site of alloantibodies, and they coined the term "aliotype" for these determinants.

Their findings received strong support from the Swedish group, who showed that the idiotypes of IgG antibodies and TcR were "similar or identical" (*196*) and provided evidence suggesting a linkage of T cell idiotypes to Ig heavy chains (*197*). Of special interest seemed to be their finding that idiotypic molecules with specificity for allogeneic rat MHC molecules could be isolated from serum or urine of normal rats, and that with the aid of Freund's adjuvant these molecules could be used to induce the production of auto-anti-idiotypic antibodies (*198*). Rats producing such antibodies were depleted of cells carrying the relevant idiotypic receptors and displayed a selective loss of reactivity against the appropriate MHC antigens as measured by graft-versus-host assays or MLC reactivity. Important from the point of view of transplantation was the demonstration that skin allograft survival times were roughly doubled in such animals. (For further critical discussion of this finding, which others had difficulty in confirming, see Chapter 6, p. 244.) Specific unresponsiveness was likewise induced when rat T lymphoblasts from one-way MLCs were used as immunogen (199), again in the presence of adjuvant. Such lymphoblasts would be expected to carry the idiotype for antigens of the strain providing the stimulator cells.

This and other experimental evidence from this group, which seemed internally consistent but which was by no means universally accepted at the time, became available before the structure of the TcR had been elucidated, and as the TcR proved not to be Ig (see below) it is difficult to comprehend its basis. It is an interesting example of the kind of cul-de-sac that science, including immunology, can enter from time to time. (The two-chain factors claimed to have been isolated by some workers from suppressor T lymphocytes are another such example.) This stricture does not, of course, apply to the many examples of long-term suppression of antibodies by anti-idiotypic antibodies directed against the BcR, which came to light in the early 1970s (200–203), for similarities between the BcR and the antibodies produced had by then been well accepted (204).

The T cell receptor – structure and function

The unraveling of the structure of the TcR is an intricate and fascinating story that deserves a book of its own, and a multi-author book on "*T Cell Receptors*" (205) has recently been published. Though it does not contain a historic account as such the reader will find detailed and up-to-date discussions in it of all structural and functional aspects, and these will be largely ignored here. Here I shall merely draw a brief sketch of the earliest events.

Several large laboratories took part in the race to clone the T cell gene and to describe the structure of its product, and it is almost invidious to credit any one group with the discovery. The work was carried out mainly in well-funded and well-equipped American laboratories able to attract bright young scientists eager to apply the latest techniques of molecular biology to this problem. In his recently published interesting as well as amusing historic account M.Davis (206) recounted how, having been on a National Institutes of Health (NIH)-sponsored visit to laboratories in China in 1983, just before to the Fifth International Congress of Immunology in Kyoto, he had the greatest difficulty in securing an air reservation to Japan and arrived only just in time after numerous crises. He was eager to get there in order to let the world know of his team's latest experiments on the identification and sequencing of a cell membrane chain isolated from a T cell clone, and although he was not officially on the program, he was given the opportunity to speak. According to Davis his talk created something of a sensation, but strangely he is not listed among the Congress participants, and his data are not included in the *Proceedings* published the following year. However, his group's data were published in two *Nature* articles in 1984.

In the first, Hedrick *et al.* (207) described how one of ten distinct DNA copies of mRNAs expressed in T but not in B lymphocytes hybridized to "a region of the genome that has rearranged in a T-cell lymphoma and several T-cell hybridomas", suggesting that "it encodes one chain of the elusive antigen receptor on the surface of lymphocytes". The genes of this particular cDNA clone (TM86) underwent somatic rearrangement in T cells but not in B cells. In the accompanying paper Hedrick *et al.* (*208*) went on to show that when comparing the sequence of the T cell-specific TM86 clone with cross-reacting cloned cDNAs isolated from a thymocyte library "the constant and joining regions were remarkably similar in size and sequence to those encoding immunoglobulin proteins". The authors concluded that the TM86 cDNA clone therefore encoded one chain of the TcR for antigen. Davis (*206*) later wrote: "I think the importance of our discovery of that first T cell receptor gene was that it gave the first glimpse of what Honjo had earlier called an 'imaginary monster'. The complete DNA sequence gave a clear snapshot of what the polypeptide would look like and how it would confer specificity . . . What was also gratifying to many people on a sociological and aesthetic level (*sic*!), was that we were this tiny little group that nobody had ever heard of working in a department with no reputation in molecular biology. We had been competing with large and well-oiled laboratories, and we had won the first round in the T cell receptor sweepstakes". Davis's team had first worked at the NIH in Bethesda and then moved to Stanford University.

T.W. Mak's Toronto group (*209*) made their attack on the TcR by cloning a human mRNA specific for mammalian T cells, and their results were published at the same time as those of the Davis team, again in *Nature*. (It is striking how this British journal has consistently tended to attract many of the most exciting scientific publications, including those from the field of immunology.) "The message was found to be expressed in human and murine T lymphoblasts, thymocytes and phytohaemagglutin-stimulated T lymphocytes," they wrote. "The protein deduced from the cDNA sequence has a molecular weight of 34,938 and shows extensive similarity to the entire length of the variable, joining and constant regions of mammalian immunoglobulin light chains." They concluded that these and other findings "suggest that the cDNA clone may correspond to a message that specifies part of the human T-cell receptor."

Thus, what turned out to be the β chains of both the mouse and human TcR were sequenced at virtually the same time. Later in 1984, S. Tonegawa's group at the Massachusetts Institute of Technology published two papers taking matters an important step forward. In the first (*210*) they described the sequencing of two "related but distinct" cDNA clones obtained from mouse cytotoxic T lymphocytes. The genes of these clones were "expressed and specifically rearranged in T cells and both have similarities to immunoglobulin variable and constant region genes." They concluded that these genes code for the two subunits of the heterodimeric antigen receptor on the T lymphocytes, deduced its complete primary structure, and provided a schematic overall structure of the receptor, which proved to be essentially correct. In their second paper Tonegawa's team described a third such gene showing clonal diversity and carrying potential N-glycosylation sites (*211*). They believed this gene to encode the α-subunit of the TcR.

Tonegawa's group acknowledged the weighty contribution that had been made by three other laboratories. Using an antibody secreted by a hybridoma of myeloma and alloantigen-sensitized spleen cells, J.P. Allison, B.W. McIntyre and D. Bloch (*212*) had isolated a tumor-specific glycoprotein antigen composed of two disulfide-bonded subunits (molecular weight 39 000 and 41 000) that was present on purified T, but not B, lymphocytes, and they suggested that it may have "the T cell equivalent of the B cell idiotype". (It was Tonegawa who was to make such a gigantic contribution to our understanding of the somatic generation of antibody diversity (213) and who became yet another immunologist to receive the Nobel Prize.) Indeed, at the Kyoto Congress a year later (1983), Allison and McIntyre (214) had proposed a crude two-chain structure for the TcR, the two chains linked by a disulfide bond, and Davies and Metzger (215) had likewise put forward a possible structure for the TcR based on X-ray crystallography. Further, the laboratory of S.F. Schlossman and E.L. Reinherz at Harvard Medical School had identified clonally restricted cell surface molecules on human cytotoxic lymphocytes consisting of subunits with a molecular weight of 49 000 and 43 000 (216), which were associated with the T3 molecule present on all human peripheral T cells. Finally, in the same volume of *The Journal of Experimental Medicine* the team of J. Kappler and P. Marrack (217) had prepared a monoclonal antibody recognizing chicken ovalbumin in association with the class II histocompatibility antigen I-Ad, which they believed to bind "to all or part of the receptors for antigen/I on the T cell hybridoma". The dimer molecule they obtained from the T hybridoma cells had a molecular weight of about 80 000 and it could be reduced to two monomers (40–44 000). Haskins *et al.* (217) concluded that "The receptor(s) for antigen/I . . . therefore includes molecules with these properties." (Note: Phillipa Marrack is the granddaughter of the English immunologist J.R. Marrack whose work is referred to on p. 23 above. She has made numerous contributions to the study of T cells and, together with a large group of others, she presented a paper at the Kyoto Congress on the application of T cell hybridomas to the study of T cell antigen receptors plus MHC (218).)

Also in 1984 – a quite remarkable year for the TcR and for immunology in general – two more contributions were published in *Nature* by the team led by M.M. Davis, now working in Stanford, California. A "new species" of TcR cDNA clone had been isolated which, according to the four potential N-linked glycosylation sites, frequency of expression and predicted molecular weight (27 800) was thought to be the α chain of the TcR (219). The second paper (220) described the analysis of three new TcR β chain variable regions; they showed "both remarkable similarities and differences" with Ig. V-β sequences proved to be "much more heterogeneous at the amino acid level than are immunoglobulin V regions and they appear to diverge between species much more quickly, apparently the result of additional hypervariable regions. Three of these . . . lie outside of the classical immunoglobulin binding site, an indication that important interactions may be occurring in these regions with polymorphic MHC determinants." Although a huge amount of work remained to be done, in which J.L. Strominger's laboratory played an important role, the basic structure of the TcR had thus been established in a remarkably short time. Within a further two years:

(1) Jones *et al.* (221) established a partial primary structure of the α and β chains of the TcR isolated from human tumor cells.
(2) Schiffer, Wu and Kabat (222) described subgroups of variable region genes of rabbit TcR β chains.
(3) Leiden and Strominger (223) provided evidence for the generation of diversity of the β chain of the human TcR.
(4) Brenner, McLean and Dialynas (224), building on earlier work of several groups

who had identified a third gene that rearranges in T cells, designated Tγ, in both mouse and humans (for refs, see 223), identified a second TcR expressing T3 glycoprotein as well as γ and δ subunits, but not α and β.

For further information the reader is referred to reference 205. It needs only to be added that the α subunit turned out to be rather more complex than had been anticipated, with considerable diversity, and that the function of the α/β TcR was shown to be in the recognition of antigen peptides in the context of MHC class I and II molecules (225). In contrast, the function of cells with the γ/δ TcR is less clear, though it is thought possible that, thanks to their more limited MHC-restriction, their wide distribution in epithelial cells, and their presence in all vertebrates they may play a special role in the body's defense against pathogens (226).

It is striking that much of the work on the elucidation of the TcR was carried out in American laboratories. One can only assume that this was brought about by the fact that there were a number of well-equipped and well-funded American laboratories staffed with senior research workers who recognized the fundamental importance of this challenge and who were able to provide the right kind of inspiration and leadership to their large research teams.

Finally, a few words need to be added about transfer factor, a material (later shown to be soluble) extracted from human blood leukocytes from individuals sensitized to streptococcal M substance and to tuberculin. H.S. Lawrence succeeded in transferring a longlasting delayed-type cutaneous hypersensitivity to tuberculin-negative volunteers with disrupted leukocytes as long ago as 1949 (see 227). Later other antigens were used successfully, including skin allografts, which were rejected more quickly if the recipients received transfer factor from deliberately sensitized donors. The notion of transfer factor was not readily accepted, mainly because similar results could not be achieved in the guinea pig – another species in which delayed-type responses can normally be easily demonstrated – and also because there was no convincing evidence as to the nature of the factor. Later experiments revealed that the active ingredient was a molecule with a molecular weight of less than 10 000 D. More recently Borkowski and Lawrence (228) have suggested that the active moiety might be an "antigen-binding proteolytic fragment of the T-cell receptor which induces and augments CMI responses by virtue of its capacity to bind to specific antigen." I believe that judgement must remain suspended. To quote the last somewhat enigmatic sentence of the review by Lawrence (229), who has pursued his elusive quarry with single-minded determination and great modesty for the best part of half a century: "When viewed with the detachment of historical perspective, the slings and arrows encountered fade into insignificance and one is indeed almost prompted to exclaim: 'What was all the fuss about?' ".

Antigen presentation

Antigen-presenting cells
The early history of the regulatory activity of macrophages in antigenic stimulation and their biologic characteristics and properties were reviewed by Z.A. Cohn (230) and E. Unanue (231) more than three decades ago. Metchnikoff's speculations about the role of phagocytic cells has already been referred to (p. 3), as has the fact

that the all-consuming interest in antibodies soon made his ideas unpopular. In the 1920s it was thought that macrophages not only ingested antigens but also made antibody against them (232), but once again interest in these cells waned, especially when Fragaeus identified plasma cells as antibody producers (see p. 29). Despite evidence indicating that macrophages were derived from blood monocytes, as for example Ebert and Florey (233) pointed out in 1939, there was much speculation that lymphocytes could transform into macrophages, a view that had to be abandoned. Although their involvement in inflammatory processes and the removal of cell debris and foreign particles such as bacteria, especially when opsonized by antibody, was well recognized their immunologic functions remained something of a mystery.

There was a brief revival of interest in macrophages as direct participants in immune responses when, in the early 1950s, Fishman (234, 235) published some astonishing data, according to which antibody secretion by lymph node cells *in vitro* was triggered by cell-free homogenates of peritoneal exudate cells (mainly macrophages) that had been incubated with the antigen (T2 bacteriophage). Fishman and Adler claimed (236) that the activity of the homogenates resided in their RNA, and they speculated that either information had been passed on by the RNA or that the RNA might have formed complexes with the antigen. Others found it difficult to confirm these results, but in the light of what is now known of the internalization, processing and presentation of antigen peptides on the macrophage cell surface these early data seem rather less surprising, especially if antigen peptides were removed together with the RNA phenol extracts. (I am indebted to M.J. Owen for this latter suggestion.) There is, however, no question that the removal by phagocytic cells of antigens from the extracellular fluids had long been appreciated, and that blockade of the reticuloendothelial system with colloidal particles and, to a lesser extent, the use of antimacrophage antisera inhibited the induction of antibody responses (see 231). In their perspicacious review of macrophages in antibody synthesis R.S. Schwartz, R.W.W. Ryder and A.A. Gottlieb (237) wrote in 1970: ". . . the macrophage, despite its common association with antigenic material, is at the center of an immunologic controversy." Yet they attributed to macrophages the immunologic equivalent of "servomechanisms" (i.e the reception and storage of signals, their amplification "by modification" (*sic*!), and the ability to influence the response to a signal by controlling its level). "Could analysis of macrophage–lymphocyte interactions in terms of servomechanisms and filtered receivers provide biologically useful information?" they asked.

The need for the participation of macrophages or other accessory cells became well defined in the 1970s. Working with guinea pigs, Seeger and Oppenheim (238) found that the removal of adherent cells by passing lymph node cells through glass-bead columns prevented the non-adherent lymphocytes from undergoing DNA synthesis after antigenic stimulation – results that were amply confirmed by others. In the mouse, Rosenwasser and Rosenthal (239) and many others found that antigenic stimulation of T cells was wholly dependent on the presence of macrophages, and human lymphocyte proliferation, too, depended on the presence of monocytes/macrophages (240). The events of the 1970s have been well reviewed by Unanue (241), who has himself made many important contributions to the rapidly growing body of knowledge of macrophage function.

The 1970s saw the remarkably rapid analysis of MHC systems in the mouse and in the human, as well as in other species, with the recognition that there were two kinds of histocompatibility antigens, class I and class II, but originally known as serologically defined and lymphocyte defined (see Chapter 4). Just before Zinkernagel and Doherty (*168, 169*) showed MHC restriction in the killing of virus-infected target cells by cytotoxic T cells, A.S. Rosenthal and E.M. Shevach (*242*) demonstrated that antigen activation of DNA synthesis by thymus-derived lymphocytes from immunized guinea pigs required MHC identity between macrophages and lymphocytes. In an accompanying paper (*243*) they took matters a vital step further. From rather complex experiments involving antigen-pulsed macrophages – the response to this antigen being Ir (i.e. class II) dependent – and responder or non-responder T lymphocytes or their hybrids, they speculated that "antigen recognition sites on the T lymphocyte are physically related to a macrophage-binding site and both are linked to the serologically determined histocompatibility antigens." (The reference to class I antigens is likely to have been an error, for they were wholly concerned with Ir-controlled responses (i.e. class II).) They finished their paper with: "We conclude from these studies that antigen recognition by the T lymphocyte is a complex multicellular event involving more than simple antigen binding to a specific lymphocyte receptor." The scene was thus set for a closer understanding of the interaction between macrophages and T lymphocytes and the role played by MHC antigens.

As Unanue has pointed out (*241*), many investigations following in the wake of those of Rosenthal and Shevach confirmed the relationship between antigen and the I-region products of macrophages in T cell–macrophage interactions, both in the guinea pig and the mouse, and with a variety of antigens. The absolute requirement of this interaction was demonstrated at an early stage by D.E. Mosier (*244, 245*), who depleted lymphoid cells of accessory cells by adhesion and showed that the antibody response to sheep red blood cells was severely impaired – a result that was rapidly confirmed by other workers. However, C.W. Pierce (*246*) found that this was true only for the primary and not for the secondary response. The role of macrophages was soon shown to be mirrored by other "accessory cells" such as:

(1) The Langerhans cells of the skin, which Stingl *et al.* (*247, 248*) found to be capable of antigen-presentation in T cell proliferation.
(2) The interdigitating cells of the lymph nodes and spleen.
(3) The "veiled" cells found in afferent lymph.
(4) The follicular dendritic cells of the spleen (*249, 250*).
(5) The more ubiquitously distributed dendritic cells (DC) first described by R.M. Steinman and Z.A. Cohn (*251, 252*), which again were rich in cell surface class II molecules (*253*).

DCs, with their extravagantly extended and mobile cell processes and high concentration of class II molecules, are antigen presenters *par excellence* and were soon shown to strongly influence the activity of lymphocytes in MLRs (*254*). Dendritic cells were later found to be important "passenger cells" in organ allotransplants. The activity of passenger cells is discussed in Chapter 2 and elsewhere in the book. Whereas the cell types just referred to constitute the "professional" antigen-presenting cells (APCs) other cells, such as endothelial cells, B lymphocytes and even activated

T lymphocytes can act as APCs provided that their class II antigens are upregulated; this usually happens in the face of an ongoing immune response. (For detailed discussions of APCs see reference *241*; follicular dendritic cells, see reference *255*; DCs, see reference *256*; Langerhans cells, see reference *257*.)

The 1960s and 1970s therefore witnessed an explosion of interest in APCs and the way they related to lymphocytes, both T and B, by virtue of their membrane class II antigens, which provided the restricting element. This was of course quite different from the restriction of cytotoxic T lymphocytes in the destruction of virus-infected cells where class I antigens were the cause of the restriction. Thus emerged a very different set of functions for these two kinds of histocompatibility antigens – class II involved in the induction of immune responses and class I with T cell cytotoxicity.

Processing of antigens by antigen-presenting cells

The next vital chapter in this story is the recognition that antigens are not only taken up by APCs but processed internally, leading to the production of peptides that are then expressed on the cell membrane via class II MHC antigens. The antigens are consequently in a form that can be recognized by the TcR. The fact that peptides need to be presented by MHC molecules immediately made sense of the phenomenon of MHC restriction.

The first hint that antigens were actively broken down into subunits within APCs came from experiments carried out in Unanue's laboratory. Thus, Ziegler and Unanue (*258*, see also *259*) discovered that accessory cells could be inhibited by agents that interfered with lysosomal function. Two approaches were followed: the use of lyso-somotropic drugs such as chloroquine that turn the normally acid intracellular vesicles alkaline, and the light fixation of macrophages in formaldehyde. Both resulted in the complete inhibition of antigen-presenting function following internalization of *Listeria monocytogenes*. They concluded that "the *Listeria* had to be internalized . . . into an acid vesicle in order for the immunogen to be recycled to the surface to be presented." Further studies with radiolabeled organisms showed that the *Listeria* were bound to a plasma membrane protein that required Ca^{2+}. This was followed by catabolism, resulting in peptides that remained associated with the membrane for long periods as well as peptides that were released into the culture medium (*260*). The membrane-bound peptides had a molecular weight of about 10 000 or less and the released peptides were larger, but curiously none seemed to be associated with Ia (class II) molecules. Yet when membrane fragments carrying peptides were fed to other macrophages these were able to present the peptides in an MHC-restricted manner.

These observations led to a great array of studies dealing with the intracellular processing of antigens and the expression of peptides on the cell surface. The reader is referred to reviews on this topic (*261–265*). It should be stressed that Townsend *et al.* (*266*) and Morrison *et al.* (*267*) recognized that some antigens, such as exogenous proteins and viral proteins, may be processed by a pathway that does not involve lysosomes although processing of viral antigens is undoubtedly required and does take place.

Major histocompatibility complex (MHC)–peptide interactions: the MHC groove

The importance of peptide presentation by class I and II MHC antigens was thus well understood by the mid-1980s. Class I molecules were generally thought to bind peptides from intracellular sources while class II molecules were known to bind peptides from extracellular antigens. What was less clear was how the association between the two molecules came about in the interior of the cell before the appearance of MHC molecules on the cell surface of APCs. Chain, Kaye and Shaw (262) had to admit in 1988 that "there is almost no evidence on which to determine the site within the cell at which processed antigen interacts with MHC molecules."

A few years later this problem had become less obscure, and Yewdell and Bennink (268), in their review of antigen processing and presentation in relation to class I MHC molecules were able to state that "Taken together, these findings from diverse systems are remarkably consistent in indicating that assembly of α chains with β_2m can occur in the absence of peptides, and that the interaction is stabilized by antigenic peptides." Both the synthesis of MHC molecules and its association with exogenous peptides are highly complex processes, the understanding of which is complicated by the possibility that the conditions of *in vitro* experiments (e.g. the concentration of peptides) do not necessarily reflect those prevailing *in vivo*. It also seems probable that exogenous peptides can enhance the expression of class I molecules on the cell surface, as first suggested by the experiments of Townsend *et al.* (269). Yewdell and Bennink (268), after a detailed examination in 1992 of the evidence for and against four possible intracellular sites for class I–peptide association, concluded: "Taken together, these findings are consistent with the idea that exogenously added peptides associate with class I molecules located in the plasma membrane. . . ."

According to the review of J.J. Monaco (270) antigens such as viral nucleoprotein, which is excluded fro.n the secretory pathway and yet effectively presented, is processed in the cytosol before it enters the exocytic system. Monaco proposed a new model of MHC class I-restricted antigen processing involving degradation of cytoplasmic proteins into peptides by a large cytoplasmic structure, the low molecular mass polypeptide complex, transporter molecules taking the peptides to the cell surface, binding of the peptides to class I molecules, and finally a conformational change in the latter.

Cresswell (265), in his review of the events accompanying the assembly, transport and function of class II molecules, has considered the question of peptide loading. He concluded that Unanue's (259) notion that the catabolism of exogenous proteins into peptides takes place in the endosomal/lysosomal system was correct, but had to leave open the question of precisely where peptide binding to MHC takes place. Likewise, it remained unclear how the class II–peptide complexes were transported to the cell surface. In their 1992 review of intracellular transport of class I molecules, Neefjes and Ploegh (271) suggested that the association between peptides and class II molecules takes place in the lysosome, where the peptides have the first opportunity to interact with the class II molecules. The complexes would then be taken to the cell surface within vesicles and anchored there, with the peptide presented extracellularly. The evidence supporting this notion is highly complex and still tentative, ultrastructural studies being hampered by the fact that visualization and quantitation of class II molecules "is fraught with the danger that different biosynthetic inter-mediates do not react equally well with the antibodies used."

The structure of peptides bound by class I and class II molecules has recently been discussed by Engelhard (272).

The discoveries leading to a detailed understanding of class I and class II molecular structures are recounted in Chapter 4, p. 147. The absolutely critical discovery, which led to a quantum leap forward in the understanding of the way MHC molecules present antigens, was made by P.J. Bjorkman *et al.* (273) when they showed by X-ray diffraction techniques applied to crystallized HLA-A2 (a class I molecule) that there was a "groove" 25 Å long and 10 Å wide between the two long helices of the α_1 and α_2 domains. The groove was near the outer aspect of the molecule and there-fore "a likely candidate for the binding site for the foreign antigen that is recognized together with HLA by a T-cell receptor". In this groove could be detected "a large continuous region of electron density" and Bjorkman *et al.* speculated that "It seems likely that the extra density is the image of the peptide or a mixture of peptides that co-purified and co-crystallized with HLA-A2." A year later the same group proposed a similar model for the class II molecule (274), the precise structure was as yet unknown, and five years later this was shown to be absolutely correct (275), when the Strominger/Wiley group discovered the three-dimensional structure of HLA-DR1. The elucidation of MHC structure was a feat to equal the elegant work on the TcR, and the extraordinarily beautiful colored three-dimensional photographs of HLA-A2 are likely to be the most ubiquitous illustrations in scientific publications and text-books in the history of immunology.

Thus came to fruition a most extraordinary decade of hectic and highly competi-tive activity in molecular immunology: the nature and physical basis of MHC restriction was at last fully comprehended, and the interaction between antigens, the MHC and the TcR had become very much clearer. Though there are many riddles left to be solved, the 1980s and 1990s did much to answer the basic question of how T cells, which are at the core of immunology, are activated to a variety of antigens. At the same time, these developments led to a better understanding of the nature of alloreactivity (see Chapter 2).

The discovery of cytokines

So far cytokines have not been mentioned – those soluble factors secreted by cells during immune activation that are important in amplifying immune responses, and in some cases, inhibiting them. It is impossible, and not intended, to give a full account of how these important mediators were discovered and where precisely matters stand at the present time. I will, however, focus on the early events, and especially those relating to the discovery of IL-1 and IL-2, two cytokines (originally called lymphokines) that are central to lymphocyte activation.

That resting lymphocytes can be activated to transform into large blast cells by plant lectins was first observed by P.C. Nowell in 1960 (276). Not many years later soluble mitogenic factors were found in the medium of cultured lymphocytes (277, 278). Although it was first assumed that this mitogenic activity merely acted as a means of augmenting antigen-triggered cellular responses, this notion was abandoned when it became clear that to be able to respond to antigens or lectins T cells had to have access to macrophages (*279–281*). Attention was therefore given to the hypothesis that T cell proliferation depends not only on the presence of a foreign antigen (signal 1) but also on a co-stimulatory signal (signal 2) in the shape of soluble factors secreted by cells of the immune system. Theories concerning these two signals have already been alluded to above (see p. 30). Once it became possible in the late 1970s to maintain T cells or T cell clones in continuous culture it became clear from the work of Gillis and Ruscetti (*282*) that the activity could be attributed to a soluble factor secreted by T cells, which was called T cell growth factor (TCGF). As macrophages associated with immune responses likewise produced soluble factors, it became possible to envisage a new model of T cell activation. This was put forward by Smith and Ruscetti (*283*) in their 1981 review of TCGF, in which they acknowledged the experimental and conceptual contributions made by several groups of workers.

The model proposed that T cell activation requires the interaction of three types of cells – accessory cells secreting lymphocyte-activating factor (LAF), the resultant release of TCGF from specific T cells, and the binding of TCGF to another T cell subset. Such a cascade would then lead to a proliferative response and clonal T cell expansion. Thus, while the antigen or mitogen triggered a specific response, its augmentation would be controlled by nonspecific, hormone-like molecules. LAF, first described by Waksman's laboratory in 1971 (*284, 285*) when working with both syngeneic and xenogeneic cell cultures, and TCGF therefore acquired a place of considerable importance in cellular immunology and were much studied. Gery and Waksman (*286*) were soon able to show that LAF emanated from mouse macrophages.

By 1979 a revised nomenclature for antigen-nonspecific T cell proliferation and helper factors was agreed in a letter to the editor signed by 34 workers in the field (*287*): LAF derived from macrophages was to be called IL-1. Gery and Handschumacher (*288*) had shown that it was a peptide with a molecular weight of about 15 000 and it was generally agreed that all macrophages were capable of secreting it in response to a variety of agents and antigens. Another factor discovered round about that time included B cell activating factor (BAF) (*289, 290*), and others followed. Because Koopman *et al.* (*291*) found no physicochemical distinction between some of the factors it was thought probable that the various activities described for the factors were manifestations of the same molecule, and at the Second International Lymphokine Workshop in 1979 (*292*) this notion was generally accepted. A review of the structure and properties of IL-1 has been written by Mizel (*293*), among others.

The nomenclature for the stimulatory factor(s) produced by helper T cells after activation by T cell mitogens or by allogeneic cells was agreed at the same workshop to be IL-2, thus replacing TCGF (*287*). IL-2 had been shown to be capable of inducing a number of cellular phenomena, from thymocyte proliferation with (*294, 295*) or without (*296*) suboptimal concentrations of T cell mitogen, to the augmented proliferation and generation of cytotoxic T cells in response to alloantigens (*296, 297*). IL-2 is secreted by T helper cells and it plays a crucial role in the formation of cytotoxic lymphocytes and in the production of antibodies by B cells. Its biology, molecular characteristics and role have been reviewed by a number of workers, including Watson and Mochizuki (*298*), Wagner *et al.* (*299*), Farrar *et al.* (*300*) and

Gillis *et al.* (*301*). A whole number of *Immunological Reviews* (*302*) has been devoted to the IL-2 receptors and their genes, and the topic has been more recently reviewed by K.A. Smith (*303*).

Since the discovery of IL-1 and IL-2 a large family of cytokines has been identified, produced by a variety of cells. Indeed, the distinction between two kinds of helper T cells, TH1 and TH2, was made by Mossmann *et al.* (*304*), mainly on the strength of the different cytokines released by them – IL-2, interferon-γ and lymphocytotoxin from TH1 cells, and IL-4 and other cytokines, including IL-10, from TH2 cells (see *305*). TH1 cells provide strong help for cell-mediated immunity (CMI) as well as help to B cells, whereas TH2 cells assist in antibody responses, but can inhibit CMI.

Conclusion

The development of immunology during the course of little over a century has been quite breathtaking and, with the exception of a relatively quiet period in the 1920s and 1930s, it has sustained the intellectual excitement of its formative years in the last two decades of the nineteenth century. It is striking how the dominance of the early German chemists faded after World War I. The reasons for this are not clear; among them could be that an outstanding immunologist like Karl Landsteiner felt it necessary to leave Germany in 1919 to settle eventually in the United States and that Nazi Germany forced most Jewish scientists to emigrate in the 1930s. The emergence of a new German school of immunology (K. Rajewski, K. Eichmann, H. Wagner, for example) did not happen until many years after World War II.

The areas I have discussed are all of considerable importance to transplantation immunology. There are, nonetheless, numerous topics that space and time have prevented me from including:

(1) The question of immunologic memory (*306*), itself of great interest in relation to the accelerated rejection of tissues and organs in presensitized individuals.
(2) Cell selection in the thymus (*307, 308*).
(3) The development of the concept of "superantigens" (*309*) (see Chapter 4) from the Mls system of antigens first described by Festenstein and his colleagues (see Chapter 4).
(4) The phenomenon of apoptosis (*310, 311*), an active, synthesis-dependent and programmed cell death resulting from cleavage of genomic DNA.
(5) The elucidation of the structure and function of complement (*312, 313*).

References

1. Silverstein, A.M. (1989) *A History of Immunology*, pp. 1–422, Academic Press, London.
2. Bibel, D.J. (1988) *Milestones in Immunology. A Historical Exploration*, pp. 1–1330, Springer-Verlag, N.Y.
3. Moulin, A.M. (1991) *Le Dernier Langage de la Médecine. Histoire de l'Immunologie de Pasteur au Sida*, pp. 1–447, Presse Univ. de France, Paris.
4. Mazumdar, P.M.H. ed. (1989) *Immunology 1930–1980. Essays on the History of Immunology*, pp. 1–307, Wall & Thompson, Toronto.

5. Gallagher, R.B., Gilder, J., Nossal, G.J.V. & Salvatore, G. (1995) *Immunology. The Making of a Modern Science*, pp. 1–246, Academic Press, London.
6. Humphrey, J.H. & White, R.G. (1970) *Immunology for Medical Students*, 3rd edn, pp. 1–34, Blackwell Scientific Publ., Oxford & Edinburgh.
7. Klein, J. (1982) *Immunology. The Science of Self–Nonself Discrimination*, pp. 1–687, John Wiley & Sons, N.Y.
8. Bibel, D.J. (1988) *Milestones in Immunology. A Historical Exploration*, p. 8, Springer-Verlag, N.Y.
9. Needham, J. (1980) *Eastern Horizon* **19**, 6.
10. Fenner, F., Henderson, D.A., Arita, I. *et al.* (1988) *Smallpox and its Eradication*, Table 5.1, World Health Org., Geneva.
11. Voltaire, F-M. (1727) In *Lettres Philosophiques*, 3rd edn. 1924, pp. 130–51, G. Lanson, Paris.
12. Fenner, F., Henderson, D.A., Arita, I. *et al.* (1988) *Smallpox and its Eradication*, p. 254, World Health Org., Geneva.
13. Maitland, C. (1922) *Account of Inoculating the Small Pox*, London.
14. Silverstein, A.M. (1989) *A History of Immunology*, p. 26, Academic Press, London.
15. Blake, J.B. (1952) *N. Engl. Quart.* **25**, 490.
16. Jenner, E. (1798) *An Enquiry into the Causes and Effects of the Variolae Vaccininae*, Sampson Low, London.
17. Pasteur, L., Chamberland, C. & Roux, E. (1880) *C.R. Hebd. Seances Acad. Sci.* **90**, 239.
18. Ehrlich, P. (1906) *Arb. Köningl. Inst. Exp. Ther. Frankf.* **1**, 77.
19. Metchnikoff, O. (1884) *Virchows Arch.* **96**, 177.
20. Metchnikoff, O. (1884) *Arch. Path. Anat. Physiol. u. Klin. Med.* **96**, 177.
21. Metchnikoff, O. (1892) *Lecons sur la Pathologie Compareé de l'Inflammation Faites a l'Institute Pasteur en Avril et Mai, 1891*, p. 239, Masson, Paris.
22. Wright, A.E. & Douglas, S.R. (1903) *Proc. Roy. Soc. B* **72**, 364.
23. Sewall, H. (1887) *J. Physiol.* **8**, 203.
24. Salmon, D.E. & Smith, T. (1886) *Proc. Biol. Soc.* **3**, 29.
25. Von Behring, E. & Kitasato, S. (1890) *Deutsch. Med. Wchschr.* **16**, 1113.
26. Ehrlich, P. (1897) *Klin. Jahrb.* **6**, 299.
27. Ehrlich, P. (1891) *Deutsch. Med. Wchschr.* **17**, 976.
28. Ehrlich, P. (1891) *Deutsch. Med. Wchschr.* **17**, 1218.
29. Pfeiffer, R. (1894) *Zeitschr. Hyg. Infektkr.* **18**, 1.
30. Kraus, R. (1897) *Wien. Klin. Wchschr.* **10**, 736.
31. Bordet, J. (1898) *Ann. Inst. Pasteur* **12**, 688.
32. Nuttall, G.H.F. (1888) *Zeitschr. Hyg. Infektkr.* **4**, 353.
33. Buchner, H. (1889) *Centralbl. Bakt. Parasitenk.* **5**, 817.
34. Buchner, H. (1889) *Centralbl. Bakt. Parasitenk.* **6**, 561.
35. Buchner, H. (1893) *Münchn. Med. Wchschr.* **40**, 449, 486.
36. Bordet, J. (1895) *Ann. Inst. Pasteur* **9**, 462.
37. Portier, P. & Richet, C. (1902) *C.R. Soc. Biol. (Paris)* **54**, 170.
38. Arthus, M. (1903) *C.R. Soc. Biol. (Paris)* **55**, 817.
39. Von Pirquet, C. & Schick, B. (1906) *Die Serumkrankheit*, Deuticke, Vienna.
40. Landsteiner, K. (1901) *Wien. Klin. Wchschr.* **14**, 1132.
41. Gibson, T. & Medawar, P.B. (1943) *J. Anat.* **77**, 299.
42. Medawar, P.B. (1944) *J. Anat.* **78**, 176.
43. Medawar, P.B. (1945) *J. Anat.* **79**, 157.
44. Owen, R.D. (1945) *Science* **102**, 400.
45. Burnet, F.M. & Fenner, F. (1949) *The Production of Antibodies*, 2nd edn., Macmillan, Melbourne, London.
46. Billingham, R.E., Brent, L. & Medawar, P.B. (1953) *Nature* **172**, 603.
47. Billingham, R.E., Brent, L. & Medawar, P.B. (1956) *Phil. Trans. B* **239**, 357.
48. Brent, L. & Medawar, P.B. (1959) In *Recent Progress in Microbiology*, p. 181, Almqvist & Wiksell, Stockholm.
49. Ehrlich, P. & Morgenroth, J. (1901) *Berl. Klin. Wchschr.* **38**, 251.
50. Donath, J. & Landsteiner, K. (1904) *Münchn. Med. Wchschr.* **51**, 1590.

51. Mackay, I.R. (1995) In Gallagher, R.B., Gilder, J., Nossal, G.J.V. *et al. Immunology. The Making of a Modern Science*, p. 49–62, Academic Press, London.
52. Witebsky, E., Rose, N.R. & Terplan, K. (1957) *J. Am. Med. Ass.* **164**, 1439.
53. Doniach, D. & Roitt, I.M. (1957) *J. Clin. Endocrinol. Med.* **17**, 1293.
54. Zinsser, H. (1921) *J. Exp. Med.* **34**, 495.
55. Dienes, L. & Schoenheit, E.W. (1929) *Am. Rev. Tuberc.* **20**, 92.
56. Landsteiner, K. & Chase, M.W. (1942) *Proc. Soc. Exp. Biol. Med.* **49**, 688.
57. Mitchison, N.A. (1953) *Nature* **171**, 267.
58. Chase, M.W. (1945) *Proc. Soc. Exp. Biol. Med.* **59**, 134.
59. Billingham, R.E., Brent, L. & Medawar, P.B. (1954) *Proc. Roy. Soc. B* **143**, 58.
60. Yoffey, J.M., Thomas, D.B., Moffatt, D.J. *et al.* (1961) In *Biological Activity of the Leucocyte*, Ciba Found. Study Group no. 10, eds G.E.W. Wolstenholme & M. O'Connor, p. 45, J. & A. Churchill, London.
61. Gowans, J.L., Gesner, B.M. & McGregor, D.D. (1961) In *Biological Activity of the Leucocyte*, Ciba Found. Study Group no. 10, eds G.E.W. Wolstenholme & M. O'Connor, p. 32, J. & A. Churchill, London.
62. Ehrich, W.E. & Harris, T.N. (1942) *J. Exp. Med.* **76**, 335.
63. Dougherty, T.F., Chase, J.H. & White, A. (1944) *Proc. Soc. Exp. Biol. Med.* **57**, 295.
64. Harris, T.N., Grimm, E., Mertens, E. *et al.* (1945) *J. Exp. Med.* **81**, 73.
65. Gowans, J.L. (1957) *J. Physiol.* **146**, 54.
66. Gowans, J.L. & Knight, E.J. (1964) *Proc. Roy. Soc. B* **159**, 257.
67. Marchesi, V.T. & Gowans, J.L. (1964) *Proc. Roy. Soc. B* **159**, 283.
68. Medawar, P.B. (1958) *Proc. Roy. Soc. B.* **148**, 159, 161.
69. Medawar, P.B. (1963) In *The Immunologically Competent Cell: Its Nature and Origin*, Ciba Found. Study Group no. 10, eds. G.E.W. Wolstenholme & J. Knight, p. 1, J. & A. Churchill, London.
70. Terasaki, P.I. (1959) *J. Embryol. Exp. Morph.* **7**, 394.
71. Simonsen, M. (1960) In *Cellular Aspects of Immunity*, Ciba Found. Symp., eds. G.E.W. Wolstenholme & M.P. O'Connor, p. 122, J. & A. Churchill, London.
72. Anderson, N.F., Delorme, E.J. & Woodruff, M.F.A. (1960) *Transpl. Bull.* **7**, 93.
73. Billingham, R.E., Brown, J.B., Defendi, V. *et al.* (1960) *Ann. N.Y. Acad. Sci.* **87**, 457.
74. Gowans, J.L. (1956) *Brit. J. Exp. Path.* **38**, 67.
75. Gowans, J.L., McGregor, D.D., Cowen, D.M. *et al.* (1962) *Nature* **196**, 651.
76. Nossal, G.J.V. & Mäkela, O. (1962) *J. Exp. Med.* **115**, 209.
77. Gowans, J.L. (1962) *Ann. N.Y. Acad. Sci.* **99**, 432.
78. McGregor, D.D., McCullagh, P.J. & Gowans, J.L. (1967) *Proc. Roy. Soc. B* **168**, 229.
79. Gowans, J.L. (1995) In *Immunology. The Making of a Modern Science*, eds. R.B. Gallagher, J. Gilder, G.J.V. Nossal & G. Salvatore, p. 65, Academic Press, London.
80. Glick, B., Chang, T.S. & Jaap, R.G. (1956) *Poultry Sci.* **35**, 224.
81. Mueller, A.P., Wolfe, H.R. & Meyer, R.K. (1960) *J. Immunol.* **85**, 172.
82. Ackerman, G.A. & Knouff, R.A. (1959) *Am. J. Anat.* **104**, 163.
83. Miller, J.F.A.P. (1991) *Immunol. Today* **12**, 43.
84. Janković, B.D. (1991) *Immunol. Today* **12**, 247.
85. Good, R.A. (1991) *Immunol. Today* **12**, 283.
86. Miller, J.F.A.P. (1996) See ref. **79**, p. 75.
87. Miller, J.F.A.P. (1961) *Nature* **184**, 1809.
88. Miller, J.F.A.P. (1961) *Lancet* **2**, 748.
89. Archer, O. & Pierce, J.C. (1961) *Fed. Proc.* **20**, 26 (Abstr.).
90. Fichtelius, K-E., Laurall, G. & Philipsson, L. (1961) *Acta Path. Microbiol. Scand.* **51**, 81.
91. Ruth, R.F. (1960) *Fed. Proc.* **19**, 579.
92. Auerbach, R. (1961) *Proc. Nat. Acad. Sci. U.S.A.* **47**, 175.
93. Woglom, W.H. (1929) *Cancer Rev.* **4**, 129, 188.
94. Miller, J.F.A.P. (1962) In *Transplantation*, Ciba Found. Symp., eds. G.E.W. Wolstenholme & M.P. Cameron, p. 384, J. & A. Churchill, London.
95. Miller, J.F.A.P. (1962) *Proc. Roy. Soc. B* **156**, 415.
96. Miller, J.F.A.P. (1962) *Ann. N.Y. Acad. Sci.* **99**, 340.
97. Billingham, R.E. & Brent, L. (1957) *Transpl. Bull.* **4**, 67.

 98. Maclean, L.D., Zak, S.J., Varco, R.L. *et al.* (1956) *Surgery* **40**, 1010.
 99. Harris, T.N., Rhoads, J. & Stokes, J. (1948) *J. Immunol.* **58**, 27.
100. Maclean, L.D., Zak, S.J., Varco, R.L. *et al.* (1957) *Transpl. Bull.* **4**, 21.
101. Archer, O.K., Pierce, J.C., Papermaster, B.W. *et al.* (1962) *Nature* **195**, 191.
102. Martinez, C., Kersey, J. & Papermaster, B.W. (1962) *Proc. Soc. Exp. Biol. Med.* **109**, 193.
103. Dalmasso, A.P., Martinez, C. & Good, R.A. (1962) *Proc. Soc. Exp. Biol. Med.* **111**, 143.
104. Martinez, C. Dalmasso, A.P. & Good, R.A. (1962) *Nature* **194**, 1289.
105. Papermaster, B.W., Dalmasso, A.P., Martinez, C. *et al.* (1962) *Proc. Soc. Exp. Biol. Med.* **111**, 41.
106. Good, R.A., Dalmasso, A.P., Martinez, C. *et al.* (1962) *J. Exp. Med.* **116**, 773.
107. Papermaster, B.W. & Good, R.A. (1962) *Nature* **196**, 838.
108. Arnason, B.G., Janković, B.D. & Waksman, B.H. (1962) *Nature* **194**, 99.
109. Waksman, B.H., Arnason, B.G. & Janković, B.D. (1962) *J. Exp. Med.* **116**, 187.
110. Janković, B.D., Waksman, B.H. & Arnason, B.G. (1962) *J. Exp. Med.* **116**, 159.
111. Arnason, B.G., Janković, B.D. & Waksman, B.H. (1962) *J. Exp. Med.* **116**, 177.
112. Warner, N.L. & Szenberg, A. (1962) *Nature* **194**, 147.
113. Warner, N.L. & Szenberg, A. (1962) *Nature* **196**, 684.
114. Claman, H.N., Chaperon, E.A. & Triplett, R.F. (1966) *Proc. Soc. Exp. Biol. Med.* **122**, 1167.
115. Miller, J.F.A.P. & Mitchell, G.F. (1968) *J. Exp. Med.* **128**, 801.
116. Mitchell, G.F. & Miller, J.F.A.P. (1968) *J. Exp. Med.* **128**, 821.
117. Nossal, G.J.V., Cunningham, A., Mitchell, G.F. *et al.* (1968) *J. Exp. Med.* **128**, 839.
118. Davies, A.J.S., Leuchars, E., Wallis, V. *et al.* (1967) *Transplantation* **4**, 438.
119. Davies, A.J.S., Leuchars, E., Wallis, V. *et al.* (1967) *Transplantation* **5**, 222.
120. Mitchison, N.A., Rajewsky, K. & Taylor, R.B. (1970) In *Developmental Aspects of Antibody Formation and Structure*, eds J. Sterzl & I. Riha, p. 547, Academia, Czechoslovakia.
121. Roitt, I.M., Greaves, M.F., Torrigiano, G. *et al.* (1970) *Lancet* **2**, 367.
122. Raff, M.C. (1969) *Nature* **224**, 378.
123. Reif, A.E. & Allen, J.M.V. (1966) *Nature* **209**, 521.
124. Cantor, H. & Boyse, E.A. (1975) *J. Exp. Med.* **141**, 1276.
125. Cantor, H. & Boyse, E.A. (1975) *J. Exp. Med.* **141**, 1390.
126. Simpson, E. & Cantor, H. (1975) *Eur. J. Immunol.* **5**, 337.
127. Arrhenius, S. (1907) Immunochemistry. *The Applications of the Principles of Physical Chemistry to the Study of the Biological Antibodies*, Macmillan, New York.
128. Landsteiner, K. (1907) *Z. Immunitätsforsch.* (Orig.) **26**, 122.
129. Landsteiner, K. (1947) *The Specificity of Serological Reactions*, pp. 1–310, Harvard Univ. Press, Cambridge, Mass.
130. Marrack, J.R. (1934) *Nature* **133**, 292.
131. Tiselius, A. & Kabat, E.A. (1939) *J. Exp. Med.* **69**, 119.
132. Porter, R.R. (1959) *Biochem. J.* **73**, 119.
133. Edelman, G.M. (1959) *J. Amer. Chem. Soc.* **81**, 3155.
134. Edelman, G.M. & Poulik, M.D. (1961) *J. Exp. Med.* **113**, 861.
135. Nisonoff, A., Wissler, F.C. & Lipman, L.N. (1960) *Science* **132**, 1770.
136. Breinl, F. & Haurowitz, F. (1930) *Z. Physiol. Chem.* **192**, 45.
137. Pauling, L. & Delbrück, M. (1940) *Science* **92**, 77.
138. Pauling, L. (1940) *J. Amer. Chem Soc.* **62**, 2643.
139. Watson, J.D. & Crick, F.H.C. (1953) *Nature* **171**, 737.
140. Crick, F.H.C. (1958) In *The Biological Replication of Macromolecules, Symp. Soc. Exp. Biol.* **12**, 138.
141. Crick, F.H.C. (1970) *Nature* **227**, 561.
142. Schweet, R.S. & Owen, R.D. (1957) *J. Cell. Comp. Physiol.* **50** (suppl. 1), 199.
143. Ehrlich, P. (1900) *Proc. Roy. Soc. B* **66**, 424.
144. Jerne, N. (1955) *Proc. Nat. Acad. Sci. U.S.A.* **41**, 849.
145. Talmage, D.W. (1957) *Annu. Rev. Med.* **8**, 239.
146. Talmage, D.W. (1959) *Science* **129**, 1643.
147. Lederberg, J. (1959) *Science* **129**, 1649.
148. Burnet, F.M. (1957) *Austr. J. Biol. Sci.* **20**, 67.
149. Burnet, F.M. (1959) *The Clonal Selection Theory of Acquired Immunity*, pp. 1–209, Cambridge Univ. Press, Cambridge.

150. Fagraeus, A. (1948) *Acta Med. Scand.* **130** (suppl. 204), 3.
151. Fagraeus, A. (1948) *J. Immunol.* **58**, 1.
152. Nossal, G.J.V. & Lederberg, J. (1958) *Nature* **181**, 1419.
153. Nossal, G.J.V. (1995) In *Immunology. The Making of a Science*, eds R.B. Gallagher, J. Gilder, G.J.V. Nossal & G. Salvatore, p. 39, Academic Press, London.
154. Talmage, D.W. (1995) In *Immunology. The Making of a Science*, eds R.B. Gallagher, J. Gilder, G.J.V. Nossal & G. Salvatore, p. 23, Academic Press, London.
155. Jerne, N. (1974) *Ann. d'Immunol.* (Paris) **125C**, 389.
156. Jerne, N. (1974) *Harvey Lect.* **70**, 93.
157. Bretscher, P. & Cohn, M. (1970) *Science* **169**, 1042.
158. Cohn, M. (1994) *Ann. Rev. Immunol.* **12**, 1.
159. Lafferty, K.J. & Cunningham, A.J. (1975) *Austr. J. Exp. Biol. Med. Sci.* **53**, 27.
160. Lafferty, K.J., Prowse, S.J. & Simenonovic, C.J. (1983) *Ann. Rev. Immunol.* **1**, 143.
161. Zinkernagel, R.M. & Doherty, P.C. (1974) *Nature* **248**, 701.
162. Doherty, P.C. & Zinkernagel, R.M. (1974) *Transpl. Rev.* **19**, 89.
163. Shearer, G.M. (1974) *Eur. J. Immunol.* **4**, 527.
164. Kinded, B. & Shreffler, D.C. (1972) *J. Immunol.* **109**, 940.
165. Katz, D.H., Hamaoka, T. & Benacerraf, B. (1973) *J. Exp. Med.* **137**, 1405.
166. Katz, D.H., Hamaoka, T., Dord, M.E. *et al.* (1973) *Proc. Nat. Acad. Sci. U.S.A.* **70**, 2624.
167. Cerrottini, J-C., Nordin, A.A. & Brunner, K.T. (1970) *Nature* **228**, 1308.
168. Zinkernagel, R.M. & Doherty, P.C. (1974) *Nature* **251**, 547.
169. Doherty, P.C. & Zinkernagel, R.M. (1975) *Lancet* **1**, 1406.
170. Zinkernagel, R.M. & Doherty, P.C. (1979) *Adv. Immunol.* **27**, 51.
171. Swain, S.L. & Dutton, R.W. (1980) *Immunol. Today* **1**, 61.
172. Dialynas, D.P., Wilde, D.B., Marrack, P. *et al.* (1983) *Immunol. Rev.* **74**, 29.
173. Townsend, A.R.M., Rothbard, J., Gotch, F.M. *et al.* (1986) *Cell* **44**, 959.
174. Maryanski, J.L., Pala, P., Corradin, G. *et al.* (1986) *Nature* **324**, 578.
175. Nagu, Z.A., Baxevanis, C.N., Ishii, N. *et al.* (1981) *Immunol. Rev.* **60**, 59.
176. Unanue, E.R. (1984) *Ann. Rev. Immunol.* **2**, 395.
177. Grey, H.M. & Chestnut, R. (1985) *Immunol. Today* **6**, 101.
178. Tansey, E.M. & Catterall, P.P. (1994) *Med. Hist.* **38**, 322.
179. Köhler, G. & Milstein, C. (1975) *Nature* **256**, 495.
180. Köhler, G. & Milstein, C. (1975) *Eur. J. Immunol.* **6**, 511.
181. Köhler, G., Hengartner, H. & Shulman, M.J. (1978) *Eur. J. Immunol.* **8**, 82.
182. Brodsky, F.M., Parham, P., Barnstable, C.J. *et al.* (1979) *Immunol. Rev.* **47**, 3.
183. Kung, P.C., Goldstein, G., Reinherz, E.L. *et al.* (1979) *Science* **206**, 347.
184. Reinherz, E.L., Kung, P.C., Goldstein, G. *et al.* (1979) *Proc. Nat. Acad. Sci. U.S.A.* **76**, 4061.
185. Gillis, S. & Henney, C.S. (1981) *J. Immunol.* **126**, 1978.
186. Cambrioso, A. & Keating, P. (1992) *J. Hist. Biol.* **25**, 175.
187. Melchers, F. (1995) *Nature* **314**, 498.
188. Goldsby, R.A., Osborne, B.A., Simpson, E. *et al.* (1977) *Nature* **267**, 708.
189. Fathman, C.G. & Hengartner, H. (1978) *Nature* **272**, 617.
190. Brown, G. & Greaves, M.F. (1974) *Eur. J. Immunol.* **4**, 302.
191. Binz, H., Kimura, A. & Wigzell, H. (1974) *Scand. J. Immunol.* **4**, 413.
192. Ramseier, H. & Lindenmann, J. (1972) *Transpl. Rev.* **10**, 57.
193. Ramseier, H. (1973) *Nature* **246**, 351.
194. Ramseier, H. (1975) *Eur. J. Immunol.* **5**, 23.
195. Ramseier, H. & Lindenmann, J. (1972) *Eur. J. Immunol.* **2**, 109.
196. Binz, H. & Wigzell, H. (1975) *J. Exp. Med.* **142**, 197.
197. Binz, H., Wigzell, H. & Bazin, H. (1976) *Nature* **264**, 639.
198. Binz, H. & Wigzell, H. (1976) *J. Exp. Med.* **144**, 1438.
199. Aquet, M., Andersson, L.C., Andersson, R. *et al.* (1978) *J. Exp. Med.* **147**, 50.
200. Cosenza, H. & Köhler, G. (1972) *Proc. Nat. Acad. Sci. U.S.A.* **69**, 2701.
201. Hart, D.A., Wang, A-L., Pawlak, L.L. *et al.* (1972) *J. Exp. Med.* **135**, 1293.
202. Hart, D.A., Pawlak, L.L. & Nisonoff, A. (1972) *Eur. J. Immunol.* **3**, 44.
203. Eichmann, K. (1974) *Eur. J. Immunol.* **4**, 296.

204. Mäkela, O. (1970) *Transpl. Rev.* **5**, 3.
205. Bell, J.I., Owen, M.J. & Simpson, E. (eds) (1995) *T Cell Receptors*, pp. 1–483, Oxford. Univ. Press, Oxford.
206. Davis, M. (1995) See ref. 153, p. 163.
207. Hedrick, S.N., Cohen, D.L., Nielsen, E.A. *et al.* (1984) *Nature* **308**, 149.
208. Hedrick, S.M., Nielsen, E.A., Kavaler, J. *et al.* (1984) *Nature* **308**, 153.
209. Yanagi, Y., Yoshikai, Y., Leggett, K. *et al.* (1984) *Nature* **308**, 145.
210. Saitoh, H., Kranz, D.M., Takasagi, Y. *et al.* (1984) *Nature* **309**, 757.
211. Saitoh, H., Kranz, D.M., Takasagi, Y. *et al.* (1984) *Nature* **312**, 36.
212. Allison, J.P., McIntyre, B.W. & Bloch, D. (1982) *J. Immunol.* **129**, 2293.
213. Tonegawa, S. (1995) See ref. 153, p. 145.
214. Allison, J.P. & McIntyre, B.W. (1984) In *Progress in Immunology* 5, eds Y. Yamamura & T. Tada, p. 755, Academic Press, Tokyo.
215. Davies, D. & Metzger, H. (1983) *Ann. Rev. Immunol.* **1**, 87.
216. Meuer, S.C., Fitzgerald, K.A., Hussey, R.E. *et al.* (1983) *J. Exp. Med.* **157**, 705.
217. Haskins, K., Kubo, R., White, J. *et al.* (1983) *J. Exp. Med.* **157**, 1149.
218. Marrack, P., Kubo, R., Haskins, K. *et al.* (1984) See ref. 214, p. 735.
219. Patten, P. Yokota, T., Rothbard, J. *et al.* (1984) *Nature* **312**, 40.
220. Chien, Y-H., Becker, D.M., Lindsten, T. *et al.* (1984) *Nature* **312**, 31.
221. Jones, N., Leiden, J., Dialynas, D. *et al.* (1985) *Science* **227**, 311.
222. Schiffer, M., Wu, T.T. & Kabat, E.A. (1986) *Proc. Nat. Acad. Sci. U.S.A.* **83**, 4461.
223. Leiden, J.M. & Strominger, J.L. (1986) *Proc. Nat. Acad. Sci. U.S.A.* **83**, 4456.
224. Brenner, M.B., McLean, J. & Dialynas, D.P. (1986) *Nature* **322**, 145.
225. Zamoyska, R. & Travers, P. (1995) See ref. 205, p. 46.
226. Hayday, A.C. (1995) See ref. 205, p. 70.
227. Lawrence, H.S. (1989) In *Immunology 1930–1980*, ed. P.M.H. Mazumdar, p. 221, Wall & Thompson, Toronto.
228. Borkowski, W. & Lawrence, H.S. (1983) In *Immunobiology of Transfer Factor*, eds. C.H. Kirkpatrick, P.R. Burger & H.S. Lawrence, p. 148, Academic Press, New York.
229. Lawrence, H.S. (1989) In *Immunology 1930–1980*, ed. P.M.H. Mazumdar, p. 221, Wall & Thompson, Toronto.
230. Cohn, Z.A. (1968) *Adv. Immunol.* **9**, 163.
231. Unanue, E. (1972) *Adv. Immunol.* **15**, 95.
232. Sabin, F.R. (1923) *Bull. Johns Hopkins Hosp.* **34**, 277.
233. Ebert, R.H. & Florey, H.W. (1939) *Brit. J. Exp. Path.* **20**, 342.
234. Fishman, M. (1959) *Nature* **183**, 1200.
235. Fishman, M. (1961) *J. Exp. Med.* **114**, 837.
236. Fishman, M. & Adler, F.L. (1963) *J. Exp. Med.* **117**, 595.
237. Schwartz, R.S., Ryder, R.J.W. & Gottlieb, A.A. (1970) *Progr. Allergy* **14**, 81.
238. Seeger, R.C. & Oppenheim, J.J. (1970) *J. Exp. Med.* **132**, 44.
239. Rosenwasser, L.J. & Rosenthal, A.S. (1978) *J. Immunol.* **121**, 2497.
240. Hersh, E.M. & Harris, J.E. (1968) *J. Immunol.* **100**, 1187.
241. Unanue, E. (1981) *Adv. Immunol.* **31**, 1.
242. Rosenthal, A.S. & Shevach. E.M. (1973) *J. Exp. Med.* **138**, 1194.
243. Shevach, E.M. & Rosenthal, A.S. (1973) *J. Exp. Med.* **138**, 1213.
244. Mosier, D.E. (1967) *Science* **158**, 1573.
245. Mosier, D.E. (1969) *J. Exp. Med.* **129**, 351.
246. Pierce, C.W. (1969) *J. Exp. Med.* **130**, 345.
247. Stingl, G., Katz, S.I., Clement, L. *et al.* (1978) *J. Immunol.* **121**, 2005.
248. Stingl, G., Katz, S.I., Shevach, E.M. *et al.* (1978) *J. Invest. Dermatol.* **71**, 59.
249. White, R.G., French, V.I. & Stark, J.M. (1967) In *Germinal Centers in Immune Responses*, eds H. Cottier, N. Odartchenko, R. Schindler & C.C. Congdon, p. 131, Springer–Verlag, N.Y.
250. Nossal, G.J.V., Abbot, A., Mitchell, J. *et al.* (1968) *J. Exp. Med.* **127**, 277.
251. Steinman, R.M. & Cohn, Z.A. (1973) *J. Exp. Med.* **137**, 1142.
252. Steinman, R.M. & Cohn, Z.A. (1974) *J. Exp. Med.* **139**, 380.
253. Steinman, R.M., Kaplan, G., Witmer, M.D. *et al.* (1979) *J. Exp. Med.* **149**, 1.

254. Steinman, R.M. & Witmer, M.D. (1978) *Proc. Nat. Acad. Sci. U.S.A.* **75**, 5132.
255. Klaus, G.G.B., Humphrey, J.H., Kunkl, A. *et al.* (1980) *Immunol. Rev.* **53**, 3.
256. Steinman, R.M. & Nussenzweig, M.C. (1980), *Immunol. Rev.* **53**, 127.
257. Stingl, G., Tamaki, K. & Katz, S.I. (1980) *Immunol. Rev.* **53**, 149.
258. Ziegler, H.K. & Unanue, E. (1982) *Proc. Nat. Acad. Sci. U.S.A.* **79**, 175.
259. Unanue, E. (1984) *Annu. Rev. Immunol.* **2**, 395.
260. Allen, P.M., Beller, D.I., Braun, J. *et al.* (1984) *J. Immunol.* **132**, 323.
261. Berzofsky, J.A., Brett, S.J., Streicher, H.Z. *et al.* (1988) *Immunol. Rev.* **106**, 5.
262. Chain, B.M., Kaye, P.M. & Shaw, M-A. (1988) *Immunol. Rev.* **106**, 33.
263. Harding, C.V., Leyva–Cobian, F. & Unanue, E. (1988) *Immunol. Rev.* **106**, 77.
264. Braciale, T.J., Morrison, L.A., & Sweetser, M.T. *et al.* (1987) *Immunol. Rev.* **98**, 95.
265. Cresswell, P. (1994) *Annu. Rev. Immunol.* **12**, 259.
266. Townsend, A.R.M., Bastin, J., Gould, K. *et al.* (1986) *Nature* **324**, 575.
267. Morrison, L.A., Lukacher, A.E., Braciale, V.L. *et al.* (1986) *J. Exp. Med.* **163**, 903.
268. Yewdell, J.W. & Bennink, J.R. (1992) *Adv. Immunol.* **52**, 1.
269. Townsend, A., Öhlen, C., Bastin, J. *et al.* (1989) *Nature* **340**, 443.
270. Monaco, J.J. (1992) *Immunol. Today* **13**, 173.
271. Neefjes, J.J. & Ploegh, H.L. (1992) *Immunol. Today* **13**, 179.
272. Engelhard, V.H.C. (1994) *Annu. Rev. Immunol.* **12**, 181.
273. Bjorkman, P.J., Saper, M.A., Samraoui, B. *et al.* (1987) *Nature* **329**, 506.
274. Brown, J.H., Jardetzky, T.S., Saper, M.A. *et al.* (1988) *Nature* **332**, 845.
275. Brown, J.H., Jardetzky, T.S., Gorga, J.C. *et al.* (1993) *Nature* **364**, 33.
276. Nowell, P.C. (1960) *Cancer Res.* **20**, 462.
277. Casacura, S. & Lowenstein, L. (1968) *J. Immunol.* **101**, 12.
278. Gordon, J. & Maclean, L.D. (1965) *Nature* **208**, 795.
279. Oppenheim, J.J., Leventhal, B.G. & Hersh, E. (1968) *J. Immunol.* **101**, 262.
280. Seeger, R.& Oppenheim, J.J. (1970) *J. Exp. Med.* **132**, 44.
281. Rosenstreich, D.L., Farrar, J.J. & Dougherty, S. (1976) *J. Immunol.* **116**, 131.
282. Gillis, K.A. & Ruscetti, F.W. (1981) *Adv. Immunol.* **31**, 137.
283. Smith, K.A. & Ruscetti, F.W. (1981) *Adv. Immunol.* **31**, 137.
284. Gery, I., Gershon, R.K. & Waksman, B.H. (1971) *J. Immunol.* **107**, 1178.
285. Gery, I., Gershon, R.K. & Waksman, B.H. (1972) *J. Exp. Med.* **136**, 128.
286. Gery, I. & Waksman, B.H. (1972) *J. Exp, Med.* **136**, 143.
287. Aarden, L.A., Burnner, T.K., Cerrottini, J.C. *et al.* (1979) *J. Immunol.* **123**, 2928.
288. Gery, I. & Handschumacher, R.E. (1974) *Cell. Immunol.* **11**, 162.
289. Schrader, J.W. (1973) *J. Exp. Med.* **138**, 1446.
290. Wood, D.D., Cameron, P.M., Poe, N.T. *et al.* (1976) *Cell. Immunol.* **21**, 88.
291. Koopman, W.J., Farrar, J.J., Oppenheim, J.J. *et al.* (1977) *J. Immunol.* **119**, 55.
292. De Weck, A.L., Kristensen, F. & Landy, M. (1980) *Biochemical Characterization of Lymphokines*, Proc. Second Intern. Lymphokine Workshop, Academic Press, N.Y.
293. Mizel, S.B. (1982) *Immunol. Rev.* **63**, 51.
294. Chen, D.M. & DiSabato, G. (1976) *Cell. Immunol.* **22**, 24.
295. Paetkau, V., Mills, G., Gerhart, S. *et al.* (1976) *J. Immunol.* **117**, 1320.
296. Farrar, J.J., Simon, P.L., Koopman, W.J. *et al.* (1978) *J. Immunol* **121**, 1353.
297. Wagner, H. & Röllinghoff, M. (1978) *J. Exp. Med.* **148**, 1523.
298. Watson, J. & Mochizuki, D. (1980) *Immunol. Rev.* **51**, 257.
299. Wagner, H., Hardt, C. Heeg, K. *et al.* (1980) *Immunol. Rev.* **51**, 215.
300. Farrar, J.J., Benjamin, W.R., Hilfiker, M.L. *et al.* (1982) *Immunol. Rev.* **63**, 129.
301. Gillis, S., Mochizuki, D.Y., Conlon, P.J. *et al.* (1982) *Immunol. Rev.* **63**, 167.
302. *Immunol. Rev.* (1986) no. **92**, 1–156.
303. Smith, K.A. (1989) *Annu. Rev. Cell Biol.* **5**, 397.
304. Mossmann, T.R., Cherwinski, H., Bond, M.W. *et al.* (1986) *J. Immunol.* **126**, 2348.
305. Mossmann, T.R. (1994) *Adv. Immunol.* **56**, 1.
306. Mackay, C.R. (1993) *Adv. Immunol.* **53**, 217.
307. Fink, P. & Bevan, M.J. (1995) *Adv. Immunol.* **59**, 99.
308. Kisielow, P. & von Boehmer, H. (1995) *Adv. Immunol.* **58**, 87.

309. Herman, A., Kappler, J.W., Marrack, P. *et al.* (1991) *Annu. Rev. Immunol.* **9**, 745.
310. Cohen, J.J., Duke, R.C., Fadok, V.A. *et al.* (1992) *Annu. Rev. Immunol.* **10**, 267.
311. Goldstein, P., Ojcius, D.M. & Young, D.E. (1991) *Immunol. Rev.* **121**, 29.
312. Müller-Eberhard, H.J. (1986) *Annu. Rev. Immunol.* **4**, 503.
313. Law, S.K.A. & Reid, K.B.M. (eds) (1995) *Complement: In Focus*, p. 1–100, I.R.L. Press, Oxford.

Biographies

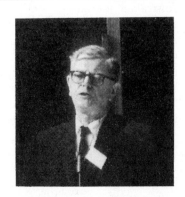

**FRANK MACFARLANE BURNET
(1899–1985)**

Macfarlane Burnet was one of the deepest thinkers immunology has produced (he began as a virologist, in fact) and his speculations and theories made a profound impact on the field, approached only by those of Niels Jerne. He was born in Victoria to parents who had emigrated from Scotland to Australia in the nineteenth century. His father was a bank manager and his mother was wholly preoccupied looking after her first child, who was born retarded and never gained normality. This, together with the fact that Burnet was badly neglected by his father, led to an unusually unloved and lonely childhood, in which he developed a love for nature and wildlife and excelled academically. He graduated in medicine from Melbourne University in 1922, took his M.D., and then earned his passage to London as a ship's doctor to study for his Ph.D. at the Lister Institute on the subject of bacteriophages in their relation to the antigenic structure of bacteria. There he was strongly influenced by the director, C.J. Martin, who encouraged him to apply for the Chair in Bacteriology at London University, but as Burnet had been offered the Assistant Directorship at the Hall Institute he decided to return to Melbourne. This he did in 1927, and thereafter, with the exception of a year at the National Institute for Medical Research, London (Sir Henry Dale was its director), he remained at the Hall Institute for the rest of his life, becoming its director in 1944. Under his powerful influence and leadership the Hall Institute became one of the most distinguished immunologic centers in the world and spawned a succession of brilliant young scientists, including Gus Nossal, who was to succeed Burnet as Director in 1965.

In 1928 he married Linda Druce, a teacher, who gave up her career to be a mother and a housewife. Burnet, in *Changing Patterns: an Atypical Autobiography* (American

Elservier, N.Y., 1969) dedicated the book "To Linda, who put up with an intolerable deal of shop and thought none the worse of me for it. Bless her!"

Although Burnet made many experimental contributions to virology he will be best remembered for two major theoretic contributions. In 1949 he published, together with Fenner, his highly influential monograph *The Production of Antibodies* (see Chapters 1 and 5), which included a discussion of self and nonself (based on R.D. Owen's experiments, to which they drew attention for the first time), and in which they postulated the existence of tolerance. The other gigantic contribution was the development of the clonal selection hypothesis, first published in an obscure Australian journal in 1957 and fully developed two years later (see Chapter 1). Burnet thus provided the theoretic foundations of modern immunology. His approach included world tours of leading laboratories and the aquisition and assimilation of the latest experimental data that seemed to fit into his theoretic constructions. (He invariably stopped off in London to visit Medawar and his team and soon got over his surprise that discussions should take place in a pub over a glass of beer!)

Burnet was widely honored and in 1960 he shared the Nobel Prize for Medicine with Medawar for his contribution to the concept of tolerance. He became a Fellow of the Royal Society in 1942, was awarded its Royal Medal in 1947 and its Copley Medal in 1959, and he received the Lasker Award and the Von Behring Prize. He was knighted in 1952 and was appointed to the Order of Merit seven years later, Knight of the British Empire in 1969, and Knight of the Order of Australia in 1978.

Burnet – now Sir Macfarlane – published many scientific papers and not a few books. He was always driven to seek out what he perceived as the truth, always looking for general biologic principles. His later excursions into the sociopolitical–philosophical realm were highly controversial and revealed his more conservative nature. A biography, *The Seeds of Time*, was published by C. Sexton in 1991 (Oxford University Press, Oxford).

JACQUES FRANCIS ALBERT PIERRE MILLER (1931–)

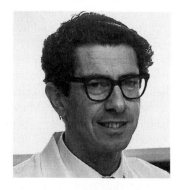

Jaques Miller was born in Nice, France. This simple statement belies an extraordinarily turbulent childhood. His mother was Fernande Eugenie Debarnot and his father Maurice Eugene Meunier, who had spent many years in China and Japan, became manager of the Franco-Chinese Bank in Shanghai, and spoke five Chinese languages as well as Japanese. His mother decided that Jacques should be born in France and therefore went to Nice in 1930, returning to China a year later to rejoin her husband. In 1935 the family moved to Switzerland because Miller's sister had contracted tuberculosis, but when the war clouds gathered they returned to Shanghai in the last boat to leave Trieste in 1939. When Pearl Harbour was bombed the family moved via Jakarta to Sydney, Australia where, penniless, his father joined the French Diplomatic Corps. The move to Australia had become possible on a false passport issued by the British authorities, with the name Meunier translated to Miller.

Before arriving in Australia at the age of ten Miller had received no formal schooling. In his school in Sydney he became friendly with a young Austrian refugee called Gus Nossal! Miller had decided long before that he wanted to become a doctor and qualified at Sydney Medical School in 1955. He married Margaret Houen, a head nurse at the Prince Alfred Hospital where Jacques was Medical Officer for a year. A cancer research scholarship took him to the Chester Beatty Cancer Research Institute, London in 1958, and he worked there for six years, in the course of which he made his fundamentally important observations on the immunologic functions of the thymus. He was initially not happy at the Institute because the search for carcinogenic compounds did not interest him, and it was through R.J.C. Harris, working in a small outpost in the north of London, that he became involved with the Gross leukemia virus. How Miller discovered that the thymus was the finishing school for the lymphocytes responsible for cell-mediated responses such as allograft rejection has been described by him in detail recently in *Immunology: The Making of a Modern Science* (1995, Academic Press, N.Y.).

His first paper on the role of the thymus was published in the *Lancet* in 1961 and the implications were so profound that some immunologists, including P.B. Medawar, remained skeptical for some time. However, others such as R.A. Good and B. Waksman very soon confirmed the data. In 1966 the Millers returned to Australia, where G.J.V. Nossal, by now Director of The Walter and Eliza Hall Institute, Melbourne, had invited him to lead the Experimental Pathology Unit. There he continued to make major discoveries in providing proof, with his Ph.D. student G.F. Mitchell, for the existence of two major lymphocyte subpopulations, T and B, with quite distinct functions. In recent years, as head of the Thymus Biology Unit, Miller and his colleagues have made significant contributions to the study of tolerance, using the transgenic approach.

His and his wife's personal life has been clouded by the death of both their young children from an undiagnosed condition. Inexplicably, his outstanding contribution to the development of modern immunology has not been recognized by the award of the Nobel Prize, but he has received many other honors. In 1970 he was elected to Fellowship of the Royal Society and the Australian Academy of Science, and in 1981 he became Officer of the Order of Australia. Among his prizes and medals are the Scientific Medal of the Zoological Society, London, the Burnet Medal, the Paul Ehrlich–Ludwig Darmstaedter Prize, the Sir William Upjohn Medal for Medicine, the Rabbi Shai Shacknai Memorial Prize, Israel, the International Saint-Vincent Prize for Medical Science, Italy, and the First Peter Medawar Prize of the Transplantation Society (1990). He became Foreign Associate of the U.S. National Academy of Sciences in 1982 and gave the Royal Society Croonian Lecture in 1992. Miller's dearest hobbies are art, music and photography.

2   The Immunologic Basis of Allograft Rejection

> *". . . the immunology of transplantation is important not merely for its bearing upon surgery and cancer research or the repair of radiation damage, but above all because it offers one of the few negotiable pathways into the central regions of biology, where immunology, genetics, embryology and the rest of them lose their identities in problems that bear upon biology as a whole".*
>
> P.B. Medawar, 1957

The Early Years

Intrepid surgeons before their time

Attempts to help patients by plastic surgery go back several centuries, at least to the sixteenth century and almost certainly to much earlier times if the evidence of Egyptian papyri and the Hindu Susruta is to be believed (1). However, in this book I am mainly concerned with the transplantation of allografts. Although the sixteenth-century Italian surgeon Gaspare Tagliacozzi who worked in Bologna has been credited with some wondrous surgical feats, including the rebuilding of noses from skin taken from the patients' slaves – thereby giving rise to the myth of the "sympathetic slave" and the "sympathetic nose", which would die only on the death of the hapless donor – he himself was healthily skeptical of the outcome of such heroic endeavors. Thus he wrote: ". . . the singular character of the individual entirely dissuades us from attempting this work on another person. For such is the force and the power of individuality, that if any one should believe that he could accelerate and increase the beauty of the union, nay more, achieve even the least part of the operation, we consider him plainly superstitious and badly grounded in physical science" (2).

How prophetic! It therefore seems all the more surprising that the Scottish pioneer anatomist, surgeon and indefatigable experimentalist John Hunter, working two centuries later, made some remarkable claims concerning the transplantation of the spurs of young cocks (3) and even a human tooth (4) into the combs of others. These gave the prevailing passion for tooth allotransplantation and even xenotransplantation a great deal of credence (see, for example, the testimony of an "eyewitness", 5). He also transplanted the testes of cocks not only into their own abdominal cavities, but also into those of hens, "where it has adhered, and has been nourished" (6). Publication of Hunter's transplantation studies was fragmentary, but some of his experimental preparations were preserved by him and incorporated into the anatomical museum he established in London. This is now the Hunterian Museum in the building of the Royal College of Surgeons of England in Lincoln's Inn Fields, and his claims of successful transplantation between individuals found their way into the literature (7). Although he had evidently convinced himself of the success of some of his transplants, he also expressed some doubts: "Although I formerly transplanted the testicles of a cock into the abdomen of a hen, and they had sometimes taken root there, but not frequently, and then had never come to perfection, yet the experiment could not, from this cause, answer fully the intended purpose (i.e. whether a male organ could grow in a female, and vice versa); there is, I believe, a natural reason to believe it could not, and the experiment was therefore disregarded" (8). Nonetheless, Hunter "made errors of interpretation and was often too generous in his speculation. He failed to distinguish between homografts and autografts, feeling that both would take readily", but his contribution in the field of transplantation "sensitized scientific minds of later years" (9). More detailed information about Hunter's transplantation experiments can be found in the Hunterian Museum and in other modern articles reviewing his contribution (9–11).

The early history of allotransplantation has been covered by several modern authors: principally by Medawar (12), Dempster (13), Woodruff's massive and well-researched 1960 tome covering surgical, clinical and immunologic aspects of transplantation (14), Hamilton's (15) more recently published and slighter chapter on the history of kidney transplantation (mainly clinical), Medawar's 1957 Harvey Lecture (16) and Silverstein's all-embracing and thoughtful A History of Immunology (17). Here I can mention only some of the publications I regard as the most significant and I have excluded those primarily concerned with techniques and clinical matters. I have read the original papers myself (mainly in German, English and French) and taken care not to follow other historians slavishly, and so it is inevitable that my evaluation of some of these early contributions should differ from theirs.

Looking back on the nineteenth and early part of the twentieth centuries it is clear, as Silverstein has pointed out, that there are two major strands of study: the work carried out by surgeons and zoologists, mainly on skin allografts but also with kidneys, and the studies carried out by tumor biologists. A third strand, represented by the investigations of geneticists, soon followed. Like Silverstein, I shall discuss these different strands separately, partly because the story can be told better that way and partly because at the time surgeons and tumor biologists did not seem to be particularly aware of each other's work; even when they were, they did not always realize that they were dealing essentially with the same phenomena.

Arguably the first systematic attempt to investigate the fate of normal allografts was made by Bert, a French biologist, in 1864 (18). He distinguished between autografts and allografts and described the events following the subcutaneous implantation of either the tip of the tail or the paw of a very young rat into another young animal, both types of graft having first been freed of the integument. The grafts apparently survived well in some recipients, showing remarkable growth, but survival was judged largely in terms of whether a graft bled when it was cut into. Bert did, however, note that in some cases elimination or slow resorption occurred. It is perhaps unfortunate that he used equally young recipients (about ten days old) and the results may have been biased by a degree of immunologic immaturity. Furthermore, the donors and recipients were "white" rats and there may have been some degree of closed colony inbreeding. His attempts at xenotransplantation (rat to guinea pig and cat to rat and in the reverse direction) met with failure and resorption and/or more or less rapid elimination was observed. Bert's experiments therefore tended to fortify those surgeons who believed that transplantation of skin allografts was a clinical possibility, and he himself advocated this. He deserves a further footnote in history because he was the first to describe the technique of para-biosis between young rats, and even between a rat and a cat. The former survived happily for two months (no graft-versus-host reaction!) and Bert believed that his xenogeneic parabiosis had been partially successful because atropine injected into the rectum of the cat caused dilatation of the partner rat's pupils four hours later.

The demonstration by the much revered French surgeon J.L. Reverdin in 1870 that small pieces of skin autografts could be used to heal chronic ulcers if placed on fresh granulating tissue (19) generated great interest in skin transplantation. Pollock in Edinburgh soon followed suit. Although he prudently confined himself mainly to autografts, with conspicuous success, he did include two small pieces of skin from a black-skinned donor in a series of autografts transplanted to a large granulating area on the buttock and thigh of an eight-year-old girl. If these grafts did indeed survive for as long as two months, as he claimed (20), this may well have been due to the debilitated state of the patient. It is of some interest that Pollock obtained his grafts by "nipping up a very small portion with a fine pair of forceps, and cutting it off close with sharp scissors". This is exactly the same method that was recommended eight decades later by Billingham and Medawar (21) when preparing "pinch" grafts in experimental animals.

Pollock at least had the donor's black pigment as an indicator of graft survival, but many nineteenth-century surgeons fooled themselves into believing that skin allo-grafts and even xenografts gave good clinical results thanks to a mixture of wishful thinking, sloppy observation, and the tendency of native epithelium to overgrow the dead dermal pad of a graft. A. Miles, a Fellow of the Royal College of Surgeons, Edinburgh, was among them (22). Once again fired by Reverdin's successes with autografts – "The astonishment and admiration with which Reverdin's comparatively brilliant results. . . . were received in 1869, have given place to a confident assurance of success in the surgeon of the aseptic era . . ." – he launched into the treatment of ulcers by transplanting skin from young dogs, rabbits, kittens and frogs, the best results being obtained with canine donors. Some patients received, at different times, grafts from a variety of dogs and kittens. He apparently carried out only one frog transplant, the details of which are not given, but he stated that "Undoubtedly the frog's skin was least satisfactory". Although he claimed that four out of ten of his cases were "perfectly successful" and four others "only partially" so, it is clear from his summary description of the scars, the loss of pigmentation, and the failure to grow hairs or regenerate sweat or sebaceous glands that his grafts had long been rejected. Another such example is provided by C.A. Ljunggren (23) who published his data two years later. He claimed to have succeeded in culturing human skin in ascitic fluid for several months. Despite some unpromising microscopic findings he sought proof of survival by transplanting some pieces to granulating wounds. Of the 22 grafts, 11 grafts allegedly survived, and his conclusion was in his view supported by microscopic examination of two biopsies, which showed mitotic figures in the epithelial cells. Unfortunately the biopsies had been taken together with granulation tissue and might well have included native epithelium.

Despite the far more critical studies of men like Lexer and Schöne (see below) it is astonishing to find that misconceptions about the fate of allografts persisted well into the twentieth century, even on the far side of the Atlantic. For example, in 1906 the American J.E. Cannady (24) claimed to have obtained remarkable results with allo- and xenografts, which included skin taken from frogs, chickens and pigs and, in one case, a common water lizard. The latter had been transplanted to the foot of an Italian "with a fair measure of success". The others had "loaned their integument to man with very good grace". And Baldwin (25) concluded just before World War I that human allografts "became permanent takes and grew almost if not equally as well as autografts" provided that the donors and recipients belonged to the same blood group – a conclusion echoed (but without acknowledgement) by his countryman J.C. Masson (26) at the end of the war, when skin donors were in great demand. He satisfied himself that "blood grouping is just as important for good results in skin-grafting as it is necessary in transfusion, and that it is governed by the same principles". If only he could have known that the blood group antigens are genetically, biochemically and antigenically quite distinct from the histocompatibility antigens! Another American, L. Sale (27), following in the footsteps of L. Loeb, studied the spread of pigment from black guinea pig skin transplanted to non-pigmented areas of the same animal, but he also performed a number of allografts. He stated quite clearly that the majority were "cast off" but noted that, if they took, there was no invasion of pigmented epithelium from the graft. (It was R.E. Billingham and P.B. Medawar who showed in the 1950s that this was a case of pigment spread rather than cellular invasion.) It is further to Sale's credit that he became aware of an infiltration of transplanted skin with "round cells", "which may lead to a partial separation and destruction of some of the transplanted cells".

This brings us to the two giants of early skin grafting, Erich Lexer and Georg Schöne – both German and both publishing in the first two decades of the twentieth century. Lexer's seminal paper (28) was published in 1911 and it has the distinction of having been described by Medawar as "one of the masterpieces of the literature of transplantation" (16). It is undoubtedly a wide-ranging review of the state of the art at that time, covering not only skin but also a variety of tissues and organs, and unlike so many papers of that period it had an extensive (if not always correct!) list of references. Despite reports to the contrary, including a review by J.S. Davis of 550 cases of skin transplants carried out at Johns Hopkins Hospital, in which he valued auto- and allografts almost equally (29): "In this series, autodermic grafts have taken somewhat better than isodermic, but my own personal experience convinces me that isodermic grafts are quite as successful as those from the same individual". Lexer concluded unequivocally from his own observations that allotransplantation of skin was invariably associated with failure. The only partial (i.e. transient) success he had encountered had been with grafts from a fresh fetus. It seems a pity that he saw fit to express the astonishingly naive view that racial differences between donor and recipient could influence the force of the rejection process merely because of his experience with a few transplants from a Polish donor to some East Prussians and a Polish child (30). Although he considered the possibility that the factors interfering with graft take may be least powerful in closely related individuals, as Schöne had shown in experimental animals (see below), Lexer was unable to confirm this using human grafts from mother to child or from daughter to father. His paper continued with a review of the transplantation of blood vessels (he reported the first apparently successful human autograft, but unfortunately the patient died on the fifth day), fascia, ligaments, bone, cartilage, whole joints ("above all technically challenging"; unfortunately his most successful transplant in a dog was destroyed when the dog bled to death after chewing off its leg . . .) and even organs (though here with not a great deal of hope). Whether with heavy sarcasm or uncharacteristic humor, Lexer added out of the blue: "Die Verpflanzung ganzer Köpfe haben wir den Americanern bisher noch nicht nachgemacht" or "We have not yet copied the Americans in the transplantation of whole heads." He wisely concluded that it is the biochemical differences of the cells and the sera that make allotransplantation so problematic (31).

Schöne published an exhaustive monograph in Berlin in 1912 in which he reviewed his and other workers' studies on the transplantation of both normal and malignant tissues (32). Silverstein gives him a great deal of credit for having summarized the rules governing the acceptance and rejection of tumor grafts and for having coined the term "transplantation immunity". Having ploughed through the 161 rather wordy and not infrequently repetitive pages I am not so sure that this credit is wholly justified. It is true that his review is astonishingly all-embracing, including learned discourses on transplantation in plants, invertebrates, the lower vertebrates such as amphibians and of course mammals; it considers auto-, allo- and xenotransplantation, and it surveys the transplantation of a plethora of tissues and organs. Anyone believing that the subject of transplantation was no more than a minority interest in those early years is encouraged to read the book and to marvel at the length of the reference list (of the order of 500), but it will require stamina! However, the reader will find that much of the book is at a descriptive level and when it comes to the mechanism of graft rejection Schöne becomes understandingly vague. Thus he is therefore unable to decide which of the following three possible causes may be the critically important one: nutritional problems (following Ehrlich's soon to be discredited notion of athrepsia, see below), primary toxicity ("it is well known that tissue juices of one animal species can be poisonous for cells of another", 33), or secondary immunity or hypersensitivity (an anaphylaxis-like reaction that could be analogous to blood transfusion incompatibility). He discusses the possibility that chemotactic influences could be involved and that toxicity for the graft could be generated from either dead or viable graft cells.

Schöne casts his net so wide that the cynic might cavil that it is hardly surprising that he managed to catch a few tasty fish! That would, I think, be unfair and some very interesting nuggets of information can be found in his monograph. He noted that skin allografts usually survive for 10–14 days and that this fitted in with the possibility of an immune reaction, and he succeeded in returning allografts to their donors after they had been on their hosts for three days but not for five. Like Lexer before him he denied that skin allografts, let alone xenografts, can be relied upon to succeed except in special circumstances (i.e. when there was a close blood rela-tionship between donor and host, such as in murine siblings, especially when they were taken from the same litter). He stated "it has long been taken as read by clinicians that transplantation between blood relatives has the best prognosis", and his own experiments with mice supported this notion. However, all Schöne's work (unlike that of some tumor workers) was carried out using non-inbred mice and "laws of transplantation" could not possibly have emerged from them except in very general terms. To his credit he suggested that studies on skin and tumor allografts might have much in common, and that tumors were for some reason able to overcome the allogeneic barrier; he was certainly conversant with some of the tumor literature, unlike many of his contemporaries, though not with some of Murphy's more telling data. He rightly pointed out that skin grafts tended to have a less favorable outcome than other types of grafts and, interestingly, he raised the possibility that in certain circumstances the graft could be deleterious to the host. This last comment arose from experiments of his in which minced allogeneic liver or spleen, or defibrinated blood, was given to mice intraperitoneally: a number of the recipients died, but Schöne had no explanation for this "toxicity". As in some of the early parabiosis experiments by Sauerbruch and Heyde (34) here perhaps was an early pointer in the direction of graft-versus-host reactivity, but as the immunologic basis of the rejection process was not understood it is hardly surprising that he did not recognize the cause of death of his cell recipients. It is, however, no feather in Schöne's cap that he blindly accepted some astonishing data of Haaland's (35), who had apparently claimed that "Frankfurt" mice, which normally accepted the Ehrlich mouse sarcoma, became resistant after they had been maintained in Norway for three months (about half the mice rejected their transplants). Schöne concluded that "we must regard it as proven that nutrition has a certain influence on the fate of tumor grafts" (36). On the positive side, he knew "from untold experiments" that the injection of xenogeneic cells and eggwhite can lead to the production of antibodies, "which can damage the cells in a specific manner" (37), and he postulated that in some cases "one finds a battle between the cellular elements of the transplant and the host," quoting v. Dungern's belief that macrophages are capable of destroying rabbit tumor allografts (38).

Schöne followed this up with another major paper four years later in which he reported on the continuation of his studies on skin graft exchanges between related mice (39). The nature of the female mice and their degree of inbreeding, if any, is not stated, but "the fathers were unknown". Skin grafts from offspring to their mothers occasionally survived for long periods – a result he was unable to confirm in a second experiment – but hardly ever in the reverse direction. Transplantation of a second graft from the same donors six months after the first was completely unsuccessful (40). This experiment should have revealed a state of sensitivity, but Schöne, unaware of the potential of the experiment, did not compare the survival times of the first and second grafts, nor are they stated. Grafts from offspring to their fathers never succeeded but the occasional graft in the reverse direction survived for some time. Schöne thought that because graft destruction always occurred suddenly in the third or at the beginning of the fourth week, "the body of the host may have produced a reaction process against the tissue of the foreign individual" (41).

Turning to the rabbit, Schöne carried out a heroic experiment (shades of P.B. Medawar in the 1940s!) in which the father, mother and six offspring received skin grafts from every other member; transplantation was to the ears, and autografts were included as controls. The latter healed-in beautifully, but none of the allografts survived. Although appropriately expressing caution about coming to general conclusions, Schöne believed that the occasional surviving graft between related mice was not accidental, but once again he thought that breeding as well as nutrition could have played a role (*42*). Although this paper is well illustrated with what I think are careful drawings of histological sections of successful grafts, they seem to be the exception rather than the rule, and my impression is that Schöne – unlike the contemporaneous tumor biologists – failed to appreciate the immunologic nature of the phenomenon he was studying. And yet he stated at one point that "if in a skin graft exchange between A and B the graft on A succeeds but not on B, one must in all probability assume that there is a chemical difference" (*43*); and he urged that allografts of glands and kidneys should be undertaken only when the problem had been resolved for skin grafts (*44*).

However, as I stated in my review of 1958 (*45*), not *all* clinical reports of successful allotransplantation should be rejected out of hand. They might have been due to close and fortuitous genetic similarity between donors and recipients or, in the case of mother-to-offspring grafting, the accidental transfer of maternal cells into the fetus, bringing about some degree of tolerance (*46*).

Notwithstanding Schöne's caution, Alexis Carrel (see biographic sketch) had already spent many years perfecting vascular surgery and especially the anastomosis of blood vessels, with a view to transplanting organs such as the kidney. His first paper on this was published in 1902 (*47*) and a stream of others followed. The reader is referred to the bibliography of Woodruff's book (*14*) for some of Carrel's early contributions. In a classic paper published in 1908 (*48*), by which time Carrel had left his native France to work at the Rockefeller Institute, he described the transplantation of kidney allografts into animals whose own kidneys had been removed as the ultimate test of whether a foreign kidney could function in its new environment. The clarity of his writing and his scientific approach come as a breath of fresh air to the historian of that period. In his introduction Carrel gives credit to others who had previously attempted kidney xeno- or allotransplantation, using protheses to unite blood vessels – principally E. Ullmann in 1902 (*49*) and A. Von Decastello in 1902 (*50*), the latter having shown that a canine allograft secreted urine for a period of 40 hours. Carrel himself had in the same year observed urine flow from several canine kidney allografts that had been anastomosed to the recipients' vessels, but none of the dogs had survived for long because of sepsis. In 1905 N. Floresco (*51*) had transplanted five allogeneic kidneys into the lumbar region of dogs, but because the recipients retained one of their own kidneys the data were of limited value; even so, one of the transplanted kidneys secreted urea-containing urine for five days but the organ was necrotic by the tenth day. Together with C.C. Guthrie, Carrel had clearly established by 1905 that a canine kidney autograft placed in the neck functioned well in terms of urine output and quality (*52*), but because it showed some abnormalities of blood flow they transplanted all subsequent kidneys into the lumbar region. A year later they described the transplantation of two kidneys from the same donor into the abdomen of a dog whose own kidneys were subsequently removed. Everything went smoothly until the ninth day, when the dog became ill, and laparotomy revealed a localized peritonitis, although the circulation of both kidneys was "found to be perfect". (For details of these and other investigations, see *48*.)

In his 1908 paper (*48*), published in the *Journal of Experimental Medicine*, thus signaling the entry of kidney transplantation into the mainstream of experimental science, Carrel described a technique that had been further improved. He reported nine technically successful kidney allografts in cats, giving detailed clinical, anatomical and microscopic information. The kidneys functioned for various periods, but all the hosts died eventually, occasionally with a kidney that had minimal lesions, though most contained inflammatory lesions. "The infiltration was composed of cells having the character of the plasma cells described by Councilman in acute interstitial nephritis, socalled". Carrel thought that this might have been secondary as it was not seen in some grafts, and that ischemia (for at least one hour), the perfusion fluid used and several other physiological factors might have had something to do with it. He concluded that kidneys from another animal could produce almost normal urine and live in good health "at least for a few weeks. This demonstrates that it is possible to reestablish efficiently the functions of transplanted kidneys."

The mold was thus broken. By 1914 Carrel published a summary of his address read at the fourth Triennial Congress of the International Surgical Society in New York entitled "The transplantation of organs" (53), in which he left no doubt that whereas autografts were always successful, allografts "although the immediate results may be excellent, are nearly always ultimately unsuccessful" and xenografts invariably failed. He stated that kidney allografts behaved normally up to the seventh day, when the appearance of albumin and kidney edema intervened. The three dogs with the longest survival all had general infections and Carrel perspicaciously observed that "General infection . . . seemed thus to prevent the reaction of the organism against the new organ." He was deeply impressed with J.B. Murphy's tumor studies (see below) and went on to say that "It is not possible to foresee whether or not the present experiments of Doctor Murphy will lead directly to the practical solution of the problem in which we are interested; but it is certain that he has contributed a very important step towards that solution."

Carrel's studies were complemented by those of Myer (54), working in St Louis, who transplanted fragments of allogeneic kidney to the ears of guinea pigs and carried out careful histologic examination of the grafts at intervals. From the ninth day marked differences were seen between the auto- and allografts in that the latter showed a more intense connective tissue invasion, a larger number of round cells, and marked destruction of tubules. He concluded that "The actual destruction of the regenerated tubules seems to be due to an invasion by round cells and connective tissue cells".

The early tumor biologists

I shall begin by considering the contribution of Leo Loeb – not because I regard him to be the greatest of innovators in this field, but because he straddled the fields of tumor and normal tissue transplantation and because he has been regarded by many as one of the great pioneers of transplantation. Thus the editor of *Transplantation Bulletin*, in an unsigned appreciation of Loeb two years after his death in 1959 (55), chose a quotation from John Ruskin to reflect great glory on Loeb: "He is the greatest artist who has embodied, in the sum of his works, the greatest number of the greatest ideas." This is indeed a handsome tribute but, alas, judged in the harsh light of history, hardly merited. Yet others who were closer to him believed that he had made "monumental contributions" (56) and he was in his time clearly held in high esteem.

Loeb left his native Germany in 1897 after completing his MD because, according to Blumenthal (56), he disapproved of the prevailing nationalism and militarism. His early work was concerned with wound healing and pigment spread. When he arrived in the United States he became involved in the transplantation of tumors and later in the transplantation of a variety of tissues. Indeed, he predated Jensen (see below) in showing that some spontaneous rat tumors are transplantable (57, 58), and he was reasonably satisfied that the tumors developed from the living cells of the implants rather than from some "infective" agent. In discussing the possibility of immunity developing in the hosts, he found it difficult to distinguish between an immunity against the tumor-producing factor and one against the cells themselves. He noted that tumor fragments could be stored on ice for up to five days without destroying their ability to grow on transplantation.

Loeb's numerous studies on tissue transplantation are fully reviewed in his book published towards the end of his active life (59). He and his colleagues transplanted many hundreds of thyroid, parathyroid, cartilage, ovarian, splenic, adrenal, testicular and pancreatic grafts, mainly into rats and guinea pigs, and he coined the terms "homoio-" and "hetero"-transplantation (which were later replaced by homo- and xeno-). He had a special interest in "syngenesiotransplantation", where donors and host were genetically related as in families of outbred animals. He became obsessed by his theory of "individual differentials", which he believed held the key to his findings, made many times over, that the survival times of syngenesiografts were intermediate between those of auto- and allografts. Therefore the fate of a graft depended upon individuality differentials between the donor and recipient. The trouble with this concept was that it deterred him from recognizing that the cause of rejection lay in the presence of inherited tissue antigens present in the graft and absent in the recipient. This lack of recognition was probably largely responsible for his inability to appreciate the immunologic nature of the rejection process. There was also a whiff of metaphysics in his theory. Loeb rigidly adhered to a baroque system of grading the survival of grafts, resulting in an average score, rather than plotting survival curves and/or calculating median survival times, and this makes appraisal of his data far from easy. He was tantalizingly close to realizing that infiltrating lymphocytes were connected with graft rejection, but he was unable to distinguish between cause and effect. His colleague Cora Hesselberg (60) got fairly close when, in concluding her study on the fate of thyroid allografts in guinea pigs, she wrote: "This destruction is not caused by a direct primary disintegration or solution of the follicles, but depends on the destructive activity of 1) the lymphocytes and 2) of the connective tissue of the host tissue. The former invade the follicles and destroy them directly. . . ." Loeb himself seemed to think that the destructive role of lymphocytes was secondary (61), following the production of "homoiotoxins by cells in the graft" (62), and he endowed the invading connective tissue with a role of equal importance. One wonders what prevented Loeb from anticipating Medawar's conclusions about the immunologic nature of allograft rejection by several decades. One factor was that although Loeb grafted some animals more than once he failed to reveal the "second-set" response for the simple reason that he worked mainly with outbred animals and the donors of first and second grafts came from different animals. However, the time was simply not ripe. Loeb's colleague L.L. Tureen (63) found that thyroid graft survival was better in very young guinea pigs (some were only four days old), with lymphocyte infiltration occurring at a later stage than in adults, but he failed to draw any general conclusions from this observation. Finally, in 1927 (a year that saw a flood of papers from Loeb's laboratory) Loeb and King (64) reported a study based on two strains of rats that had been subjected to a fairly rigorous inbreeding program for 38 and 48 generations respectively. Tissues grafted within the strains were rejected almost as rapidly as between the strains, and the strain inbred for the longer period showed, perversely, the more intense reactions. In this paper they demonstrated a hierarchy in graft survival, with liver, spleen and bone marrow being most vulnerable and cartilage least – a finding that has stood the test of time.

As a result of reading Loeb's papers I felt very negative about his overall contribution. I was therefore almost relieved to come across a paper by the respected American geneticist C.C. Little on "The genetics of tissue transplantation in mammals" (65), published in 1924. In it he devastatingly criticizes Loeb's concept of individuality differentials, mainly because it was based on the supposition that such differentials are adapted to their normal environment and that in other environments they can act as "syngenesio-, homoio- or hetero-differentials." Little goes on to explain that Loeb established these categories on the basis of pedigree relationship alone and that this can be very misleading, as for example in Loeb's conclusion that grafts exchanged between related individuals provide results that are intermediate between auto- and allotransplantation. "... The indefiniteness of the above statements will without doubt be apparent. It is largely the product of the use of stocks of unknown genetic make-up. ... It is also clear that no adequate genetic analysis of his material can be made, because its genetic constitution is unknown or ignored. No controls are therefore available and no experiments to test genetic similarity or differences can be planned. ... It is especially unfortunate that the genetics of the transplantation of tissues will be the first acquaintance many well-meaning medical men will have with that field of biology. Even if their contact with genetics is first made through the work of over-ardent eugenic field workers it may, through irritation, survive the shock more readily than if it becomes submerged in a maze of experiments and facts collected on the basis of pedigree relationship." I doubt that it is possible to be more dismissive.

I do not propose to describe the early history of tumor transplantation in detail, but I am intrigued by the fact that the immunologic nature of the resistance to allogeneic tumor implants was understood long before an immunologic mechanism of allograft rejection was accepted. Curiously – and almost certainly because tumor biologists and surgeons tended to inhabit separate worlds – the former did not have the impact upon the latter that might have been expected. Readers interested in the early years of tumor transplantation are advised to read the reviews of Tyzzer (66), Woglom (67) and Little (68).

The Danish veterinarian bacteriologist C.O. Jensen is often credited with the realization that the resorption or take of tumors is determined by heredity: thus, a spontaneously arisen carcinoma was transplantable to other members of a closed colony of mice but not to other mice (69). Indeed, he managed to "passage" the tumor through as many as 19 generations of white mice, with a 40–50% success rate. Jensen also had some promising preliminary curative results in mice using an antiserum prepared against the tumor in a rabbit, but he stressed that it would be unwarranted on the basis of animal experiments to hold out hope for the treatment of human cancer by antibody transfer. Jensen's findings were quickly confirmed by Bashford (70) and others working in the laboratories of the Imperial Cancer Research Fund (I.C.R.F.), London, but the term "immunity" was not used in their scientific reports until 1908, when Russell (71) expressed the view that "there must be present in the resistant animals, either in the circulating fluids or in the tissues, something which inhibits this chemiotaxis". He believed that the immunity was "directed against chemiotactic influences exerted by the tumor cells on the connective tissue of the host". He went on: "Owing to the absence of any evidence which could justify an analogy with the antitoxins or antibodies to infective organisms, we refrain from the use of these terms." However, four years later Woglom (72) continued the series of reports from the I.C.R.F. with a most telling histologic study of a tumor transplanted in rats, from which he concluded that the early appearance of polymorphonuclear cells merely "prepared the soil for other cell types", the large numbers of lymphocytes around the inoculation site had an "intimate connection with the development of immunity", these lymphocytes must be "derived by a process of diapedesis from the bloodstream", and that plasma cells had "an intimate relationship with the development of immunity", whereas macrophages arrived later as scavengers. Mast cells and fibroblasts were of no importance. Woglom's conclusions received ample confirmation in mouse studies by the Italian Da Fano (73), again working at the I.C.R.F., whose paper was published in German and was clearly strongly influenced by Woglom's previous experiences. These data were greatly reinforced by Baeslack's subsequent finding (74) that a transplantable mouse carcinoma caused a shift in the number of blood white cells from polymorphonuclear leukocytes to small lymphocytes, and that this was associated with a cessation of growth or spontaneous regression of the tumors.

Paul Ehrlich was without doubt one of the founders of immunology. He was a dominant force around the turn of the century and he left his marks on many facets of the field, from his theory of antibody formation to the neutralizing power of antitoxins and the passive transfer of antibodies from mother to offspring (see Chapter 1). In 1906, only a few years after enunciating his side chain theory of antibody formation, he wrote a long and rather tedious paper on the transplantation of a mouse carcinoma into rats, in which he put forward his "athrepsia" theory (75). He observed that the implants grew for about eight days before they became necrotic and that he could rescue them by returning them before the eighth day. This "zigzag" procedure could be continued through many passages, persuading Ehrlich to suggest that each species provides its tissues with substances required for growth and survival, but that these were used up by the eighth day in a foreign host and followed by death unless replenished in the species of origin. The hypothesis was soon discredited, but in fairness to him he did go on to say that there was an additional phenomenon, an "active rat immunity", for when a rat received a second mouse tumor inoculum after regression of the first there was no growth at all. "The failure of the second vaccination can only be explained by an actively acquired immunity, established on the formation of antibodies resulting from resorption of the tumor mass" (77).

Before I turn to the remarkable contributions made by J.B. Murphy at the Rockefeller Institute, New York, I must mention two other significant contributions:

H. Apolant's finding that splenectomy prevented or reduced the active resistance of the host against transplanted foreign tumors (77); and Uhlenhuth, Händel and Steffenhagen's observation (78), confirmed by Bindseil (79), that radical removal of a growing tumor leads to immunity against a second tumor implant from the same strain, the immunity lasting in Bindseil's experiment for at least 127 days.

Of all those studying the rejection of tumors or normal tissues in the first two decades of the century it was J.B. Murphy who had the clearest understanding of the direct causal relationship between allograft rejection and the presence of host lymphocytes in the graft. He published most of his studies in the *Journal of Experimental Medicine* between 1913 and 1925, but republished his full output in 1926 (80) "for the convenience of the reader". His findings may be briefly summarized as follows:

(1) When transplanting a rat sarcoma to the chorioallantoic membrane of the chick embryo, its growth could be prevented if adult chicken spleen or bone marrow was implanted close to the graft (81). At this point he was still not sure whether the lymphoid cells were causally connected with graft failure but "Certainly a large preponderance of evidence points in that direction" (82).

(2) Resistance to allogeneic tumors, induced by previous inoculation of defibrinated blood from the tumor donors, "is accompanied in every case by a definite lymphoid crisis in the blood", (i.e. lymphocytosis) (83). He went on to say that "All the evidence points, therefore, towards the lymphocytes as a necessary factor in the immunity processes" (84). He quoted in support Apolant's finding (77) that previous splenectomy interfered with the development of immunity and mentioned that a role for antibodies in cancer immunity had not been found. "We are not prepared, however, at the present time to discuss the mechanism of the lymphoid reaction in cancer immunity" (85).

(3) Mice that were normally resistant to an allogeneic tumor became susceptible by previous exposure to X-rays (86). Because he and others had demonstrated that X-rays primarily affect the cells of the lymphoid system and that the reduction in lymphocytes was the most striking manifestation (87), he stated that ". . . lymphocytes are a potent factor in the immunity to cancer".

(4) Murphy and Sturm found that exposing mice to dry heat led to a decline in the blood lymphocytes followed by a rapid rise to values far above normal (88) and that this "brings about a high degree of immunity to certain transplantable tumors" (89).

(5) In confirming the previous finding of Y. Shirai (90) that xenogeneic tumors grow well when injected into the brain of rats, Murphy (91) noted that a) it was true only when the implant was not in contact with the ventricle, in which case there was a cellular reaction; b) tumor growth could be prevented by the addition of autologous spleen fragments; and c) tumors inoculated into the brain of mice previously immunized by subcutaneous inoculation of the tumor failed to grow. Murphy suggested two possibilities to account for these findings – either host cells could not migrate beyond the perivascular spaces or else lymphoid cells found the brain "an uncongenial environment". He thought the data confirmed "his earlier views on the association of cellular reaction with the resistance mechanism in respect of heteroplastic grafting".

These and other studies (he extended his observations to the etiology of tuberculosis, for example, again implicating lymphocytes) provide a formidable array of evidence that lymphocytes are a causal factor in graft rejection. It is therefore surprising that his studies did not have more influence on those who studied the mechanism of graft rejection several decades later. Murphy was clearly an excellent experimentalist who was loathe to speculate on the wider significance of his data, and one wishes that he had included experiments with tissues other than tumors. Even in his grand summary of his work in 1926 (80) he appeared cautious in his interpretation and unwilling to extend his ideas to the transplantation of normal tissues.

Although direct proof was not available, a connection had nonetheless been made between lymphocytes and rejection of both normal and malignant allografts. At the same time the evidence favoring the participation of antibodies was, at best, weak and in the hands of Tyzzer, for example, non-existent, the passive transfer of sera from immune mice having failed to influence adversely the fate of transplanted tumors (66). In reviewing the evidence for the participation of antibodies, Woglom stated in 1929: "It may be concluded that except for a few isolated observations which run contrary to the general evidence, no sign of the existence of agents similar to antibodies . . . has yet been discovered in connection with cancer" (67).

The contribution of the geneticists

Woglom (67) had little to say about the nature of the antigens that incite the recipient of a tumor graft to reject it, most of his discussion on this topic being taken up with the question of whether the tissue eliciting immunity had to be dead or alive. The consensus of opinion at that time was that dead tissues were unable to provoke immunity; but see below. Instead, some attention had been focused on the factors that determined "natural immunity". They were generally thought to be at least in part hereditary, and much of the evidence came from C.C. Little, E.E. Tyzzer and their colleagues in the United States though Loeb (57, 58) had set the ball rolling with his observation at the turn of the century that a tumor from a strain of Japanese waltzing mice was accepted by all mice of that strain, but failed to grow in an unrelated non-waltzing strain. Tyzzer (92) studied the genetics of this and concluded that susceptibility to a particular carcinoma was inherited but not according to Mendelian rules, for an apparent Mendelian dominance in the F1 generation had vanished in the F2 generation. Little (93), a few years later, put forward the notion that Tyzzer's data could in fact be explained in Mendelian terms by postulating the existence of more than one gene, and calculated that the percentage of takes declines with an increase in the number of Mendelizing susceptibility genes. By 1915 Little and Tyzzer (94) believed from their further genetic studies that the number of genes could be as large as 12–14, and in his review a year later Tyzzer (66) stated that susceptibility to a tumor depended on "the presence of a large number of independently inherited factors". In this review Tyzzer raised the possibility that susceptibility and resistance might, additionally, owe something to the "foreignness" or "incompatibility" of the tumor and he pointed out that this was true regardless of whether the tumor or the animal host was the constant factor in a transplantation experiment. "Although the degree of foreignness is not sufficient for the production of markedly cytotoxic or cytolytic sera, as when different species are employed, it appears probable that an immune body is formed which, in the presence of the antigen – or living tumor – excites an inflammatory reaction around the tumor so that the latter is isolated and eventually destroyed" (95). This is a very clear statement of the immunologic basis of tumor allograft rejection, though an understanding of its antigenic basis had to await the later studies of G.D. Snell and P.A. Gorer.

In this connection, it is hugely to C.C. Little's credit that having become President of the University of Maine he founded the Jackson Memorial Laboratory at Bar Harbor, Maine, in 1929. This institute was to become the power house of research on the genetic basis of tissue transplantation after G.D. Snell (see biographic sketch, Chapter 4) joined its staff in 1935, the field having waned in the 1920s and 1930s.

However, it was P.A. Gorer (see biographic sketch, Chapter 4) who was the first to demonstrate that tumor transplantation between mouse strains was governed by antigens present in the donor's tissues but absent in the recipient's, and that rejection was usually associated with the appearance of isoantibodies that could be identified by agglutination and other methods. In 1937 (96) he showed that a sarcoma that had arisen in, and was specific for Strong's albino A strain, grew in susceptible members of an F2 cross (and backcross generations) between the A strain and the resistant C57 Black strain, and that all susceptible animals possessed an antigen that had been derived from their albino ancestors. This antigen, called by Gorer "antigen II", was present on red blood cells and could be identified by isoagglutinins in the blood of mice that had either been immunized or had recently regressed tumors. A year later (97) he provided evidence showing that the isoagglutinins were formed as the result of a specific response of the tumor host to antigenic factors present in the tumor cells, which came from either a sarcoma or a leukemia. The anti-II antibody could be produced in C57 black mice by sarcoma or leukemic tissue as well as by blood from the A strain, and maximal titers corresponded with the time of complete tumor regression. "Experiments with hybrids justify the deduction that the iso-antibody specific for albino cells reacts with the same antigen as sera from immunised rabbits (antigen II)", he declared, and he found that the malignant tissues absorbed the isoagglutinating sera and contained more antigen II than red blood cells. He also found another antibody, "consistent with the previously obtained genetic evidence that two genes govern the transplantability of the tumor and with the hypothesis that both genes determine iso-antigenic differences".

A decade later Snell (98) called what proved to be a complex of dominant genes determining the transplantability of tumors the "histocompatibility antigens", and the genetic locus discovered by Gorer became known as H-2. This was one of many that were subsequently discovered, but which almost by definition proved to be much the strongest in terms of the level of immunity incited by its allelic antigens. The development of today's understanding of the H-2 complex was initially largely due to the pioneering work of Snell and Gorer and their colleagues, and I shall consider this critically important advance in detail in Chapter 4 on immunogenetics.

Because Gorer and his colleagues continued to work with dissociated tumors such as leukemias, for which they had no difficulties in demonstrating not only agglutinating but also cytotoxic and protective antibodies, the "Gorer school" became vociferous advocates of the humoral destruction of allografts, a point on which they were opposed by the "Medawar school", which favored cellular mechanisms in the

destruction of skin allografts and other normal tissues. This conflict became something of a cause célèbre and will be discussed further below (p. 74).

Enter P.B. Medawar: skin transplantation brought to a fine art

In his autobiographic book (99), Medawar relates how he came to become embroiled
with the problem of skin transplantation. It began with some futile attempts to help
a British airman whose plane had crashed early in World War II near Medawar's
home in Oxford and who had suffered extensive body burns. He was encouraged
by a colleague to "lay aside my intellectual pursuits and take a serious interest in
real life"! Having visited some patients with extensive burns and having attempted
to "grow" their own skin from small epidermal fragments he felt that the solution
lay elsewhere. "I guessed that if one could use what were then known as 'homografts' . . . the treatment of war wounds would be transformed." He wrote a memorandum to the War Wounds Committee of the Medical Research Council, later
published in 1943 (12), entitled "Notes on the problem of skin homografts", in
which he reviewed the literature. He concluded that the blood group theory favored
by some was unsatisfactory and that "the balance of evidence turns against a theory
of natural immunity". In contrast, he found "powerful circumstantial evidence" in
favor of the theory of active immunity although "direct evidence is feeble or wanting".
He was dismissive of Loeb's cellular theory because it was difficult to appraise because
of its vagueness and because it was too histological. "There is, for example, a great
deal of doubt about what lymphocytes do. On the other hand, any immunity hypothesis must account satisfactorily for the inflammatory reaction," and he went on to
say such a reaction could have the character of a local anaphylaxis (i.e. something
akin to the Arthus phenomenon). He was attracted to the notion that relatively few
genes may control tissue compatibility, and he pointed out that blood polymorphism
and tissue incompatibility evolved "hand in hand, and that the same type of genetic
differentiation underlies them both". He did not refer to Murphy's salient experiments implicating lymphocytes and was clearly unaware of them.

Medawar's memorandum impressed the committee. A grant was found and thus
began an astonishingly successful career during the course of which Medawar was
to dominate the field of experimental transplantation. In order to gain some background information of the practical problems involved he was sent to the Burns Unit
of the Glasgow Royal Infirmary for a few months, where he became acquainted with
T. Gibson, a surgeon. There followed a collaborative project involving the first truly
scientific study of human skin allografts, in which Gibson performed the surgery
using pinch grafts, and Medawar carried out the histological analysis. The results
were published in the *Journal of Anatomy* in 1943 (100). A single patient with extensive burns had received 52 autografts and 50 allografts from her brother, and at
each dressing biopsy specimens were removed from both sets. A second set (note
the introduction of this term, which has become firmly entrenched in the literature
even when it refers to only a single graft) of allografts from the same donor was
transplanted 15 days after the first. The results were clear: the autografts grew in
size and coalesced, whereas the first set allografts – though initially showing some
epidermal outgrowth – began to degenerate by day 15 and were necrotic by day 23.
The second set grafts, in contrast, showed no outgrowth and "dissolution" was far

advanced by the eighth day. Strangely, rejection was not accompanied by a "local reaction on the part of lymphocytes or other mesenchyme cells". They concluded that "the destruction of the foreign epidermis was brought about by a mechanism of active immunisation".

This demonstration of the accelerated rejection of a second graft from the same donor was convincing evidence in favor of the notion that allograft rejection is an immunologic phenomenon. However, Medawar immediately set out to repeat these observations on a large scale and with detailed histologic investigations in outbred rabbits, and the results were described in two papers that have become classics.

The first of these papers, published in 1944 (101), contains a detailed morphologic and histologic description of auto- and homografts at sequential stages, with the latter undergoing an acute inflammatory phase characterized by "a massive invasion of the grafts by lymphocytes and monocytes of native origin through the walls of the vessels within them". Medawar noted that the entire process of graft breakdown, once it began to manifest itself, took four days. He was the first to apply statistical analysis and the use of median survival times to graft survival, which was 10.4 ± 1.1 days for first set and 6.0 ± 0.6 days for second set grafts from the same donor. Significantly, this accelerated rejection "did not necessarily extend with equal vigour" to second set grafts from another donor, therefore introducing the concept of specificity. Survival times were dose-dependent (the smaller the graft, the longer the survival time), and the immune state was mainly systemic rather than mainly local. Because "the rabbit is peculiarly susceptible to anaphylactic inflammation (the Arthus reaction)" he thought that the inflammation in the allografts was probably of an anaphylactic type. He realized, however, that as an Arthus response the reaction was atypical, the usual polymorph infiltration having been substituted by an invasion of lymphocytes. Medawar concluded that "the mechanism by which foreign skin is eliminated belongs to the general category of actively acquired immunity", but his thoughts were entirely preoccupied by the possibility that antibodies were the mediator, in line with the analogy with the Arthus reaction.

Medawar's second study was published a year later (102). It confirmed his previous observations, especially the second set response – this time with fitted rather than free grafts – and the systemic nature of the immunity incited by the first set. He concluded that differences in the survival times of grafts from different donors were "an expression of the antigenic relationship between donor and recipient". The homograft reaction was governed by "*at least* seven antigens freely combined among *at least* 127 skin transplantation groups", and the working hypothesis was put forward that skin homografts generated antibody that "specifically prevents the completion of nuclear division in the cells of the homografted skin". "This interpretation may be wholly incorrect; but it . . . lends itself without very great difficulty to experimental refutation or proof."

Thus, although Medawar incisively laid the foundations for the immunologic basis of allograft rejection with these two papers, his thoughts were dominated by humoral antibodies. Ignorant as he was of Murphy's much earlier studies, he failed at that time to understand the significance of the lymphocytic infiltrate. However, by the time he gave his Harvey Lecture in 1957 (16) he was clearly well acquainted with the work of Murphy and Da Fano, for he wrote that "one need only mention the beautiful experiments which led J.B. Murphy to believe that the destruction of foreign tissue was carried out by the hostile activities of the recipient's lymphoid cells – by them, that is to say, rather than by a conventional antiserum. Perhaps Da Fano was the first to give reasonable grounds for thinking that lymphocytes and plasma cells were the chief accomplices of the host's reaction against homografts, and the wealth of circumstantial evidence amassed by Leo Loeb in researches extending over many years has given that interpretation added weight. All we have now to regret is that these authors believed a 'cellular' theory ... to be incompatible with an immunological theory". At the same time, the elegance of Medawar's skin graft studies convinced many of those who, encouraged by his pioneering work, entered the field in ever increasing numbers to use skin rather than tumor grafts for further analysis. Thus began (as Medawar himself pointed out many years later) the era of "the tyranny of the skin graft", an era that came to an end only in the late 1960s when kidney transplantation in the rat became feasible. This, strangely, happened to coincide roughly with Medawar's first and disabling brain hemorrhage, as a result of which he was no longer able to carry out experiments with his own hands.

It is of some interest that, in an anecdotal sort of way, Medawar's antibody-mediated interpretation of skin allograft rejection had already been anticipated by two earlier workers, both American. H.L. Underwood observed as early as 1914 (103) that large numbers of skin allografts transplanted sequentially to a badly burnt patient from a variety of donors, including the brother, first survived but then "melted", and later grafts also failed. Furthermore, some of the patient's own epithelium growing over the granulation tissue became "mushed" and the patient's heart beat became weak and irregular. Underwood wrote: "so far as I am aware there has been no effort to identify the reaction accompanying repeated skin grafting over large areas with that of anaphylaxis, yet it seems clear that they are closely related if not identical".

E. Holman's clinical experience ten years later was not dissimilar (104). A young boy with major lacerations received 151 small pinch grafts from his mother; all of them "took" and their epithelium had begun to spread by the fourth week, when a further 168 maternal grafts were transplanted. A month later the leg had become almost completely epithelialized, but after a further two weeks the patient developed a widespread exfoliative dermatitis involving not only the grafted area but also other parts of his skin. ". . . It occurred to me that the general dermatitis was most probably a phenomenon of anaphylaxis or protein intoxication, and a manifestation of sensitiveness to the foreign protein of the mother." Removal of all grafts led to a great improvement in the patient's condition and the dermatitis rapidly disappeared. A second attempt at allotransplantation was made using two donors, one but not the other belonging to the same blood group. Both sets of grafts were destroyed within a few weeks, and a second set of grafts from one of the donors never took. Holman concluded that this failure "calls one's attention very forcibly to Lexer's emphatic statement that the success of isografts (= allografts) may be relegated to mythology". He noted some specificity in the rejection of grafts from different donors, an observation that led Holman to think with great prescience that "each group of grafts develops its own antibody which is responsible for the subsequent disappearance of the new epidermis". Both these surgeons were thus very much ahead of their time and Gibson and Medawar were aware of their publications.

A somewhat curious footnote to all this is that Gibson published a case history in 1986 (*105*), 43 years after the event, of a two-year-old child who had received a large number of pinch grafts from the father, the second group 13 days after the first. All grafts, regardless of when transplanted, lost their epithelium in the fourth week after the first operation. "It seemed that we were dealing with an antigen–antibody reaction of some kind", Gibson wrote, though with the benefit of hindsight. He had undertaken this clinical experiment before Medawar had joined him in Glasgow and had been keen to publish the case on his own; in the event he was conscripted into the army and the data were allowed to languish.

Another human study, though of a different kind, was published in 1927 by the German surgeon K.H. Bauer (*106*), working in Göttingen. Having been convinced by Lexer of the futility of using allografts, he proceeded to transplant skin between identical twins whose bilateral syndactyly of the little and ring fingers was being repaired. He also used an autograft as a control. Both types of grafts took equally well and the operation was wholly successful. Bauer was in no doubt about the importance of his observation that individuality was the decisive factor in deciding whether an allograft failed or succeeded, and he saw no reason why even organs should not be transplanted between uniovular twins, as eventually happened in the case of the human kidney some 30 years later (see Chapter 7).

Silverstein has posed the question as to "why so much work was forgotten and why Medawar's studies in the 1940s were received as 'new' disoveries". He suggested that for several reasons – the unwillingness of the kidney surgeons to contemplate whole body X-irradiation to enable human grafts to survive, and the disenchantment of the tumor biologists in their quest to solve the cancer problem – the science of tissue transplantation had run out of steam by the late 1930s, and that it needed "new data, new technologies and, above all, a new point of view to rekindle . . . interest . . ." (*107*). Silverstein also noted that no professional immunologists had been involved and that immunologic textbooks and reviews of the period had failed to refer to the study of tumor or normal tissue transplantation. Although these points are valid there is, nonetheless, one other reason why Medawar's experiments immediately made their mark: they were carefully designed, rigorously controlled and executed with painstaking care; above all, the results were utterly incisive and left no doubt that the rejection of a normal tissue like skin is mediated by immunologic mechanisms. Biologists and immunologists alike needed just this stimulus, which was further enhanced by the subsequent demonstration of immunologic tolerance (Chapter 5). Immunologists were therefore encouraged to enter a field that provided them with a considerable new challenge.

Medawar, like his later colleagues R.E. Billingham and L. Brent and many others entering the field at that time, was a zoologist by training and by profession (see Medawar's biographic sketch, Chapter 5), and it was as biologists that they carried out their early studies. Only in the mid-1950s did the immunologic community accept that their investigations were relevant to the main stream of immunology and they themselves began to regard themselves first and foremost as immunologists.

Rejection Mechanisms

Humoral versus cellular: a controversy

Although the early tumor biologists generally failed to associate the regression of allogeneic tumors with the appearance of specific antibodies, Gorer had shown in 1942 (*108*) that tumor allografts not only incited the production of hemagglutinating antibodies but that leukemic cells suspended in sera from immunized mice before transplantation were greatly retarded in their growth and often failed to grow at all. These sera contained both hemagglutinating and protective antibodies, and by absorption experiments Gorer concluded that the two were distinct and acting quite independently although "there are reasons for supposing that they react with the same antigens". This observation was confirmed and extended by both Gorer and his colleagues on many subsequent occasions, always working with pure inbred strains of mice. For example, by 1950 (*109*) Gorer had further discovered an antibody in the serum of immunized mice that in the presence of unheated human serum brought about the lysis of cells and proved to be protective to mice given the tumor *in vivo*. In 1955 (*110*) he showed that very low titers of specific hemagglutinating antibody could be demonstrated in mice after the transplantation of skin allografts, although the donor strain red blood cells had to be suspended in absorbed human serum to make the cells sticky enough to form clumps with the antiserum. This sensitive method (*111*) was subsequently widely adopted and, together with Billingham and Sparrow, in Medawar's group at University College, Gorer's team used it to reveal the formation of antibodies after transplantation of allogeneic epidermal cells (*112*). Isoantibodies were detected not only as hemagglutinins but also as cytotoxins (*113*), hemolysins (*114*) and leukoagglutinins (*115*). Numerous workers found alloantibodies after skin transplantation and Hildemann and Medawar (*116*) showed that they also formed in mice that had been sensitized with crude cell-free nuclear fractions prepared from mouse spleens. These observations made good sense in the light of Medawar's earlier finding that skin and blood leukocytes share antigens (*117, 118*). He had demonstrated this important link through the accelerated destruction of rabbit skin allografts after the recipients had received several intradermal inoculations of purified blood leukocytes from the skin donors. He failed to find a similar antigenic overlap with red blood cells, and it was later shown that the representation of transplantation antigens on red cells was an anomaly of the murine species. In his 1946 paper Medawar (*118*) pointed out that although in his experience the intravenous route was far less effective in bringing about a state of sensitization than the intradermal route (and this was amply confirmed subsequently by many workers), the presence of potentially immunogenic antigens on blood leukocytes had implications for the practice of blood transfusion.

The formation of antibodies during and following allotransplantation was therefore not at all in doubt. The ensuing controversy was engendered by the question of whether these antibodies were causally connected with graft rejection or whether their production was an epiphenomenon. The Gorer school believed the former to be true and in this they were opposed by Medawar and his colleagues, as well as many others. The controversy undoubtedly gave a certain edge to Gorer and Medawar's intellectual relationship. In his biographic memoir of Peter Gorer, written for the Royal Society after Gorer's premature death, Medawar wrote (*119*): "We at University College began by thinking that humoral antibodies were of secondary importance, and that the homograft reaction was mediated through the action of sensitized lymphoid cells, with the antibodies as lookers-on. Gorer, naturally enough, attached great importance to antibodies, and took some convincing of the importance   of N.A. Mitchison's work on cellular components of the reaction. In the outcome each recognized the importance of the other's ideas . . ." (*120*). This controversy recalls the much more vitriolic one towards the end of the nineteenth century when the giants of the nascent immunology were daggers drawn in their evaluation of the importance of macrophages (Metchnikoff) and humoral factors (E. von Behring, S. Kitasato, H. Buchner, R. Pfeiffer, J. Bordet, R. Koch, P. Ehrlich, to name but a few) in the body's defense against micro-organisms – a debate that was resolved to the satisfaction of most scientists by A.E. Wright and S.R. Douglas' demonstration that opsonizing antibodies facilitate phagocytosis by macrophages (*121*). A full account of this interesting episode is given in Silverstein's book (*122*).

So what *was* the evidence against the humoral interpretation and in favor of cellular mediators? It began with experiments published by Medawar in 1948 (*123*) in which he put the humoral hypothesis to the test, with entirely negative results. Thus the culture of skin from adult rabbits in the presence of serum "heavily and specifically immunized against it" did not in any way prejudice its survival or the ability of the epidermal epithelium to migrate or to undergo cell division, causing Medawar to write: "With certain stated qualifications, it has therefore been concluded that the occurrence of free antibodies is not a sufficient explanation of the regression of skin homografts *in vivo*." However, this paper, which it must be said was not presented with Medawar's characteristic lucidity, did not further the cellular cause either, for the inclusion of various lymphoid tissues from the sensitized rabbit likewise failed to prejudice the survival of the skin. There was still no mention of Murphy's work linking tumor regression with lymphocytic infiltrates (see above).

It was N.A. Mitchison's experiments on what he called the "passive transfer of transplantation immunity" that provided vital evidence in favor of the hypothesis that lymphoid cells are directly responsible for allograft destruction (*124–126*). Having shown that the rejection of a mouse lymphosarcoma was considerably faster in non-susceptible mice that had already rejected a tumor graft or been immunized with normal tissues from animals of the tumor donor strain, he transferred the draining lymph nodes from immune mice into normal syngeneic animals, followed by the implants of the tumor. This procedure conferred immune status on the recipients, whereas the transfer of serum, peritoneal exudate and lymphocyte suspensions of non-draining nodes did not. Surprisingly, the power to transfer immunity lasted only a short time following implantation of the tumor. Mitchison, who performed these studies in Oxford as part of his Ph.D. thesis, for which Medawar was one of his supervisors, wrote: "The conclusion can therefore be drawn . . . that transplantation immunity is transferred with greater facility by cells rather than by antibody in solution, if transferred by the latter at all." He added that his results were analogous to those working with different antigenic systems, sensitization to simple chemical compounds (*127*) and tuberculin (*128*) having already been achieved by the transfer of sensitized cells but only exceptionally with serum.

Billingham, Brent and Medawar (129) immediately set out to repeat these studies using skin allografts as the target, and they confirmed and greatly extended Mitchison's data; they too used inbred mouse strains – a critically important device because it allowed the transferred cells to survive in the "secondary" hosts – and they coined the term "adoptively acquired immunity" to distinguish cellular transfer from passive transfer with antibody. This term has been in use ever since. They confirmed that the regional lymph node fragments were most effective, though with their more sensitive system they also established a lesser role for the spleen. "The regional nodes are therefore held to be the principal but not the only seat of the reaction against skin homografts", they wrote, and they showed that extirpation of the regional nodes after skin graft rejection did not impair the host's capacity to produce a secondary response. Likewise, extirpation of regional nodes before skin grafting did not significantly reduce the power of the primary response because, they postulated, new pathways were opened up. They argued that the transfer results could not be explained by the passive transfer of antibodies because killed lymph nodes and nodes transplanted subcutaneously rather than intraperitoneally were ineffective, as were massive doses of blood, blood leukocytes or serum. Significantly, they succeeded in abolishing neonatally induced tolerance by transferring regional lymph node fragments, thus eliminating the alternative explanation of active immunization by antigenic matter within the nodes. The immunity of the primary hosts was durable in that transfer could still be brought about 30 days after rejection of the grafts of the primary hosts, and this was in keeping with the longevity of the immune state in actively sensitized mice. Billingham, Brent and Medawar concluded that "The fact that transplantation immunity can be adoptively but not passively acquired argues in favour of its similarity to the tuberculin reaction and to sensitisation reactions of the delayed type" – a conclusion that has stood the test of time.

It should be added that the notion of transferring the capacity for antibody production with sensitized lymphoid tissues goes as far back as 1899, when Deutsch (130) found antityphoid antibodies in the sera of guinea pigs that had been given splenic tissue from immune donors. Others confirmed this and S. and T.N. Harris made a detailed study of it in the 1950s, using rabbits. The first of a series of papers was published in 1954 (131) in which they showed that after lymph node transfer, antibody production peaked in these outbred animals at three days and then declined rapidly. Their studies were summarized and concluded in 1960 (132) when they felt able to state that "antibody found in the recipient animals is produced by a mechanism of antibody formation transferred in the lymph node cells, and . . . the synthetic process is continued within the transferred cells". It should be added that the adoptive transfer of normal or sensitized cells was used very successfully by Davies and Cole (133) in breaking tolerance to skin grafts induced by the inoculation of allogeneic bone marrow cells into lethally irradiated allogeneic recipient mice.

The adoptive transfer of immunity by Mitchison and by Billingham, Brent and Medawar not only revealed that lymphoid cells play a key role in allograft destruction but also provided an experimental design for the analysis of allograft responses that continues to be used to the present day. At that time the physiology and function of lymphocytes was still far from clear; thus Rich (134), in his treatise on the pathogenesis of tuberculosis, was moved to state: "The lack of more adequate information regarding the function of the lymphocyte is one of the most lamentable gaps in medical knowledge." Together with the older literature already quoted and primed by the data obtained from adoptive immunity studies, precise data on the function of lymphocytes did not become available until Gowans had shown that not all lymphocytes are shortlived end cells and that they could initiate graft-versus-host reactions, and Miller and others had carried out their important studies pointing to the thymus as the provider of those lymphocytes participating in alloreactivity (see Chapter 1, pp. 13–14 and below).

Much of the subsequent experimental evidence favored the cellular hypothesis. Further systematic attempts by Billingham and Brent (135) to transfer immunity passively to skin allografts using antisera failed completely; insofar as there was an effect at all it tended to be in the direction of *prolonging* graft survival. Indeed, alloantisera were soon shown to be the mediators of the phenomenon of enhancement of tumor allograft survival (see Chapter 6), that is, they were shown to be protective to many tumors. One dissenting voice was raised by Stetson and Demopoulos (136) who, working with skin grafts, found that sera from mice sensitized with donor strain spleen cells emulsified with Freund's complete adjuvant passively immunized secondary recipients – a study the Medawar group (137) could not confirm. Very relevant to the debate were the studies of Algire, Weaver and Prehn (138, 139) with tissues enclosed in diffusion chambers made of membranes with pores fine enough to prevent the passage of cells through them while allowing metabolites and other substances in solution, such as antibodies, to gain entry by diffusion. Such diffusion chambers were implanted into the body cavity of mice and the fate of a variety of allogeneic tissues within them was monitored: survival always far exceeded the survival times obtained by direct implantation into the hosts, even when the hosts had been specifically presensitized. By contrast, xenogeneic tissues known to be vulnerable to the cytotoxic action of antibodies were promptly destroyed, and the authors concluded that the destruction of allogeneic tissue did not require the participation of circulating antibodies.

Nonetheless, Gorer's (108) observation that cytotoxic (or protective) antibodies can be raised against a mouse leukemia were confirmed by others, notably by Mitchison and Dube (140) with a mouse sarcoma, Mitchison (141) with a lymphoma, and Amos and Day (142) with several mouse leukoses. Evidently tumor cells in suspension are highly vulnerable to antibody, especially in the presence of added complement, and Gorer and Boyse (143) extended this concept to normal cells such as thymus and bone marrow cells in suspension. The resolution of the humoral versus cellular debate therefore came from the realization that isolated tumor (especially leukemic) or normal cell suspensions are vulnerable to the action of cytotoxic antibodies whereas tissues such as skin and solid tumors require the direct participation of lymphoid cells.

A further important qualification must, however, be made, for it was shown in the 1960s – a decade later – that the hyperacute rejection of human kidney allografts in presensitized individuals was brought about by pre-existing antibodies, even though normal rejection is usually associated with lymphocyte infiltrates. This disastrous form of rejection happens within minutes or hours of completion of the vascular anastomosis between the kidney and the recipient and it is always linked with either presensitization or major blood group incompatibility (i.e. natural antibodies), neither of which should have occurred once transplant surgeons were alerted to the danger.

Although Terasaki, Marchioro and Starzl (*144*) alluded to a patient with antidonor antibodies whose kidney was immediately rejected, the first clear demonstration of this phenomenon was provided by the Dane Kissmeyer-Nielsen and his colleagues (*145*), who published their data in the *Lancet* in 1966 and who coined the term "hyperacute rejection". Both their patients had been "heavily isoimmunised by blood transfusions and pregnancies", and both possessed complement-fixing thrombocyte and kidney antibodies as well as leukocyte agglutinins before they received their kidneys. These authors believed "that these humoral antibodies played a decisive part ...", and the teams of Williams (*146, 147*) – who included D.M. Hume and, in the 1968 paper, P.J. Morris and F. Milgrom – and Starzl *et al.* (*148*) soon provided confirmation, drawing attention to the similarity with the Schwartzman reaction. Williams *et al.* (*147*) were forthright in stating that "humoral antibodies to histocompatibility antigens may be responsible for hyperacute graft rejection" and they suggested how cross-matching between donor and recipient should prevent it. Hyperacute rejection of kidneys was subsequently shown to occur in a variety of experimental animals though many strains of rat proved to be relatively refractory. Detailed references may be found in the 1975 review of Brent and Porter (*149*).

The cellular hypothesis of primary rejection of solid allografts has stood the test of time, and soon after the events described above it was greatly strengthened by evidence from three areas: the similarity between the allograft reaction and delayed-type hypersensitivity (DTH), the participation of lymphocytes in alloreactivity, and the *in vitro* demonstration of direct cytotoxicity of lymphocytes (see below).

The allograft reaction as a variant of delayed-type hypersensitivity

Burnet and Fenner (*150*), in their highly influential 1949 monograph, discussed the possible relationship between transplantation immunity and DTH – the class of immunologic reactions, exemplified by the tuberculin reaction, which are revealed as a delayed skin response when the appropriate antigen is injected intradermally into presensitized individuals. Such reactions, as they pointed out, are usually associated with lymphocytic accumulations at the reaction site and an apparent lack of circulating antibody. They believed that sensitization in DTH "is always a result of the production and liberation of antibodies which are either identical with classical circulating antibodies ... or differ only in the greater ease with which they are taken up by cells" (*151*). Accordingly, they thought that the passive transfer of tuberculin hypersensitivity with cells may have been the result of antibody production by these cells in their new hosts. The concept of "cell-bound antibodies", which prevailed in the 1950s and 60s until the T cell receptor became fully understood, was given support by the finding in 1958 by Berrian and Brent (*152*) that lymphoid cells from animals that had been sensitized with allogeneic tissues were specifically able to absorb solubilized histocompatibility antigens – a result that predated recognition of the T cell receptor and suggested a mechanism for the action of lymphoid cells in transplantation immunity.

With great prescience Burnet and Fenner went on to point to the analogy between these two phenomena, listing the absence of detectable antibodies, the systemic nature of the sensitization process, and the necessity for intradermal as opposed to intravenous immunization with leukocytes in rabbits as features of the allograft reaction (see *117, 118*). "A working hypothesis is that the mechanism involved is similar to that postulated for tuberculin hypersensitivity." Some years later the American immunologist C.B. Favour (*154*) developed these arguments further in a short but well-argued annotation in which he allocated a central role to the lymphocyte and which ended with the conclusion that "information from the field of immunology supports the thesis that the rejection of homografts ... is a complex homeostatic response involving the specific function of both the tuberculin type allergy and anaphylactic immunity as well as non-specific inflammatory processes which these reactions set in motion and which predominate in transplant sites at the time of graft rejection".

A successful attempt to prove this concept experimentally was made by Brent, Brown and Medawar (*155, 156*). Working with the guinea pig, a species that was well known for its ability to display inflammatory cutaneous hypersensitivity reactions, this group sensitized animals with skin grafts from known donors and tested the resultant sensitivity by the intradermal inoculation of semi-soluble extracts prepared from the donor's spleen. They were thus able to show that alloreactivity could manifest itself as a typical DTH response in terms of the tempo and appearance of the skin lesions and the cellular infiltrate. This cutaneous response was called the "direct reaction" to distinguish it from the "transfer reaction". The latter was brought about by the intradermal inoculation of cells from the regional lymph nodes of the sensitized animal into the skin graft donor, setting up a cutaneous reaction that resembled the direct reaction but tended to be more intense. It could not be invoked with either immune serum or by heat-killed lymphoid cells. "The evidence ... thus supports the analogy long since drawn between the homograft and tuberculin reactions, and upholds the contention that the 'second set' homograft reaction reveals a pre-existing and not a re-awakened (anamnestic) sensitivity" (*156*). Brent and Medawar (*157*) went on to show that the intradermal transfer of normal blood lymphocytes excited a similar delayed inflammatory reaction (the normal lymphocyte transfer reaction) which, they suggested, could be used as a means of typing prospective human organ donors and recipients. Using inbred guinea pigs they went on to prove that this reaction was essentially one by the donor cells against host antigens, that is, a graft-versus-host reaction (*158, 159*).

As the majority of the cells infiltrating allografts in adoptive transfer of sensitivity are of host origin (*160, 161*) there appears to be a degree of non-specificity. This was shown to be the case by Prendergast (*162*), further emphasizing the similarity between allograft responses and cutaneous hypersensitivity reactions in general. As these responses are quite specific this remained something of a puzzle until it was shown that the nonspecific recruitment of lymphocytes comes about in response to the release of lymphokines from specifically activated cells (*163*).

The participation of lymphocytes in alloreactivity

The adoptive transfer of immunity to tumor skin allografts showed clearly enough that lymphoid cells are involved in allograft rejection, and the same was equally true of graft-versus-host reactions in the chick embryo (*164*) and in the neonatal mouse (*165*). The demonstration that lymphocytes, and small lymphocytes in particular, constitute the immunologically competent cells came somewhat later. It was, incidentally, Medawar (*166*) who coined the term "immunologically competent cell" in his Croonian Lecture of 1958 to distinguish immunologic capability from performance and to describe a cell that is "fully qualified to undertake an immunological response" of a specific kind.

The first clear indication that lymphocytes are responsible for graft-versus-host disease (GVHD) came in 1960. Both Billingham *et al.* (*167*) and Anderson, Delorme and Woodruff (*168*) found that rat thoracic duct cells, which Gowans (*169*) had previously shown to comprise 95% small and 5% large or medium lymphocytes, induced GVHD when inoculated into allogeneic newborns. This result had already been foreshadowed by other workers such as Simonsen (*164*), Terasaki (*170*) and Terasaki, Cannon and Longmire (*171*) when inducing GVHD with blood white cells. (Terasaki, Cannon and Longmire had used chicken blood lymphocytes with a purity of 99% to bring about GVHD.) The question of whether the thoracic duct cells responsible were small lymphocytes was, however, left open, both groups (*167, 168*) having expressed considerable reservations about the capacity of small lymphocytes, which at that time were regarded as "end cells", to perform such a major role. Nonetheless, Simonsen (*172*) found the "guilty" cells to be rapidly dividing and he concluded that they must belong to "the mononuclear lines". Gowans, Gesner and McGregor (*173*) and Gowans (*174*) soon provided conclusive proof. Having shown that the inoculation of parental strain thoracic duct lymphocytes (TDL) into relatively young F1 hybrid rats led to a virtually 100% mortality from GVHD they compared this with the effect of cell suspensions that consisted predominantly of large lymphocytes harvested by late drainage of the thoracic duct: their recipients did not die. Conversely, small lymphocyte preparations that excluded large cells were fully operational. These authors therefore concluded that the small lymphocyte was the immunologically competent cell of thoracic duct lymph, and they provided evidence for the development of such cells into large pyroninophilic cells capable of dividing in their allogeneic hosts.

Such a conclusion was likewise reached by another British group when Porter, Chapuis and Freeman (*175*) reported their investigations into the causes of death in rabbit radiation chimeras established by treatment with allogeneic blood and bone marrow cells: ". . . it is tempting to . . . suggest that it is the small lymphocytes (in the blood) . . . that are harmful . . .", and these workers provided evidence based on radiolabeling that some small lymphocytes transformed into large pyroninophilic cells in their allogeneic hosts.

Of considerable corroborative significance was the finding by Gowans, McGregor and Cowen (*176*) that normal small syngeneic lymphocytes transferred adoptively to tolerant rats bearing healthy allogeneic skin grafts led to destruction of the grafts and, conversely, that thoracic duct cells obtained from tolerant rats were incapable of inducing GVHD, thus mirroring the earlier work by Medawar's group, which had used crude suspensions of lymphoid cells such as splenic and lymph node tissues with similar results. These findings were subsequently confirmed by many others (for example, Billingham, Silvers and Wilson (*177*) implicated blood lymphocytes in the adoptive transfer of sensitivity) and the status of the small lymphocyte as the prime mediator of allograft reactivity and many other immunologic responses was no longer in doubt.

A dissenting voice came from the Australians Szenberg and Warner (*178*), whose experiments on GVHD after implantation of blood cells on the chorioallantoic membrane of chick embryos led them to conclude that it was the large and not the small lymphocyte that was the cause of the lesions. Darcy (*179*), in an even earlier histologic study in 1952, dismissed plasma cells as prime suspects in the destruction of rabbit allografts but was almost equally skeptical of a role for lymphocytes.

It was later shown that small lymphocytes comprise T (thymus-derived) and B (bone marrow-derived, antibody precursor) subpopulations. T cells could then be further subdivided into functionally different CD4-positive and CD8-positive cells, the former being involved predominantly in antigen recognition and induction of immune responses, and the latter primarily as cytotoxic effectors of responses to virus infections and allograft rejection (see below and Chapter 1). The "cellular" school of transplantation immunology therefore received strong support, though sight must not be lost of the fact that in certain circumstances, for example in xenoreactivity, antibodies can likewise be crucially important.

In vitro *reactivity of lymphocytes*

Direct cytotoxicity
The participation of lymphocytes in allograft responses was the pressing topic in the 1950s. The next decade saw further advances when it became clear that lymphocytes could be cytotoxic *in vitro*. (The separation of lymphocytes into the two major subgroups, T and B, came somewhat later and at this time they were regarded as a single entity.) The first demonstration of this was by the Belgian A. Govaerts (*180*), working with kidney allografts in dogs. Blood lymphocytes taken from dogs that had rejected their kidneys were found to have a specific cytotoxic effect on cultured renal cells of the donor, while serum was entirely innocuous, an observation that he believed reinforced the concept of "cellbound antibodies" as proposed by Berrian and Brent (*152*). Rosenau and Moon (*181, 182*) at the University of California followed hard on his heels when studying the effect of sensitized mouse lymphocytes on allogeneic L cells: they described a sequence of lymphocyte clustering around their targets, followed by cytopathic changes and eventually cell death. They concluded that "Close contact between sensitized lymphocytes and homologous cells seems essential for the cytolytic reaction" (*181*) and they followed this up by showing that cytotoxicity could be achieved with almost pure lymphocyte populations (*183*). Others confirmed these observations, notably Brondz (*184*) in Prague, who also found that immune lymphocytes could be "adsorbed" by donor target cells, but only if there was complete antigenic conformity between them.

More detailed *in vitro* studies were reported by D.B. Wilson (*185, 186*), working in Billingham's department at the Wistar Institute and using inbred rats that had been sensitized with allogeneic skin. By developing a sensitive quantitative assay he found that the degree of target cell survival was inversely related to the number of sensitized lymphocytes and that the exponential nature of his graphic plots suggested a "single-hit" mechanism (*185*). He computed that as many as 1–2% of the lympho-cytes participated and he confirmed Rosenau and Moon's observation that clustering after seven hours' incubation preceded cytolysis at 20 hours. Serum or an extract of sonicated sensitized cells were ineffectual, as were cells that were kept at arm's length from their targets by a millipore membrane. Like Rosenau and Moon he concluded that close apposition of the cells was "apparently required" and that, if cell-bound substances were involved, these could not be easily detached from the lymphocytes. From his follow-up paper (*186*), in which he described the inhibition of cytotoxicity with a derivative of the drug 6-mercaptopurine, it became clear that RNA-dependent protein synthesis on the part of the sensitized cells was necessary for the destructive interaction. H. Ginsburg in Israel (*187*) carried out extensive studies on the adhesive and lytic powers of lymphocytes using cultured allogeneic monolayers; because the cells looked like transformed blast cells and their exact nature was not ascertained he gave them the functional name of "lysocytes", and he captivated audiences in the 1960s with his time-lapse cinematography showing lysocytes killing target cells and then moving on to others.

Enter Brunner's laboratory in Lausanne. Adopting a quantitative method of measuring cell lysis developed by A.R. Sanderson (*188–190*) using antibody and complement and labeling the target cells with chromium-51 and counting the radioactive supernatant at the end of the reaction time, Brunner's group (*191*) measured cell-mediated lysis. Having shown that thymus cells (*192*) and thymus-derived lymphocytes (*193*) (identifiable by the θ alloantigen) from sensitized inbred mice were specifically cytotoxic to allogeneic target cells, Brunner *et al.* (*194*) established a quantitative *in vitro* cytotoxicity assay in 1970 that soon became the standard method for assessing the capacity of lymphocytes to kill targets *in vitro* (cell-mediated lympholysis, or CML). It is used, with minor modifications, to this day and it has become an invaluable tool in the assessment of cytotoxic cell function. In the same year the same group (*195*) studied the conditions required for maximal cytotoxicity, and established that deoxyribonucleic acid (DNA) synthesis was not required, trypsinization of the effector cells temporarily inhibited cytotoxicity, and anti-target cell antisera blocked the response only when they were directed at part or the whole of the H-2 complex. Like the technique of adoptive transfer of sensitivity the cytotoxic assay became one of the vital tools used in the dissection of alloreactivity and of other *in vitro* immunologic responses such as antitumor and antiviral reactivity. It ushered in a new era of immunology in which *in vitro* studies took their place alongside the more traditional investigations with whole animals. For example, *in vitro* cytotoxicity was used to great effect in 1974, when Zinkernagel and Doherty (*196–198*) made their critically important observations concerning the major histocompatibility complex (MHC)-restricted nature of T lymphocyte cytotoxicity against virus-infected cells, and Shearer (*199*) implicated the mouse MHC in the cytotoxicity of spleen cells against trinitrophenyl-modified syngeneic cells. The importance of these papers lay in the fact that they alerted the immunologic world to the true function of the histocompatibility antigens – that their primary role is one of controlling cell-to-cell interactions, in this case between the cytotoxic T lymphocyte and the virus-infected or hapten-modified target cells.

It was subsequently shown that cytotoxic alloreactive lymphocytes could be generated *in vitro* by culturing lymphoid populations together with allogeneic simulator cells (i.e. after mixed lymphocyte culture, MLC). The MLC and the cytotoxic cells generated by it therefore came to be seen as the *in vitro* counterpart of alloreactivity and it was almost immediately applied to the problem of tissue typing (see below and Chapter 4). Its antecedents lay in the observation by P.C. Nowell (*200*) in 1960 that blood leukocytes, which he had prepared for culture with the aid of a plant extract called phytohemagglutin (PHA), went into mitosis as a result of contact with the extract, which therefore became known as a mitogenic agent and has since been used widely as a nonspecific activator of T lymphocytes. A year later Hastings *et al.* (*201*), with K. Hirschhorn as one of the co-authors, described a method of culturing blood lymphocytes with a 95–99% purity, based on this observation. The lymphocytes formed large clusters and mitoses were formed within the clusters, which prompted the authors to speculate that the mitogenic action of the PHA was due to cluster formation that provided the lymphocytes with a congenial environment for cell division.

The mixed lymphocyte culture assay

In 1964 Bach and Hirschhorn (*202*), working at the New York School of Medicine, published their seminal experiments on the culture of blood lymphocytes from two unregulated individuals, this time without the use of PHA. They found that after 7–8 days some of the cells underwent a morphological transformation to large cells, which then divided. Both blast cell formation and mitoses were estimated quantitatively by microscopic observation of fixed smears. A study of three individuals whose probable sharing of histocompatibility antigens had been determined by their colleagues (F.T. Rapaport *et al.*) in the Department of Surgery, using skin transplantation, showed that the individuals who were most strongly cross-reactive had the lowest *in vitro* percentage of large cells and mitoses. Bach and Hirschhorn therefore suggested that it might be practicable to develop mixed cell cultures as a typing test for potential recipients and donors of kidney allografts, and they proposed intra- and inter-family studies to prove their point. Almost concomitantly they published a paper in the same volume of *Science* (*203*) in which they applied the technique to two prospective patients and relatives who were potential kidney donors. One patient's cells responded very poorly to her mother's lymphocytes and the mother's kidney was transplanted; the other patient's cells responded poorly to her mother and somewhat more strongly to her father and sister; however, because of "other considerations the father was chosen as the kidney donor". Although at the time of publication the kidneys had been transplanted for only three and four months, both had shown "minimal evidence of graft rejection" on immunosuppression with azathioprine, prednisolone and puromycin. The conclusion that "This technique of lymphocyte culture offers a new approach to the problem of . . . typing for renal homotransplantation" was, however, complicated by the fact that two-way stimulation had been measured (i.e. reactivity of the recipient against the donor and vice versa). It was only later, following a suggestion from L. Brent while sharing a taxi in New York and graciously acknowledged in Bach's recent recollections (*204*)), that the reactivity of only the recipient's cells was assessed, the activity of the potential donor's cells having been blocked by previous treatment with mitomycin C (*205*) or X-irradiation (*206*).

Quite independently and possibly even predating these important developments (for their paper appeared in *Blood* in January 1964, the month in which the first papers from the Bach–Hirschhorn group were submitted to *Science*, and an abstract had appeared in mid-1963 (*207*)), Bain, Vas and Lowenstein (*208*), hematologists working in Montreal, reported their studies on "The development of large immature mononuclear cells in mixed lymphocyte cultures". They too cultured blood leukocytes from unrelated individuals and found that some of them transformed into "large basophilic cells that can synthesize DNA and undergo mitosis", resembling the cells that "develop *in vivo* in lymph nodes and spleen in response to injection of soluble antigens and following skin homografting". They established that the effect stemmed from the presence of two sets of leukocytes rather than red blood cells, plasma or platelets, and their preliminary comparison of pairs of identical and non-identical twins led them to conclude that "genetic factors may be involved". It was this group that coined the term MLC and they suggested, rather cautiously, that the reaction "may be related to homograft immunity" and that it might "prove to be valuable in predicting the compatibility between the prospective donor and recipient of a homograft". Their starting point had been the incidental observation by Schrek and Donelly (209) that, under certain conditions, human leukocytes cultured in the absence of PHA transformed and went into mitosis, and they used the uptake of tritiated thymidine from the culture fluid as a measure.

Bain and Lowenstein (210) then published a second paper in the same year in which they confirmed their previous data and in which they reported on the reactivity of 15 non-identical sibling pairs against each other and against unrelated individuals: most of the siblings reacted less strongly against their sibling, and the authors concluded that:

(1) Fraternal twins and siblings did not differ in their behavior in MLC.
(2) The results were "compatible with the laws of inheritance".
(3) The MLC test (also described by them as the mixed leukocyte reaction, MLR) "may be particularly useful as an indicator of compatibility between siblings".

Lowenstein's group soon returned to conventional hematology and he died within a few years; as a result his and Bain's very significant contributions in the mid-1960s tend to be overlooked. However, Bach and his colleagues went on to use the MLR to great effect in the identification of the so-called lymphocyte-defined histocompatibility antigens – the antigens that were undetectable by conventional serologic assays. This development in the understanding of histocompatibility antigens is considered in Chapter 4.

An important consequence of the early work on the MLR was the discovery in 1970 that lymphocytes generated in mixed cultures were cytotoxic to cells of the stimulator. This was shown by both Häyry and Defendi (211) and Hodes and Svedmyr (212) in mice, and by Solliday and Bach (213) with human cells. The wheel had thus come full circle and *in vitro* alloreactivity became fully identified with *in vivo* graft rejection. The MLR was now seen as representing activation of the immune response and the CML as the cellular effector arm.

Other lines of evidence linking allograft reactivity with delayed type hypersensitivity

At the beginning of the 1950s W.J. Dempster, B. Lennox and J.W. Boag made the important observation that the response to skin allografts (214), like the tuberculin reaction (215) – that archetypal manifestation of hypersensitivity – could be partially inhibited by a sublethal dose of whole-body X-irradiation. Others long before them had, however, observed that X-irradiation suppressed antibody production against bacteria (216–219). As lymphocytes were well known to be especially vulnerable to irradiation this further strengthened the belief that the allograft response had an immunologic basis, as well as the role of lymphocytes as likely effector cells.

Dempster was a perceptive transplant surgeon working at the Hammersmith Hospital, London, who made some valuable contributions in the early 1950s to our understanding of kidney allograft rejection in dogs and in patients and who wrote several early reviews on the allograft reaction. His work is discussed further in Chapters 7 and 8.

Another pioneering paper on the suppression of reactivity to skin allografts came from Billingham, Krohn and Medawar (220) when they demonstrated in 1951 that daily administration of cortisone to rabbits lengthened the life of the grafts three or four-fold, though it had little effect in presensitized rabbits. They attributed the finding to a systemic effect on the immune system and quoted, as the only precedent, Whitelaw's (221) observation that adrenocorticotropic hormone (ACTH) prolonged the survival of skin allografts in a patient. Their findings further underpinned the immunologic nature of the allograft response and marked the beginning of the quest to curb the response by hormones and drugs.

A novel approach linking alloreactivity to DTH was that of H.S. Lawrence and his colleagues (222) who used a protocol based on Lawrence's earlier transfer of tuberculin hypersensitivity from hypersensitive to normal individuals (223). They brought about the accelerated rejection of human skin allografts by local or systemic administration of blood leukocyte extracts from individuals who had been specifically sensitized to the graft donors. Serum from sensitized and cell extracts from normal individuals had no such effect, and the authors stated that "This finding fulfills a critical criterion relating delayed hypersensitivity (DTH) of the tuberculin type to homograft sensitivity". The basis of this transfer has never been adequately explained and although it has been extended to other antigenic systems (see Chapter 1), subsequent attempts to confirm the human allograft data in experimental animals have on the whole been unsuccessful.

The effectors of allograft rejection

The 1970s were marked by an explosion of research in basic immunology and this was also true for transplantation immunology. The explosion has continued unabated and our understanding of immunologic processes has been vastly increased. However, whereas transplantation immunology had, in the previous three decades, led the way in several areas it was now largely carried along by major advances in basic immunology. I have already referred to the pioneering studies (196–199) that led to the realization that MHC antigens play a vital part in the recognition by, and mode of action of, T lymphocytes. The phenomenon of MHC restriction for viral antigens was subsequently shown to apply likewise to the allograft response against minor histocompatibility antigens (see Chapter 4). Much interest centered on the receptors of B and T cells that enable them to recognize antigens, and with the help of highly specific monoclonal antibodies the structure of these receptors was worked out in detail in the 1980s, providing the key to the vexing question of how specific recognition of antigens comes about and why MHC recognition is an integral part of it. These developments also provided forceful evidence in favor of the clonal selection hypothesis and laid the foundations for the concept of antigen presentation. The elucidation of the structure of MHC antigens and their ability to bind foreign (and self) peptides came as a quantum leap forward. Many of the pieces of The Great

Immunologic Puzzle thus came together and the foundations for immunology in the twenty-first century were firmly laid. Although many of these developments were initiated outside the field of transplantation, it was nonetheless powerfully affected and frequently provided basic immunologists with assays and experimental strategies. It is hardly possible in this historic account to do justice to all this, but some of the exciting developments in basic immunology have already been discussed in Chapter 1.

It became possible to pinpoint the effectors of allograft rejection once cell surface markers had been described for T lymphocytes and their subpopulations. Initially this had to be done with relatively crude antisera directed against these markers, but as soon as monoclonal antibodies with their exquisite specificity for single antigenic determinants became available it was possible to dissect the role of cells with great precision. The mouse led the way in the characterization of lymphoid cell surface antigens and this field, before the advent of monoclonal antibodies, was exhaustively reviewed in 1979 by McKenzie and Potter (224).

The first antigen that allowed the analysis of effector cells to proceed was the theta (later called Thy-1) antigen described by Reif and Allen in 1964 – an antigen restricted to thymocytes (225) and thymus-derived leukemic lymphocytes (226). It was M. C. Raff (227), using antisera with a fluorescent label, who realized that Thy-1 was only present on lymphocytes that were immunoglobulin-negative and who therefore proposed that Thy-1 was a defining marker for T cells, while cell surface immunoglobulin was characteristic of B cells. Monoclonal antibodies subsequently allowed more precise cellular characterization and led to the identification of T lymphocyte subpopulations, notably the helper (h) and cytotoxic/suppressor (c/s) subsets and the Th1 and Th2 subpopulations, the former characterized phenotypically (CD4, CD8) as well as functionally, and the latter by a characteristic pattern of cytokine production (228).

Because the analogy between *in vitro* cytotoxicity and *in vivo* allograft rejection seemed to be so convincing it was taken for granted by many that the Tc was the main effector cell. This rather lazy assumption was challenged in 1981 by the Australians Loveland et al. (229) when they showed that the cells best able to restore reactivity to thymectomized, irradiated and syngeneic bone-marrow-reconstituted mice – the so-called B mice – belonged to the Th rather than the Tc subpopulation. Nonetheless, their conclusion that ". . . cytotoxic T cells are not responsible for skin graft rejection" was somewhat premature, as D. Steinmuller (230) pointed out in his excellent 1985 overview, because of a technical deficiency in one of the monoclonal antibodies they used. They rectified this in subsequent experiments reported a year later (231) and by further showing that DTH responses to alloantigens were likewise mediated in B mice by Th cells (232).

Soon after, the Oxford group of Dallman et al. (233) reported similar results in the rat using non-overlapping monoclonal antibodies against rat Th and Tc, but they also found substantial Tc infiltrates in skin allografts undergoing rejection. Subsequent investigations on this issue have been well summarized by Steinmuller (230), Mason and Morris (234), Hall and Dorsch (235) and, more recently, Shelton et al. (236): evidence has clearly accumulated in favor of *both* Th and Tc. For example, a series of papers by Lowry et al. (237–239) involving the adoptive transfer of sensitivity with selected subpopulations suggested that both Th and Tc were effective in causing rejection of hearts and kidneys, though Th were more efficient on a numerical basis. Their observations that Tc played a leading role when the vascularized heart targets possessed class I antigens only (240) indicated that the nature of the target antigens was one of the important factors. Heidecke *et al.* (212) likewise found evidence in support of both subpopulations. Although sensitized Tc were less effective on their own, even when interleukin-2 (IL-2) was added, Th acted most powerfully in the presence of Tc and exogenous IL-2. This result was confirmed by Palladino *et al.* (242).

Snider and Steinmuller (243) added to the controversy by showing that cytotoxic T lymphocytes (CTL) extracted from allografts and their draining lymph nodes lysed donor target cells *in vitro* and brought about tissue damage when injected intradermally. In this case the target antigen was a non-MHC antigen (Epa-1) expressed on mouse epidermal cells, but poorly represented on lymphocytes (244).

The prolongation of rat cardiac allografts with an anti-Th antibody (245) seemed to lend further support to the notion that the Th was mainly responsible for allograft rejection. However, the work of Sprent *et al.* (246, 247) made it clear that the nature of the target MHC antigens was critically important in skin grafts, with Th cells reacting to class II but not class I targets whereas the reverse was found to be true for Tc. Similarly, Rosenberg *et al.* (248), using athymic "nude" mice, found that Tc reconstituted such mice for reactivity against a class I disparity on skin allografts whereas Th cells were "neither necessary nor sufficient", but proved to be highly effective against grafts bearing class II histocompatibility antigens (249). These workers were able to demonstrate *in vivo* collaboration between these two kinds of cells and they concluded that "the ability to reject skin allografts is neither unique to a specialized subset of T cells ... nor unique to a specialized subset of helper-independent effector T cells with so-called dual function capability. Rather, skin allograft rejection can be mediated by *in vivo* collaborations between T-inducer cells and T-effector cells. .. " Thus some sort of resolution of seemingly conflicting evidence seems to have come about and this was supported by the study of Cobbold and Waldmann (250), when they showed in the same year that although Th cells were sufficient to reject skin grafts in Tc-depleted mice, Tc could nonetheless become involved in graft rejection in intact mice; this was presumed to have come about by cooperation with Th cells.

A more recent paper from the Washington University School of Medicine (236) underlines the potential dual nature of the cellular response. Using mice suffering from the severe combined immunodeficiency syndrome (scid) and therefore lacking all forms of immunologic response, they were able to induce skin allograft reactivity by the adoptive transfer of either Th (CD4-positive) or Tc (CD8-positive) lymphocytes, which functioned without detectable numbers of cells of the other subset. These authors raised the possibility that CD8-positive cells were functional in their experimental system because of the presence of IL-2-secreting CD8-positive cells.

Before leaving the topic of effector cells it is appropriate to mention the earlier contributions of P. Häyry and his colleagues in Finland. Together with P.J. Roberts (251) he developed an ingenious cellulose sponge matrix filled with fibroblasts of one inbred mouse strain which was then implanted in small pieces into the body cavity of allogeneic mice. On recovery of the sponges 6–8 days later the infiltrating host cells were expressed by compression, with a 90% recovery. They were therefore able to identify the host cells, which comprised blast cells, lymphocytes, monocytes/ macrophages and granulocytes. These cells, unseparated, gave specific cytolytic responses against the relevant allogeneic targets that were greater than those of the host spleens or draining lymph nodes. The activity of these cells was directly correlated with the presence of idiotypic receptors on their membranes (252). It was Häyry's group (253–254) in Finland that uncovered evidence in favor of peripheral sensitization of lymphocytes within kidney allografts undergoing rejection. This became possible when fine needle apiration cytology had been developed (255) for the diagnosis of acute renal rejection episodes in patients.

The role of cytokines and their receptors in transplantation has recently been reviewed by Dallman and Clark (256).

Other cells such as natural killer (NK) cells and macrophages probably play some role in graft rejection. However, the most important effectors identified within three decades of the first demonstration that lymphoid cells were intimately involved in the adoptive transfer of sensitivity were T lymphocytes of both Th and Tc sub-populations. This became possible by the advent of monoclonal antibodies and the use of both traditional assays such as adoptive transfer, reconstitution of irradiated animals and graft prolongation with antibodies directed against one or other sub-population, as well as by analysis of allograft rejection in nude or scid mice.

The chemical nature of alloantigens

The discovery of the genetic basis of the histocompatibility antigens, and therefore of alloreactivity, has already been alluded to (p. 68) and will be described in greater detail in Chapter 4. Each species possesses an MHC that codes for a large number of antigens, both class I (recognized by Tc) and class II (recognized by Th) antigens, and these antigens have very different functions. Each MHC is made up of a large number of highly polymorphic loci, and the total number of antigens is very large. In addition each species has a number of other genetic loci independent of the MHC that code for the so-called minor antigens – antigens that compared with the MHC antigens are relatively weak, though they can incite strong alloreactivity if several are present in the graft donor but absent in the recipient.

The distribution of class I and II antigens is quite different, class I being found on most tissue cells (in the mouse, but not man, including the red blood cells) whereas class II antigens are restricted to certain cell types such as antigen-presenting cells, B lymphocytes and activated T cells. Both class I and II antigens can, however, be upregulated or newly expressed during the course of allograft rejection.

The antigens playing a role in rejection used to be called, for obvious reasons, "transplantation antigens", even though transplantation biologists had always suspected that their primary functions had to be concerned with basic physiologic processes because their evolution could hardly have been driven by the need to develop graft rejection mechanisms. The data of Zinkernagel and Doherty (196) and many others following them provided an insight into their true function – the provision of class I signals that enable antiviral Tc to be cytotoxic for virus-infected cells. It was later shown that class II antigens gave important signals leading to the activation of Th. This led to the formulation of "MHC restriction" for both viral and minor antigens, and led to the abandonment of the term transplantation antigens in the mid-1970s in favor of histocompatibility antigens. This term had been coined by Snell much earlier in relation to the histocompatibility genes controlling their phenotypic expression (see above).

Until the mid-1950s it had been widely believed that only living cells could incite alloreactivity – a belief that had been based on the fact that allogeneic cells killed *in vitro* by a variety of methods lost their ability to sensitize animals. However, a paper published in *Nature* in 1956 by Billingham, Brent and Medawar (257) exploded this notion by showing that "the powers of cells to elicit transplantation immunity depends neither upon their being alive nor upon their structural integrity in any anatomical sense". These workers showed that mouse spleen cells totally disintegrated by ultrasonic irradiation retained their power to bring about the accelerated rejection of skin allografts when inoculated into the recipients 3–5 days before skin grafting, and that this power was abolished by precisely those methods that had previously been used to make the case for the involvement of living cells. The antigens were found to be insoluble in salt solutions but soluble in water, from which they could be precipitated with calcium chloride; and they could be extracted from nuclei by treatment with 2M sodium chloride. Because neither ribonuclease nor trypsin had a deleterious effect on the sensitizing powers of nuclear preparations, whereas they were destroyed by desoxyribonuclease, Billingham, Brent and Medawar concluded that it was "probable that the antigens responsible . . . are desoxyribonucleoproteins". This conclusion was, however, disowned by the same group (258, 259) two years later, as well as by others (260, 261), when it was shown that DNA and DNA-protein was not a necessary ingredient, and that on the contrary the determinants of the transplantation antigens seemed to be related to the human blood group substances (i.e. mucopolysaccharides). This agreed with the work of Kandutsch and Reinert-Wenck (262–263), who had made the same suggestion for extracted antigens with the capacity of enhancing (i.e. prolonging) the survival of allogeneic tumors.

In 1961 Brent, Medawar and Ruskiewicz (264, see also 265) demonstrated that cell-free alloantigens extracted by treating cells with water and ultrasound elicited the formation of alloantibodies. When used in semisoluble form these extracts inhibited the agglutination of red cells with the appropriate alloantibody raised by conventional means. Because the preparation and properties of these extracted antigens were the same as for extracts that caused the accelerated rejection of skin grafts and DTH skin reactions the authors concluded that "These results do not therefore uphold the distinction (266) between 'T-antigens' that sensitize and 'H-antigens' that provoke the formation of humoral antibodies or inhibit their action *in vivo*." Because polysaccharides with Forssman affinities had "some discernible effect" in inhibiting red cell agglutination with specific alloantisera they saw this as further evidence for the complicity of carbohydrate moieties in the antigenicity of extracted histocompatibility antigens.

It was soon shown that active antigenic extracts could be prepared not only from lymphoid tissues but also from non-lymphoid tissues such as epidermal cells (267). Medawar then demonstrated that crude semisoluble extracts could be used to induce tolerance in mice compatible for H-2 MHC but incompatible at minor loci, provided they were administered intravenously (268). In the same year (1963) Martinez *et al.* (269) found that skin graft survival could be prolonged even across the H-2 barrier, though large doses of extracts had to be used and the effects were highly erratic.

These extracts therefore had potent biologic actions, the physical form and route of injection dictating whether they induced sensitization (265). The use of extracted antigens in inducing cutaneous hypersensitivity reactions in guinea pigs has already been described (see p. 79).

Professional biochemists now took over from the amateurs, providing new methods of extraction and more precise characterization of the extracted antigens. Early in the field were Davies and his colleagues in Porton, England, who used as their starting point mouse ascites tumor cells or fluid (270–272) or tumor cell ghosts (273). They concluded that the antigens were lipoproteins and were a structural part of the cell membrane, as had also been suggested by Manson, Foschi and Palm (274). However, this hypothesis was discarded when the glycoprotein suggestion of the early workers was upheld. The group of Mann, Corson and Dammin (275), working in Boston, likewise provided early confirmation of the data of Medawar's group: having demonstrated that the antigens were unaffected by 2M sodium chloride, they used this salt concentration in the extraction process (276). They also extracted antigens with the aid of sucrose (277) and were able to freeze-dry the extracts without any significant loss of biologic activity, and they established a quantitative method for the evaluation of in vivo sensitization using extracts obtained with sucrose and ethylenediaminetetraacetic acid (EDTA) (278). A veritable flood of papers describing different methods of extracting soluble antigens, including organic solvents such as butanol, detergents, proteolytic digestion, cobra snake venom and ultrasound, was a marked feature in the 1960s. Apart from those already mentioned, principal workers included R.A. Reisfeld, B.D. Kahan, A.R. Sanderson and S.G. Nathenson and their numerous associates.

This early mouse work with relatively crude preparations led to subsequent studies elucidating the structure of the murine histocompatibility antigens, their molecular weight, and the basis of their specificity. These issues will be covered in Chapter 4. They facilitated the successful extraction and characterization of the human HLA antigens (see below), culminating in the extraordinary insight into their structure and function when it became possible in 1987 to elucidate their three-dimensional structure using crystallographic techniques (279; see also Chapters 1 and 4). Experimental animals, especially the mouse, led the way but, in the end, it proved to be an HLA antigen that was used for crystallography. Two American workers, Kahan and Reisfeld (280), published a detailed review of the very diverse studies carried out up to 1969.

Probably the earliest attempt to apply some of the lessons learned from experimental animals to humans was made by Rapaport et al. (281). They disrupted human blood leukocytes by repeated freezing and thawing and then isolated subcellular components by differential centrifugation. Some of these sensitized human volunteers, causing skin allografts from the leukocyte donors to be rejected in an accelerated fashion, but they were particulate rather than soluble. Others reported their preliminary results on soluble preparations in 1967 at the Third Conference on Histocompatibility Testing. For example, Batchelor and Sanderson (282) solubilized human spleen cells by water extraction followed by autolysis and used extracts to inhibit the cytotoxicity of specific antisera and complement. Metzgar, Flanagan and Mendes (283) extracted soluble antigen from cultured human or chimpanzee lymph node cells with the aid of sodium deoxycholate and dialysis and found that it inhibited both leukocyte agglutination and a rather complex assay known as the mixed agglutination reaction. Bruning et al. (284) isolated soluble preparations from human placental tissue that were lyophilized and used in the dry state to absorb antibodies from group-specific sera.

As for the mouse antigens, these early studies with far from pure HLA extracts paved the way for the more sophisticated techniques used by subsequent workers. By 1968 Sanderson and Batchelor (285) had produced partially purified HLA antigens with papain and ion exchange chromatography, and Kahan et al. (286) had successfully applied gel filtration on Sephadex G-200 and discontinuous electrophoresis on polyacrylamide. Davies et al. (287), using highly purified HLA antigens, showed in the same year that "the isolated HLA and mouse H-2 antigens are molecules with closely similar over-all composition" and that HLA and H-2 were genetic homologes, both HLA and H-2 being glycoproteins with an approximate molecular weight of 50 000 (288). A similar conclusion had already been arrived at by Mann, Rogentine and Fahey (289), and it was backed up by the finding that antibodies against H-2 and HLA could cross-react (290). Of considerable interest was the finding by Mann et al. (291), based on a comparison of the amino acid composition of extracts prepared from two cell sources with different HLA specificities, that there was "a general similarity in amino acid content"; the authors concluded that "the HLA-alloantigen-carrying molecules have a similar fundamental structure". Later it was shown that there were indeed structural similarities between HLA and H-2 and between the histocompatibility molecules and the immunoglobulins, suggesting a common evolutionary pathway for the supergene family (see Chapter 4).

The driving force behind the avalanche of papers in the 1960s and 1970s describing extraction procedures for the histocompatibility antigens and their purification and characterization was three-fold.

(1) It was hoped that it would lead to an understanding of their structure and, hence, their precise function and mode of action.
(2) It was assumed that soluble antigens would provide a tool for studying the function of the effector cells involved in graft rejection.
(3) Bearing in mind that it proved to be relatively easy to induce specific tolerance in adult animals to soluble protein antigens (292, 293), there was the hope that solubilized histocompatibility antigens would facilitate the induction of transplantation tolerance – not only in animals, but also clinically.

The first two aspirations were undoubtedly realized; the third was largely fulfilled experimentally but unfortunately not clinically.

Immunogenicity, the concept of the passenger leukocyte, and antigen presentation

The problem of "antigenic strength"
The question of what constitutes "antigenic strength" has been debated for well over two decades; there is still no simple answer to it though knowledge of the structure of MHC antigens has provided more plausible hypotheses. The question arose when it was realized in the 1960s that different tissues and organs incite allograft reactions of variable ferocity and that the MHC generally speaking codes for strong antigens,

while loci for the minor antigens tend to incite much weaker responses. (For the history of the MHC and the minor loci see Chapter 4.) The question was discussed at some length by both Hildemann (294) and Simonsen (295) in 1970.

One very puzzling issue arose from the finding that MHC-induced allograft responses engage an unexpectedly high proportion of the lymphocyte pool, which seemed to be inconsistent with the clonal selection hypothesis. Using chromosomal markers in a graft-versus-host assay (splenomegaly), Nisbet, Simonsen and Zaleski (296) estimated a minimum of 1–2%, a comparable figure to that of Wilson, Blythe and Nowell (297), based on quantitative studies of MLCs. From considerations concerning the "factor of immunization" Simonsen (285) went so far as to suggest that MHC responses might engage as many as 50% of the lymphocyte pool. (The factor of sensitization was a term introduced by Simonsen (298) to describe the finding that in a GVHD assay the presensitization of MHC-incompatible donor cells leads to a very small increment of lymphocyte activity compared with normal cells, whereas presensitization of donor cells differing from the hosts only for minor antigens usually results in a marked increase.) Even if the number of allo-reactive cells against any one combination of MHC antigens is "only" of the order of 1–12%, as later workers showed (299–301), it is nonetheless an astonishingly high figure compared with that for conventional antigens. It should be said that Skinner and Marbrook's estimation of the frequency of precursor cytotoxic cells specific for an allogeneic mastocytoma using the limiting dilution technique was much lower (302), though other workers came up with figures varying from 1 to 10%, depending on the source of the cells. Much seemed to depend on the purity of the cell populations.

So what were the notions concerning antigenic strength that were floated in 1970? They were clearly limited by the fact that the structure of MHC antigens had not yet been elucidated and knowledge of the organization of MHC complexes was incomplete. H-2 restriction had not been thought of and there was still some doubt, certainly in Simonsen's mind, as to whether lymphocytes were pluri- or unipotential – that is, capable of responding to only one or to more than one antigen. Hildemann (294) concluded that: "Many antigenic specificities determined by alleles of complex H-loci such as HL-A in man may commonly be intermediate or even weak in strength. However, given the multiplicity of antigens associated with each allele, additive immunogenicity may frequently occur." In other words, he believed that the MHC antigens were strong because of their complexity and the fact that any one haplo-type involved a number of distinct antigens. Such a view had been advocated earlier by J. Klein (303). So far as the minor loci are concerned, he suggested that "the interallelic combinations of many H-loci, singly or additively, will turn out to have the most influence on allograft survival times".

"Dr. Hildemann has just been moving from facts to beliefs. I shall go the opposite way", wrote Simonsen (294). He believed that "the strength of the transplantation antigens is essentially a direct function of the number of immunologically competent (antigen sensitive) cells which can recognize the antigen as foreign and react against it", a concept that he felt to be equally valid for graft-versus-host and host-versus-graft reactions. The strength of this hypothesis lay, in his view, in its consistency with the clonal selection hypothesis: "it may even be seen to represent Clonal Selection itself, if the latter sets out to explain the fact that antigens differ in strength" (surely something of a tautology!). Thus, the larger the clone of potentially reactive cells, the stronger the response.

Another possibility considered by Simonsen was that antigenic strength depended on the density of antigenic molecules on the target cell, thus perhaps explaining why different organs and tissues tend to be rejected at widely varying speeds. That this could not represent the whole truth was suggested to him by the fact that it was possible to convert the graft-versus-host reaction of weak antigens into a strong one by presensitization of the donor, an increase in the size of the cell clone being a more likely explanation. This notion was resurrected and developed 14 years later by Bevan (*304*), who proposed that "the alloreactive determinant is a sequence or conformational determinant contributed entirely by the foreign MHC molecule in isolation, which is expressed at high density on the antigen-presenting cell". He did not mention the earlier speculations and wrote his article before the relationship between MHC molecules and peptides had been fully elucidated, but well after MHC restriction had been established as a basic phenomenon of T cell function (see above). His modern high determinant density theory was based on the realization that T lymphocytes do not recognize foreign antigens in isolation, but recognize and respond to them only when they are associated with MHC antigens on antigen-presenting cells, and on "the widely held view ... that alloreactive T cells and the T cells that respond to self-MHC plus foreign antigen (self plus X) are one and the same pool of cells and ... that the same T-cell receptor is used in both responses". Bevan argued that the complex between self-MHC and antigen X was by no means stable, probably depending on a transient low-affinity interaction between two molecules on the same cell membrane, suggesting that the density of the determinant on antigen-presenting cells that is recognized is considerably lower than the density of the MHC molecules themselves. This led him to speculate that if the determinant recognized is on the MHC molecule itself it would be available on antigen-presenting cells at a far higher density, enabling even T cells with low-affinity receptors to respond to the foreign MHC. It should be added that a self plus X hypothesis was originally propounded by Lawrence in his excellent 1959 review of "homograft sensitivity" (*305*), in which he drew on ideas discussed by Thomas (*306*) and by Burnet and Fenner (*150*) in their influential monograph on *The Production of Antibodies*.

A second major hypothesis to account for the fact that alloantigens stimulate a disproportionate percentage of T lymphocytes was enunciated by Matzinger and Bevan (*307*) in the late 1970s. In essence they suggested that lymphocytes responding to MHC antigens on other cells recognize not only the MHC as foreign, but also "a multitude of other surface components" that interact with them. According to this hypothesis, and unlike Bevan's later attempt to explain alloreactivity, foreign MHC molecules are "seen" by T lymphocytes not in isolation, but as "interaction antigens" involving a multitude of other cell surface components. The number of such complex antigens would be large and sufficient to account for the disproportionately large number of cells activated by them. This idea was strongly influenced by the discovery of MHC restriction (i.e. that cytotoxic T lymphocytes specific for non-MHC molecules must recognize not only the non-MHC component but also the MHC molecule with which it is associated). It anticipated the discovery of peptide-binding by MHC molecules by many years and modern variants of the Matzinger–Bevan hypothesis have recently been proposed.

Some vital observations based on studies with influenza nucleoprotein (NP) were made by Townsend *et al.* (*308, 309*) when they showed that short synthetic peptides corresponding to antigenic sites of NP could make uninfected target cells susceptible to lysis by NP-specific class I-restricted cytolytic T cells. This suggested that class I-restricted T cell recognition was dependent on processed antigen. Maryanski *et al.* (*310*) demonstrated that this phenomenon applied equally to antigens that are an integral part of the cell membrane, such as MHC molecules: thus, HLA-negative mouse cells were lysed by syngeneic anti-HLA cytotoxic T cells in the presence of a synthetic HLA peptide. Further direct support for the concept that peptide binding by the cleft found on MHC molecules (*279*) plays an integral part in alloantigen presentation and recognition has been provided by Marrack and Kappler (*311*), who showed that molecules specific for B lymphocytes combine with I–E (a murine class II gene product) to form the allogeneic ligand for mouse B-β17a receptors.

Finally, Strominger's group (*312*) has further strengthened support for the modern version of the Matzinger–Bevan hypothesis based on their work with HLA. They found that recognition of HLA class I antigens by a self-restricted CD8-positive T cell receptor came about through the accommodation by the receptor of a few amino acid differences in the MHC molecule, suggesting cross-recognition. These authors concluded that alloreactivity is the result of the presence in the foreign antigen-binding site (i.e. the cleft) of the allogeneic MHC molecule of unusual self-peptides, and that reactivity against these had not been eliminated by negative selection in the thymus. The fact that each MHC molecule can evidently present a variety of peptides would explain why allogeneic differences stimulate more than the expected number of T lymphocytes.

Lechler *et al.* (*313*) have recently reviewed the molecular basis of alloreactivity and have come out in support of the Matzinger–Bevan model, this time on the strength of experiments carried out with HLA class II molecules and CD4-positive lymphocytes. According to them, the binary complexes (interaction antigens) envisaged by Matzinger and Bevan "would consist of an array of different peptides, derived by the internalization and processing of endogenous proteins, in the antigen-binding groove of the allogeneic MHC molecule. Each of these peptide–MHC complexes could then stimulate a separate population of T cells, and hence account for the high precursor frequency of alloreactive cells." It is of considerable interest in this context that it has very recently become possible to identify the octamer peptide responsible for the H-2-restricted rejection of male skin grafts transplanted to female mice (*314*) (see also Chapter 4), which is controlled by a gene coding for the minor antigen H–Y. Thanks to the molecular biology revolution we have come a very long way since the early speculations on alloreactivity – a problem that is so central to transplantation immunology – a quarter of a century ago!

The concept of passenger leukocytes

In 1957 G.D. Snell published a review (*315*) in which the notion of passenger leukocytes was first floated. Snell had been struck by an observation made by Stoerk (*316*) a few years earlier that some organs and tissues taken from cortisone-treated rats and transplanted to allogeneic recipients were far less immunogenic than organs taken from normal donors. Snell felt that the data implied that cortisone had reduced the number of leukocytes in the donor's organs and that donor leukocytes therefore played an important role in the sensitization process. Although direct supporting evidence for this hunch did not become available for many years it has proved to be entirely valid.

It is Steinmuller (317) who is usually credited with providing the first evidence ten years later, though he seems to have been unaware of Snell's speculations and the term "passenger leukocyte" was not coined until a year later by some other American workers, Elkins and Guttmann (318). Steinmuller induced tolerance to allogeneic donors in neonatal mice by the time-honored method of inoculating hybrid spleen and bone marrow cells (see Chapter 5) and then transplanted skin from the tolerant animals to syngeneic recipients. Such isografts, as they were called at that time, would normally have been expected to survive indefinitely, and so they did; however, they sensitized the recipients to skin allografts from the cell donor strain. Steinmuller concluded that allogeneic leukocytes from the tolerance-inducing inoculum had made their way into the skin of the tolerant mice in sufficient numbers to incite an allograft response in the syngeneic recipients. Although the concept of cellular chimerism in tolerant animals was by no means new, Billingham *et al.* having demonstrated a decade earlier that chimeric cells could sensitize secondary recipients (319) (see also Chapter 5), this was the first time that it had been demonstrated with skin, which was considered to contain very few migrating cells. Having considered several possible interpretations of his findings Steinmuller concluded: "If the leukocyte containment hypothesis is correct, it raises the question of the extent to which the immunizing ability of skin graft in general is dependent on contained leukocytes".

In 1968 Elkins and Guttmann (318) reported an ingenious experiment involving a local graft-versus-host reaction. They transplanted rat kidneys into F1 hybrid recipients in which they would not be expected to incite an allograft response, and a day later some syngeneic spleen cells were inoculated under the capsules of the transplanted kidneys. Histologic examination eight days later revealed "invasive–destructive lesions" in the transplanted kidneys where the spleen cells had been deposited, with all the hallmarks of a local GVHR. The authors concluded that activation of the spleen cells had been brought about by immunogenic migrant cells from the hybrid hosts (passenger cells) and they postulated that interactions of this kind – this time between host lymphocytes and graft passenger cells – could be an important factor in the response against organ allografts. The site of such interactions could be either in the graft or in the regional lymph nodes, and Elkins and Guttmann suggested that "rigorous attempts to eliminate such cells might be of value in clinical practice". They further suggested that the *in vitro* mixed lymphocyte reaction (MLR) might represent a cognate phenomenon. This suggestion was supported later by Lafferty, Misco and Cooley in Australia (320), who showed that lymphocytes inactivated by ultraviolet light cannot stimulate allogeneic lymphocytes in MLR.

It is of interest that in the same year that Elkins and Guttmann published their data, a letter by Dempster (321) appeared in the *Lancet*. In this letter he pointed out, in a rather different context, that a dog kidney allograft returned to its donor after three days' residence in an allogeneic host was "apparently rejected by the same kind of cellular process which produces acute rejection" – an observation that had first been made by Simonsen (322) many years earlier. This is probably another example of a reaction against passenger cells, though Dempster did not attempt to distinguish between the possibility of "rejection by self antibodies or by plasma cells from the former recipient or the donor itself".

After publication of the papers by Steinmuller and by Elkins and Guttmann (see above) there followed a flood of papers in support of the passenger leukocyte concept, underlining the importance of these cells in the induction of allograft responses. Especially cogent were the data of Steinmuller and Hart (323), who showed with the aid of radiation chimeras that "the parenchyma of skin allografts contributes little or nothing to their immunogenicity during the first few days and that skin allograft immunity is induced by the rapid release of passenger leukocytes into the graft bed and regional lymphatics".

Billingham (324) published a careful review of the literature up to 1971, but it is impracticable for me to follow this through except to say that the concept has been validated in many experimental systems. However, one particular line of evidence should be mentioned because it has some bearing on later attempts to reduce the immunogenicity of human kidneys. Having shown that the immunogenic stimulus of kidney allografts consisted largely of drug-sensitive cells of hematopoietic derivation, Guttmann and his colleagues in Boston (325, 326) found that pretreatment of rat kidney donors with one of several immunosuppressive drugs markedly reduced the allograft rejection pattern in a number of untreated recipients. Later attempts to reduce the immunogenicity of human kidneys by perfusion with an anti-CD45 monoclonal antibody directed against passenger cells succeeded in reducing the number of rejection crises, but not in improving long-term graft survival (327), but this is an area that probably deserves further exploration.

Two other facets of research on the topic of passenger leukocytes deserve mention. The first concerns the transplantability of thyroid and pancreatic islet allografts after the elimination of passenger cells bearing Ia (class II) antigens. Following sensational claims by Summerlin and his colleagues (328–330) that the culture of mouse and human skin for 1–6 weeks led to permanent survival when the cultured skin was transplanted to allogeneic recipients – claims that his senior colleagues were subsequently unable to confirm (331) and which seem to have involved some fraudulent activity – Lafferty and his team in Canberra took up this approach by applying it to thyroid and pancreatic islet allografts. They were aware that Jacobs and Huseby (332) had already described the unhindered growth of allogeneic tumors after the tumors had been cultured for 1–4 weeks, although these workers had not formulated any clear hypotheses to account for this reduction in immunogenicity. By culturing the lobes of mouse thyroids for 12 days before transplantation under the kidney capsule of H-2 incompatible recipients, Lafferty et al. (333) found that survival times were significantly extended. Such a result fitted into the theoretic framework of alloreactivity that Lafferty, Prowse and Simeonovic (334) later formulated, namely that histocompatibility antigens are not strong antigens capable of inciting alloreactivity unless accompanied by an allogeneic stimulus emanating from metabolically active and immunocompetent cells. They were influenced in this by the two-signal model of cell activation proposed by Bretscher and Cohn (335, 336) and postulated that engagement of the T cell receptor by histocompatibility antigens (signal 1) was not sufficient for activation unless signal 2, emanating from a stimulator cell providing an inductive molecule with costimulatory powers, was also present. This theory, which was treated by some transplantation immunologists with some reserve, has been fully discussed, with supporting evidence, in their 1983 review of the passenger leukocyte concept (338). In modern language, signal 1 would be provided by peptides presented by antigen-presenting cells such as dendritic cells and Langerhans' cells, and signal 2 would come from the release of cytokines such as IL-2 from the stimulator cells. One gains the impression from reading Lafferty's papers that a certain lack of clarity may have contributed to the fact that it has taken a long time for his ideas to become accepted.

At any rate, working with a group in the United States Lafferty (337) soon followed up his thyroid work with the demonstration that long-term survival of allogeneic mouse thyroids could be achieved by previous *in vitro* culture for 20–27 days or by cobalt-60 irradiation of the donor. Rejection was initiated when the recipients received viable peritoneal exudate cells (comprising mainly macrophages) that were syngeneic with the donor strain. Thereafter Lacy and his team in St Louis (338) extended observations of this kind to islets of Langerhans: seven days of culture and a single dose of antilymphocyte serum administered to the diabetic rat recipients immediately after transplantation allowed the islets to survive for long periods in a functional state, although freshly transplanted islets were promptly destroyed. Pretreatment of donor rats with irradiation and silica, followed by transplantation of "handpicked" islets cultured for only one or two days, led to the survival of the islets in MHC-compatible rats without further immunosuppression. The same result was obtained in an MHC-incompatible combination provided that a single dose of antilymphocyte serum was administered to the recipients. These workers stressed the importance of handpicking the islets to prevent contamination with more immunogenic cells. Even xenogeneic islets (rat to mouse) could be made to survive for long periods by these means (339). The concept of passenger cells providing the principal immunogenic stimulus therefore became firmly established and it was subsequently corroborated by numerous workers.

The key to the concept was provided when it was shown that islets lack Ia (class II) antigens (340) and that islets treated with an anti-Ia serum and complement survive indefinitely in allogeneic recipients (341). This lack of Ia antigens could be made good by inoculating donor strain spleen cells into the islet-bearing recipients, thus bringing about rejection of the grafts (341). A similar finding was reported by Serie and Hegre (312), who had succeeded in bringing about the indefinite survival of allogeneic rat islets by previous culture of neonatal islets without any form of immunosuppression.

The fact that responsiveness could be restored by inoculating lymphoid cells from the donor strain would argue against the possibility that allogeneic islets induce tolerance in the recipients. This was supported by the inability of islet-bearing mice to sustain donor strain skin grafts or freshly transplanted islets (343). Yet there were suggestions that the prolonged residence of cultured islets eventually led to at least a partial "adaptation" (344) – a concept first introduced by Woodruff (345) in 1950 – or tolerance. Thus Lafferty's team (346) claimed that islets that had been in residence in their allogeneic hosts for more than 100 days became less vulnerable to rejection and that the tolerant hosts accepted uncultured islets from the same strain. More recently tolerance has likewise been induced by cultured thyroids, the recipients displaying reduced *in vivo* and *in vitro* responses to donor strain antigens (347). As islets express class I antigens, tolerance induction to those antigens is perfectly possible but it is more difficult to account for the fact that the tolerance should also extend to class II antigens.

What emerged from these studies is that class I antigens on their own, unaccompanied by class II-bearing passenger cells, are relatively non-immunogenic and possibly tolerogenic. This principle had been established earlier, when it was shown that mouse red cells, which carry only class I H-2 antigens, do not sensitize allogeneic recipients to skin grafts (265). Batchelor's group (348) failed to incite primary responses with rat blood platelets, which likewise lack class II antigens. Further support for the notion that histocompatibility antigens *per se* are poor alloantigens was provided by Batchelor *et al.* (349) when they compared antibody and cellular responses following immunization of rats with cell membranes or viable cells. They were unable to induce primary responses with membranes, which nonetheless carried MHC antigens. They concluded that primary responses depend on both the presentation of alloantigen and a second signal, which they believed to be provided by intact viable lymphocytes that were not necessarily capable of division. Such a signal was redundant for secondary responses. They therefore gave strong support to the ideas first expressed by Lafferty and his colleagues (see above).

Conclusive evidence for the passenger leukocyte hypothesis came from studies involving rat kidney allografts by Batchelor's group, at that time working in East Grinstead, Sussex. They set out to show that long-surviving, passively enhanced kidneys carrying MHC antigens are poorly immunogenic when retransplanted to hosts syngeneic with the recipient's strain – a possibility that had already been raised by the earlier work of others (350, 351). In an elegant series of experiments Batchelor, Welsh and Burgos (352) found that kidneys retransplanted after 1–3 months into normal secondary recipients induced only feeble alloresponses and survived in their new hosts for long periods, a finding they attributed to the absence of passenger leukocytes.

It has been established that the passenger cells *par excellence* in organs such as the kidney are the dendritic cells (see review by R.M. Steinman (353), who has made major contributions to this topic), and in skin grafts they are the Langerhans cells (see 354). That they are of great importance has been demonstrated by many groups, foremost among them Streilein's group (355), who found that the removal of most Langerhans cells from mouse skin by tape-stripping considerably reduced their immunogenicity, as well as by J.L. McKenzie's group (356), who showed that cardiac allografts had prolonged survival if the dendritic cell population had been reduced to less than 5% following pretreatment of the donors with cyclophosphamide and X-irradiation.

The concept of passenger cells has therefore stood the test of time extremely well: such cells are clearly excellent at presenting alloantigens. Even so, very recent studies suggest that even kidney parenchymal cells (357) are capable of presenting class I antigens to alloreactive T cells, and that Langerhans cell-depleted epidermis is not totally bereft of immunogenicity (358). As Fabre (359) has pointed out, upregulation of MHC antigens is a notable feature of allograft responses, whether in cardiac allografts (360) or in skin keratinocytes (361), thus allowing a variety of other cell types to present antigens "non-professionally". This is especially true for the vascular endothelium of organ grafts.

Direct versus indirect antigen presentation

In the MLR Ia-positive glass-adherent cells provide the dominant stimulatory signals (*362*) and purified responder lymphocytes require the presence of donor dendritic cells for activation (*363*). Thus, Knight *et al.* (*364*) were able to induce host-versus-graft responses in parental strain mice by inoculating small numbers of F_1 hybrid dendritic cells into the footpads. Attention was therefore focused in the 1980s on the efficacy of donor antigen-presenting cells in the activation of alloresponsiveness.

Lechler and Batchelor (*365*), working at the Royal Postgraduate Medical School, London, investigated this question with some decisive *in vivo* studies. Having secured the long-term survival of rat kidney allografts by conventional enhancement procedures they showed that the survival of the kidneys when retransplanted into syngeneic recipients could be severely prejudiced by inoculating very small numbers of donor dendritic cells (DC), but not donor strain blood or much larger numbers of T or B lymphocytes. These workers concluded that "intrarenal DC provide the major immunogenic stimulus of a kidney allograft" and that "the antigenic strength of MHC-incompatible tissue correlates with the content of donor strain dendritic cells". Because in some strain combinations passenger cell-depleted kidneys are rejected rapidly (*344*) Lechler and Batchelor proposed two distinct routes of allo-sensitization: the *direct* route via donor dendritic cells, which would bypass the need for further antigen processing and presentation, and the *indirect* route, according to which alloantigens are processed and presented by the graft recipient's own accessory cells. The former would be applicable only where incompatibility involves class II antigens and the latter would resemble the handling and presentation of conventional protein antigens and minor histocompatibility antigens.

Initially, evidence in support of the indirect route was confined to *in vitro* studies. Thus, allogeneic cell membranes or liposomes containing class I molecules induced secondary cytotoxic T lymphocytes in the absence of donor antigen-presenting cells (*366*), and responder as well as stimulator antigen-presenting cells were able to facilitate the development of cytotoxic T cells. The responder (*367*) but not the donor (*368*) antigen-presenting cells were dependent on antigen-processing, and Lechler and Batchelor's two-route hypothesis was therefore strongly underpinned.

In vivo evidence for the indirect route was first provided by Sherwood, Brent and Rayfield (*369*), who showed that host antigen-presenting cells could present both class I and class II antigens to syngeneic lymphocytes, thus triggering skin allograft rejection. In the light of their data Sherwood *et al.* suggested that "Attempts to deplete human organ allografts of antigen-presenting cells to render them non-immunogenic could therefore be disappointing."

Fabre's group at the Institute of Child Health, London, have recently strongly advanced the claims made for the indirect route as a major form of cell activation.

(1) They succeeded in stimulating a CD4-positive cellular response by sensitizing rats with an isolated pure class I molecule (*370*).

(2) Isolated denatured chains of class I and II rat MHC antigens inoculated into allogeneic recipients produced alloantibodies and the accelerated rejection of skin allografts (*371*).

(3) Sensitization of rats with allogeneic peptides in Freund's adjuvant led to good CD4 responses (*372*).

(4) Sensitization with pure class I peptides established strong primary and secondary antibody responses, T cell proliferative responses, and accelerated skin graft rejection (373).

Very recently Fabre's group took matters one further step forward by demonstrating that immunization of rats with class I synthetic allogeneic peptides led to the rapid destruction of kidney allografts that had first been depleted of donor interstitial dendritic cells (374).

Both direct and indirect antigen presentations have therefore been shown to play an important role in the induction of alloresponses. As Sayegh, Watschinger and Carpenter (375) have pointed out in their recent review, the two pathways need not be mutually exclusive if it is true that they are mediated by different sets of T cells. In this article they also refer to "the original hypothesis" for the high frequency of alloreactive T cells by Jerne (376) and Von Boehmer, Haas and Jerne (377), which was based on the assumption that the T cell receptor undergoes somatic mutation – an assumption that was later shown to be unwarranted.

Immunologically privileged sites

This topic has been extensively reviewed by Barker and Billingham (378). Brent (379), in a more recent review, wondered who had first coined this term. "Many authors imply that it was Medawar in his 1948 paper (380) . . . Indeed, the term has a distinct Medawarian ring to it. Nonetheless . . . to my knowledge, the term was first used by Billingham and Boswell (381) five years later, in a paper in which they proved beyond doubt that the cornea is every bit as immunogenic as the skin, and that the survival of corneal grafts cannot be ascribed to an absence of histocompatibility antigens."

Transplantation of the cornea to the eye

The history of corneal transplantation can be said to have begun towards the middle of the nineteenth century, when Bigger (382), an Irish surgeon, transplanted the first successful allogeneic cornea to a pet gazelle belonging to some nomadic Arabs who had taken him captive. The early history of corneal transplantation can be found in Woodruff's tome (383), published in 1960. I shall concern myself entirely with its immunology, except to point out that a highly successful human case was described in 1906 by a German surgeon, E. Zirm (384). Although it became a well-established procedure, even in 1954 B.W. Rycroft (385) failed to list rejection among the six factors influencing the fate of grafts. However, it was subseqently shown that a significant proportion of corneal grafts undergo rejection crises that are frequently reversible with topical steroids (386) and that HLA matching can be beneficial (387).

The cornea certainly possesses histocompatibility antigens capable of invoking alloresponses, as Billingham and Boswell (381) made clear in the early 1950s when they transplanted corneal allografts to the chest of rabbits. However, one factor operating in its favor is that it lacks Langerhans cells and therefore Ia (class II) antigens (388), which are the more potent in activating T cells. The most important factor accounting for the immunologic privilege of the anterior surface of the eye is, however, the fact that normally it lacks both lymphatic drainage and a vasculature, one or both of which are needed if the host response is to be triggered, as Medawar pointed out in 1948 (380) (see below). It is therefore the corneal grafts that for one reason or another become vascularized that undergo rejection crises or outright rejection (389).

The anterior chamber of the eye

Several, for example Greene (390), showed that allografts and even xenografts often survived for long periods in the anterior chamber of the eye. However, it was Medawar in 1948 (380) who fully analyzed the reasons for this apparent dispensation in rabbits, and found that although small fragments of allogeneic skin survived well, previous and specific systemic sensitization led to destruction provided that the grafts had been vascularized. They can and do, however, often survive in an avascular state and this, together with the absence of lymphatic drainage, prevents them from activating the immune system. Medawar concluded that the unvascularized corneal transplant "cannot succumb to an immune reaction even if it can initiate one".

Medawar's observations were confirmed in mice by Sonoda and Streilein (391) some three decades later; furthermore, according to these workers, the highest rate of rejection occurred in strain combinations differing at multiple minor histocompatibility loci. Of considerable interest is the observation by Streilein and his colleagues (392, 393) that allografts in the anterior chamber induce a systemic unresponsiveness, which they described as a form of immunologic deviation.

The brain

A Japanese worker, Y. Shirai (394), was the first to show that allogeneic tissues implanted into the brain survive for long periods without encountering rejection, and this was confirmed by Murphy (395) and Tansley (396). What was far from clear, however, was whether the tissues failed to provoke an immune response or whether they were protected from it in some way. This question was addressed by Medawar (380) in what proved to be yet another influential paper. He showed beyond doubt that as in the anterior chamber of the eye, tiny skin allografts transplanted to the brain are rejected in specifically presensitized rabbits. Medawar concluded that ". . . a lymphatic drainage is required to create a state of immunity but not necessary to enforce a response to it" and skin allografts transplanted to the brain "submit to but cannot elicit an immune state". Such conclusions were of special importance because most previous workers had used tumor allo- or xenografts, which are known to be able to override immunologic responses. Medawar also introduced rigorous controls, which in earlier studies had frequently been conspicuously absent.

Those following Medawar reported evidence both to support and refute his findings with a great variety of tissues and in several species (378, 379). Among those whose findings supported Medawar's conclusion one can single out the studies by Head and Griffin (397) using parathyroid allografts, and Mason, Charlton and Jones (398), who analyzed the importance of MHC and non-MHC histocompatibility antigens of neural tissues transplanted to the third ventricle and who found that a combination of these antigens produced the least favorable outome. These workers found that class I antigens were upregulated after transplantation and that the density of antigens was related to the vigor of the immune response. The fact that graft rejection in the brain comes about more slowly than one would expect in strongly presensitized animals suggests that activated lymphocytes traverse the blood–brain barrier with some degree of difficulty.

Although the normal brain lacks classic lymphatics it has nevertheless been shown that tracer substances injected into the parenchyma can pass to the deep cervical lymph nodes (399), and particles injected into the caudate nucleus are cleared by lymphatics (400). What is more, antigens inoculated intracerebrally have been found to induce antibody formation (401, 402). Although the brain may lack conventional dendritic cells it possesses several types of cells with the potential for antigen presentation (see 399). Despite these and other features, which make the brain potentially reactive, "the brain is beyond doubt a privileged site for grafts, when privilege is defined as a prolonged graft survival . . . The reason for this is still unclear" (399). In view of this, and especially when it became apparent that brain implants of dopamine-rich mesencephalic tissue from fetal rats reduced the symptoms of a 6-hydroxy-dopamine-induced parkinsonian syndrome in adult animals (403, 404), attempts were made in recent years to treat patients with severe Parkinson's disease and other movement disorders with allogeneic fetal neural grafts, with or without immunosuppression. The first trial was described by a Swedish group in 1985 (405) and others in Mexico, Sweden, China, the United States, Cuba and the United Kingdom have followed (for references, see 406, 407), some involving neural and others adrenal fetal allografts. Results have been extremely variable and the long-term value of this form of treatment remains to be proved. Thus M.S. Fiandaca, in reviewing the literature (406), writes: "The future of transplantation therapy for Parkinson's disease continues to appear promising, although the initial enthusiastic hysteria has been sobered somewhat by the recent objective analyses of the clinical results."

Other immunologically privileged sites

Two of the three sites I have briefly considered have turned out to have clinical implications, a point that the early pioneers could hardly have anticipated. Thus, corneal transplantation has become a routine method for restoring sight and transplantation into the brain at least raises the hope that it might yet become the treatment of choice for conditions such as Parkinson's disease. There are, nonetheless, several other immunologically privileged sites that seem of little clinical interest but which have thrown some light on the special conditions that confer immunologic privilege.

The testis.   This organ, which possesses a blood–testis barrier around the seminiferous tubules preventing the escape of antigenic material (408), has been known since the 1940s to sustain allografts and even xenografts for considerable periods. Greene (409) was the first to show that the rabbit Brown–Pearce carcinoma could be successfully transplanted to the testis of several laboratory species, although the success rate was lower than when using the anterior chamber of the eye. The grafts regressed quite variably, and regression was followed by resistance when the same tumor was reimplanted. The subsequent literature up to 1977 has been reviewed by Barker and Billingham (378). Billingham's group at the University of Texas (he emigrated to the United States in 1957) has analyzed allotransplantation to the testis. Thus, Head, Neaves and Billingham (410) established that privilege was not due to a lack of lymphatic drainage and although the mechanism was far from clear, they believed (411) that local immunosuppression by steroid-producing Leydig cells and by the spermatozoa themselves were possibly the critical factors. However, the privilege extended to skin or parathyroid allografts was at best partial, and it is improbable that the testis as a privileged site holds more than passing theoretic interest.

The cheek pouch of the Syrian hamster.   This is another rather puzzling site that permits both allo- and xenografts to survive and, if they are tumors, to grow. Lutz *et al.* (*412, 413*) led the way in the early 1950s, using this site to measure the growth of tumor grafts, the semitransparent membrane of the cheek pouch making it relatively easy to observe the implant by reflected light. Cancer research workers therefore hoped to exploit this site for the study of human tumors which, as H. Toolan (*414, 415*) had demonstrated, could otherwise only be grown in corti-sone-treated or X-irradiated hosts – with all the disadvantages of a highly abnormal milieu. Some further early references to such early work can be found in Woodruff's book (*383*).

Cohen (*416*) took this topic further in 1961 by comparing the fate of auto-, allo- and xenografts of normal skin, the latter having been obtained from adult rabbits. He also investigated whether systemic treatment with cortisone acetate was benefi-cial. A majority of all three kinds of grafts survived for at least six weeks in both conditioned and unconditioned hosts, but in the former the lymphocytic infiltration of grafts undergoing rejection or in long-surviving xenografts was reduced. He wrote: "One is struck by the seeming impotence of these lymphocytes and plasma cell infil-trations amid the proliferating cheek pouch implants." Evidently the nature of the immunologic privilege was different here from that in the anterior chamber.

The mechanism underlying this privilege was much studied by Billingham and his team in the 1960s. Billingham and Silvers (*417*) found from some ingenious exper-iments that although some allografts of cheek pouch skin survived for very long periods when transplanted to the chest of recipients, even well-established grafts became susceptible when the recipients were systemically sensitized. Normal skin allografts "inlaid" into a bed provided by a long-surviving pouch skin graft had prolonged survival times. They concluded that the privileged status of pouch skin as a transplant and as a site "derive from properties of the connective tissue", which "appears to impede the escape of transplantation antigens". Nonetheless, there is also a marked absence of lymphatics in the cheek pouch (*418, 419*), and the fact that ordinary skin allografts inlaid into a long-surviving pouch graft survive (*420*) can probably be explained on that basis. An additional factor that may be relevant is the finding that pouch tissue has a paucity of class II-bearing cells (*421*). Why the privilege of the hamster pouch should be of benefit to the species has never been adequately explained, but as it is a site used for food storage it could conceivably reduce the danger of allergic responses to food allergens.

The alymphatic skin flap or pedicle.   Although this is an experimental artefact it should be included because it underscores the crucial importance of lymphatic drainage in the destruction of allografts. In 1968 the ever inventive team of Barker and Billingham (*422*) devised an alymphatic flap in the guinea pig by cutting a full-thickness disc on the flank of an adult animal and raising it on a stalk consisting of a vein and artery, but lacking any discernible lymphatics. A small allograft trans-planted onto the flap, which was housed in a plastic capsule, survived far beyond the expected time; systemic sensitization of the host nonetheless led to its rapid rejection. By contrast, Tilney and Gowans (423), using a similar approach in the rat, found skin allografts were rejected, though more slowly than in a conventional site – a finding that they interpreted as having been brought about by a form of peripheral sensitization as postulated by Medawar (424).

As an amusing observation, though not wholly devoid of medical implications, was the finding that ground squirrels hibernating at a temperature of 4°C rejected skin allografts only when the animals had woken up and become active (425). The reason for this is that the grafts were not fully vascularized at low temperature. A somewhat different explanation underlies the earlier striking finding by Hildemann in 1957 (426) that allogeneic scale grafts in goldfish have survival times directly related to the ambient temperature, demonstrating conclusively for the first time that the allograft response is, like other metabolic activities, temperature-dependent. Quite clearly, although this history is largely concerned with mammals, immunologic and allograft responses are by no means the prerogative of mammals and they have evolved partly as defense mechanisms and partly as a form of communication between cells, since chordates first appeared (see 427).

Are invertebrates capable of allograft reactivity?

It has been argued that primitive immunologic mechanisms and the ability to distinguish between self and non-self are present in many invertebrate phyla and species. Interest in invertebrate immunology arose mainly in the 1970s when the groundwork had been laid for mammals and other vertebrates. Many biologists or immunobiologists like W.H. Hildemann and E.L. Cooper devoted much time and effort to the study of such mechanisms, especially those leading to what appeared to be the rejection of allo- or xenografts. It is not practicable for me to go into the detailed literature and I refer the reader to Hildemann's 1979 review (428) of what had, by then, become a much studied topic. Although recognizing a certain skepticism prevailing at that time by notable immunologists such as Burnet (429) and Marchelonis (430), he believed that evidence for immunologic competence had been uncovered in a variety of invertebrate groups, from sponges, coelenterates, sea anemones, corals, annelid worms, molluscs and echinoderms to insects. Hildemann defined immunologic competence as having three components:

(1) Selective or specific reactivity.
(2) Cytotoxic or antagonistic reactions following sensitization.
(3) Inducible memory or selectively altered reactivity on secondary contact – criteria with which most immunologists would concur.

He cited species of sea anemones in which "acute or hyperacute allogeneic incompatibility is the rule", and experiments in corals showing that syngeneic (intracolony) grafts are always compatible and xenografts or intercolony allografts are invariably incompatible. Immunologic memory (accelerated destruction of grafted tissue) persisted for at least four weeks. The mechanisms responsible for these phenomena were, admittedly, less clear, though "leukocytes" capable of destroying both xeno- and allogeneic targets were described in sipunculid worms, and earthworms were said to possess functionally heterogeneous leukocytes, able to respond to three different mitogens. Hildemann concluded that "Extensive allogeneic polymorphism of cell surface macromolecules is a characteristic shared by all animals from proto-zoans to mammals. ... The beginnings of both cell-mediated immunity and of the major immunogene complex of higher vertebrates are suggested by the finetuned, and often acute, primary allograft reactions at this lower invertebrate level of phylogeny." He went on to say that ". . . the products of H loci, including the major immunogene complex or its precursors, probably serve as essential recognition molecules in all metazoans", and to express the conviction that it was wrong to interpret immunologic competence in the narrower sense applicable to mammals (i.e. in terms of T and B lymphocytes and immunoglobulins).

Lest I be accused of having ducked the issue I will give two examples, both from Hildemann's laboratory in Los Angeles, of alloreactivity and memory in two groups of invertebrates. First, he and his colleagues (431) presented evidence for transplan-tation immunity with a specific memory component in a species of coral. Intracolony grafts (isografts) were always compatible (i.e. there was soft tissue fusion within 3–5 days and complete reconstitution "indistinguishable from normal ungrafted coral" by 24–30 days). By contrast, first set allografts – after a latent period of 2–3 weeks – underwent antagonistic reactions with progressive blanching and loss of soft tissue in the contact area by 19–25 days. Second set grafts showed accelerated and inten-sified cytotoxic reactions in 9–14 days. "Third party" grafts from a geographically distant population transplanted to colonies that had undergone rejection reactions exhibited a variety of rejection times from normal to "sensitized", thus revealing some degree of specificity and an "impressive antigenic polymorphism of H markers". No lymphocytic- or phagocytic-type cells could, however, be identified.

Second, Hildemann's group (432) found that primitive alloreactivity was detectable in "the lowest metazoan phylum", the sponges. Working with a large tropical sponge they demonstrated that intracolony grafts (the equivalent of syngeneic transplants) became firmly fused after 2–3 days and "persisted thereafter in compatible conflu-ence without exception". Allogeneic parabionts invariably failed to fuse even though they had been brought into intimate contact. After a latent period "interfacial soft tissue death developed". When a second attempt was made with tissue from the same donor colony, accelerated cytotoxicity occurred. "We now conclude," wrote Hildemann et al., "that exquisite immunorecognition of subtle differences among allogeneic markers is a characteristic of essentially all major groups of multicellular animals".

Not all immunobiologists agreed with this notion, and a decade later Klein (433) published a provocative review in which he stated his conviction that "it does not make sense trying to apply the knowledge and methodology acquired from studying vertebrate immune responses to invertebrates". He argued that as some of the most primitive chordates such as amphioxus and the tunicates lack lymphoid tissue alto-gether, sea-living organisms did not need the kind of immune system encountered in vertebrates. One argument strikes this reader as somewhat specious, namely that "most invertebrates cannot afford to lose so many cells to a function that for them is not really critical". Klein believed that the observed reactions in invertebrates "merely mimic anticipatory responses but in reality are fundamentally different from immune responses as we know them from vertebrate studies", and he made the point that – as for example in insects – accelerated secondary responses can also occur in non-anticipatory systems. He predicted that "invertebrate 'lymphocytes' will turn out to be totally unrelated to true lymphocytes" and that true lymphocytes "will turn out to be vertebrate (chordate) inventions", as would T cell receptors, MHC molecules and antibodies.

A stout defense was put up by Cooper *et al.* (*434*) when they published a review in 1992 in the *Scandinavian Journal of Immunology*. They considered the problem in the light of what was then known of cell receptors, gene rearrangements, and other vertebrate immunologic mechanisms. They recognized the danger of proposing a close evolutionary kinship between invertebrates and vertebrates in that, for example, the former do not possess variable region molecules as in vertebrate immunoglobulins and T cell receptors. They argued that, quite apart from phagocytosis, many of the other mechanisms available to invertebrates, for example cytotoxicity, allogeneic/xenogeneic recognition and inducible antimicrobial peptides, allow the assertion that primitive immunologic defense mechanisms do exist in invertebrates. According to these authors, the by now well-delineated receptor-mediated responses involving rearranged clonally distributed antigen-specific receptors and other recognition receptors "need not force upon invertebrates the organization, structure and adaptive functions of vertebrate immune systems. Thus, we can freely delve into the unique aspects of the primitive immune mechanisms of invertebrates." Although Cooper conceded that neither immunoglobulins nor T cell receptors had been identified in invertebrates, there were nevertheless "proteins related to the immunoglobulin superfamily – molecules which mediate the discrimination between self and non-self". They concluded that "The ferment of research on recognition and subsequent activation of immune responses in invertebrates may be relevant to connections between immune defence in invertebrates and vertebrates."

In the year after Klein's critique another partial rebuttal had come from Marchelonis and Schluter (*435*) in the form of an editorial in the same journal. "It would be patent nonsense to try to suggest that contemporary invertebrates were ancestral to vertebrates or that their defence mechanisms are directly ancestral to vertebrate immune mechanisms. It is not nonsensical, however, to point out that these living forms have similar problems of recognition and defence and thus the lessons learned from studying vertebrates can provide a basis for studying the solutions adopted by these animals. . . . The ability to recognize some sort of foreignness seems universal to all living forms." And they stressed that "vertebrates have retained ancient defence mechanisms of sensitized phagocytosis involving lectins such as C-reactive protein and lectin-type molecules". Marchelonis and Schluter concluded that "much can be learned about primordial defence and cellular recognition mechanisms by studying invertebrates, despite the fact that the vast majority of these lack a vertebrate-type immune response".

An honorable draw? Probably. Bill Hildemann, who died prematurely, would have relished this lively debate. He was another American scientist who, having studied for his PhD with Ray Owen at the California Institute of Technology, had spent a year in Medawar's department at University College in the late 1950s and had been much influenced by that experience, both scientifically and in other respects. Politically conservative and having served in the Korean War he found the preponderance of left-wing debate in Medawar's department (though this did not include Medawar himself) something of a shock, but to the surprise of many he later embraced the ethos of "flower power" in the 1960s.

References

1. Bennett, J.P. (1983) *J. Roy. Soc. Med.* **76**, 152.
2. Tagliacozzi, G. (1597) *De Curorum Chirurgia*, Chapter 18, 61 (translated by M.T. Gnudi & J.P. Webster). In *The Life and Times of Gaspare Tagliacozzi* (1950), p. 285, H. Reichner, N.Y.
3. Palmer, J.F. (1841) *The Complete Works of John Hunter*, vol. 3, part 3, p. 264, Haswell, Barrington & Haswell, Philadelphia.
4. Hunter, J. (1771) *Treatise on the Natural History and Diseases of the Human Teeth*, J. Johnson, London.
5. Irvine, W. (1771) Letter reproduced in the *Lancet* (1928), **1**, 359.
6. Palmer, J.F. (1841) *The Complete Works of John Hunter*. vol. 2, part 1, p. 58, Haswell, Barrington & Haswell, Philadelphia.
7. Anonymous (1950) *Bull. Hist. Med.* **24**, 482.
8. Palmer, J.F. (1841) *The Complete Works of John Hunter*, vol. 3, part 3, p. 273, Haswell, Barrington & Haswell, Philadelphia.
9. Martin, C.E. (1970) *Surg. Gynec. Obstet.* **131**, 306.
10. Forbes, T.R. (1949) *Endocrinol.* **41**, 329.
11. Turk, J.L. (1993) *J. Roy. Soc. Med.* **86**, 65.
12. Medawar, P.B. (1943) *Bull. War Med.* **4**, 1.
13. Dempster, W.J. (1951) *Brit. Med. J.* ii, 1041.
14. Woodruff, M.F.A. (1960) *The Transplantation of Tissues and Organs*, pp. 1–777, Charles C. Thomas, Springfield, Ill.
15. Hamilton, D. (1988) In *Kidney Transplantation*, ed. P.J. Morris, 3rd edn., p. 1, W.B. Saunders Co.
16. Medawar, P.B. (1957) *The Harvey Lectures*, p. 144, Academic Press, N.Y.
17. Silverstein, A.M. (1989) *A History of Immunology*, pp. 1–422, Academic Press, N.Y.
18. Bert, P. (1864) *J. Anat. Physiol.* **1**, 85.
19. Reverdin, j.L. (1870) *Bull. Soc. Chir., Paris*, 2nd ser. **10**, 511.
20. Pollock, G.D. (1871) *Trans. Clin. Soc. Lond.* **4**, 37.
21. Billingham, R.E. & Medawar, P.B. (1951) *J. Exp. Biol.* **28**, 385.
22. Miles, A. (1895) *Edinb. Hosp. Rep.* p. 647.
23. Ljunggren, C.A. (1897) *Dtsch. Zeit. Chir.* **47**, 608.
24. Cannady, J.E. (1906) *J. Amer. Med. Ass.* **46**, 1681.
25. Baldwin, H.A. (1913) *Med. Res.* **98**, 686.
26. Masson, J.C. (1918) *J. Amer. Med. Ass.* **70**, 1581.
27. Sale, L. (1913) *Arch. Entwicklmechn.* **3**, 248.
28. Lexer, E. (1911) *Arch. Klin. Chir.* **95**, 287.
29. Davis, J.S. (1910) *Johns Hopkins Hosp. Rep.* **15**, 307.
30. Lexer, E. (1911) *Arch. Klin. Chir.* **95**, 832.
31. Lexer, E. (1911) *Arch. Klin. Chir.* **95**, 849.
32. Schöne, G. (1912) *Die Heteroplastische und Homöoplastische Transplantation*, pp. 1–161, Springer–Verlag.
33. Schöne, G. (1912) *Die Heteroplastische und Homöoplastische Transplantation*, p. 27, Springer–Verlag.
34. Sauerbruch, F. & Heyde, M. (1909) *Z. Exp. Path. Ther.* **6**, 33.
35. Haaland, M. Quoted by Schöne, G. (1912) *Die Heteroplastische Homöoplastische Transplantation*, p. 255, Springer-Verlag.
36. Schöne, G. (1912) *Die Heteroplastische und Homöoplastische Transplantation*, p. 62, Springer–Verlag.
37. Schöne, G. (1912) *Die Heteroplastische und Homöoplastische Transplantation*, p. 31, Springer–Verlag.
38. v. Dungern, E. (1909) *Münchn. Med. Wschr.* 56i, 1099.
39. Schöne, G. (1916) *Beitr. Klin. Chir.* **99**, 233.
40. Schöne, G. (1916) *Beitr. Klin. Chir.* **99**, 238.
41. Schöne, G. (1916) *Beitr. Klin. Chir.* **99**, 246.
42. Schöne, G. (1916) *Beitr. Klin. Chir.* **99**, 249.
43. Schöne, G. (1916) *Beitr. Klin. Chir.* **99**, 254.

44. Schöne, G. (1916) *Beitr. Klin. Chir.* **99**, 263.
45. Brent, L. (1958) *Progr. Allergy* **5**, 271.
46. Brent, L. (1958) *Progr. Allergy* **5**, 275.
47. Carrel, A. (1902) *Lyon Méd.* **98**, 859.
48. Carrel, A. (1908) *J. Exp. Med.* **10**, 98.
49. Ullman, E. (1902) *Wien. Klin. Wschr.* **15**, 281.
50. Von Decastello A. (1902) *J. Physiol. Paln. Gén.* **7**, 47.
51. Floresco N. (1905) *Science* **22**, 473.
52. Carrel A. & C.C. Guthrie (1905) *Science* **22**, 473.
53. Carrel, A. (1914) *N.Y. Med. J.* **99**, 839.
54. Myer, M.W. (1913) *Arch. Entwickmech.* **38**, 1.
55. Unsigned (1961) *Transpl. Bull.* **27**, 85.
56. Blumenthal, H.T. (1960) *Science* **131**, 907.
57. Loeb, L. (1901) *J. Med. Res.* **6**, 28.
58. Loeb, L. (1902) *J. Med. Res.* **8**, 44.
59. Loeb, L. (1945) *The Biological Basis of Individuality*, pp. 1–711, C.C. Thomas, Baltimore.
60. Hesselberg, C. (1915) *J. Exp. Med.* **21**, 164.
61. Loeb, L. (1918–19) *J. Med. Res.* **39**, 39.
62. Loeb. L. (1926) *Amer. J. Path.* **2**, 111.
63. Tureen, L.L. (1927) *Amer. J. Path.* **3**, 501.
64. Loeb, L. & King, H.D. (1927) *Amer. J. Path.* **3**, 143.
65. Little, C.C. (1924) *J. Cancer Res.* **8**, 75.
66. Tyzzer, E.E. (1916) *J. Cancer Res.* **1**, 125.
67. Woglom, W.H. (1929) *Cancer Rev.* **4**, 129.
68. Little, C.C. (1941) In *Biology of the Laboratory Mouse*, ed. G.D. Snell, p. 279, Dover Publ. N.Y.
69. Jensen, C.O. (1903) *Centrbl. Bakteriol. Parasitenk. Infektionskr.* Abt. 1, Orig. **34**, 28 & 122.
70. Bashford, E.F. (1905) *Sci. Rep. Imp. Cancer Res. Fund* **1**, 1.
71. Russell, B.R.G. (1908) *Sci. Rep. Imp. Cancer Res. Fund* **3**, 341.
72. Woglom, W.H. (1912) *Sci. Rep. Imp. Cancer Res. Fund* **5**, 43.
73. Da Fano, C. (1910) *Sci. Rep. Imp. Cancer Res. Fund* **17**, 219.
74. Baeslack, F.W. (1914) *Zeitschr. Immunitätsforsch.* Orig. **20**, 421.
75. Ehrlich, P. (1906) *Arb. Königl. Inst. Exp. Ther. Frankf.* **1**, 77.
76. Ehrlich, P. (1906) *Arb. Königl. Inst. Exp. Ther. Frankf.* **1**, 85.
77. Apolant, H. (1913) *Zeitschr. Immunitätsforsch.* Orig. **17**, 219.
78. Uhlenhuth, Händel, & Steffenhagen (1910) *Immunitätsforsch.* Orig. **654**.
79. Bindseil (1913) *Immunitätsforsch.* Orig. **17**, 639.
80. Murphy, J.B. (1926) *Monogr. Rockef. Inst. Med. Res.* **21**, 1–168.
81. Murphy, J.B. (1914) *J. Exp. Med.* **19**, 13.
82. Murphy, J.B. (1914) *J. Exp. Med.* **19**, 520.
83. Murphy, J.B. (1915) *J. Exp. Med.* **22**, 204.
84. Murphy, J.B. (1915) *J. Exp. Med.* **22**, 210.
85. Murphy, J.B. (1915) *J. Exp. Med.* **22**, 211.
86. Murphy, J.B. & Taylor, H.D. (1918) *J. Exp. Med.* **28**, 1.
87. Taylor, H.D., Witherbee, W.D. & Murphy, J.B. (1919) *J. Exp. Med.* **29**, 53.
88. Murphy, J.B. & Sturm, E. (1919) *J. Exp. Med.* **29**, 1.
89. Murphy, J.B. & Sturm, E. (1919) *J. Exp. Med.* **29**, 25.
90. Shirai, Y. (1921) *Jap. Med. World* **1**, 14.
91. Murphy, J.B. (1923) *J. Exp. Med.* **23**, 183.
92. Tyzzer, E.E. (1909) *J. Med. Res.* **21**, 519.
93. Little, C.C. (1914) *Science* **40**, 904.
94. Little, C.C. & Tyzzer, E.E. (1915) *Science* **33**, 393.
95. Tyzzer, E.E. (1916) *J. Cancer Res.* **8**, 150.
96. Gorer, P.A. (1937) *J. Path. Bact.* **44**, 691.
97. Gorer, P.A. (1938) *J. Path. Bact.* **47**, 231.
98. Snell, G.D. (1948) *J. Genetics* **49**, 87.
99. Medawar, P.B. (1986) *Memoir of a Thinking Radish*, pp. 76, Oxford Univ. Press, Oxford.

100. Gibson, T. & Medawar, P.B. (1943) *J. Anat.* **77**, 299.
101. Medawar, P.B. (1944) *J. Anat.* **78**, 176.
102. Medawar, P.B. (1945) *J. Anat.* **79**, 157.
103. Underwood, H.L. (1914) *J. Amer. Med. Ass.* **63**, 775.
104. Holman, E. (1924) *Surg. Gynec. Obstet.* **38**, 100.
105. Gibson, T. (1986) *Brit. J. Plast. Surg.* **39**, 96.
106. Bauer, K.H. (1927) *Beitr. Klin. Chir.* **141**, 442.
107. Silverstein, A.M. (1989) *A History of Immunology*, p. 284, Academic Press, N.Y.
108. Gorer, P.A. (1942) *J. Path. Bact.* **54**, 51.
119. Gorer, P.A. (1950) *Brit. J. Cancer* **4**, 372.
110. Gorer, P.A. (1955) *Ann. N.Y. Acad. Sci.* **59**(3), 365.
111. Gorer, P.A. & Mikulska, B.M. (1954) *Cancer Res.* **14**, 651.
112. Amos, D.B., Gorer, P.A., Mikulska, Z.B. et al. (1954) *Brit. J. Exp. Path.* **35**, 203.
113. Gorer, P.A. & Gorman, P. (1956) *Transpl. Bull.* **3**, 142.
114. Hildemann, W.H. (1957) *Transpl. Bull.* **4**, 148.
115. Amos, D.B. (1953) *Brit. J. Exp. Path.* **34**, 464.
116. Hildemann, W.H. & Medawar, P.B. (1959) *Immunology* **2**, 44.
117. Medawar, P.B. (1946) *Nature* **157**, 161.
118. Medawar, P.B. (1946) *J. Exp. Path.* **27**, 15.
119. Medawar, P.B. (1961) *Biogr. Mem. Fellows Roy. Soc.* **7**, 95.
120. Medawar, P.B. (1961) *Biogr. Mem. Fellows Roy. Soc.* **7**, 104.
121. Wright A.E. & Douglas, S.R.
122. Silverstein, A.M. (1989) *A History of Immunology*, p. 46, Academic Press, N.Y.
123. Medawar, P.B. (1948) *Quart. J. Microscop. Sci.* **89**, 239.
124. Mitchison, N.A. (1953) *Nature* **171**, 267.
125. Mitchison, N.A. (1954) *Proc. Roy. Soc. B,* **143**, 58.
126. Mitchison, N.A. (1955) *J. Exp. Med.* **102**, 157.
127. Landsteiner, K. & Chase, M.W. (1942) *Proc. Soc. Exp. Biol.* **49**, 688.
128. Chase, M.W. (1945) *Proc. Soc. Exp. Biol.* **59**, 134.
129. Billingham, R.E., Brent, L. & Medawar, P.B. (1954) *Proc. Roy. Soc. B* **143**, 58.
130. Deutsch, L. (1899) *Ann. Inst. Pasteur* **13**, 689.
131. Harris, S., Harris, T.N. & Farber, M.B. (1954) *J. Immunol.* **72**, 148.
132. Harris, T.N. & Harris, S. (1960) In *Cellular Aspects of Immunity*, Ciba Found. Symp., eds G.E.W. Wolstenholme & M. O'Connor, p. 172, J. & A. Churchill, London.
133. Davies, W.E. & Cole, L.J. (1961) *J. Natl. Cancer Inst.* **27**, 1341.
134. Rich, A.R. (1951) *The Pathogenesis of Tuberculosis*, 2nd edn, p. 600, Charles C. Thomas, Springfield, Ill.
135. Billingham, R.E. & Brent, L. (1955) *Brit. J. Exp. Path.* **37**, 566.
136. Stetson, C.A. & Demopoulos, R. (1958) *Ann. N.Y. Acad. Sci.* **73**, 687.
137. Brent, L., Brown, J.B. & Medawar, P.B. (1959) In *Biological Problems of Grafting*, p. 64, Congr. Colloq. Univ. Liege, Blackwell Sci. Publ., Oxford.
138. Algire, G.H., Weaver, J.M. & Prehn, R.T. (1954) *J. Natl. Cancer Inst.* **15**, 493.
139. Weaver, J.M., Algire, G.H. & Prehn, R.T. (1955) *J. Natl. Cancer Inst.* **15**, 1737.
140. Mitchison, N.A. & Dube, O.L. (1955) *J. Exp. Med.* **102**, 179.
141. Mitchison, N.A. (1955) *Transpl. Bull.* **2**, 93.
142. Amos, D.B. & Day, E.D. (1954) *Ann. N.Y. Acad. Sci.* **64**, 851.
143. Gorer, P.A. & Boyse, E.A. (1959) In *Biological Problems of Grafting*, p. 193, Congr. Colloq. Univ. Liége, Blackwell Sci. Publ., Oxford.
144. Terasaki, P.I., Marchioro, T.L. & Starzl, T.E. (1965) In *Histocompatibility Testing*, p. 83, Nat. Acad. Sci. – Nat. Res. Council, Washington.
145. Kissmeyer-Nielsen, F., Olson, S., Petersen, V. et al. (1966) *Lancet* **2**, 662.
146. Williams, G.M., Lee, H.M., Weymouth, R.F. et al. (1967) *Surgery* **62**, 204.
147. Williams, G.M., Hume, D.M., Hudson, R.P. et al. (1968) *New Engl. J. Med.* **279**, 611.
148. Starzl, T.E., Lerner, R.A., Dixon, F.J. et al. (1968) *New Engl. J. Med.* **278**, 642.
149. Brent, L. & Porter, K.A. (1975) In *Clinical Aspects of Immunology*, 3rd edn, eds R.R.A. Coombs & P.J. Lachmann, p. 507, Blackwell Sci. Publ., Oxford.

150. Burnet, F.M. & Fenner, F. (1949) *The Production of Antibodies*, 2nd edn, Macmillan & Co. Ltd, London.
151. Burnet, F.M. & Fenner, F. (1949) *The Production of Antibodies*, 2nd edn, p. 117, Macmillan & Co. Ltd, London.
152. Berrian, J.H. & Brent, L. (1958) *Ann. N.Y. Acad. Sci.* 73, 654.
153. Brunel, F.M. & Fenner, F. (1949) *The Production of Antibodies*, 2nd edn, p. 117, Macmillan & Co. Ltd., London.
154. Favour, C.B. (1954) *Transpl. Bull.* 1, 145.
155. Brent, L., Brown, J.B. & Medawar, P.B. (1958) *Lancet* 2, 561.
156. Brent, L., Brown, J.B. & Medawar, P.B. (1962) *Proc. Roy. Soc. B* 156, 187.
157. Brent, L. & Medawar, P.B. (1963) *Brit. Med. J.* 2, 269.
158. Brent, L. & Medawar, P.B. (1964) *Nature* 204, 90.
159. Brent, L. & Medawar, P.B. (1966) *Proc. Roy. Soc. B* 165, 281.
160. Najarian, J.S. & Feldman, J.D. (1962) *J. Exp. Med.* 115, 1083.
161. Billingham, R.E., Silver, W.K. & Wilson, D.B. (1963) *J. Exp. Med.* 118, 397.
162. Prendergast, R.A. (1964) *J. Exp. Med.* 119, 377.
163. Dumonde, D.C., Wolstencroft, R.A., Panayi, G.S. *et al.* (1969) *Nature* 224, 38.
164. Simonsen, M. (1957) *Acta Path. Microbiol. Scand.* 40, 480.
165. Billingham, R.E. & Brent, L. (1957) *Transpl. Bull.* 4, 67.
166. Medawar, P.B. (1958) *Proc. Roy. Soc. B* 148, 159 & 161.
167. Billingham, R.E., Brown, J.B., Defendi, V. *et al.* (1960) *N.Y. Acad. Sci.* 87, 457.
168. Anderson, N.F., Delorme, E.J. & Woodruff, M.F.A. (1960) *Transpl. Bull.* 7, 93.
169. Gowans, J.L. (1957) *Brit. J. Exp. Path.* 38, 67.
170. Terasaki, P.I. (1959) *J. Embryol. Exp. Morph.* 7, 394.
171. Terasaki, P.I., Cannon, J.A. & Longmire, W.P. (1959) *Proc. Soc. Exp. Biol. Med.* 100, 639.
172. Simonsen, M. In *Cellular Aspects of Immunity*, Ciba Found. Symp., eds. G.E.W. Wolstenholme & M. O'Connor, p. 122, J. & A. Churchill Ltd., London.
173. Gowans, J.L., Gesner, B.L. & McGregor, D.D. (1961) In *Biological Activity of the Leucocyte*, Ciba Found. Study Group no. 10, eds G.E.W. Wolstenholme & M. O'Connor, p. 32, J. & A. Churchill Ltd, London.
174. Gowans, J.L. (1962) *Ann. N.Y. Acad. Sci.* 99, 432.
175. Porter, K.A., Chapuis, G. & Freeman, M.K. (1962) *Ann. N.Y. Acad. Sci.* 99, 456.
176. Gowans, J.L., McGregor, D.D. & Cowen, D.M. (1963) In *The Immmunologically Competent Cell*, Ciba Found. Study Group no. 20, eds. G.E.W. Wolstenholme & M. O'Connor, p. 20, J. & A. Churchill Ltd., London.
177. Billingham, R.E., Silvers, W.K. & Wilson, D.B. (1962) *Lancet* 1, 512.
178. Szenberg, A. & Warner, N.L. (1962) *Brit. J. Exp. Path.* 43, 123.
179. Darcy, D.A. (1952) *Phil. Trans. B* 236, 463.
180. Govaerts, A. (1960) *J. Immunol.* 85, 516.
181. Rosenau, W. & Moon, H.D. (1961) *J. Natl. Cancer Inst.* 27, 471.
182. Rosenau, W. & Moon, H.D. (1962) *J. Immunol.* 89, 422.
183. Janowski, D.S., Rosenau, W. & Moon, H.D. (1964) *Proc. Soc. Exp. Biol. Med.* 115, 77.
184. Brondz, B.D. (1968) *Folia Biol. (Praha)* 14, 115.
185. Wilson, D.B. (1965) *J. Exp. Med.* 22, 143.
186. Wilson, D.B. (1965) *J. Exp. Med.* 22, 167.
187. Ginsburg, H. (1970) *Adv. Cancer Res.* 13, 63.
188. Sanderson, A.R. (1964) *Nature* 204, 250.
189. Sanderson, A.R. (1964) *Brit. J. Exp. Path.* 45, 398.
190. Sanderson, A.R. (1965) *Transplantation* 3, 557.
191. Brunner, K.T., Mauel, J., Cerrottini, J.C. *et al.* (1967) *Immunology* 14, 181.
192. Cerrottini, J.C., Nordin, A.A. & Brunner, K.T. (1970) *Nature,* 227, 72.
193. Cerrottini, J.C., Nordin, A.A. & Brunner, K.T. (1970) *Nature* 228, 1308.
194. Brunner, K.T., Mauel, J., Rudolf, H. *et al.* (1970) *Immunology* 18, 501.
195. Mauel, J., Rudolf, H., Chapuis, B. *et al.* (1970) *Immunology* 18, 501.
196. Zinkernagel, R.M. & Doherty, P.C. (1974) *Nature* 248, 701.
197. Zinkernagel, R.M. & Doherty, P.C. (1974) *Nature* 251, 547.

198. Zinkernagel, R.M. & Doherty, P.C. (1979) *Adv. Immunol.* **27**, 51.
199. Shearer, G.M. (1974) *Eur. J. Immunol.* **4**, 527.
200. Nowell, P.C. (1960) *Cancer Res.* **20**, 462.
201. Hastings, J., Freedman, S., Rendon, O. *et al.* (1961) *Nature* **192**, 1214.
202. Bach, F. & Hirschhorn, K. (1964) *Science* **143**, 813.
203. Rubin, A.L., Stenzel, K.H., Hirschhorn, K. *et al.* (1964) *Science* **143**, 815.
204. Bach, F.H. (1964) In *Histocompatibility of HLA: Ten Recollections*, ed. P.I. Terasaki, p. 191, UCLA Typing Laboratory, Los Angeles.
205. Bach, F.H. & Voynow, N.K. (1966) *Science* **153**, 545.
206. Bach, F.H. & Bach, M.L. (1972) *Nature New Biol,* **235**, 243.
207. Bain, B., Vas, M.R. & Lowenstein, L. (1963) *Fed. Proc.* **22**, 428 (abstr.).
208. Bain, B., Vas, M.R. & Lowenstein, L. (1964) *Blood* **23**, 108.
209. Schrek, R. & Donelly, W.J. (1961) *Blood* **18**, 561.
210. Bain, B. & Lowenstein, L. (1964) *Science* **145**, 1315.
211. Häyry, P. & Defendi, V. (1970) *Science* **168**, 133.
212. Hodes, R.J. & Svedmyr, E.A.F. (1970) *Transplantation* **9**, 470.
213. Solliday, S. & Bach, F.H. (1970) *Science* **170**, 1406.
214. Dempster, W.J., Lennox, B. & Boag, J.W. (1950) *Brit. J. Exp. Path.* **31**, 670.
215. Lennox, B., Dempster, W.J. & Boag, J.W. (1952) *Brit. J. Exp. Path.* **33**, 380.
216. Hektoen, L. (1915) *J. Infect. Dis.* **17**, 414.
217. Hektoen, L. (1915) *J. Infect. Dis.* **33**, 380.
218. Murphy, J.B. & Sturm, E. (1925) *J. Exp. Med.* **141**, 245.
219. Craddock, C.G. & Lawrence, J.S. (1948) *J. Immunol.* **60**, 241.
220. Billingham, R.E., Krohn, P.L. & Medawar, P.B. (1951) *Brit. Med. J.* **1**, 1157.
221. Whitelaw, M.J. (1951) *J. Amer. Med. Ass.* **145**, 85.
222. Lawrence, H.S., Rapaport, F.T., Converse, J.M. *et al.* (1960) *J. Clin. Invest.* **39**, 185.
223. Lawrence, H.S. (1949) *Proc. Soc. Exp. Biol. N.Y.* **71**, 516.
224. McKenzie, I.F.C. & Potter, T. (1979) *Adv. Immunol.* **27**, 179.
225. Reif, A.E. & Allen, J.M.V. (1964) *J. Exp. Med.* **120**, 413.
226. Reif, A.E. & Allen, J.M.V. (1966) *Cancer Res.* **26**, 123.
227. Raff, M.C. (1969) *Nature* **224**, 378.
228. Mosmann, T.R., Gherwinski, H., Bond, M.W. *et al.* (1986) *J. Immunol.* **136**, 2348.
229. Loveland, B.E., Hogarth, P.M., Ceredig, R. *et al.* (1981) *J. Exp. Med.* **153**, 1044.
230. Steinmuller, D. (1985) *Transplantation* **40**, 229.
231. Loveland, B.E. & McKenzie, I.F.C. (1982) *Transplantation* **33**, 411.
232. Loveland, B.E. & McKenzie, I.F.C. (1982) *Immunology* **46**, 313.
233. Dallman, M.J., Mason, D.W. & Webb, M. (1982) *Eur. J. Immunol.* **12**, 511.
234. Mason, D.W. & Morris, P.J. (1986) *Annu. Rev. Immunol.* **4**, 119.
235. Hall, B.M. & Dorsch, S.E. (1984) *Immunol. Rev.* **77**, 31.
236. Shelton, M.W., Walp, L.A. & Basler, J.T. (1992) *Transplantation* **54**, 278.
237. Lowry, R.P., Gurley, K.E. & Forbes, R.D.C. (1983) *Transplantation* **36**, 391.
238. Gurley, K.E., Lowry, R.P. & Forbes, R.D.C. (1983) *Transplantation* **36**, 401.
239. Lowry, R.P. & Gurley, K.E. (1983) *Transplantation* **36**, 405.
240. Lowry, R.P., Forbes, R.D.C., Blackburn, J. *et al.* (1985) *Transpl. Proc.* **17**, 227.
241. Heidecke, C.D., Kupiec-Weglinski, J.W., Lear, P.A. *et al.* (1984) *J. Immunol.* **133**, 582.
242. Palladino, M.A., Welte, K., Carroll, A.M. *et al.* (1984) *Cell. Immunol.* **86**, 299.
243. Snider, M.E. & Steinmuller, D. (1985) *Transpl. Proc.* **17**, 596.
244. Burlingham, W.J., Snider, W.N., Tyler, J.D. *et al.* (1984) *Cell. Immunol.* **87**, 553.
245. Madsen, J.C., Peugh, W.N., Wood, K.J. *et al.* (1987) *Transplantation* **44**, 849.
246. Sprent, J., Schaffer, M., Lo, D. *et al.* (1986) *J. Exp. Med.* **163**, 998.
247. Sprent, J., Schaffer, M., Lo, D. *et al.* (1986) *Immunol. Rev.* **91**, 195.
248. Rosenberg, A.S., Mizuochi, T. & Singer, A. (1986) *Nature* **322**, 829.
249. Rosenberg, A.S., Mizuochi, T., Sharrow, S.O. *et al.* (1987) *J. Exp. Med.* **165**, 1296.
250. Cobbold, S. & Waldmann, H. (1986) *Transplantation* **41**, 634.
251. Roberts, P.J. & Häyry, P. (1976) *Cell. Immunol.* **26**, 160.
252. Binz, H., Wigzell, H. & Häyry, P. (1976) *Nature* **259**, 401.

253. Pasternack, A., Virolainen, M. & Häyry, P. (1973) *J. Urol.* **109**, 167.
254. Häyry, P. & Von Willebrand, E. (1981) *Scand. J. Immunol.* **13**, 87.
255. Pasternack, A. (1968) *Lancet* **2**, 82.
256. Dallman, M.J. & Clark, G.J. (1991) *Curr. Opin. Immunol.* **3**, 729.
267. Billingham, R.E., Brent, L. & Medawar, P.B. (1956) *Nature* **178**, 514.
258. Billingham, R.E., Brent, L. & Medawar, P.B. (1958) *Transpl. Bull.* **5**, 377.
259. Medawar, P.B. (1958) *Nature* **182**, 62.
260. Hašková, V. & Hrubešová, M. (1958) *Nature* **182**, 61.
261. Castermans, A. & Oth, A. (1959) *Nature* **184**, 1224.
262. Kandutsch, A.A. & Reinert-Wenck, U. (1957) *J. Exp. Med.* **105**, 125.
263. Kandutsch, A.A. (1957) *Ann. N.Y. Acad. Sci.* **64**, 1002.
264. Brent, L., Medawar, P.B. & Ruszkiewicz, M. (1961) *Brit. J. Exp. Path.* **42**, 464.
265. Brent, L., Medawar, P.B. & Ruszkiewicz, M. (1962) In *Transplantation*, Ciba Found. Symp., eds G.E.W. Wolstenholme & M.P. Cameron, J. & A. p. 6, Churchill, London.
266. Medawar, P.B. (1959) In *Biological Problems of Grafting*, p. 6, 19, Blackwell, Oxford.
267. Lejeune-Ledant, G.N. & Albert, F.H. (1960) *Ann. N.Y. Acad. Sci.* **87**, 308.
268. Medawar, P.B. (1963) *Transplantation* **1**, 21.
269. Martinez, C., Smith, J.M., Blaese, M. *et al.* (1963) *J. Exp. Med.* **118**, 743.
270. Davies, D.A.L. & Hutchison, A.M. (1961) *Brit. J. Exp. Path.* **42**, 587.
271. Davies, D.A.L. (1962) *Nature* **193**, 36.
272. Davies, D.A.L. (1962) *Biochem. J.* **84**, 307.
273. Haughton, G. & Davies, D.A.L. (1962) *Brit. J. Exp. Path.* **43**, 488.
274. Manson, L.A., Foschi, G.V. & Palm, J. (1962) *Proc. Natl. Acad. Sci.* **48**, 1816.
275. Mann, L.T., Corson, J.M. & Dammin, G.J. (1960) *Nature* **187**, 774.
276. Mann, L.T., Corson, J.M. & Dammin, G.J. (1962) *Nature* **193**, 168.
277. Mann, L.T., Corson, J.M. & Dammin, G.J. (1962) *Nature* **199**, 499.
278. Mann, L.T., Corson, J.M. & Dammin, G.J. (1967) *Transplantation* **5**, 465.
279. Bjorkman, P.J., Saper, M.A., Samraoui, B. *et al.* (1987) *Nature* **329**, 506.
280. Kahan, B.D. & Reisfeld, R.A. (1969) *Science* **164**, 514.
281. Rapaport, F.T., Dausset, J., Converse, J.M. *et al.* (1965) *Transplantation* **3**, 490.
282. Batchelor, J.R. & Sanderson, A.R. (1967) In *Histocompatibility Testing 1967*, eds E.S. Curtoni, P.L. Mattiuz & R.M. Tosi, p. 139, Munksgaard, Copenhagen.
283. Metzgar, R.S., Flanagan, J.F. & Mendes, N.F. In *Histocompatibility Testing 1967*, eds E.S. Curtoni, P.L. Mattiuz & R.M. Tosi, p. 307, Munksgaard, Copenhagen.
284. Bruning, J.W., Masurel, M. Bent, V.D. *et al.* In *Histocompatibility Testing 1967*, eds E.S. Curtoni, P.L. Mattiuz & R.M. Tosi, p. 303, Munksgaard, Copenhagen.
285. Sanderson, A.R. & Batchelor, J.R. (1968) *Nature* **219**, 184.
286. Kahan, B.D., Reisfeld, R.A., Pellegrino, M.A. *et al.* (1968) *Proc. Natl. Acad. Sci. U.S.A* **61**, 897.
287. Davies, D.A.L., Manston, A.J., Viza, D.C. *et al.* (1968) *Transplantation* **6**, 571.
288. Summerell, J.M. & Davies, D.A.L. (1968) *Biochim. Biophys. Acta* **207**, 92.
289. Mann, D.L., Rogentine, G.N. & Fahey, J.L. (1968) *Nature* **217**, 1180.
290. Götze, D., Ferrone, S. & Reisfeld, R.A. (1972) *J. Immunol.* **109**, 439.
291. Mann, D.L., Rogentine, G.N., Fahey, J.L. *et al.* (1969) *J. Immunol.* **103**, 282.
292. Dresser, D. W. (1962) *Immunology* **5**, 378.
293. Mitchison, N.A. (1968) *Immunology* **15**, 509.
294. Hildemann, W.H. (1970) *Transpl. Rev.* **3**, 5.
295. Simonsen, M. (1970) *Transpl. Rev.* **3**, 22.
296. Nisbet, N.W., Simonsen, M. & Zaleski, M. (1969) *J. Exp. Med.* **129**, 459.
297. Wilson, D.B., Blythe J.C. & Nowell, P.C. (1968) *J. Exp. Med.* **128**, 1157.
298. Simonsen, M. (1962) In *Transplantation*, Ciba Found. Symp., eds G.E.W. Wolstenholme & M.P. Cameron, p. 185, J. & A. Churchill, London.
299. Bach, F.H., Block, H., Graupner, K. *et al.* (1969) *Proc. Natl. Acad. Sci. U.S.A.* **62**, 377.
300. Ford, W.L., Simmonds, S.J. & Atkins, R.C. (1973) *J. Exp. Med.* **141**, 681.
301. Atkins, R.C. & Ford, W.L. (1975) *J. Exp. Med.* **141**, 664.
302. Skinner, M.A. & Marbrook, J. (1976) *J. Exp. Med.* **143**, 1562.

303. Klein, J. (1967) In *Histocompatibility Testing*, eds E.S. Curtoni, P.L. Mattiuz, & R.M. Tosi, p. 21, Munksgaard, Copenhagen.
304. Bevan, M.J. (1984) *Immunol. Today* 5, 128.
305. Lawrence, H.S. (1959) *Physiol. Rev.* 39, 811.
306. Thomas, L. (1959) In *Cellular and Humoral Aspects of the Hypersensitive States*, ed. H.S. Lawrence, p. 529, Hoeber, New York.
307. Matzinger, P. & Bevan, M.J. (1977) *Cell. Immunol.* 29, 1.
308. Townsend, A.R.M., Gotch, F.M. & Davey, J. (1985) *Cell* 42, 457.
309. Townsend, A.R.M., Rothbard, J., Gotch, F.M. *et al.* (1986) *Cell* 44, 959.
310. Maryanski, J.L., Pala, P., Corradin, G. *et al.* (1986) *Nature* 324, 578.
311. Marrack. P. & Kappler, J. (1988) *Nature* 332, 840.
312. Santos-Aquado, J., Crimmins, M.A.V., Mentzer, S.J. *et al.* (1989) *Proc. Natl. Acad. Sci. U.S.A.* 86, 8936.
313. Lechler, R., Lombardi, G., Batchelor, J.R. *et al.* (1990) *Immunol. Today* 11, 83.
314. Scott, D.M., Ehrmann, I.E., Ellis, P.S. *et al.* (1995) *Nature* 376, 695.
315. Snell, G.D. (1957) *Ann. Rev. Microbiol.* 11, 439.
316. Stoerk, H.C. (1953) *Ann. N.Y. Acad. Sci.* 56, 742.
317. Steinmuller, D. (1967) *Science* 158, 127.
318. Elkins, W.L. & Guttmann, R.D. (1968) *Science* 159, 1250.
319. Billingham, R.E., Brent, L. & Medawar, P.B. (1956) *Phil. Trans. B* 239, 357.
320. Lafferty, L.J., Misco, I.S. & Cooley, M.A. (1974) *Nature* 249, 275.
321. Dempster, W.J. (1968) *Lancet* 1, 145.
322. Simonsen, M. (1953) *Biological Incompatibility in Kidney Transplantation in Dogs*, Copenhagen.
323. Steinmuller, D. & Hart, E.A. (1971) *Transpl. Proc.* 3, 673.
324. Billingham, R.E. (1971) *Cell. Immunol.* 2, 1.
325. Guttmann, R.D., Lindquist, R.R. & Ocker, S.A. (1969) *Transplantation* 8, 472.
326. Guttmann, R.D. & Lindquist, R.R. (1969) *Transplantation* 8, 490.
327. Brewer, Y., Palmer, A., Taube, D. *et al.* (1989) *Lancet* 2, 935.
328. Summerlin, W.T., Broutbar, C., Foanes, R.B. *et al.* (1973) *Transpl. Proc.* 5, 707.
329. Summerlin, W.T., Charlton, E. & Karasek, M. (1970) *J. Invest. Dermatol.* 55, 310.
330. Summerlin, W.T. (1973) *Clin. Immunol. Immunopath.* 1, 372.
331. Ninnemann, J.L. & Good, R.A. (1974) *Transplantation* 18, 1.
332. Jacobs, B.J. & Huseby, R.A. (1967) *Transplantation* 5, 410.
333. Lafferty, K.J., Cooley, M.A., Woolnough, J. *et al.* (1975) *Science* 188, 259.
334. Lafferty, K.J., Prowse, S.J. & Simeonovic, C.J. (1983) *Ann. Rev. Immunol.* 1, 143.
335. Bretscher, P. & Cohn, M. (1966) *Nature* 220, 444.
336. Bretscher, P. & Cohn, M. (1970) *Science* 169, 1042.
337. Talmage, D.W., Dart, G., Radovich, J. *et al.* (1976) *Science* 191, 385.
338. Lacy, P.E., Davie, J.M., Finke, E.H. *et al.* (1979) *Transplantation* 27, 172.
339. Lacy, P.E., Davie, J.M., Finke, E.H. *et al.* (1980) *Science* 209, 283.
340. Faustman, D., Hauptfeld, V., Davie, J. *et al.* (1980) *J. Exp. Med.* 151, 1563.
341. Faustman, D., Hauptfeld, V., Lacy, P. *et al.* (1981) *Proc. Natl. Acad. Sci. U.S.A.* 78, 5156.
342. Serie, J.R. & Hegre, O.D. (1985) *Transplantation* 39, 684.
343. Morrow, C.E., Sutherland, D.E.R., Steffes, M.W. *et al.* (1983) *Transplantation* 36, 691.
344. Hart, D.N.J., Winnearls, C.G. & Fabre, J.W. (1980) *Transplantation* 30, 73.
345. Woodruff, M.F.A. (1950) *Phil. Trans. B.* 234, 559.
346. Donohoe, J.A., Andrus, L., Bowen, K.M. *et al.* (1983) *Transplantation* 35, 62.
347. La Rosa, F.G., Smilek, D., Talmage, D.W. *et al.* (1992) *Transplantation* 53, 903.
348. Welsh, K.I., Burgos, H. & Batchelor, J.R. (1977) *Eur. J. Immunol.* 7, 267.
349. Welsh, K.I., Burgos, H. & Batchelor, J.R. (1978) *Nature* 273, 54.
350. Stuart, F.P., Bastien, E., Holter, A. *et al.* (1971) *Transpl. Proc.* 3, 461.
351. Fabre, J.W. & Morris, P.J. (1972) *Transplantation* 14, 634.
352. Batchelor, J.R., Welsh, K.I. & Burgos, H. (1979) *J. Exp. Med.* 150, 455.
353. Steinman, R.M. (1981) *Transplantation* 31, 151.
354. Streilein, J.W. & Bergstresser, P.R. (1980) *Transplantation* 30, 319.
355. Streilein, J.W., Lonsberry, L.W. & Bergstresser, P.R. (1982) *J. Exp. Med.* 155, 863.

356. McKenzie, J.L., Beard, M.E.J. & Hart, D.N.J. (1984) *Transplantation* **38**, 371.
357. Hadley, G.A., Linders, B. & Mohanakumar, T. (1992) *Transplantation* **54**, 537.
358. Rouabhia, M., Germain, L., Belanger, F. *et al.* (1993) *Transplantation* **56**, 259.
359. Fabre, J.W. (1988) *Transpl. Int.* **1**, 165.
360. Milton, A.D. & Fabre, J.W. (1985) *J. Exp. Med.* **161**, 98.
361. Niederwieser, D., Aubick, J., Troppmair, J. *et al.* (1988) *J. Immunol.* **140**, 2556.
362. Minami, M. & Shreffler, D.C. (1981) *J. Immunol.* **126**, 1774.
363. Steinman, R.M., Inaba, K., Schuler, G. *et al.* (1986) *Progr. Immunol.* **6**, 1013.
364. Knight, S.C., Mertin, J., Stackpoole, A. *et al.* (1983) *Proc. Natl. Acad. Sci. U.S.A.* **80**, 6032.
365. Lechler, R.I. & Batchelor, J.R. (1982) *J. Exp. Med.* **155**, 31.
366. Weinberger, O. (1981) *Eur. J. Immunol.* **11**, 405.
367. Golding, H. & Singer, A. (1984) *J. Immunol.* **133**, 597.
368. Finnegan, A., Needleman, B.W. & Hodes, R.J. (1985) *J. Immunol.* **134**, 2960.
369. Sherwood, R.A., Brent, L. & Rayfield, L.S. (1986) *Eur. J. Immunol.* **16**, 569.
370. Parker, K.E., Dalchau, R. & Fowler, V.J. (1992) *Transplantation* **53**, 918.
371. Dalchau, R., Fangmann, J. & Fabre, J.W. (1992) *Eur. J. Immunol.* **22**, 669.
372. Dalchau, R., Fangmann, J. & Fabre, J.W. (1992) *Eur. J. Immunol.* **22**, 1525.
373. Fangmann, J., Dalchau, R. & Fabre, J.W. (1992) *J. Exp. Med.* **175**, 1521.
374. Benham, A.M., Sawyer, G.J. & Fabre, J.W. (1995) *Transplantation* **59**, 1028.
375. Sayegh, M.H., Watschinger, B. & Carpenter, C.B. (1994) *Transplantation* **57**, 1295.
376. Jerne, N.K. (1971) *Eur. J. Immunol.* **1**, 1.
377. Von Boehmer, H., Haas, W. & Jerne, N.K. (1978) *Proc. Natl. Acad. Sci. U.S.A.* **75**, 2439.
378. Barker, C.F. & Billingham, R.E. (1977) *Adv. Immunol.* **25**, 1.
379. Brent, L. (1990) In *Pathophysiology of the Blood–Brain Barrier*, eds B.B. Johansson & H. Widmer, p. 383, Elsevier Science Publ.
380. Medawar, P.B. (1948) *Brit. J. Exp. Path.* **29**, 58.
381. Billingham, R.E. & Boswell, T. (1953) *Proc. Roy. Soc. B* **141**, 392.
382. Bigger, S.L. (1837) *Dublin Quart. J. Med. Sci.* **11**, 408.
383. Woodruff, M.F.A. (1960) *The Transplantation of Tissues and Organs*, p. 400, Charles C. Thomas, Springfield, Ill.
384. Zirm, E. (1906) *Albrecht v. Grafes Arch. Ophthal.* **64**, 580.
385. Rycroft, B.W. (1954) In *Preservation and Transplantation of Normal Tissues*, eds. G.E.W. Wolstenholme & M.P. Cameron, Ciba Found. Symp., p. 210, J. & A. Churchill Ltd., London.
386. Sanfillipo, F., McWueen, M., Vaughn, W. *et al.* (1968) *New Engl. J. Med.* **315**, 29.
387. Batchelor, J.R., Casey, T.A., Douglas, C. *et al.* (1976) *Lancet* **1**, 551.
388. Streilein, J.W., Toens, G.B. & Bergstresser, P.R. (1979) *Nature* **282**, 326.
389. Volker-Dieben, H.G., Kok-van Alphen, C.C., Landsbergen, Q. *et al.* (1982) *Acta Ophthalmol.* **60**, 190.
390. Greene, H.S.N. (1943) *Cancer Res.* **3**, 809.
391. Sonoda, Y. & Streilein, J.W. (1992) *Transplantation* **54**, 694.
392. Kaplan, H.J. & Streilein, J.W. (1978) *J. Immunol.* **120**, 689.
393. Whittum, J.A., Niederkorn, J.Y. & Streilein, J.W. (1982) *Transplantation* **34**, 190.
394. Shirai, Y. (1921) *Jap. Med. World* **1**, 14.
395. Murphy, J.B. (1926) *Monogr. Rockef. Inst. Med. Res.* **21**.
396. Tansley, K. (1946) *J. Exp. Med.* **22**, 221.
397. Head, J.R. & Griffin, W.S.T. (1985) *Proc. Roy. Soc. B.* **224**, 375.
398. Mason, D.W., Charlton, H.M. & Jones, A.J. (1987) *Science* **235**, 772.
399. Widner, H. & Brundin, P. (1988) *Brain Res. Rev.* **13**, 287.
400. Szentistvanyi, F., Patlak, C.S., Ellis, R.A. *et al.* (1984) *Amer. J. Physiol.* **246**, F835.
401. Widner, H., Johansson, B.B. & Möller, G. (1985) *J. Cerebr. Blood Flow Metab.* **5**, 88.
402. Widner, H., Johansson, B.B. & Möller, G. (1988) *Scand. J. Immunol.* **28**, 563.
403. Björklund, A. & Stenevi, U. (1979) *Brain Res.* **177**, 555.
404. Perlow, M.J., Freed, W.J., Hoffer, B.J. *et al.* (1979) *Science* **204**, 643.
405. Backlund, E-O., Granberg, P-O., Hamberger, B. *et al.* (1985) *J. Neurosurg.* **62**, 169.
406. Fiandaca, M.S. (1991) *Transplantation* **51**, 549.
407. Several authors. In *Intracerebral Transplantation in Movement Disorders*, eds O. Lindvall, A. Björklund & H. Widner, part II, Elsevier.

408. Neaves, W.B. (1977) In *The Testis*, vol. 4, eds A.D. Johnson & W.R. Gomes, Academic Press, N.Y.

409. Greene, H.S.N. (1940) *J. Exp. Med.* **71**, 305.

410. Head, J.R., Neaves, W.B. & Billingham, R.E. (1983) *Transplantation* **35**, 91.

411. Head, J.R., Neaves, W.B. & Billingham, R.E. (1983) *Transplantation* **36**, 423.

412. Lutz, B.R., Fulton, G.P., Patt, D.I. *et al.* (1950) *Cancer Res.* **10**, 231.

413. Lutz, B.R., Fulton, G.P., Patt, D.I. *et al.* (1951) *Cancer Res.* **11**, 64.

414. Toolan, H.W. (1951) *Proc. Soc. Exp. Biol. Med.* **77**, 572.

415. Toolan, H.W. (1953) *Cancer Res.* **13**, 389.

416. Cohen, S.N. (1961) *Proc. Soc. Exp. Biol. Med.* **106**, 677.

417. Billingham, R.E. & Silvers, W.K. (1962) In *Transplantation*, eds G.E.W. Wolstenholme & M.P. Cameron, Ciba Found. Symp., p. 90, J. & A. Churchill, London.

418. Shepro, D., Cohen, P. & Kula, N. (1964) *J. Immunol.* **93**, 925.

419. Shepro, D., Kula, N. & Halkett, J.A.E. (1963) *J. Exp. Med.* **117**, 749.

420. Barker, C.F. & Billingham, R.E. (1971) *J. Exp. Med.* **133**, 620.

421. Bergstresser, P.R., Fletcher, C.R. & Streilein, J.W. (1980) *J. Invest. Dermatol.* **74**, 77.

422. Barker, C.F. & Billingham, R.E. (1968) *J. Exp. Med.* **128**, 197.

423. Tilney, N.L. & Gowans, J.L. (1971) *J. Exp. Med.* **133**, 951.

424. Medawar, P.B. (1958) *Proc. Roy. Soc. B.* **149**, 144.

425. Billingham, R.E. & Silvers, W.K. (1960) *Ann. Surg.* **152**, 975.

426. Hildemann, W.H. (1957) *Ann. N.Y. Acad. Sci.* **64**, 775.

427. Weissman, I.L., Saito, Y. & Rinkevich, B. (1990) *Immunol. Rev.* **113**, 227.

428. Hildemann, W.H. (1979) *Transplantation* **27**, 1.

429. Burnet, F.M. (1976) In *Receptors and Recognition*, eds. P. Cuatrecasas & M. Greaves, p. 35, Chapman & Hall, London.

430. Marchelonis, J.J. (1977) *Immunity in Evolution*, p. 238, Arnold, London.

431. Hildemann, W.H., Raison, R.C., Cheung, G. *et al.* (1977) *Nature* **270**, 219.

432. Hildemann, W.H., Johnson, I.S., Jokiel, P.L.C. *et al.* (1979) *Science* **204**, 420.

433. Klein, J. (1989) *Scand. J. Immunol.* **29**, 499.

434. Cooper, E.L., Rinkevic, B., Uhlenbruck, G. *et al.* (1992) *Scand. J. Immunol.* **35**, 247.

435. Marchelonis, J.J. & Schluter, S.F. (1990) *Scand. J. Immunol.*, **32**, 13.

Biographies

**JAMES LEARMONTH
GOWANS (1924–)**

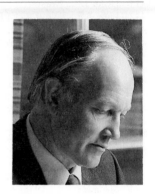

James Gowans (Jim to his friends, even after he received his Knighthood) was born in Sheffield, England. He was an academic high flyer from the beginning, having qualified with honors as a doctor at King's College Hospital, London in 1947 and obtained a first class degree in physiology at Oxford University a year later. His father had been a technician in a hospital pathology laboratory and it was perhaps no accident that the young Gowans should have opted to work for his higher degree (the D.Phil.) at the Sir William Dunn School of Pathology, Oxford, which at the time was under the direction of the eminent Australian pathologist, Howard (later Lord) Florey. It was Florey who suggested to Gowans that he should work on lymphocytes, especially with a view to discovering what caused these cells, whose function was unknown at the time, to have such a high turnover in the blood. Thus began an outstanding research career that was to make a profound impact on the postwar development of immunology.

The presence of lymphocytes in inflammatory reactions, delayed-type hypersensitivity responses, bacterial diseases such as tuberculosis and in allografts undergoing rejection had been widely documented, but because the small lymphocyte had been regarded as an end cell with a very short lifespan, its central role as a mediator of many immunologic responses was not appreciated. The vital contribution of Gowans was to show that some of the small lymphocytes taken from the thoracic duct of rats were not short-lived and had the capacity to circulate from the blood into the lymph nodes and back again into the blood; and he and his colleagues showed precisely how this came about. His close contact with P.B. Medawar came later, when Gowans wanted to design an experiment that would reveal something of the functional ability of small lymphocytes. It was Medawar who encouraged him to transfuse lymphocytes from sensitized or normal donors into recipients of inbred strains, and Gowans and his team soon discovered that these cells could induce graft-versus-host reactions and destroy skin grafts on rats that had been made tolerant neonatally. By contrast, the lymphocytes of tolerant rats did not transfer adoptive immunity. "So Peter had nothing to do with my becoming a 'lymphomaniac' but he did, of course, introduce me to transplantation biology," Gowans told me. Gowans' many contributions thus led to a clear understanding of the physiology and function of small lymphocytes and this vitally important advance has been recognized by the conferment of many honors, from election to Fellowship of the Royal Society in 1963, a Knighthood in 1982, to several College Fellowships at Oxford University. Gowans has been awarded numerous honorary degrees from British and American universities and honorary membership of several societies, including the Foreign Associateship of the U.S. National Academy of Sciences. His prizes include, appropriately, the first Medawar Prize (shared with J.F.A.P. Miller) in 1990.

To the dismay of the immunologic world he gave up active research in 1977 to become Secretary of the Medical Research Council (M.R.C.), a post that he held for a decade in what proved to be a financially trying time for the M.R.C. Gowans has been a member of the councils or boards of many scientific institutions and in 1989 he became Secretary-General of the Human Frontier Science Program based in Strasbourg, France.

On a personal note, Gowans' intellectual sharpness combined with his great height made him a somewhat forbidding figure to some, though he was unfailingly courteous and helpful to junior scientists. He married Moira Leatham in 1956 and they have a son and two daughters. His interests outside science have been "unremarkable", according to him, and he may be unique in not listing any in *Who's Who*; he does, however, admit to enjoying gardening.

**NICHOLAS AVRION MITCHISON
(1928–)**

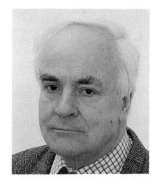

Avrion Mitchison was born in London into a distinguished family. His father was a barrister and Member of Parliament, his mother a novelist and farmer, who became the "mother" of the Bakgatla tribe in Botswana, and his uncle the geneticist J.B.S. Haldane. Av, as his friends and collegues know him, read zoology at New College, Oxford University, where his tutor was P.B. Medawar who, like his uncle, was to become a considerable influence in his scientific life. In 1948 he gained a first class degree in zoology and his doctoral degree followed in 1952. His thesis was in part devoted to the adoptive transfer of immunity to tumors, an assay that Medawar and his colleagues soon applied to skin allografts and which proved to be one of the most valuable analytic tools in transplantation immmunology. (His postdoctoral supervisor had been Medawar and his examiner P.A. Gorer. The latter at first declined to recommend the thesis for acceptance because of some literary deficiencies, thus causing a temporary rift between the two great men!)

After completion of his doctorate Mitchison went to Indiana University and to the Jackson Laboratory, Bar Harbor as a Commonwealth Fund Fellow. In the years that followed he carried out research and lectured in the Department of Zoology of Edinburgh University, and it was Mitchison who imported several strains of inbred mice from Bar Harbor to the United Kingdom, some of which he passed on to other groups such as Medawar's. He also visited Harvard and Stanford Universities for extended periods. In 1957 he married Lorna Martin and they had two sons and three daughters.

In 1962 Mitchison left Edinburgh to become head of the Division of Biology at the National Institute for Medical Research, London, at a time when Medawar was the Institute's Director, and his presence helped to turn the institute into a renowned center of immunology. It was there that he carried out his important studies on low zone tolerance and cooperation between T and B lymphocytes. He left Mill Hill in 1971 to fill the Jodrell Chair of Zoology at University College, which had previously been occupied by Medawar, and he became honorary Director of the Imperial Cancer Research Fund's Tumor Immunology Unit. Mitchison wrote to me: "What I am most proud of is having shared in the discovery of cellular immunity to tissue transplants, of low zone tolerance, of cooperation between T and B cells, and of the immunoregulatory function of T-cell clusters (*European Journal of Immunology* 20, 699, 1990). The first three are part of the history of immunology, but the last needs further explanation. The T cell areas of lymph nodes are composed of many clusters of T cells, each arranged round a dendritic cell to which they adhere. The discovery to which I refer is that T cells profoundly influence the behavior of their neighbours within the cluster, by secreting cytokines (or so it seems). The cross-talk within a cluster enables a majority decision to be reached, rather as a Member of Parliament is chosen in a British election. The opinions of the minority get completely discounted, as is only fitting among cells responsible for tolerance of self."

Mitchison has been one of the most distinguished and most imaginative immunologists in Britain and his clear intellect combined with his endearing eccentricities (such as wearing slippers at meetings and apparently falling asleep during sessions, only to ask searching questions during the discussions) won him admirers throughout the scientific community. He and his wife kept open house in London, and Lorna was never quite certain where she had met people before when they presented themselves for breakfast. He has published over 200 research papers and received many honors, among them Fellowship of the Royal Society (1967), the Scientific Medal of the Zoological Society of London, and the Paul Ehrlich Prize. After retiring from his Chair at University College in 1991 he went to Berlin to become the Scientific Director of the Deutsches Rheuma Forschungszentrum.

3 Blood Transfusion, Blood Groups, and Hemolytic Disease of the Newborn

*"Philosophy and common sense, though often parted, have
long agreed about the uniqueness of individual man . . . It is a truism
that if inborn diversity and genetic individuality were to be extinguished . . .
then selection would have nothing to act on, and the species would
be left without evolutionary resource."*

P.B. Medawar, 1956

This topic is briefly covered for several reasons.

(1) Blood transfusion (BT) can and should be considered to be a highly successful transplant, although it is normally transient in nature.
(2) The ABO blood group system is of importance in renal transplantation, as it is in blood transfusion.
(3) Landsteiner's discovery of the human ABO blood groups marked the beginning of the field of immunogenetics, which is considered in detail in Chapter 4.
(4) The prevention of hemolytic disease of the newborn is the first successful immunoregulatory strategy applied to human beings and should be of interest to those who have attempted immunoregulation in the context of histocompatibility antigens (Chapter 6).
(5) BTs have been known to be associated with graft-versus-host reactions (Chapter 8).
(6) The longstanding controversy and schism engendered by the Rh nomenclature is likely to have served as a lesson, however subconsciously, to those immunogeneticists who have grappled with the complexities of nomenclature relating to both mouse and human histocompatibility antigens and who so conspicuously avoided that kind of controversy by timely international agreement.

Blood Transfusion Before the Birth of Immunology

Although there are references to BT dating back to classical times, the ancient Egyptians and the Old Testament (1), it was taken up in Europe only towards the middle of the seventeenth century, after W. Harvey (2) had described the circulation of the blood in 1628. The physicians who pioneered this treatment, which became something of a panacea for all manner of conditions, were rightly worried about the problems of transfusing blood directly from human donors to their patients at a time before anticoagulants had been discovered. They therefore turned their attention to the use of animal blood donors, and some early attempts with xenogeneic blood are described in Chapter 9. Although miraculous cures were claimed, the procedure soon fell into disrepute and was banned in both France and England, where it had been largely pioneered. It was not to make a comeback until the middle of the nineteenth century, thanks to the advocacy of the English physician J. Blundell (3), who turned to the use of human blood by syringe rather than by the direct transfusion technique that had been in vogue earlier. But interest in BT again waned until the middle of the nineteenth century, when the use of defibrinated blood was proposed in order to overcome the problem of coagulation. However, the modern and successful application of BT had to await the twentieth century, following the discovery of the ABO blood groups by Landsteiner and the use of sodium citrate and later heparin as effective anticoagulants.

Karl Landsteiner's Vital Discoveries

The ABO blood groups

Landsteiner's seminal paper was published in 1901 (4). In it he described the serologic reactions between sera and red blood cells from healthy individuals, previous studies having focused more on sera from sick patients. He showed that the antibodies involved occurred naturally (i.e. that they did not depend on immunization protocols). Natural antibodies to micro-organisms and to xenogeneic red blood cells had already been described by the early immunologists (see Chapter 1) and the concept of naturally occurring antibodies had been essential to Ehrlich's side-chain theory of antibody formation (see Chapter 1).

Landsteiner's huge contribution was to study sera from a panel of normal people (mainly drawn from his own laboratory) and to allow them to react with the blood of other members of the panel on the subsequently much used checkerboard principle. His method was to mix equal volumes of serum and blood diluted in salt solution and to observe the reaction between them in hanging drops or in test tubes. He used material from healthy adults, from healthy women in labor and from the umbilical cord, and among his observations were the following. All sera from healthy adults reacted with some blood samples, and a clear pattern emerged in that the sera fell into three distinct classes. A few (group A) reacted with cells from another group (B), but not with cells obtained from group A; and conversely, group B sera reacted with cells from group A, but not with B group cells. The sera of individuals of the third group (C) agglutinated both A and B cells but, in contrast, C cells were not agglutinated by either A or B sera. He concluded that there were two kinds of agglutinins, one present in A and the other in B, and both in C. Several sera prepared from cord blood seemed to lack agglutinins. Landsteiner was rather taken aback by his findings and considered one or two alternative interpretations. He also showed that redissolved dried sera did not lose their power to agglutinate blood cells, stated that the technique might be of use in forensic medicine to recognize the non-identity of blood, and concluded that his observations helped to explain the differing consequences of therapeutic human blood transfusion.

A year later Landsteiner's colleagues V. Decastello and A. Sturli (5) confirmed and extended his data. They showed that only four of 155 individuals over the age of six months failed to have isohemagglutinins, that their health was of no consequence, that neonates and infants of less than six months often behaved atypically and that the physiologic or pathologic destruction of red cells was not a cause of the serologic interactions.

The reasons for the occurrence of natural anti-A and anti-B antibodies did not become apparent until it was shown half a century later by Springer and his colleagues (6–8) that antigens resembling A and B are present on many microbial cells and that exposure to such microbes was the probable cause of "natural" antibody in humans. The serology, genetics, tissue distribution and molecular biology of the ABO system have recently been reviewed by R. Oriol (9) and detailed information about the A and B subgroups is to be found in P.L. Mollison's standard text (10).

The fact that the A and B antigens are also expressed on many tissue cells makes the presence of natural antibodies to them of great consequence in organ transplantation, where A and B incompatibility is studiously avoided. Mollison also described the many other blood groups, such as Rh, H and Lewis, which were subsequently discovered. Fortunately none of these have to be taken into account in organ transplantation. It should be stressed that the blood group determinants are oligosaccharides, unlike the histocompatibility antigens, which are glycoproteins (see Chapter 4). These two kinds of molecules are quite distinct genetically, structurally and in their tissue distribution.

Landsteiner's discovery, for which he was awarded the Nobel Prize in 1930, together with technologic developments in the prevention of coagulation of blood and its storage and in transfusion techniques, soon established BT as a routine life-saving procedure in times of both peace and war (11). For detailed information the reader is referred to P.L. Mollison's authoritative and much-revised book (10) as well as to the multi-author book by L.D. Petz and S.N. Swisher (12).

The total number of blood group antigens identified is of the order of 600 and it would be astonishing if they did not serve a biologic function, as do the histocompatibility molecules (see Chapter 4). Although blood group determinants are involved in many pathologic conditions it would appear that a wholly convincing biologic role has not yet been found for them. Some associations with human diseases have, however, been demonstrated. This question has recently been discussed by G. Garratty (13).

Serologic specificity

Even before Landsteiner left his native Vienna to live and work in the United States not long after the end of the First World War he had become deeply embroiled in the study of serologic specificity, his interest having been aroused from his work on the ABO blood groups. His book *The Specificity of Serological Reactions* (14), published in revised form posthumously in 1947, was a remarkable if densely written review of his own studies and those of others. He was especially interested in the way chemical modification of molecules led to changes in specificity. Thus he and his colleagues studied the influence exerted by small radicals attached in different positions of the benzene ring in giving rise to altered specificities that incited the formation of different and specific antibodies; and they examined the immunologic properties of proteins that had been subtly altered with the aid of acetylation and methylation. For example, while still in Vienna he found that methylation of horse serum albumin elicited antibodies in rabbits with a distinct serologic specificity and that methylation brought about some erosion of species specificity (15). Landsteiner's monumental work was therefore instrumental in establishing the modern basis of immunologic specificity.

Graft-Versus-Host Reactions After Blood Transfusion

Graft-versus-host reactions (GVHR) occur when tissues or organs containing signifi-cant numbers of viable T lymphocytes are transplanted to recipients who are either immunologically immature, incompetent or immunosuppressed (see Chapter 8). Because the cells are not rejected in such circumstances they are activated by the recipient's histocompatibility antigens and, if present in adequate numbers, induce severe pathologic complications known collectively as graft-versus-host (or runt) disease (GVHD). This can be lethal and it remains to this day one of the major problems to overcome in bone marrow transplantation (see Chapter 8).

The first description of GVHD after multiple BTs was that of Hathaway et al. (16) in 1965. Two infants, just over three months and eight months old, respectively, received multiple BTs to treat vaccinia necrosum following routine smallpox vacci-nation a month or so earlier. The first infant was given "three 250 ml transfusions of fresh, leukocyte-rich plasma from recently vaccinated donors". Various symptoms became evident between 10 and 17 days: a diffuse macular erythematous rash, hepatomegaly, and severe pancytopenia, followed by convulsions, respiratory problems, and mild congestive heart failure. The patient died on the twentieth day. The autopsy revealed generalized icterus and multiple ecchymoses in the skin, mucosal ulceration of the stomach mucosa, focal lesions in the lungs, small lymph nodes without recognizable lymphoid nodules, an absence of lymphocytes from the malpighian corpuscles of the spleen, and a dearth of hematopoietic cells in the bone marrow. The thymus was small and lacked Hassal's corpuscles and lymphocytes, and the small intestine too was devoid of lymphoid tissue.

The second infant received ten 500 ml units of fresh citrated whole blood by exchange transfusion as well as vaccinia immune globulin. Although the vaccinia lesions showed some improvement, hepatosplenomegaly was observed on the tenth day, together with a diffuse erythematous macular rash. Pancytopenia developed rapidly and a bone marrow sample revealed only a few histiocytes. This patient died 17 days after admission. The histopathologic report after autopsy was similar to that of the first patient.

The authors concluded that both infants must have been immunologically deficient because of their abnormal response to smallpox vaccination. In the second case the initial finding of agammaglobulinemia and lymphopenia, together with a family history with immunologic deficiencies, suggested to them that there may have been thymic alymphoplasia or Swiss-type agammaglobulinemia with alymphocytosis. This was, however, not the case for the first patient. The authors rightly concluded that the symptoms and pathologic findings were closely similar to those previously described in GVHD induced in experimental animals, either in newborns or in lethally irradiated adults who had received allogeneic spleen, whole blood or bone marrow cells (see Chapter 8). "These observations suggest that runt disease may occur in the human infant, and that this possibility should be considered in clinical situations in which large amounts of viable leukocytes are transfused into patients who potentially are immunologically deficient", they wrote.

K. Sazama and P.V. Holland (17) have recently reviewed the incidence of GVHD after BT. According to them, some 115 cases had been reported in the English literature by 1992. The majority resulted from the transfusion of fresh blood or blood that had been stored for only a few days. Such blood would be expected to have a near-normal number of viable lymphocytes. The threshold dose of lymphocytes large enough to induce GVHD in patients is thought to be of the order of ten million per kg body weight (18), though the number would be smaller in immunodeficient or immunosuppressed recipients. As lymphocytes stored for up to three weeks remain capable of mitosis in vitro (19), buffy-coat-depleted blood has been used in many centers, but gamma-irradiation of blood is now considered to be safer. Whereas in immunologically normal adults allogeneic lymphocytes can be expected to be eliminated within ten days, this is not necessarily the case in patients whose immune responses are deficient or compromised.

It hardly needs to be emphasized that the number of cases of GVHD after BT is miniscule compared to the vast number of BTs administered. It is, however, possible that mild and transient GVHRs occur more frequently and that they are either unrecognized or unreported.

The Discovery of the Rh System and Hemolytic Disease of the Newborn

Although the discovery of the ABO blood groups was without doubt Landsteiner's, the situation concerning the Rh system was rather more complicated. Indeed, it became the focus of a bitter controversy between the two chief protagonists involving, to a degree, Landsteiner himself.

In 1939 P. Levine, a pathologist working at Mount Sinai Hospital in New York, published together with R.E. Stetson (20) the serologic data of "an unusual case of intra-group agglutination". A woman of blood group O and in her second pregnancy gave birth to a 36-week-old stillborn fetus. She was given a BT from her husband, like her belonging to blood group O. Within ten minutes she suffered an acute transfusion reaction, but was given two more. Nineteen hours after the first BT she voided some bloody urine. To the authors' astonishment her serum agglutinated not only her husband's red blood cells, but also those of most people belonging to blood group O. The patient was given six more BTs from "carefully selected professional donors". The red blood cells of only eight of 50 group O donors failed to react with her serum, and just 21/104 were found to be compatible. These reactions were shown to be independent of blood groups M, N and P. Unaccountably, Levine and Stetson did not give the putative blood group a designation: it might have saved some acrimony had they done so!

In the following year A.S. Wiener and H.R. Peters (21), working at the Jewish Hospital in Brooklyn, New York, described three cases in which hemolytic reactions were observed after the transfusion of blood from the homologous group and for which the same agglutinogen seemed to be responsible. They recounted that ever since Landsteiner's definition of the ABO system BT had become safe, but that occasionally transfusion reactions had been encountered. These were usually, they thought, caused by mistaken blood grouping or indiscriminate use of "universal" donors. Reactions when the donor and recipient were indisputably of the same blood group did sometimes occur, but were rare. Here, however, they described three such reactions after repeated BTs, two of them with fatal consequences. The isoagglutinin found in their serum was designated as "anti-Rh" because "Remarkably, the reactions of the anti-Rh sera corresponded with those of immune rabbit sera prepared by Landsteiner and Wiener by the injection of rhesus blood. The frequency distribution of agglutinogen Rh in the general population is approximately 85% Rh-positive and 15% Rh-negative." Of postpartum patients who experienced a transfusion reaction after having been given blood of the correct group they wrote: ". . . these should belong to the same category as the patients immunized by repeated blood transfusion, if the theory suggested is correct; antigens shared by fetus and blood donor (usually the husband) but absent from the patient's body."

The work Wiener and Peters had referred to was almost certainly a study published by Landsteiner and Wiener (22) in 1937, which showed that some sera from rabbits immunized with rhesus monkey blood reacted with human blood cells bearing agglutinogen M. Indeed, in 1940 Landsteiner and Wiener (23), in a communication occupying a single page, went on to show that such rabbit anti-rhesus sera retained their activity after absorption with "selected bloods", for example blood of group OM, and that this activity was independent of M, N and P blood groups. They wrote that "The results are of some interest in that they suggest a way of finding individual properties in human blood, namely, with the aid of immune sera against the bloods of animals."

The decisive blows implicating anti-Rh antibodies as the cause of hemolytic disease of the newborn (erythroblastosis fetalis) were struck by Landsteiner's former colleague P. Levine in 1941 when he and his team published three papers clarifying the issue. In the first of these (24) they analyzed 12 cases of atypical agglutinins in obstetric patients with histories of repeated abortions, miscarriages and stillbirths. They were struck by the fact that out of five women with such agglutinins, three had given birth to babies suffering from erythroblastosis. This and other clinical observations led them to conclude that "It is probable that there is a connection between the occurrence of these complications and the presence of immune agglutinins in the mother . . . The hypothesis of isoimmunization can readily explain the familial incidence of this condition . . . Most of these serums contain an agglutinin which parallels the anti-Rh agglutinin of Landsteiner and Wiener". And, finally, "In view of the fact that the blood of many of the patients studied does not contain the Rh antigen, a list of Rh-negative donors should be available".

In the second paper (25) Levine's group demonstrated that:

(1) In 93% of cases investigated, erythroblastosis fetalis resulted from immunization of a Rh-negative mother by the Rh-positive father.
(2) In the remaining cases blood factors other than Rh were involved.
(3) Agglutinin tests were of value for diagnosis.
(4) The pathologic manifestations were produced by the intrauterine interaction of maternal immune isoagglutinins with the susceptible red blood cells of the fetus.

They concluded that "It is probable that iso-immunization is also the cause of a certain proportion of natural abortions and stillbirths", and that "Intra-group blood transfusion accidents associated with pregnancy can now be prevented by the use of Rh-negative donors and by means of a modified cross-matching test".

Finally, Levine et al. (26), in a paper published in *Nature*, provided statistical evidence in favor of their hypothesis. Thus, of the 111 mothers who had given birth to infants suffering from erythroblastosis fetalis, 91% were Rh negative whereas 100% of the 60 husbands studied were positive. Likewise, all affected infants were Rh positive. They wrote: "The results ... provide striking evidence to support the importance of the Rh factor in the etiology of erythroblastosis foetalis ... According to the concept of isoimmunization, the mother's immune agglutinins pass through the placenta and exert lytic action on the susceptible fetal blood. However, this could not occur if the Rh factor had a wide distribution in tissue cells and fluids, which could specifically bind the anti-Rh agglutinins". Because the Rh antigen had not been found in saliva (unlike the AB blood groups), seminal fluid and sperm, they assumed that it was present only on red blood cells. They finished by stating "That the Rh factor is inherited as a Mendelian dominant property was recently demonstrated by Landsteiner and Wiener (pers. comm.)".

By 1943 Wiener and Landsteiner (27) felt able to discuss the genetic theory of the Rh blood types. They proposed that according to the reactions with two varieties of anti-Rh agglutinins, there were three sorts of Rh-positive blood, Rh1, Rh2 and Rh', and that they were controlled by triple allelic genes. Wiener (28) enlarged on this by showing that the three varieties of antisera – anti-Rh (standard), anti-Rh1 and anti-Rh2 – agglutinated the red cells of 85%, 70% and 35%, respectively, of the white population of New York, and he designated sera with anti-Rh and anti-Rh2 specificity as anti-Rh', and those with anti-Rh and anti-Rh2 specificity as anti-Rh'''. By means of three types of Rh agglutinins, he claimed, one could recognize five varieties of Rh agglutinogen – Rh1, Rh2, Rh, Rh' and Rh''. These in combination gave rise to eight Rh blood types, including Rh negative.

In 1944 the English blood group geneticist R.R. Race, working in the Medical Research Council Blood Transfusion Service, and his colleagues G.L. Taylor and M.N. McFarlane entered the fray (29). They compared the Wiener terminology (30) with their own, which was based on three anti-Rh sera recognizing 68% of genotypes in the population, with five identified allelomorphs. They were closely similar "but for the gene Wiener calls Rh (Rh1, bar) we prefer Rho, for Rh has for so long had a far wider meaning". "The two schemes show complete agreement save that Wiener has not met the Rhy allelomorph because he has not had an St serum. The results are so strikingly similar that the probability of their being correct must be very high", they wrote.

R.A. Fisher, the eminent English geneticist, and Race published further observations in 1946 (31) when they discussed the gene frequency for Rh in Britain. "The genetics of the Rhesus Factor have turned out to be so complex and our understanding of it has advanced so rapidly that it is difficult for many to arrive at a clear picture of the situation now substantially established", they wrote. "The notation has been frequently changed, and we feel that only a notation which designates unambiguously the antibodies, the genes or gene-complexes, and the antigens with which these antibodies react can avoid widespread confusion."

Yet further changes to the notation were later introduced (see *10, 32, 33*). An important simplification was the introduction by Fisher and Race of the CDE nomenclature, D (Rho) having been the first antigen to be identified and being by far the most important. Those working in the field of histocompatibility antigens avoided the potential pitfalls and schisms of nomenclature by organizing a series of regular international workshops based on the exchange of sera and typing cells, and during the course of these workshops the many reagents used by a large number of laboratories in many parts of the world were fastidiously and rigorously compared. The first of these workshops was held in 1964 at Duke University Medical Center and organized by B.D. Amos and others under the aegis of the American National Academy of Sciences and the National Research Council (see Chapter 4, p. 138). Although J. Dausset, Rose Payne and J.J. Van Rood had given the human leukocyte antigens (HLA) identified by them their own and parochial designations, these were changed to a uniform and generally accepted system of designations as a result of these workshops. That the Rh story had been a formative influence is implicit in the preface to the second Histocompatibility Testing Conference and Workshop held a year after the first, when Amos and van Rood wrote: "The first few years after the discovery of the Rh factor were of intense activity in the elucidation of new knowledge of red cell antigens. Similar developments are now occurring with white cell antigenic systems".

Both Levine (*34*) and Wiener (*35*) later laid claim to the discovery of Rh polymorphism and the controversy, with was to be reflected in the difficulties encountered in adopting a common terminology for what proved to be a complex antigenic system, simmered on. R.E. Rosenfield (*36*), who was trained by Levine and who had been a friend of both the protagonists, recently wrote about "*Who discovered Rh?*". It is a complex, sad and salutory story.

The Prevention of Hemolytic Disease of the Newborn

This story is fascinating, involving as it does genetic variability in butterflies, the overnight hunch of the wife of one of the medical scientists involved, and experiments in Sing Sing prison, if the account by J. Jewkes, D. Sawers and R. Stillerman (*37*) is to be believed. The idea was conceived in Britain and in the United States at roughly the same time, but the British team based in Liverpool published their data well ahead of the American group. Briefly (and leaving out the more colorful aspects researched by Jewkes, Sawers and Stillerman) the story is as follows.

The British group had been influenced by Levine's 1943 observation (*38*) that there was a deficiency of ABO mating types in the parents of offspring affected by hemolytic disease of the newborn, and by the demonstration in 1956 by K. Stern, I. Davidsohn and L. Masaitis (*39*) that Rh sensitization in male volunteers came about more readily if the injected blood was ABO compatible. Furthermore, H.R. Nevanlinna and T. Vainio (*40*) had demonstrated by means of a family study that once sensitization to Rh had occurred, ABO incompatibility between mother and fetus was no longer protective. The Liverpool group confirmed this in 1958: in 14 ABO incompatible matings in which the ABO group of the sensitizing fetus could be established this always turned out to be compatible with that of the mother (*41*). The implication was that when fetal Rh-positive cells entered the Rh-negative mother's circulation they were eliminated through ABO incompatibility before sensitization to Rh could commence, as had been suggested by R.R. Race and R. Sanger (42). Finn (43) confirmed this by studying a number of families with Rh-negative mothers in which at least four children had been born without any sign of either maternal sensitization or hemolytic disease: in those families where the husband was Rh positive there was a preponderance of ABO-incompatible matings compared with the general population. These considerations prompted the Liverpool group to initiate experimental studies on the influence of ABO incompatibility on the prevention of Rh hemolytic disease, the results of which they published in 1961 (44). They found that:

(1) Fetal cells could be detected in the blood of 11.7% of 256 postpartum women.
(2) Rh antibodies developed in two out of three women who had experienced large fetal bleeds and in only one out of 75 in whom no fetal cells could be detected.
(3) Fetal cells were never found in the mother when there was ABO incompatibility.
(4) Most significantly, injection of radiolabeled Rh-positive blood into six Rh-negative male volunteers led to the more rapid elimination of the cells when they were given intravenous anti-Rh (anti-D) antibody 30 minutes later.

Furthermore, they showed that some of the donor cells still circulating were coated with the antibody. Finn et al. concluded this landmark paper by writing: "Our results suggest it may be possible to prevent most cases of Rh sensitization, and thus eliminate Rh haemolytic disease".

This conclusion was borne out by further studies by the same group (45) in which a large number of Rh-negative male volunteers (made up partly of blood donors and partly of inmates of the Maryland State Penitentiary) were given Rh-positive blood and anti-D plasma. Provided a large enough dose of anti-D was administered only three out of 21 treated men made their own antibodies, compared with 11 out of 21 in the control group. Preliminary work suggested that anti-D gammaglobulin given intramuscularly was more effective than "the most powerful plasma we have used". They cautioned, nonetheless, that further experimental work was necessary before clinical application, but expressed the hope that "the technique will prevent most cases of Rh immunization and thus in time help to eliminate Rh haemolytic disease of the newborn".

Two years later (1965) Woodrow et al. (46) carried out further studies on post-menopausal Rh-negative women and showed that treatment with 5 ml of anti-D gamma2-globulin given intramuscularly was highly effective in clearing Rh-positive cells from their circulation. They also concluded from the study of positive cells in women before and after delivery that in the majority of cases the cells entered the woman's circulation as a result of transplacental hemorrhage during labor or shortly before it. The Liverpool group proceeded to outline the design and organization of a clinical trial still in progress, and some preliminary results. "At the time of writing . . . the three-month follow-up shows that none of the six protected cases has any evidence of immune-antibody formation, while three out of eight untreated controls have produced immune anti-D."

The Americans V.J. Freda and J.G. Gorman working at Columbia University, New York, became interested in the same problem quite independently and roughly at the same time as the Liverpool group. Their suggestion that it might be possible to prevent sensitization of Rh-negative mothers by giving them Rh antibody was first made in 1962 (47), and two years later they published a report on the successful prevention of experimental Rh sensitization with an anti-Rh gamma2-globulin antibody preparation (48). Their colleague W. Pollack was an Englishman working with the Ortho Research Foundation in New Jersey and he had prepared a sterile 16% solution of gamma2-globulin from the plasma of donors with high anti-Rh titers who had been plasmapheresed repeatedly. The nine experimental subjects were unsensitized group O, Rh-negative male "volunteers" from Sing Sing Prison who were given five monthly intravenous doses of Rh-positive blood. Four of them were passively protected with 5 ml of the globulin preparation 24 hours before each aliquot of blood. It took the antibody three months after the last inoculation to disappear, and none of the four subsequently made anti-Rh antibody in their own right. In contrast, four of the five controls became strongly sensitized after the fourth inoculation. Freda, Gorman and Pollack wrote: "If there are no data forthcoming to show conclusively that the delivery event is not an important factor in Rh sensitization by pregnancy, and if additional studies should confirm the safety and effectiveness of this experimental antibody preparation, then it would be ready for a prompt clinical trial". In an addendum they provided additional data for an expanded group of prisoners, essentially confirming the reported results.

By 1966 Freda, Gorman and Pollack (49) had carried out their own clinical trial, using anti-Rh gamma-G globulin to prevent active immunization of Rh-negative mothers: 107 mothers had been followed for periods of 6–18 months after delivery, about half of them treated and the remainder serving as controls. None of the treated mothers became sensitized, compared with seven of the control group. The authors concluded that ". . . the outlook is fairly promising that gamma-G globulin to the Rh factor will soon become a practical public health measure for the prevention of of Rh hemolytic disease of the newborn".

In contrast to the Wiener–Levine controversy over the discovery of Rh, both the Liverpool and the New York groups gave full credit to the other for its contribution. Indeed, Clarke and Sheppard (50), in a letter to the Lancet, acknowledged the superiority of gamma globulin over plasma and reported that as soon as they had become aware of the work by Freda, Gorman and Pollack they had abandoned plasma. They also drew attention to the fact that a leading article in the Lancet (51) had failed to mention the contribution of the New York group.

In 1994 C.A. Clarke (now Sir Cyril) and R.M. Hussey (52) were able to write in a review of the decline in deaths from Rh hemolytic disease of the newborn: "Giving anti-D immunoglobulin postnatally to Rh negative women to prevent Rhesus haemolytic disease of the newborn in future pregnancies has reduced the incidence of this disease in the U.K. to such low levels that younger doctors are no longer familiar with it".

Although the strategem described here is perhaps not an example of immunoregulation in the strictest sense, it is reminiscent of attempts in the context of tissue and organ transplantation to render the graft less immunogenic, either by culturing endocrine tissues before transplantation or by the removal of passenger cells from organs (see Chapter 6).

References

1. Oberman, H.A. (1981) In *Clinical Practice of Blood Transfusion*, eds. L.D. Petz & S.N. Swisher, p. 9, Churchill Livingstone, New York.
2. Harvey, W. (1628) *Exercitatio Anatomica de Motu Cordis et Sanguinis in Animalibus*, Francofurti sumptibus, Guilielmi Fitzeri.
3. Blundell, J. (1819) *Med. Chir. Trans.* **10**, 296.
4. Landsteiner, K. (1901) *Wien. Klin. Wchnschr.* **14**, 1132.
5. v. Decastello, A. & Sturli, A. (1902) *Münch. Med. Wchnschr.* **49**, 1090.
6. Springer, G.F. (1956) *J. Immunol.* **76**, 399.
7. Williamson, P. & Springer, G.F. (1959) *Fed. Proc.* **18**, 604.
8. Springer, G.F., Horton, R.E. & Forbes, M. (1959) *J. Exp. Med.* **110**, 221.
9. Oriol, R. (1995) In *Blood Cell Biochemistry*, vol 6 (*Molecular Basis of Human Blood Group Antigens*), eds. J–P. Cartron & P. Rouger, p. 37, Plenum Press, New York, London.
10. Mollison, P.L. (1993) *Blood Transfusion in Clinical Practice*, 9th edn, pp. 1–1015, Blackwell Sci. Publ., Oxford.
11. Whitby, L. (1945) *Lancet* **1**,1.
12. Petz, L.D. & Swisher, S.N. (1981) *Clinical Practice in Blood Transfusion*, pp. 1–856, Churchill Livingstone, New York.
13. Garratty, G. (1993) In *Immunobiology of Transfusion Medicine*, ed. G. Garratty, p. 201, Marcel Dekker, New York.
14. Landsteiner, K. (1947) *The Specificity of Serological Reactions*, rev. edn, pp. 1–310, Harvard Univ. Press, Cambridge, Mass.
15. Landsteiner, K. (1917) *Zschr. Immunforsch.* (Orig.) **26**, 122.
16. Hathaway, W.E., Githens, J.H., Blackburn, W.R. *et al.* (1965) *New Engl. J. Med.* **273**, 53.
17. Sazama, K. & Holland, P.V. (1993) In *Immunobiology of Transfusion Medicine*, ed. G. Garratty, p. 631, Marcel Dekker, New York.
18. Leitman, S.F. (1989) *Transfus. Sci.* **10**, 219.
19. McCullough, J., Yunis, E.J., Benson, S.J. *et al.* (1969) *Lancet* **2**, 1333.
20. Levine, P. & Stetson, R.E. (1939) *J. Am. Med. Ass.* **113**, 126.
21. Wiener, A.S. & Peters, H.R.C. (1940) *Ann. Int. Med.* **13**, 126.
22. Landsteiner, K. & Wiener, A.S. (1937) *J. Immunol.* **33**, 19.
23. Landsteiner, K. & Wiener, A.S. (1940) *Proc. Soc. Exp. Biol. Med.* **43**, 223.
24. Levine, P., Katzin, E.M. & Burnham, L. (1941) *J. Am. Med. Ass.* **116**, 825.
25. Levine, P., Newark, N.J., Burnham, L. *et al.* (1941) *Am. J. Obstet. Gynec.* **42**, 925.
26. Levine, P., Vogel, P., Katzin, E.M. *et al.* (1941) *Nature* **94**, 371.
27. Wiener, A.S. & Landsteiner, K. (1943) *Proc. Soc. Exp. Biol Med.* **53**, 167.
28. Wiener, A.S. (1943) *Proc. Soc. Exp. Biol Med.* **54**, 316.
29. Race, R.R., Taylor, G.L. & McFarlane, M.N. (1944) *Nature* **153**, 52.
30. Wiener, A.S. (1944) *Science* **99**, 532.
31. Fisher, R.A. & Race, R.R. (1946) *Nature* **157**, 48.
32. Issitt, P.D. (1993) In *Immunobiology of Transfusion Medicine*, ed. G. Garratty, p. 111, Marcel Dekker, New York.
33. Cartron, J-P. & Agre, P. (1995) In *Blood Cell Biochemistry*, vol 6 (*Molecular Basis of Human Blood Group Antigens*), eds. J–P. Cartron & P. Rouger, p. 189, Plenum Press, New York, London.
34. Levine, P. (1984) *Vox Sang.* (Basel) **47**, 187.
35. Wiener, A.S. (1954) *Rh–Hr Blood Types*, p. 15, Grune & Stratton, New York.
36. Rosenfield, R.E. (1989) *Transfusion* **29**, 355.
37. Jewkes, J., Sawers, D. & Stillerman, R. (1969) *The Sources of Invention*, 2nd edn, p. 348, Macmillan, London.
38. Levine, P. (1943) *J. Hered.* **34**, 71.
39. Stern, K., Davidsohn, I. & Masaitis, L. (1956) *Am. J. Clin. Path.* **26**, 833.
40. Nevanlinna, H.R. & Vainio, T. (1956) *Vox Sang.* (Basel) **1**, 26.
41. Clarke, C.A., Finn, R., McConnell, R.B. *et al.* (1958) *Int. Arch. Allergy* **13**, 380.
42. Race, R.R. & Sanger, R. (1950) *Blood Groups in Man*, 1st edn, Blackwell, Oxford.
43. Finn, R. (1961) Ph.D. Thesis, Univ. Liverpool.

44. Finn, R., Clarke, C.A., Donohoe, W.T.A. *et al.* (1961) *Brit. Med. J.* **1**, 1486.
45. Clarke, C.A., Donohoe, W.T.A., McConnell, R.B. *et al.* (1963) *Brit. Med. J.* **1**, 979.
46. Woodrow, J.C., Clarke, C.A., Donohoe, W.T.A. *et al.* (1965) *Brit. Med. J.* **1**, 279.
47. Freda, V.J. & Gorman, J.G. (1962) *Bull. Sloane Hosp. Women* **8**, 147.
48. Freda, V.J., Gorman, J.G. & Pollack, W. (1964) *Transfusion* **4**, 26.
49. Freda, V.J., Gorman, J.G. & Pollack, W. (1966) *Science* **151**, 828.
50. Clarke, C.A. & Sheppard, P.M. (1965) *Lancet* **2**, 343.
51. Leading article (1965) *Lancet* **1**, 1311.
52. Clarke, Sir Cyril & Hussey, R.M. (1994) *J. Roy. Coll. Phys.* **28**, 310.

4 Immunogenetics: Histocompatibility Antigens – Genetics, Structure and Function

"You may think that our recent history entitles us to feel pretty pleased with ourselves. Perhaps: but then we felt pretty pleased with ourselves twenty-five years ago, and in twenty-five years' time people will look back on us and wonder at our obtuseness."

P.B. Medawar, 1961

The Seminal Influence of Gorer and Snell

The term immunogenetics was almost certainly first coined in 1936 by the geneticist M.R. Irwin, when he and L.J. Cole (*1*) were studying species hybrids in doves and they separated species-specific substances in backcross generations. He continued to use it in this sense and also applied it to the study of the human blood groups. Some ten years later his former student R.D. Owen (*2*) used the term when he described his seminal experiments on the "immunogenetic consequences" of the vascular anastomosis between bovine twins (see Chapter 5) and thereafter it was widely applied to the antigenic systems of red blood cells as well as tissue cells.

In Chapter 2 (p. 68) I refered to the contributions of the early pioneers, foremost among them two American geneticists, E.E. Tyzzer and C.C. Little. They were active in the first few decades of the twentieth century and their researches were largely directed at the genetics of the cellular substances triggering the regression of allogeneic tumors. Reviews of this era include thoses of Bittner (*3*), Little (*4*), Hauschka (*5*) and Snell (*6*). It was Little (*7*) and Little and Tyzzer (*8*) who were the first to suggest a Mendelian explanation to account for susceptibility and resistance to allogeneic tumors, a theory that was to have a profound effect on subsequent workers. However, here I shall make P.A. Gorer my starting point.

Gorer (see biographic sketch, p. 176) was a pathologist working first in the Lister Institute and later in cramped conditions at Guy's Hospital, London, where for many years he ploughed a lone furrow. Inspired by the speculations of his mentor, J.B.S. Haldane, he made several critically important observations in the 1930s, which led directly to the discovery of the first major histocompatibility locus to be identified – H-2 in the mouse. He published two papers in 1936 (*9, 10*) in which he described sera capable of distinguishing between the red blood cells of several strains of inbred mice that Haldane had imported from Bar Harbor, and with the help of absorption tests he found that he could identify two kinds of mice. Using a first generation cross between different strains (or stocks, as he called them) he felt able to state that the strong serologic reaction between natural antibodies present in his own group A serum and mouse red cells was due to a single dominant gene in the red cell donors (*9*). In the second paper (10) he described how he immunized rabbits with red cells from three different lines of mice (the lines had been brother-sister-mated for 25 generations and were therefore virtually homogeneous) and how, again with absorption experiments, he succeeded in identifying several antigens. Thus the albino mice (later known as Strong A) had antigens I and II, but antigen II was relatively unique for that strain. Comparison of the data obtained with his own serum led him to conclude that the human serum had identified yet another antigen (antigen III). He considered four possible explanations for his data, but felt that they "cannot yet be distinguished from another". These possible causes included quantitative differences, differences in determinant groups, and cross-reactivity.

Haldane had earlier suggested to Gorer that tumor resistance factors might be very similar to blood group antigens and, having drawn an analogy between the regression of allogeneic tumors and the destruction of mismatched blood cells in blood transfusion, Gorer now proceeded to put this hypothesis to the test and in 1937–1938 he published several papers on this. I have already summarized these studies in Chapter 2 (p. 69) and I shall merely state here that it allowed him to conclude that two genes governed the transplantability of an A strain sarcoma in C57 Black mice, that antibody formation against antigen II was associated with rejection, and that such antibodies could also be incited by immunization of animals with normal blood. Although J. Klein (11, 12), in his highly recommended books, leans towards 1936 as having seen the birth of the H-2 locus, I am inclined to think that it would be more appropriate to credit this important discovery to the following year, or possibly even to the year 1948 (see below). Not that it matters!

From Gorer's work the notion became firmly established that the "histocompatibility genes", as Snell later called them (13) – the genes determining whether mice were susceptible to allogeneic tumor grafts – were identical to those determining the presence of antigens on the red blood cells and on other tissues of normal individuals of the pure strain in which the tumor had arisen. There can be no doubt that Gorer's discovery proved to be one of the most significant in the development of immunology in the twentieth century.

Meanwhile G.D. Snell had entered the fray (for biographic sketch, see p. 177). Snell was another important pioneer who was to receive the Nobel Prize in 1980, an honor that Gorer would surely have shared had he not died prematurely. Snell joined the Jackson Laboratory at Bar Harbor in 1935, an Institute run by C.C. Little and where Little strongly encouraged him to immerse himself in mouse genetics. Indeed, it was there that Snell edited an authoritative book on the Biology of the Laboratory Mouse (14), which was to become the bible for a rapidly growing band of biologists and immunologists who used the mouse as an experimental subject, taking advantage of the existence of an ever increasing number of highly inbred strains. Because Snell believed that there were many genes controlling resistance, he proceeded to establish coisogenic resistant lines (later called congenic) – lines of mice created by repeatedly backcrossing the progeny between two strains and selecting in each generation animals that were resistant to a particular tumor. The outcome of such backcrosses is to create lines of mice differing at only one or very few genetic loci. Snell (13) described the procedures he was to adopt in 1948. This innovation led to the production of large numbers of such lines, each carrying its particular gene and gene product, and it gave the study of histocompatibility antigens in the mouse a huge impetus. Others, among them D.C. Shreffler and J.H. Stimpfling, added to the burgeoning 'library' of congenic strains.

By the mid-1940s Snell and Gorer had become familiar with each other's investigations and in 1946 Gorer joined Snell in Bar Harbor for joint experiments using some of the available congenic lines. This resulted in the publication of a crucially important paper in 1948 in the *Proceedings of the Royal Society* (*15*), appropriately enough communicated by J.B.S. Haldane. They used six inbred strains – A, CBA, C57 black and dba (subline 2), P and CA, and their backcrosses. The latter strain was homozygous for the gene 'fused,' resulting in a grossly deformed tail. Combining Snell's tumor transplantation approach with Gorer's red cell agglutination technique, they found that:

(1) The gene coding for tumor resistance was closely linked with the gene 'fused.'
(2) The tumor resistance gene in the A strain was identical with the gene coding for Gorer's antigen II.
(3) Serologic testing was on the whole preferable to tumor inoculation in identifying genotypes.

They called the gene coding for antigen II 'H' and they were able to assign a genotype for each of the six strains. Because A strain tumors could elicit antibodies other than anti-II they concluded that "a tumour (sic) may give a single-gene ratio but contain more than one antigen". They finished their paper by stating: "It was shown some time ago (Gorer 1936) that the CBA strain also contained an antigen related in a similar manner to II. Recently, this has been shown to be true of the C3H strain as well. All these antigens differ from one another so there may be a long series of alleles at this locus. Tentatively we suggest that the dba gene studied should be considered an allele and designated H". Although H was later changed to H-2 this historic paper established H-2 as the first major histocompatibility locus or complex, and the assumption that it possessed "a long series of alleles" was subsequently proved to be prophetic.

As Dunn and Caspari (*16*) had identified the gene 'fused' on the ninth chromosome it was clear that H-2 was likewise present on that chromosome. Although clearly excited by their discovery, Gorer and Snell cannot possibly have guessed at the complexity of the genetic locus they had identified or at the overriding importance of its gene products in the activation and execution of the immune response. That only became clear three decades later.

Snell's personal recollections (*17*) are to be found in Terasaki's *History of Transplantation*; they are written with the modesty and understatement typical of this softly spoken New Englander.

H-2: Its Complexity Unraveled

Although both Gorer and Snell continued to develop their ideas, the explosion of research into the structure and function of H-2 did not come about until several years after their joint 1948 paper. This might have been due to two reasons, though neither seem very convincing. First, the papers they published were not easy to read and absorb by biologists and immunologists who lacked a sound knowledge of genetics, and thus their huge significance was not immediately self-evident. Second, Gorer was by no means the most lucid of communicators when giving talks or lectures at scientific meetings, only partly because – being a chain smoker – he invariably had a cigarette dangling from the corner of his mouth! It is striking that neither Gorer nor Snell read papers at the first Ciba Foundation Symposium devoted to transplantation in 1954 (18) although Medawar had been instrumental in its organization. Even in his prestigious Harvey Lecture of 1957 Medawar (19) gave them but a passing reference, though he did ackowledge that "we are especially indebted to G.D. Snell and P.A. Gorer and their respective colleagues" for the genetic evidence showing that "the antigens which can cause transplantation immunity are numerous and under an uncompromising genetical control". However, the Ciba Foundation Symposium on transplantation held in London in 1961 was dedicated to Gorer, who had died that year, and in his opening remarks Medawar (20) paid tribute to Gorer's huge contribution: "Although Peter Gorer's discoveries and ideas will pervade all our discussions, now and for many years to come, we shall miss him grievously as a colleague and a friend. Gorer had for many years been the world's leading authority on the serology and serological genetics of homograft reactions." It was Medawar (21) who wrote Gorer's biographic memoir for the Royal Society.

Gorer became interested in the antibody response to allogeneic tumors – his strong support for the humoral destruction of allografts is mentioned in Chapter 3 – and several technical advances enabled him to measure hemagglutinating antibodies quantitatively. Thus he found that the use of suitably absorbed human serum facilitated the detection of mouse alloantibodies (22) and he was able to conclude that a tumor's ability to grow in a foreign strain is due to "a high resistance to the action of antibodies". A few years later he and Mikulska (23) used such a red cell-absorbed human serum and mouse isoantibodies diluted in a high molecular weight dextran in a method of isoagglutination that was sensitive enough for analyzing humoral allograft responses to both neoplastic and normal tissues, which became widely used. Shortly afterwards Gorer and O'Gorman (24) described a cytotoxicity test for nucleated cells based on the uptake of trypan blue by dead cells, and this soon replaced the leukocyte agglutination test previously established by Amos (25).

Meanwhile Snell (26) had continued his genetic analysis by showing that the H-2a allele expressed at least two antigens, but the work of Hoecker, Counce and Smith (27) and Amos, Gorer and Mikulska (28) made it clear that the H-2 alleles identified at that time coded for several antigens, usually four or five. By 1953 Snell, Smith and Gabrielson (29) had identified as many as nine H-2 alleles and Allen (30), likewise working in Bar Harbor, described a tenth two years later; but this proved to be merely the tip of the iceberg. As Gorer (31) pointed out in his 1956 review of tumor immunity, the number of mice used in such experiments, though large, "represent a very small random sample of the species as a whole. Therefore any generalizations concerning the frequencies of various H-2 combinations and individual antigens must be made with some reserve". Many more were to be described and thus, in a relatively short time, the extraordinary polymorphism of the H-2 complex was revealed. Each allele was given a lower case superscript designation (H-2a, b and so on).

It is quite impossible here to give a blow by blow account of the detailed dissection of the H-2 complex and the reader is referred to the historic reviews in the two books devoted to H-2 by Jan Klein (11, 12), who later made numerous important contributions himself. To quote from his 1975 book (12): "By the late 1960s, the H-2 system consisted of approximately 24 different haplotypes, over 30 antigens, and six histocompatibility regions. Because of this system's forbidding complexity, the H-2 workers soon found themselves relatively isolated, and although they continued to probe deeply into the system, they found little outside interest in their accomplishments. The H-2 system was often considered an exotic curiosity detached from reality", I believe this statement to contain more than a germ of truth: for those who did not belong to the H-2 fraternity, listening to expert discussions on H-2 tended to be like listening to people speaking a foreign language.

Several important developments occurred in the 1960s and 1970s. First, Shreffler and Owen (32) discovered a genetic locus comprising two alleles (Ss), which was "closely linked to or a part of the H-2 region in the ninth linkage group" and coded for a specific serum protein, which was later shown to have two allotypic forms (33). Shreffler (34) placed this locus right in the middle of the H-2 complex, with H-2 alleles on either side, and it became fashionable thereafter to describe H-2 as a system rather than a complex.

In 1973 Demant et al. (35), working in Hašek's Institute in Prague, identified the function of the Ss alleles as controlling the production of one of the proteins of the complement cascade, a finding that they felt "strengthens the hypotheses on evolutionary and functional interrelationships between components of the major histocompatibilty complex", and they cited both Snell (36) and Ivanyi (37) in this context. These interrelationships and the evolutionary significance of the presence of the Ss locus within H-2 were illuminated when it later became clear that the same was true for the human major histocompatibility complex (MHC; human leukocyte antigens, HLA), and here it fell to Meo, Krasteff and Shreffler (38) to identify the serum protein involved as the fourth complement component (C4), Fu et al. (39) already having found yet another close association between HLA and a locus controlling complement C2 deficiency. Meo et al. (40) were able to locate the C2 locus, made up of codominant alleles, within the HLA complex. "It has been suggested that all genes of MHC are related in origin, and thus in function, being derived from one or a few ancestral genes according to Darwinian 'descent with modification'. Furthermore, they have been kept together during evolution in a limited chromosomal area by natural selection", they wrote, and they quoted Ceppellini – the theoretic mastermind of the histocompatibility fraternity. It was about this time (the mid-1970s) that one of the vital functions of MHC antigens became understood (see Chapter 2 and below) and one of these functions involved the ability of T lymphocytes to kill virus-infected cells. The close association between the MHC and complement, which are both vital in the defense against viruses, suddenly seemed less esoteric, though still difficult to explain. Even in 1995 the MHC complex presents some baffling features, prompting the question "What is the MHC?" (41).

It is conceivable that the enthusiasm of the H-2 workers might have declined in the 1960s had it not been for the discovery of the human MHC (HLA). The development of this will be described below but once it became apparent that the overall structure of the MHCs for mouse and man were extraordinarily similar, interest became even more intense: clearly these complexes had been conserved, to a degree, during the course of evolution and that suggested that they were serving some basic functions unconnected with the role of their antigens in transplantation. This was further emphasized by two observations. First, Lilly, Boyse and Old (42) revealed a link between a gene closely associated with H-2 and susceptibility to infection with the Gross virus, and this gene was later shown to be within the H-2 complex. It was to be the forerunner of the numerous associations later described between HLAs and diseases of various kinds. Second, there was the vitally important demonstration by McDevitt and Tyan (43) that the antibody response in mice to synthetic poly-peptide antigens was linked to the H-2 complex (and hence localized in the ninth linkage group) and this was soon confirmed for three such antigens (44). To quote McDevitt and Chinitz (44): "the response ... appears to vary independently with respect to ability to respond to the other two synthetic polypeptide antigens. Such a picture is compatible either with multiple loci controlling the ability to respond to these antigens (all closely linked to the H-2 locus) or with multiple alleles (five or more) at a single locus controlling the immune response to these antigens". It was subsequently shown that these "immune response (Ir) genes" control all kinds of responses, from graft rejection and delayed-type hypersensivity to antibody produc-tion to a large number of different antigens (45); and the work of McDevitt et al. (46) also made it clear that the Ir-1 gene, although it appeared to be distinct from the H-2 genes (but see below), was located right in the middle of the H-2 complex. Some of these early studies and the even earlier observations on high and low responder strains of mice and guinea pigs were well reviewed by McDevitt and Benacerraf in 1969 (47). As it turned out, the immune response genes proved to be the class II histocompatibility genes (see below). Although Benacerraf was to share the Nobel Prize with Snell and Dausset in 1980, the omission of McDevitt, who had done so much to discover the immune response genes, from a prize dedicated to histocompatibility and immune response genes, was surprising.

The Two Locus Model of H-2: Controversy and Resolution

The hunt was now on – and we are now in the late 1960s, but mainly in the 1970s – for a closer understanding of the structure and organization of H-2. A large number of independent workers and their colleagues contributed to this, and it will not be possible to give all of them full credit. Most were American, but several Czechs who had fled from their country, among them J. Klein, P. Demant and V. Hauptfeld, made important contributions. The Americans included, apart from Snell himself, C.S. David, D.C. Shreffler and J.H. Stimpfling, as well as B.D. Amos and E.A. Boyse, though the latter two had emigrated from Britain, having originally come from Gorer's stable in London. G. Hoecker from Chile and H. Festenstein (a South African who had escaped from the oppressive apartheid regime to Britain) likewise made significant contributions.

In 1971 the Norwegian immunogeneticist, E. Thorsby (48), suggested a "tentative new model" for the organization of the H-2 system. Drawing on his knowledge of the human HLA system, with its closely linked subloci named at that time LA and Four (see below), he proposed that the complexities of H-2 – with its 17 alleles and about 30 apparently different antigens – could be most easily accommodated by postulating that they consisted of two segregant series, K and D, with the Ss locus between them. It was based on the assumption that, as for HLA, each H-2 allele determined only one antigen and that the other H-2 specificities, based largely on serologic evidence, were brought about by cross-reacting antibodies. Thorsby believed that such a model "amplifies the homology between the H-2 and HL-A systems" – a point he developed further in the same year (49).

The concept of homology between H-2 and HL-A was, as Thorsby acknowledged, not new. As far as I am able to ascertain, it was first mooted in 1968 by an Anglo-French group led by Davies (50), who based their arguments on the structural similarity between H-2 and HL-A molecules and on their finding that the extraction procedures were virtually the same for both. This met with the briefest, but nonetheless interested, response from M.F.A. Woodruff (51), who raised one clear difference between the two systems: the expression of H-2 on mouse red blood cells but the absence of HLA on human red corpuscles. In replying to this implied criticism, Davies et al. (52) pointed out that human reticulocytes do carry certain HLA and that there are considerable differences between species and even between different mouse strains in the ease with which red cells agglutinate. They finished their letter by stating: "The question will be settled only when analyses are available of demonstrably homogeneous H-2 and HL-A preparations. . . We will wager a bottle of Scotch on the outcome, having in mind Sir Michael's knowledge of the best sources". I don't know whether that wager was ever accepted or, if so, kept!

Thorsby's proposal met nonetheless with a robustly worded response from Klein and Shreffler (53), who produced a detailed critique and claimed that Thorsby's interpretation of serologic data has "confused and confounded the interpretation with the system of notation used to represent serologic findings". They were critical of the "complex-simple" model (54) favored by Thorsby, according to which "each H-2 molecule carries only a single antigenic site which is recognized by a heterogenous population of cross-reacting antibodies". Klein and Shreffler preferred the "simple-complex" hypothesis, which postulates that "each H-2 molecule carries more than one antigenic site and the multiple sites are recognized by specific antibodies". However, the homology between H-2 and HLA and the MHC systems of other species later became firmly established and Thorsby's (49) conclusion that "HL-A and H-2 are not only homologous but very similarly organized, no matter which model is ultimately shown to be correct", has stood the test of time. In fact, in the same year in which Thorsby published his "tentative new model" of H-2 Snell, Cherry and Demant (55) showed that the "private" H-2 specificities could be arranged in two mutually exclusive systems, "possibly homologous with two subsystems of HL-A". These two allelic series appeared to be at the two ends of the H-2 crossover map, and these private specificities induced especially high titers of cytotoxic antibodies compared with the "public" specificities, which were shared by different H-2 phenotypes. Thus Thorsby's hypothesis received strong support from the H-2 guru himself – his "cross-reacting antibodies" almost certainly directed at public as opposed to private antigens.

Klein (12) and Klein and Shreffler (56) very soon accepted the two locus model, but a third locus had to be added: the Ir region coding for a separate set of antigens (the Ia or 'immune response associated' antigens) with quite different properties and functions (see below). Indeed, in his 1972 paper with Shreffler (56) Klein provided supporting evidence for the two-gene model rather than for the hitherto accepted model postulating multiple regions controlling histocompatibility antigens. Their evidence was derived from skin transplantation studies of 14 well-defined H-2 crossovers, and they felt that, in addition, "the genetic, serological and biochemical findings ... can be more readily explained by the assumption that there are only two histocompatibility regions (loci) in the H-2 system, H-2D and H-2K, which are separated by loci controlling serum proteins (Ss-Slp), immune response (Ir-1), and perhaps others".

The Early History of HLA

Before considering the Ia genes and the discovery of non-H-2 loci (the minor loci), the early history of HLA will be considered, for in many ways studies on these two MHC systems began to run in parallel, with one influencing the other. Those working on HLA undoubtedly benefitted greatly from the knowledge already accumulated on H-2 and progress was therefore remarkably rapid. One other factor accounted for the rapid progress and for the fact that, unlike the blood group serologists in the 1930s, the HLA fraternity avoided the pitfalls of rival nomenclatures. This factor was the inception of regular (biannual) workshops, always published rapidly under the title of *Histocompatibility Testing*, which were attended by HLA workers and those working on the MHC of other species. At these workshops, the specificity of the plethora of new antibodies and the antigens they defined was searchingly tested, numbers were allocated to antigens, and the theoretic implications of new findings were discussed. This is where the big guns of the burgeoning HLA fraternity – J. Dausset, J.J. Van Rood, R. Ceppellini, P. Terasaki, R. Payne, B.D. Amos, E. Thorsby, R. Walford, F. Kissmeyer-Nielsen, W. Bodmer, R.J. Batchelor, H. Balner, E. Albert and their colleagues, among many others – met in closed session to make sense of the latest findings. These workshops also provided quality control for anti-HLA sera and helped to train workers in newly created tissue typing laboratories. The man who must be credited for this important innovation is B.D. Amos, who has described the genesis of the workshops (57) and who organized the first of a long series in 1964 in Durham, North Carolina. This first conference comprised a symposium as well as a workshop (58) and it set the pattern for subsequent meetings. Some idea of the explosive interest in HLA may be gained from the length of the published proceedings: 192 pages in 1964, 288 at the Leiden workshop a year later, 432 plus workshop report in Torino in 1967, and 658 in the United States in 1970. A further development of considerable importance was the creation of The Transplantation Society in 1968, which succeeded the series of New York conferences organized by the American surgeon J.M. Converse under the auspices of the New York Academy of Sciences. This took under its wing not only histocompatibility in humans and animals, but the whole range of experimental and clinical transplantation, thus uniting all interests in its biannual congresses. Amos was again instrumental in launching this international society, which proved to be a powerful catalyst in the development of transplantation.

The foundations for the HLA complex may be said to have been laid in the same year – 1958 – by three individuals working in hematology laboratories: Jean Dausset in Paris, Rose Payne at Stanford University and Jon Van Rood in Leiden. In 1952 Dausset and Nenna (59) had described some antileukocyte antisera detectable by agglutination, the sera having come from patients who had received multiple blood transfusions. Other workers, including Payne (60), subsequently encountered febrile blood transfusion reactions that were clearly not attributable to blood group incompatibility. Dausset, Nenna and Brecy (61) and Whyte and Yee (62), with the Rh analogy in mind, had wondered whether fetal leukocytes could induce antibodies like that in the mother, but Killmann (63) had failed to establish a connection between pregnancy and the formation of leukocyte agglutinins.

Three important papers were published in 1958. First, Dausset (64) (for biographic sketch see p. 179), using an agglutination technique, identified a leukocyte antigen that he called 'MAC' in individuals whose cells had been exposed to a panel of antisera from patients who had received multiple blood transfusions. Having typed a group of individuals with the antiserum he found that the cells of three of them were rarely agglutinated. He assumed that these three lacked an antigen that was widely prevalent in the French population and, somewhat perversely, the name MAC was made up from the first letters of the names of the three non-reacting individuals. Dausset satisfied himself that the antigen was not a conventional blood group antigen. MAC turned out to be present in about 60% of the French population. Dausset again emphasized that transfusion reactions should be avoidable by the use of blood from which leukocytes had been largely removed. The paper was written in French and although the names of some other workers were mentioned there was, surprisingly, no reference list.

The second set of observations came from Rose Payne. She had been visited by Dausset in 1956 and they had discussed their mutual interest in transfusion reactions and antileukocyte antisera. She subsequently found that febrile reactions could occur even after a single transfusion, but only in women who had given birth to more than one child. Such mothers seemed to be reacting against fetal leukocyte antigens inherited from the father, and she published her data with M.R. Rolfs in 1958 (65). Thus they found leukocyte agglutinins in 17% of the 144 multiparous women tested even though none had previously received a blood transfusion. Furthermore, the maternal sera agglutinated the leukocytes of 10 out of 12 of their newborn infants and 12 out of 13 of their husbands, "suggesting the inheritance by the offspring of the father's leukocyte factor". They noted that "The search for distinct and separate leukocyte types has been attempted with limited success" and went on to say that "A most interesting possibility arises from the finding of leukoagglutinins in non-transfused women. This particular kind of antileukocyte serum may provide the tool necessary for the separation of the different human leukocyte antigens".

Van Rood, Van Leeuwen and Eernisse in Leiden (66, 67) were evidently on the same track when they published their paper, again in 1958, in Vox Sang. Having quoted W. Spielman (68) as the first to describe a leukocyte antibody-mediated transfusion reaction (Dausset and Nenna had in fact anticipated him by three years), they described investigations that had been in progress since 1955: the systematic identification of complete leukocyte antibodies in the sera of patients with febrile transfusion reactions. They came across one woman who underwent a severe reaction after a transfusion given to counter the effects of postpartum bleeding, the woman having had six previous pregnancies. They went on to examine 40 sera from pregnant women that had been stored at low temperature, and after testing them against a panel of cells from 12 normal people, detected antileukocyte antibodies in six. Their preliminary data (67) had been published in *Nature* and there they speculated that the need for a relatively large panel of cell donors was possibly due to "the different antigenic structure of leukocytes... Little is known at present about the clinical significance of these antibodies, except that they produce transfusion reactions". In their fuller paper (66) they were able to state, like Payne and Rolfs, that the agglutinins were present on the leukocytes of the husbands and some of the children, that the sera made it possible to recognize leukocyte groups, and that the relevant antigens were present not only on leukocytes but also on thrombocytes and in placental tissue, though not on erythrocytes. These observations took matters a big step forward. Van Rood, Van Leeuwen and Eernisse concluded their paper by writing: "Although there is still much that is obscure about the leukocyte groups, they may eventually be of some use in forensic medicine and in bone marrow transplantation" – quite the most far-sighted pronouncement made in that fateful year, for HLA typing has remained to this day an absolutely vital ingredient in the successful transplantation of allogeneic bone marrow.

The discovery of the first HLAs must therefore be attributed to the independent observations of Dausset, Payne and Van Rood, though Dausset was the first to identify a particular antigen (i.e. MAC). The significance of these antigens for transplantation was at that time still quite obscure and only subject to conjecture.

The implications of these discoveries were only slowly understood by those working on organ and tissue transplantation even after the HLA concept had been developed. Thus the American transplant surgeon B.O. Rogers (69), in a lengthy review in 1963 entitled "*Genetics of Transplantation in Humans*", discussed the histocompatibility genes of the mouse but seemed to be totally ignorant of the nascent HLA story. Instead, he devoted considerable space to the question of whether blood group antigens played a role in clinical transplantation. He did, however, give prominence to a 1954 paper by Gorer's and Billingham's groups (70) in which they had described the formation of antibodies in mice after skin graft rejection that reacted with red cells as well as with leukocytes of the skin graft donor strain. They had concluded, he wrote, that "It is therefore possible that we might greatly prolong the life of human homografts if we could match them for a relatively small (sic!) number of major antigens".

Further Development of the Human Leukocyte Antigen System

I have so far mainly referred to the 'HL-A' or 'HLA' locus, though it should be said that it was originally designated 'Hu-1' by Dausset, Ivanyi and Ivanyi (71) at the second Histocompatibility Workshop in 1965, by which time ten antigens had been identified. The term HL-A (human leukocyte antigen) was agreed at the third Histocompatibility Workshop in Torino (72) after careful consideration by an international *ad hoc* committee whose recommendation was later endorsed by a formally appointed nomenclature committee. (A verbatim account of the first meeting of the nomenclature committee in 1968 has been published by R.L. Walford (73) and it might afford some amusement to those interested in how its members grappled with the thorny problems confronting them!) The designation was subsequently changed to HLA when the two subloci LA and Four were identified and designated as HLA-A and B, respectively. It is thanks to the unparalleled international cooperation that characterized the Histocompatibility Workshops and the formation of a nomenclature committee that HLA escaped the damaging controversies associated with the Rh nomenclature.

The three "serologically defined (SD)" subloci

Three technical innovations greatly facilitated the analysis of the large number of human histocompatibility antigens that were to be identified. First, Van Rood and his team (74, 75) developed a sophisticated technique for computer analysis of highly complex serologic data. This made it possible to discern patterns in the serologic reactions against large panels of cell donors and allowed conclusions to be drawn from what might otherwise have remained a jumble of meaningless data.

Second, Terasaki and McClelland (76) described a microdroplet assay of human cytotoxic antibodies that required minute amounts of reagents and was relatively quick to carry out; it was further refined a few years later (77, 78) and became the standard method in tissue typing, especially after Terasaki's tissue typing laboratory in Los Angeles had issued its plastic microcytotoxicity tray, which became and has remained a vital tool in the comparative analysis of data throughout the world. It was R. Ceppellini who was evidently the first to see it as a great advance when it was demonstrated at the first Histocompatibility Workshop in 1964 (79, 80) and who was the first to adopt it. It is no exaggeration to say that these two purely technical contributions markedly speeded up the unraveling of the HLA system. It should be added that Sanderson and Batchelor (81) had previously compared the cytotoxic assay read by dye exclusion and with the aid of chromium-51 labeled cells and found the latter to be comparable and preferable.

Third, the fine dissection of the HLA system (as well as the MHC systems of other species) was later, from the mid-1970s onward, greatly facilitated by the advent of monoclonal antibody technology (see Chapter 1).

Although Van Rood's laboratory had originally identified four possible leukocyte antigens, which they designated the numbers 1–4, the first three proved to be erroneous and they were left with a single antigen, "4", with alleles 4a and 4b (82), with a gene frequency of 0.38 and 0.62 respectively. This identified one sublocus that was detectable serologically. A year later Payne et al. (83), who had adopted Van Rood's computer approach and who had the benefit of W. Bodmer's extensive experience as a population geneticist, published evidence for the existence of a separate sublocus, which they called LA, three antigens (LA1, 2 and 3) having been identified. Theirs was later to be called HLA-A and that of the Leiden group HLA-B, with Dausset's MAC antigen subsumed by the former as HLA-A2. Thus a 2-sublocus model of HLA, with independently segregating alleles, became accepted; it received strong support from the genetic and statistical studies of Kissmeyer-Nielsen, Svejgaard and Hauge (84), who provided the first evidence in its favor. Some highly personal (and far from objective!) accounts by some of the HLA pioneers can be found in Terasaki's book on the history of HLA (85). Although the level of international cooperation was of an exceptionally high order, predominantly because of the continuing series of Histocompatibility Workshops, the HLA arena was inhabited by some powerful personalities and, not surprisingly, there was a strong competitive edge to many publications and discussions (73).

The early 1970s saw an extraordinary increase in activity in HLA research, and to accommodate the vast number of papers being published two new journals were formed, *Tissue Antigens* (1971) and *Immunogenetics* (1974). *Transplantation*, the major journal for experimental and clinical transplantation, expanded but even so it was necessary to add yet another journal, *The Journal of Immunogenetics*, in 1974. The *Proceedings* of the *Congresses of The Transplantation Society*, under the genial editorship of F.T. Rapaport, likewise expanded, congress after congress, and eventually became multivolume publications, despite a strict limit on pagination.

As early as 1969 a team led by Dausset (86, 87) had suggested that there might be yet a third sublocus coding for serologically detectable HLA antigens, but the evidence was not conclusive. Likewise, Mickey, Singal and Terasaki (88) believed that they had suggestive evidence for a third sublocus. Walford *et al.* (89) took matters a step further by detecting some additional antigens that could not be accommodated by a two subloci hypothesis. Further highly suggestive evidence came from Thorsby's laboratory (90) a year later, after they had subjected a putative new antigen, which they called AJ and which had been detected in sera from multiparous women, to population and family studies. Conclusive evidence from the same group (Solheim *et al.*, 91) materialized three years later, when they demonstrated that lymphocyte capping (92) of the AJ antigen occurred independently of the antigens of the known two subloci. This new sublocus eventually became known as HLA-C; again it turned out to be polymorphic though not as highly as HLA-A and B, but its antigens did not prove to be of any great importance in clinical organ transplantation.

Lymphocyte-defined Antigens: H-2IA and HLA-D

The discovery in the mid-1960s of the mixed lymphocyte reaction (MLR), resulting from the culture of lymphoid cells or purified lymphocytes of different genetic constitution and expressing itself in terms of cell replication and its sequelae, has been described in Chapter 2 (p. 83). It was made by two independently working groups in the United States – Bain and Lowenstein on the one hand, and Bach and his associates on the other. Initially a two-way reaction, with each set of lymphocytes responding to the histocompatibility antigens of the other, it was converted into a one-way reaction by treating one set of cells with X-irradiation or an antimitotic drug (93). It was thus possible to regard one set of cells as the stimulators and the other as the responders, and the assay could be applied more meaningfully to establish the level of reactivity of a putative transplant recipient against a panel of potential donors. Although both the serologically identifiable antigens and the MLR were predictive of skin graft survival between siblings (see below), it was initially not clear whether the two approaches identified different transplantation antigens. Certainly Amos and Bach (94), though reporting several exceptions – including two sisters with identical HL-A genotype who responded to each other in cell-mediated lympholysis (CML) – to the generally good correlation between MLC identity and serologic identity, saw no reason in 1968 to postulate a separate sublocus coding for antigens responsible for MLR activity.

Students of the mouse MHC now took up the running in identifying yet another sublocus controlling the antigens responsible for the MLR. By 1972 the conception of H-2 was of a highly complex system consisting of K and D ends, each highly polymorphic, with the Ss-Slp and Ir loci closely associated with them. "It was natural," Bach *et al.* wrote in 1972 (95), "that since MLC (mixed lymphocyte culture) activation was dependent on MHC differences, SD (serologically detected) antigen differences were responsible for stimulation." As these authors, who included J. Klein, themselves showed (95), this proved to be a gross oversimplification, for by using congenic mouse strains carrying recombinant MHC chromosomes they were able to demonstrate that the strongest MLC activation was associated with Ir region differences, H-2K or H-2D differences alone causing very weak stimulation or none at all. Indeed, they confirmed this remarkable finding by showing that in strain combinations that were identical for H-2K and D antigens there could nonetheless be MLC activation (96, 97). Bach *et al.* therefore began to think in terms of serologically-defined (SD) and lymphocyte-defined (LD) antigens and they believed that the genes controlling the LD antigens lay within the Ir region. They speculated that the Ir product could be the T cell receptor, a suggestion that was to be a non-starter. They concluded their paper (95): "The findings presented in this paper force us to reevaluate the genetic and immunological complexity of the major histocompatibility complex. The possibility that the MLC test can be used to detect the Ir loci products or alternatively define yet other loci of this region present exciting possibilities for future research". That turned out to be very true. The concept of SD and LD defined antigens was enthusiastically accepted by those working in the field. It is worth noting that whereas most investigators were concerned with either H-2 or HLA, it was fortunate that both Amos and Bach straddled the divide.

Close on their heels there followed a paper by Sachs and Cone (98), which took matters a big step forward. They used as their springboard previous studies showing that humoral responses across species included the production of antibodies against the MHC antigens of the donor animal – an observation that Sachs, Winn and Russell (99) had first made and others had confirmed. Rats hypersensitized with mouse lymphoid tissue produced an antiserum that should have contained antibody to only one weak specificity (H-2.31) but which was highly cytotoxic. Using appropriate congenic strains, they produced alloantisera that likewise detected the same specificity, and to their surprise Sachs and Cone found that the new antigen thus identified, which they called beta, was expressed preferentially on B lymphocytes. Finally, they were able to show that the determining gene was linked to the K-end of H-2, probably "in or to the left of the Ir-1 region". "The strain distribution of this antigen indicates that it is probably part of an allelic system and we are presently attempting to define other alleles." They noted that the percentage of lymph node cells killed by anti-beta and complement varied in different strains, a finding that they attributed to differences between the cell types in the lymph nodes of different strains. The beta antigen proved to be the first of many Ia antigens to be identified (they were later called class II antigens) and it was subsequently shown that their special activity was concerned with T lymphocyte activation and MLC stimulation. The Ia antigens proved to have a wider distribution than just on B lymphocytes: they were found on antigen-presenting cells such as macrophages, activated T lymphocytes and epidermal cells, and even on spermatozoa (*100*). The finding that Ia antigens were serologically detectable gave a great boost to the study of the Ir region in the mouse and the equivalent D region in humans, both coding for class II antigens.

In the same year – 1973 – two further important contributions were made in the study of antigens controlled by the Ir region of H-2. First, Hauptfeld, Klein and Klein (*101*) found that reciprocal immmunization of congenic lines differing only in the middle of the H-2 system, where the Ir region was known to reside, produced an antibody against an antigen that they called Ir-1.1. Like the beta antigen (but unlike other H-2 antigens) it had a restricted tissue distribution, being present on a subpopulation of lymphocytes found in lymph nodes and spleens, but absent in bone marrow and thymus. Based on experiments with mice that had been thymectomized at birth they arrived at the tentative conclusion that the cells carrying Ir-1.1 were probably T and not B lymphocytes. This was diametrically opposed to the conclusion of Sachs *et al.* that antigens determined by the Ir region are present on B lymphocytes and must have been due to a technical flaw or an error of interpretation.

Second, David, Shreffler and Frelinger (*102*), using recombinant mouse strains, detected an antigen "Lna" (lymph node antigen) by serologic means. Its gene was once again mapped in the Ir region between H-2K and Ss-Slp. Although the antigen was present on lymph node cells it was also found on peripheral blood cells, splenocytes and thymocytes; yet only about half of lymph node cells succumbed to a highly cytotoxic antibody. Two allelic forms of the antigen were defined, each associated with a different H-2 haplotype. The authors noted "sufficient parallels between Lna and Ir/MLR systems to raise the question whether the so-called lymphocyte-detected antigens of the H-2 system may not also be serologically detected", but they could not be certain whether the antigen was the product of Ir or MLR genes or "independent genes that happen to map in the same chromosomal region".

Evidence for an Ir-associated region now came thick and fast. For example, Klein, Hauptfeld and Hauptfeld (*103*) found that mouse strains identical for H-2K and D and differing only in part of the Ir region rejected skin allografts very rapidly. They proposed the term H-2I for this third locus, which they mapped as being within the Ir region, close to H-2K. In the same year and in the same journal the three groups that had reported Ir-associated antigens (see above) got together and agreed on a notation, according to which the genes controlling these antigens and the antigens themselves (Ir-1.1, beta and Lna) were to be known as Ia (I-region associated antigens) (*104*). This was a considerable simplification that turned out to be wholly justified. Thus the mouse MHC comprised H-2 K, Ia, Ss-slp, and D – a structure very similar to the MHC of other species and of humans.

Meanwhile there had been stirrings within the HLA fraternity, and others likewise concluded that there must be a separate locus coding for the antigens important in MLC activation. The first demonstration by Amos and Bach (*94*) that there can be anomalous reactions between well-matched siblings was confirmed by others. The observations of several groups of workers (*105–108*) that MLC activation occurred between HLA-identical siblings and HLA-identical unrelated individuals suggested that the HLA subloci involved in serotyping were not the only ones important in the MLR. Further evidence for a separate MLC locus was soon provided by Mempel, Albert and Burger (*109*), working in Munich: one sibling showed strong stimulation with three HLA-identical siblings but failed to stimulate the lymphocytes of a sister who differed by one haplotype. "The best explanation for our case seems to be a separate MLC locus closely linked to the HL-A region" and they seemed to think that it was probably closely linked to the second ('Four') locus. By 1975, the year of the sixth Histocompatibility Conference and Workshop (*110*), the situation had become clear. The MLC locus coding for LD antigens had been named the D locus and six antigens had been provisionally identified. This compared with 20 specificities for the A locus, 20 for B, and five for C, though many of these were still provisional and subject to further comparative studies. In many ways 1975 can be regarded as the zenith of the HLA story, for:

(1) The overall structure of the system had been mapped (though subloci of D, DR, DQ and DP, had yet to be identified).
(2) Population studies had been carried out in many countries beyond Europe and the United States showing considerable variations in the frequency of some of the alleles.
(3) Many associations had been uncovered between HLA specificities and diseases (see below).
(4) The controversy about tissue typing and its place in organ transplantation went on unabated.
(5) There was the first glimmer of the true function of MHC antigens (see below).
(6) The D region had been mapped to the left of B so that the linear map now read: D, B, C and A, the letters reflecting chronology rather than location.

The enormous interest in HLA and its role was reflected in the unusually fat *Proceedings* volume of the 1975 Histocompatibility Meeting (*110*) which ran to 1000 pages plus appendices, 74 laboratories from 31 countries having participated. Two years later (*111*) the situation had not changed profoundly, although the number of specificities of the B locus had increased to 33 (20 of them still provisional). The D locus had, however, been subdivided into D (11 specificities identified by cell typing) and DR (seven specificities found on B lymphocytes by serologic methods). Further subloci of the D region – DP and DQ – had yet to be uncovered. HLA was shown to be located on the short arm of chromosome six and to represent approximately one thousandth of the human genome, an astonishingly large proportion, reflecting the many vital functions of MHC antigens.

Meanwhile similar progress had been made in the unraveling of the complexities of the H-2 system of the mouse, in which as many as six SD and five I region loci had been located, though not all of them were to stand the test of time as distinct entities. The remarkable feature of MHC systems – and they have been found in all vertebrate species studied, including the toad *Xenopus laevis* (*112*) – is their unique polymorphism. The study of wild mice by J. Klein and his colleagues (*113–117*) proved to be instructive: a larger number of alleles were present at the two SD loci (K and D) studied than in inbred mice though at a lower frequency, and there was a high degree of heterozygosity. Some of the alleles closely resembled those found in laboratory strains but there were many new specificities. As many as 56 K locus alleles and 45 D alleles were identified, suggesting as many as 2500 possible combinations at these two loci alone. As Klein (*113*) remarked: "...the variability of natural populations at this complex is extraordinary". In his exhaustive book on the mouse MHC Klein (*11*) discussed the possible reasons for this. He cited evidence for supposing that it is not necessarily required for the survival of a wild population as in both the Syrian hamster and the Norway rat MHC polymorphism is minimal. Of the two possible causes of MHC polymorphism he considered genetic drift and natural selection by pathogens and concluded that both probably play a role.

One other development is worthy of mention. In 1966 Festenstein (*118*) described some strong MLC unidirectional reactions between two strains of mice that appeared to have the same H-2 haplotypes; however, when stimulators and responders were reversed using the same strains, there was no stimulation. Festenstein and his colleagues subsequently showed that the determinants triggering this MLR were controlled by a non-MHC locus, which they initially called M (*119*) and subsequently the Mls (mixed lymphocyte stimulation) locus (*120*), and its alleles were identified. Unlike the Ia antigens, the Mls determinants, having triggered an MLR, did not cause the formation of cytotoxic T lymphocytes (*121, 122*) and the rejection of skin (*123*) and cardiac (*124*) allografts, and they did not induce lethal graft-versus-host disease (*125*). However, very feeble graft-versus-host reactions were measurable by a local assay concerned with cell proliferation (*126, 127*).

No equivalent of Mls has so far been uncovered in man and the biologic function of these antigens remained mysterious until very recently, when Marrack and Kappler and their associates (*128, 129*) drew attention to the similarity between the properties of bacterial toxins and Mls products. Both are presented by class II antigens (see below) and both stimulate T lymphocytes bearing Vβs receptors. Mls antigens are now known to cause the intrathymic deletion of all cells bearing Vβs with which they can interact. Although considered to be endogeneous superantigens the Mls products do not appear to be harmful to the mice expressing them and they do not appear to predispose them to disease. Marrack, Kappler and their colleagues (*130, 131*) have suggested that "mice use structures analogous to toxins to protect themselves from the toxic effects of the bacterial superantigens" (*129*). In favor of this notion they quoted the fact that mice lacking T cells bearing toxin-reactive Vβs are resistant to the pathologic effects of the toxins (*132*). Festenstein, who had discovered the mysterious Mls antigens 20 years earlier, unfortunately died prematurely in 1989, just before the analogy between Mls and bacterial toxin superantigens had been made.

Class I and II Antigens

In 1977 Klein (*133*) suggested a great simplification in terminology that at the same time created far greater conceptual clarity. He proposed that all SD antigens controlled by H-2K and D and by HLA-A, B and C should be called class I antigens, and those controlled by the H-2I and HLA-D regions class II antigens. The same was to apply to the antigens of the MHCs of other species. What prompted his proposal was that the structure of class I and II antigens had by then been ascertained and found to be quite different. The terminology, which he used in his review of 1979 (*134*), became widely accepted by the immunologic community. The term class III was reserved for the proteins coded by the genes of the Ss and Slp locus of the mouse and the complement genes of humans.

Chemical structure: enter the biochemists and molecular biologists

Class I antigens

The pioneering work on the extraction of histocompatibility antigens up to 1969 is described in Chapter 2 (p. 88) and has been reviewed by Kahan and Reisfeld (135). The 1970s and 1980s saw a huge surge of activity directed at determining the structure and composition of the antigens, facilitated by developments in molecular biology. Thus it became possible to purify the extracted soluble antigens and to establish the structure of their chains, their molecular weight and their amino acid composition. Hundreds of workers participated in this enterprise and it is possible to mention only some of the more important developments here.

There is no doubt that the biochemists grappling with the isolation, purification and characterization of MHC antigens in the 1960s and early 1970s had to make do with techniques and equipment that were insufficiently sophisticated to enable them to reach definitive conclusions. Even so, it became clear that different H-2 molecules carried only one kind of specificity, and by 1969 ten different molecular species had been distinguished (136). Likewise, it was shown with HLA antigens that different specificities were present on separable molecules (137, 138). H-2 and HLA SD antigens were thought to have a molecular weight of about 50 000 or less (139–142), and Sanderson, Cresswell and Welsh (142) considered it possible that the carbohydrate moiety of HLA molecules might be involved in determining specificity. They thought that HLA-2 had "a remarkable similarity" to fragments of the immunoglobulin heavy chain. Sanderson and Welsh (143) demonstrated that HL-A2 and A7 antigens had their epitopes represented only once on the solubilized molecules, and they went on to calculate the number of determinant sites per peripheral human lymphocyte – approximately 7000 (144).

This was roughly the state of the art when the new breed of molecular biologists stepped in, foremost among them L. Hood at the California Institute of Technology, J.L. Strominger at Harvard University, and P.A. Peterson in Uppsala, Sweden, and their colleagues. By 1977 the picture had become a great deal clearer even though the detailed sequencing of the MHC chains had not yet been done. A two-chain structure had been established for both human and mouse SD antigens, composed of a glycoprotein heavy chain with a molecular weight of about 44 000 closely associated with β_2-microglobulin (molecular weight about 12 000). As the β_2-microglobulin (light chain) was invariant, the variability accounting for different specificities clearly resided in the heavy chain, which was thought to show structural homology with immunoglobulins. The LD antigens, on the other hand, comprised two heavy chains of slightly unequal molecular weight. References to these advances may be found in the paper by Terhorst et al. (145), who themselves further emphasized the similarity between the HLA-B7 heavy chain and immunoglobulins, considerable homology of amino acid sequences having been found. The possibility of such a relationship had already been hinted at much earlier on far less secure evidence (see above), and Peterson et al. (146) had argued in favor of a common evolutionary origin of these two kinds of molecules because of structural similarities. Thus the concept of the supergene family was initiated. Evidence for MHC homology between even very distantly related species, the mouse and the chicken, had also been presented (147).

With the advent of amino acid analyzers, sequencing became widespread and the hunt was on for the complete sequencing of MHC molecules, both class I and II. The first partial sequence was established in 1978 for mouse H-2K and D antigens (*148*): they were found to be homologous, but differed from each other by multiple amino acid substitutions. Their amino acid sequence, however, differed from that of immunoglobulins. Partial sequencing of rat MHC (AgB) antigens was reported a year later and rat antigens were found to be substantially homologous to those of the mouse, human and guinea pig (*149*). The first complete sequence, for the heavy chain of HLA-B7, was determined by Strominger's laboratory in 1979 (*150*): it consisted of a polypeptide of 271 residues with two loops marked by disulfide bonds. "Significant homology" was found between a portion of the molecule and immuno-globulin constant domains as well as β_2-microglobulin. Comparison of the HLA-B7 and HLA-A2 sequences indicated a 74% homology (*151*), but two stretches of greater variability were encountered in two clusters that were thought to be the sites of alloantigenic specificity and polymorphism. Within a year the complete sequence for H-2Kk had been elucidated by Rothbard *et al.* (*152*), who emphasized that it closely resembled H-2Kb, with a mere 11 differences in the heavy chain. These two allelic antigens, with an 88% identity, were more closely related than to either HLA-B7 or A2 (about 70% homology). Complete sequences for HLA-A, B and C antigens were described in 1980 (*153*). Their primary structure encompassed two immunoglobulin-like bisulfide loops and the site for a single carbohydrate moiety was identified. The COOH-terminal one-third of the sequence (called H3) showed a statistically signif-icant homology with immunoglobulins, but not with the rest of the molecule (H1 and 2).

In sequencing the whole of H-2Kb, comprising a 346-residue polymorphic glyco-protein subunit (molecular weight 45 000) covalently linked with a 99-residue constant β_2-microglobulin subunit, Coligan *et al.* (*154*) took a further step forward. By now it had become clear that the COOH-terminal of the heavy chain was anchored in the cell membrane, with the remainder of the molecule extending outside the cell. The heavy chain was organized in three domains (α_1, α_2 and α_3) and the β_2-microglobulin formed the fourth domain. Crystallization and X-ray diffraction studies suggested that the pairing was between α_1 and α_2 and between α_3 and β_2-microglobulin (*155*). Having compared the structure of the mouse H-2Kb molecule with that of other mouse H-2 and with HLA molecules, Coligan *et al.* (*154*) had been struck by the possibility that all these molecules had a common ancestor way back in evolutionary history. The H-2Db molecule was fully sequenced by two groups (*156*, *157*) by 1982.

Class II antigens

The intense interest in the structure of class I antigens was concomitantly extended to the class II molecules, which turned out to have a very different structure. By 1977 incomplete sequences had been established for HLA-DR (*158*), H-2IE (*159*, *160*) and H-2IA (*161*) molecules. The molecular weights of these different molecules were similar: the two non-covalently associated sialoglycoprotein subunits that made up the Ia molecules had molecular weights of 29 000 and 34 000 – which were virtually the same as those of the H-2I-E chains (*160*) – and although they had different amino acid sequences there were also considerable similarities in other parts.

Springer *et al.* (*158*), who had obtained their molecules from human B lymphocytes, reported that the two-chain structure of their glycoprotein was similar to that found for mouse and guinea pig Ia molecules. Once again homology seemed to be the order of the day, suggesting, as for class I molecules, a common ancestry. Silver *et al.* (*162*) compared the I-E chains (α and β) of two strains of mice with human DR molecules. Eα and DRα and the Eβ and DRβ chains showed a high degree of sequence homology with each other "provided a gap is inserted at position 1 of the DRα chain". There were several differences in N-terminal sequences between the two chains of the two strains of mice and the authors concluded that it was likely that the polymorphism of I-E and, by implication, DR molecules resided in the lighter β chain.

In 1982 Kaufman and Strominger (*163*) published a paper in *Nature* in which they were able to propose a more complete structure for human class II antigens, one that is closely in accord with the modern view. Thus the extracellular region of the light (β) chain consisted of two domains, each with a bisulfide loop, the amino-terminal domain bearing the carbohydrate moiety and being polymorphic, whereas the carboxy-terminal domain was "relatively conserved" and with "significant homology with immunoglobulin". On the basis of these findings and similar observations for the heavy chain of DR they were able to propose a model for HLA-DR that has, in its essentials, retained its validity, with both chains anchored in and projecting through the plasma membrane. A year later it became clear that the chain of DR existed as a family, seven β chains having been identified (*164*). In contrast, Walker *et al.* (*165*) were unable to find any differences in the amino-terminal domains of the chains of HLA-DR1 and DR2; differences were, however, discernible in two regions of the chains, each comprising about six amino acids. It was thought "conceivable" that one or both of these regions were responsible for the polymorphism of DR antigens.

Equally impressive advances were made in the analysis of the histocompatibility antigens of other species, especially those of non-human primates and the rat, guinea pig and chicken, for which MHC systems had also been unraveled (*11*, *12*).

Although these advances owed a great deal to impressive technologic innovations I have nonetheless given them some prominence, for two reasons. First, they give a glimmer of the remarkable rapidity with which knowledge of the histocompatibility antigens increased in the 1970s and 1980s, the intelligence and single-mindedness applied and the high level of competition prevalent at that time between laboratories. Such rapid progress was possible because the research groups became larger and larger; in this field, at least, gone were the days when research could be carried out by a single scientist (*vide* Gorer, Medawar or Snell) or even by small groups armed by the simplest technical tools. (I write "glimmer" because only the tip of the iceberg has been considered here.) Second, these studies were clearly of the greatest importance in elucidating the function of histocompatibility molecules. They led directly to the crowning glory of molecular immunology – the determination of the precise three-dimensional structure of these molecules (see below), which more than anything else was to provide a physical basis for speculations on their function in antigen presentation.

The three-dimensional structure of class I and II molecules

In October 1987 *Nature* published two papers by the Strominger/Wiley group that, not surprisingly, the editors of the journal accepted with great alacrity. They created a huge stir in the world of immunology. The first, by Pamela Bjorkman *et al.* (*166*), described how the group had purified HLA-A2 after solubilization with papain (the enzyme used by most investigators) and, having obtained 3–4 mg of protein from 200 liters of cultured cells, how they went on to crystallize the protein. Bjorkman was a young crystallographer recruited from Stanford University and she proceeded to subject the crystals to X-ray diffraction techniques. An electron density map was then calculated to 3.5 Å resolution. "Due to the poor quality of the heavy atom derivatives, the map was not fully interpretable, although the molecular outline and the two immunoglobulin-like domains of α_3 and β_2-microglobulin were evident. Subsequent electron density maps derived from many cycles of model building, phase combination and CORELS refinement permitted the complete structure of a α_3 and β_2-microglobulin to be determined, and about 80% of the main chain of α_1 and α_2 to be fit (*sic*) as segments of polyalanine." To quote their brief summary verbatim: "The class I histocompatibility antigen from human cell membranes has two structural motifs: the membrane-proximal end of the glycoprotein contains two domains with immunoglobulin-folds that are paired in a novel manner, and the region distal from the membrane is a platform of eight antiparallel β-strands topped by α-helices. A large groove between the α-helices provides a binding site for processed foreign antigens. An unknown 'antigen' is found in this site in crystals of purified HLA-A2."

The deep groove was about 25 Å long and 10 Å wide and it ran between the two long helices of the α_1 and α_2 domains. The groove, being located on the top surface of the molecule, "is therefore a likely candidate for the binding site for the foreign antigen that is recognized together with HLA by a T-cell receptor. The dimensions of the site are consistent with the expectation that class I molecules bind a processed antigen, probably a peptide". Bjorkman *et al.* found "a large continuous region of electron density" in this site and, the density level being comparable to that of the protein, they speculated that "most or all of the crystalline HLA molecules have a molecule(s) bound in the proposed antigen binding site. It seems likely that the extra density is the image of a peptide or a mixture of peptides that co-purified and cocrystallized with HLA-A2," and they went on to consider possible sources of such peptides, including "endogenous self peptides created during normal recycling and degradation of cellular proteins". The accompanying paper by the same authors (*167*) considered the implications of these findings for MHC-restriction and antigen presentation and these matters will be considered below.

Within a year the same group with several new co-authors (*168*) proposed "a hypothetical model of the foreign antigen binding site of class II molecules" although the crystal structure of these molecules remained unknown. They did this by comparing the patterns of conserved and polymorphic residues of 26 class I and 54 class II amino acid sequences. The model included a groove or cleft, as for class I molecules, between the C-terminal α-helices of its polymorphic α_1 and β_1 domains, with the bottom of the cleft formed by the N-terminal β-strands of each domain. They believed that "the hypothetical model provides a framework for generating testable models for peptide binding", but concluded by warning that "any hypothetical model derived from even closely related sequences may differ from the true structure in important details and should be thought of only as an imperfect guide for experiments".

The composition and conformation of the putative processed peptide could not be "unambiguously determined", but the fact that the material had remainded attached to the groove throughout the purification and crystallization procedures suggested to the authors that it may indicate that "a conformational change is required to release bound peptide". This remarkable paper was illustrated with exquisitely beautiful color photographs of the electron density maps – photographs that have become the most frequently reproduced in the literature of immunology and cell biology.

It was five years before this hypothetic model could be proven, appropriately enough by the Strominger/Wiley group. Thus Brown et al. (169) found the three-dimensional structure obtained after X-ray crystallography of HLA-DR1 to be similar to that of class I HLA-A2. "Peptides are bound in an extended conformation that projects from both ends of an 'open-ended' antigen-binding groove. A prominent non-polar pocket into which an 'anchoring' peptide side chain fits is near one end of the groove. A dimer of the class II$\alpha\beta$ heterodimers is seen in the crystal forms of HLA-DR1, suggesting class II HLA dimerization as a mechanism for initiating the cytoplasmic signalling events in T-cell activation." They found the electron density in the binding groove to be "straight and thin as expected for a peptide in an extended conformation", and they believed the peptides to be "a collection of endogenous peptides from human lymphoblastoid cells", the cells from which the molecules had been isolated. They believed the electron density of the material in the groove to be consonant with about 15 peptide residues, which was "consistent with the average length of the most abundant peptides bound to DR1 from LG2 cells" – the cells from which the DR1 had been obtained. Brown et al. also made a detailed comparison of the internal structure of the groove (binding site) in class I and II molecules and found some significant differences; for example, a critical binding pocket of DR1 was found to be near one end of the groove, "before the location where the class I groove begins". However, the paper firmly established peptide binding by class II molecules to be similar to that of class I molecules, thus providing a physical basis for the well-known fact that such molecules act as powerful initiators of the immune response.

A mere half century has passed since Gorer's discovery of antigen II in the mouse. It is extraordinary that in that interval we have seen such a flowering of the science of histocompatibility antigens, culminating in the elucidation of their molecular structure.

The Function of Histocompatibility Antigens

In transplantation

Ever since the discovery of antigen II by Gorer, followed by the tumor transplantation studies of Snell and Gorer and their colleagues (see p.131), it was clear that murine tumor donors bearing this antigen (soon to be subsumed by the H-2 system), but absent in the recipient strain, were likely to reject tumor allografts with great vigor. This was made plain by the early work of Snell's group (170) showing that the H-2 alleles carried by donor and host strains were the decisive factor in determing whether or not there was resistance to an allogeneic tumor. Furthermore, it was found in the 1950s that the antigens responsible for the phenomenon of tumor enhancement – the progressive growth of a tumor in a normally resistant recipient – depended on pretreatment of the recipient with H-2 antigens of the donor, either in the form of living or non-viable cells or cell extracts (see Chapter 6).

The importance of H-2 antigens was also amply demonstrated in the induction of neonatal tolerance (see Chapter 5), in which the tolerizing inoculum had to share all the histocompatibility antigens of the test skin graft.

Finally, the role of H-2 antigens in skin allograft rejection was demonstrated in adult mice when Billingham, Brent and Medawar (171) established precise median survival times of grafts transplanted between inbred strains of mice, intrastrain skin grafts being invariably accepted. This observation was to be confirmed by a host of other laboratories (see 172). It soon became apparent that the "strength" of the different subloci i.e. their ability to incite responses against allografts in the (MLR 173) and in graft-versus-host reactions (174) was unequal, the response elicited by H-2D antigens being weaker than that of H-2K antigens. Klein (175) investigated this question with skin allografts using several intra-H-2 crossovers and he came to the same conclusion. He considered several explanations for this, one of them being the possibility that the K sublocus could be linked to a third, as yet unknown and serologically undetectable sublocus. It is quite possible that this may have been the I region. Because of the existence of many scores of inbred and congenic strains and the ease with which allografts could be transplanted the importance of the H-2 antigens was never in any doubt, and that is why they quickly became known as "transplantation antigens" even though Snell had proposed the name "histocompatibility antigens" way back in 1948 (13).

Similar correlations between MHC antigens and allograft reactivity have been established in other experimental species such as the rat and the chicken. With human MHC antigens it was, however, a far more difficult matter to prove that they were important in skin or organ graft rejection, especially as organ transplantation was invariably accompanied by systemic immunosuppression that could so easily obscure the finer aspects of incompatibility. Nonetheless, the fact that identical twins accepted each other's skin (see Chapter 3) and kidney (see Chapter 7) grafts, together with evidence from other species, made it highly probable that the HLA system had to be regarded as the controlling factor in human allotransplantation.

In the mid-1960s J. Dausset, the discoverer of the first human transplantation antigen (MAC) and F.T. Rapaport, who together with J.M. Converse had made the study of human skin allografts his special interest at New York University Medical Center (176), joined forces to establish whether such tissue antigens exerted any influence over the outcome of skin allotransplantation. Ironically, Rapaport et al. (177) had considered some issues bearing on the question of tissue typing and had stated at the first Conference on Histocompatibility Testing in 1964: "It must be emphasized that it is by no means certain that tissue types exist in man. Grave questions have been raised on this subject, particularly in view of the uniform rejection of all skin homografts performed between unrelated or even related individuals, with the exception of those exchanged between identical twins". Dausset *et al.* (*178*) nonetheless published their first study a year after this historic meeting, showing that incompatibility for Van Rood's 4a/4b antigens (later to become members of the HLA-B series) "appeared to have some bearing" on the length of survival of skin grafts. The difference between 'compatible' and 'incompatible' grafts was very small (about two days), as was the number of experimental subjects.

A year later the same group (*179*) extended their observations to volunteers who had been typed for ten putative antigens, but this time the graft recipients were pre-immunized and then grafted with skin from donors who were either compatible or incompatible with the individuals whose tissues were used for immunization. This time the differences were greater, most of the compatible grafts having a more or less normal rejection time (8–12 days) whereas the majority of the incompatible grafts were rejected in accelerated fashion (4–6 days). The authors concluded that "It was demonstrated that Hu-1 leukocyte (tissue) antigens are transplantation antigens". And they confirmed together with H.S. Lawrence that, as Medawar (*180*) had demonstrated in the rabbit, human leukocytes and skin grafts share transplantation antigens (*181*). Van Rood's team (*182*) reported results at the same meeting that were remarkably similar to those of Dausset *et al.* (*179*): individuals who had been presensitized against antigens 6c and 6b rejected skin grafts more quickly if the skin graft donors carried the two antigens. They concluded that these antigens were, by definition, "relatively strong".

These data were strongly confirmed and extended by Amos *et al.* (*183*), who studied graft donor selection based on single locus (haplotype) analysis within families. In a group of 80 sibling transplants the 'compatible' skin grafts survived for more than 15 days (mean = 23) whereas 'incompatible' grafts where uniformly rejected in less than 15. Ceppellini (*184*) came to very similar conclusions and they were entirely upheld by later studies (*185–187*). Thus, by 1969 it was clear that even with the limited number of antigens that had been identified, the transplantation antigens of the HLA system did influence the outcome of skin allograft rejection. Indeed, Thorsby and Kissmeyer-Nielsen (*188*) successfully used human skins allografts to produce potent antisera containing antibodies with limited specificity.

Tissue typing and renal transplantation
In 1964 D.B. Amos organized the first of what proved to be a long and productive series of conferences and workshops on histocompatibility testing and its related problems (*58*). It was to give tissue typing both intellectual standing as a new discipline and a unique opportunity for the comparison and standardization of reagents and data. L. Brent (*189*) had been asked to make "some remarks on the present state of the problem of tissue typing" and he began by stating that although "a valiant attempt was made to evaluate the results obtained at some of the chief clinical centers" by J.E. Murray (*190*), "enthusiasts as well as skeptics have no doubt derived some support from the data presented, for although there have been some notable successes, the longterm survival of patients . . . is still depressingly low". Basing himself on the speculative calculations of I.J. Good (*191*) and D.R. Newth (*192*), he thought that the number of loci controlling transplantation antigens lay

between five and 20 and the number of antigens between 20 and 50, lending "support to the thesis that it would be entirely unreasonable to expect any typing test, no matter how refined, to solve all our problems in one clean stroke". At that time there was no satisfactory serologic typing test, and for that reason he and Medawar (193) had devised a cellular typing test based on the intradermal transfer of normal allogeneic lymphocytes (NLT) in guinea pigs (i.e. on a local graft-versus-host reaction). Gray and Russell (194, see also 195) reported at the same conference that they had applied the test to human volunteers who had then been challenged with skin grafts to assess the efficacy of the test. They concluded that "At the present time we consider that the test has some value". Van Rood et al. (182) had come to similar conclusions, the correlation between graft outcome and NLT response existing "only when the NLT test is considered to be an expression of GVH reactivity". However, with the rapid advances made in serologic testing, with all its advantages over an in vivo test, the NLT test was soon abandoned for clinical use.

Early attempts to prove retrospectively that tissue matching could influence the outcome of kidney allograft survival and function were made by two transplant centers, each using the expertise of P.I. Terasaki (the doyen of tissue typing) and his colleagues from the University of California. The first involved, among many others, T.E. Starzl in Denver, then a young, bright and enthusiastic surgeon (he remained bright and enthusiastic into his mature years. . ., see biographic sketch, p. 342), who had decided to make his career in organ transplantation and who appears in various guises in this history. Among the co-authors was K.A. Porter, an expert histopathologist from St Mary's Hospital, London with whom Starzl developed a long and fruitful collaboration. Thus Starzl et al. (196) published a comprehensive study of 64 patients who were given renal allografts from living donors, both related and unrelated, but excluding identical twins. The standard immunosuppressive treatment then comprised azathioprine; 36 of the patients were alive 13–30 months after transplantation. The paper included a thorough description of the histopathology and the effect of adult thymectomy was monitored. However, here we are concerned with early attempts at tissue typing: 102 crude antisera were used, many of them presumably against the same antigens. "When both members of a pair reacted the same to an antiserum, or if the antigens not represented in the donor were demonstrable in the recipient, a mismatch was not considered to be present." It is hardly surprising that on this crude basis "the correlation of the immunologic rating with the clinical results was imperfect in individual cases, many patients with poor matches have done well and two with good matches have had late difficulty. Furthermore, the extent of donor–recipient incompatibility in the entire group was less than would have been predicted by indiscriminate pairing. These results suggest that the antigens being measured may have some relation, if only indirect, with histocompatibility". The second study yielding suggestive results was published in the same year by Vredevoe et al. (197), this time based on data from Boston.

Further support for tissue typing came from the same group (198) when one year later they tried to assess the possible connection between long-term survival of cadaveric kidneys, protected by the prevailing immunosuppression, and compatibility with the recipients. Typing had advanced and seven putative antigens were typed for. Of 36 kidneys, 21 had survived for 2–3 years despite incompatibility for one or two "major leukocyte antigens", although 15 grafts given to recipients without a mismatch were "clinically superior" to those with antigen incompatibilities in terms of function, survival and histopathology. They concluded that the major leukocyte antigens were indeed transplantation antigens and that "since survival can be attained at times despite mismatches . . . the antigens are intermediate in strength and kidney homograft rejection may occur if excessive numbers of antigens are incompatible or if particular combinations of antigens are mismatched". Here then was an affirmative answer, if qualified, to the question of whether tissue typing could be beneficial. The study was, however, retrospective.

The same group (199) next applied serologic typing prospectively using 32 patients treated in Denver between 1964 and 1965, but the controls were historic, relating to previous results with cadaveric kidneys that had not been matched. Survival at four months was significantly better in the matched group, although survival rates at one year were blurred by three deaths in the matched group. The authors concluded from a very detailed study that "coincidental to matching for provisional leukocyte types, an improved early clinical outcome was obtained with respect to survival and minimization of pathologic changes associated with rejection. Whether the improvements are attributable to the matching procedure or to other unrecognized factors . . . could not be determined". In 1967, Van Rood, Van Leeuwen and Bruning (200), in testing the leukocyte groups 'Four' (ten antigens) and 'Five' (two antigens), provided convincing confirmatory evidence with skin grafts that they were transplantation antigens in the accepted sense and that, in renal transplantation between siblings, survival was "significantly increased if donor and recipients are sibs and their leukocyte groups are identical". This was not the case when the donors were parents.

Further support for the notion that tissue typing had a distinctly beneficial effect was scattered throughout the literature, especially when it became possible to type for both HLA-A and B antigens. The case for tissue typing had been made particularly convincingly for living related donor kidneys. For example, Singal, Mickey and Terasaki (201) analyzed the data from a number of transplant centers and found that leukocyte matching was "highly significantly correlated with the clinical outcome and survival among sibling transplants", with a mean graft survival time for matched donors of more than 90% at four years compared with only just over 40% for unmatched kidneys. For parent to child grafts the results, although statistically significant, were much less impressive. "If the HL-A locus is to be considered the principal histocompatibility locus in man, it is clear that with kidney transplantation utilizing current immunosuppressive therapy an incompatibility for a single allele having any of the five antigens studied is not invariably deleterious. Thus the HL-A antigens are not 'strong' antigens but rather can be thought of as 'intermediate' in strength." In the same year (1969), Patel and Terasaki (202) showed conclusively that crossmatch tests could avoid the disastrous consequences of transplanting cadaveric kidneys into patients with preformed cytotoxic antibodies directed against the graft.

Additional support for tissue typing of cadaveric kidneys came from a British group in the same year. Batchelor and Joysey (203), in analyzing the tissue match of 52 cadaveric renal transplants from three centers in the United Kingdom, found a clear correlation between compatibility for up to seven antigens and clinical outcome. "It is concluded that prospective HL-A typing . . . should be carried out whenever possible, so that multiple incompatibilities can be avoided." Furthermore, Batchelor and Hackett (204) showed that well-matched skin allografts transplanted to badly burnt patients survived consistently longer than poorly matched grafts.

There now occurred one of the more bizarre episodes in the history of transplantation. At the Third International Congress of The Transplantation Society in the Hague in 1970 Terasaki's group presented several papers on histocompatibility matching. One of them was devoted to the problems of reproducibility of the available serologic tests, correlation with clinical outcome and the possibility of new matching procedures. In it (205) Terasaki and M.R. Mickey (his longstanding collaborator and statistical expert) once again stressed the overwhelming case for matching sibling donors, but also referred to difficulties they had encountered in establishing correlations for other donor–recipient combinations. They concluded by stressing "the necessity for worldwide sharing of histocompatibility data with respect to outcome". However, another paper presented at the same Congress, in which they reported some negative correlations, raised such a storm that it was not included in the *Proceedings*, an unprecedented occurrence in a non-refereed journal, and it had to be published, after reassessment, in the journal *Tissue Antigens* (206) – to the credit of its editor, F. Kissmeyer-Nielsen, though he felt it necessary to run an editorial warning the reader of the paper's possible pitfalls. "The paper underscored the lack of correlation between HLA matching with the results of cadaver donor transplants and drew attention because by 1970 tissue typing had reached its pinnacle", to use Terasaki's own words in his much later recollections (207). In particular, Terasaki's group had drawn attention with scrupulous honesty to the fact that some patients with well-matched kidneys fared badly whereas others with badly matched kidneys showed good survival, a point that others had already noted and that was difficult to explain without undermining the status of tissue typing. It is for this reason that not a few transplant surgeons have consistently chosen to ignore typing results, believing that it was more important to get patients off waiting lists and to provide them with kidneys that were in good condition. However, all this was happening at a time when only the HLA-A and B loci had been identified and by no means all of their antigens were known; as for DR typing, that had yet to come. Looking back it seems that the incident was blown up out of all proportion and stances were adopted prematurely, even though the dispute between the pro- and anti-typing factions grumbles on to the present day. For Terasaki's laboratory it had, however, some unfortunate consequences in that within months of the Congress and after a site visit from representatives of the National Institutes of Health his research contract was ended (207). Happily, Terasaki's Tissue Typing Laboratory survived from the income derived from selling its HLA reagents and microtest trays throughout the world as well as with the help of grants from other institutions.

In 1971 the *Proceedings* of an International Symposium on Histocompatibility were published. In their editorial Dausset and Rapaport (208) made it clear that the symposium had been called in an attempt to clarify the confused situation resulting from the controversies at the Hague Congress. "This question is clearly one of the most pressing issues in clinical transplantation today", they wrote. Groups from nine countries had contributed, with virtually all major centers represented, including Terasaki's. The overall view seemed to be (209) that tissue typing was useful, even for cadaveric kidneys, and that there was a clear tendency for the best matched patients to have better graft survival and function than poorly matched patients.

By 1974 the situation had not changed greatly so far as cadaveric donors were concerned, although Opelz, Mickey and Terasaki (*210*) put up a spirited defense for the principle of HLA typing insofar as it related to siblings, cross-matching and the identification of low responders. They were unable to confirm the reports of two other laboratories (*211, 212*) that the second HLA focus (B) influenced organ transplantation more than the first (A). Thus, tissue typing for cadaveric donors went into a state of limbo, having its supporters as well as detractors. Most proponents of typing for renal transplantation found 10–15% differences in the survival of kidneys after two years in the era of HLA-A and B typing, differences that the detractors felt were too small to justify the inevitably longer waiting period for patients. Three factors were to influence such data in future years:

(1) The addition of serologic DR typing, which proved to be an important innovation.
(2) The institution of blood transfusion policies in many centers (see Chapter 7), which tended to obscure the beneficial effect of typing.
(3) The advent of the powerful immunosuppressive drug cyclosporin (see Chapter 7) in the early 1980s, which greatly improved kidney graft survival and tended to minimize the benefits of both typing and blood transfusion (see Chapter7).

An MLR determining locus (later known as DR) associated with HLA, close to the 'Four' locus, was identified by Eijsvoogel *et al.* (*213*) (see above) in family studies in 1972. They postulated that it might be of considerable importance in determining organ graft rejection, a suggestion that seemed to be borne out by the earlier experimental studies of Bildsoe *et al.* (*214*) when they found a clear correlation in rats between serologic typing and MLC reactivity on the one hand, and kidney and heart allografts on the other. Both Ceppellini *et al.* (*215*) and Russell, Nelson and Johnson (*216*) found some suggestive evidence for the notion that MLC stimulation provided advance information about the speed with which human individuals rejected skin allografts, and Bach and Kisken (*217*) confirmed this in family studies. It was, however, a cumbersome test taking several days and therefore not easily applied to cadaver donors. Using a computer, Van Rood and Eijsvoogel (*218*) screened 500 unrelated individuals for HLA antigens ("Four" and "LA" series of antigens), and two pairs were selected for further study because they proved to be phenotypically identical. Only one pair was found to be non-reactive in MLC, "so it is clear that blind testing of unrelated individuals will rarely reveal a pair which does not stimulate in the test". This was confirmed by Bach, Day and Bach (*219*) who additionally found cases where the individual, though serologically HLA-identical, responded in cell-mediated lympholysis (CML).

The serologic identification of some of the human MLC determinants (later designated DR) was first made by Van Rood's group in Leiden (*220*) in 1975; the determinants were found to be present on B lymphocytes and macrophages, and this was rapidly confirmed by Thorsby's group in Norway (*221*) and by others. In the 1977 Histocompatibility Workshop (*111*) eight HLA-D-related B cell specificities were provisionally agreed on (Dw1–7 and WIA8), and Albrechtsen *et al.* (*222*) soon showed that they were "excellent markers for the HLA-D determinants, which can thus be typed for by serologic means"; and they proved to their satisfaction that HLA-D "has great value in predicting the outcome of MLCs". In the same year

(1978) Ting and Morris (223) took a further step forward by retrospectively typing 84 donors and recipients of cadaveric renal allografts and establishing a pecking order in terms of clinical results: the grafts with two DR identities performed better than those with only one, and the latter did better than those with none.

Hard on the heels of Ting and Morris came a prospective DR typing study by Albrechtsen *et al.* (224) revealing very significantly improved kidney graft survival in D-compatible recipients, irrespective of matching for HLA-A and B. Further confirmatory evidence was provided by Persijn *et al.* (225) when reporting the results of a Eurotransplant study: patients well matched for DR had a graft survival that was about 25% better than for mismatched patients two years after transplantation. This group also found quite a strong effect for HLA-A/B matching though the two effects were not additive. Moen *et al.* (226) yet again confirmed the benefit of DR typing in a single center study, though the relatively small numbers prevented the data from being more than statistically just significant. Thus the value of DR typing came to be largely accepted (227). Modern tissue typing involves both HLA-A/B and DR matching, with DR arguably the most influential. However, by 1986 a Scandinavian group (228) reported that, with the introduction of cyclosporine as the main immunosuppressive agent, the HLA-DR typing effect was largely lost.

Nonetheless, the efficacy of tissue typing continued to be questioned by many transplant surgeons and the issue has never been wholly resolved to everyone's satisfaction. Dick *et al.* (229) fired an early warning shot across the bow of the tissue typing enthusiasts by showing in 1972 that a kidney from an HLA-identical brother against whose antigens the patient had not responded in MLC underwent two severe rejection episodes four and six weeks after transplantation. The patient was, admittedly, on a reduced regimen of immunosuppressive therapy at the time.

From the vast and often confusing literature on this controversial topic I will single out one or two more recent contributions, if only to illustrate that the debate has by no means ended. First, a recurrent topic in the "Current Controversies" of the congresses held under the auspices of The Transplantation Society has been the problem of tissue typing. For example, in 1987 Van Rood (230) argued at length why he believed that prospective HLA typing is "helpful" in cadaveric renal transplantation, stressing that the quality of the typing methods was critically important. His opponent in the debate was M.A. Hardy (231) who, in presenting his case, began by stating that to argue against Van Rood was rather like "peeing against the wind (Roumanian proverb)"! He concluded his critique by saying that "... it was not intended to recommend the abandonment of tissue typing, but to encourage its revitalization along more practical and efficient lines, and to point out its present fallibilities".

Second, in 1989 the Leiden group (232) felt it necessary to present the case in favor of A, B and DR matching once again, and they argued that matching "yields a significant beneficial influence on renal allograft survival even in cyclosporin-treated recipients, even five years after transplantation". Survival was, in fact, best in patients treated with this drug even though the drug diminished the difference between well and poorly matched individuals.

Third, two years later, Opelz (233), a former colleague of Terasaki's and now working in Heidelberg, Germany, presented some extensive data based on a Collaborative Transplant Study in which 279 transplant centers in 40 countries had participated. It involved thousands of patients and showed "a stepwise decline in (kidney) graft survival rates with an increase in the number of HLA mismatches". Typing was for HLA-A, B and DR, so that the "best" match was for six antigens. He asked: "With the facts being so overwhelmingly in favor of HLA matching, why is there a controversy?" and concluded that "the answer must be related to the sample size of the patients that were analyzed".

Finally, at the same congress E. Möller (234) argued that conventional typing methods were inadequate and advocated the use of new methods, including genomic typing with cDNA probes for class II genes, cDNA being visualized by autoradiography and restriction fragment length polymorphism (RLFP). Such a technique had been used by Carlsson et al. (235) and had indicated a greater DR and DQ polymorphism than had been revealed by serologic methods. She also pointed out that the binding of peptides by MHC molecules was a further potent complication and that "the identity of MHC-bound peptides and the level of peptide variability that will influence MHC-directed alloreactivity has to be evaluated". The RLFP method of typing is now being used in some transplant centers and differences between this approach and serologic typing have come to light. Opelz et al. (236) found the difference to be as high as 25%, though others (237) found them to be somewhat less. That RFLP typing is superior to serologic typing seemed to be indicated by the observation by the Opelz group that there was almost a 20% difference in terms of kidney graft survival at one year, with 87% of kidneys transplanted to DNA-typed patients surviving. A recent report from the Collaborative Transplant Study found the differences to vary widely from one center to another. It would seem that the technique has yet to be fully mastered by tissue typing laboratories. However, other DNA methodology has already been developed and largely replaced RFLP.

A considerable amount of space has been given to tissue matching, partly because it became a major preoccupation of a large number of geneticists, immunologists and transplantation surgeons in the second half of the century, and partly because – despite the fact that its impact on organ transplantation has not wholly fulfilled expectations – it is of the greatest importance to living related organ donation and to bone marrow transplantation. There is the hope that more sophisticated typing techniques will yet prove to be valuable. Typing has also been an indispensable tool in tracking down HLA associations with numerous diseases (see below) and in research directed at elucidating the role of MHC antigens in immunologic phenomena such as MHC restriction and antigen presentation (see below and Chapter 1). In view of the fact that tolerance induction is generally easier in experimental animals for which the donor is MHC-identical it is probable that any attempts to induce tolerance in patients will have to involve tissue matching. The unraveling of the fine structure of the HLA system, laborious as it has proved to be, has therefore been entirely justified. It is doubtful that without the vast effort expanded on mapping the MHC systems – initially in relation to tissue typing and later to disease associations (see below) – the real significance of MHC molecules in the functioning of the immune system would have come to light.

Human leukocyte antigens and disease: mapping associations

This topic is largely beyond the scope of this book. However, in view of the fact that detailed knowledge of the HLA system has permitted such associations to be made and the likelihood that they will increasingly shed light on the genetics and pathogenesis of such diseases, it is appropriate that this topic should receive at least a mention. What is more, disease associations also underline the general importance of the HLA system and provide pointers to its evolution. The great impact made by monoclonal antibody technology on the fine dissection of the HLA system has been reviewed by Brodsky *et al.* (*238*).

Once again the mouse and its MHC led the way. In 1964, Lilly, Boyse and Old (*239*) published data in the *Lancet*, which was to become the favored journal for others who followed them, from which they concluded that "The susceptibility of mice to the induction of leukaemia by Gross virus is strongly influenced by H-2 type". Their paper finished with the perceptive observation that "This close relation between a histocompatibility factor and susceptibility to the development of leukaemia in the mouse suggests the possibility of similar associations in other species, including man". A few years later Nandi (*240*) made a similar observation for the Bittner virus, a blood-borne form of mammary tumor virus: susceptibility to infection depended strictly on the H-2 alleles carried by the recipient strain of mouse. Although he did not at the time have experimental evidence relating to it, Nandi speculated that the virus may have been "coated with, or associated with, H-2 alloantigens of the host".

The hunt was now on, and it was to lead to an avalanche of papers demonstrating disease–HLA associations in humans. The first came from J.L. Amiel (*241*), working in Villejuif, France, when he compared the HLA profile of patients with Hodgkin's disease with that of normal individuals, using a battery of 45 sera from multiparous women. One antigen (number "5 of Dausset or 4c of Payne") had a prevalence about twice as great in patients as in the controls, but Van Rood, Van Leeuwen and Schippers (*242*) were unable to confirm this. Van Rood (*243*) later explained their failure by suggesting that in the Dutch population there might be linkage disequilibrium between the predisposing Hodgkin gene and the relevant HLA gene. In 1970, Forbes and Morris (*244*), at that time working in Australia, confirmed Amiel's correlation between Hodgkin's disease and the antigen that had previously been designated 4c and which involved an increased frequency to an included antigen, W5 (HL-A5). They considered several possible explanations, including linkage between a disease-determining gene and W5 or cross-reactivity between an oncogenic virus and W5. Several years later the Dutch group (*245*) were able to confirm the association in the Dutch population using more sophisticated typing methods.

A large number of disease associations with different HLA alleles have been described – from 21-hydroxylase deficiency, rheumatoid arthritis, multiple sclerosis, celiac disease, psoriasis, chronic active hepatitis to numerous other autoimmune or infectious diseases. The literature has been exhaustively reviewed (*246–253*), and I will confine myself to the case of ankylosing spondylitis, for which the association with HLA-B27 is so extraordinarily high that presence of the antigen is used diagnostically. The original discovery was made quite independently by two groups, one in the United Kingdom and the other in the United States, and they were published in different journals in the same month of 1973. Using the standard microcytotoxicity technique for tissue typing, Brewerton *et al.* (*254*) found that 72 of 75 (96%) patients with ankylosing spondylitis carried B27 (its later designation) compared with 4% of normal controls, with 52% of first-degree relatives carrying the antigen. The results by Schlosstein *et al.* (*255*) were very similar, the figures being 88% and 8% respectively. "The association . . . is so marked that it is possible to assume either very close genetic linkage of a specific immune responsiveness gene to the disease or perhaps a strong immunologic cross-reaction between W27 and the etiologic agent involved." Brewerton (*256*) later established that a person with B27 was 40 times more likely to develop peripheral arthritis after contracting urethritis, and 50 times more likely to develop a reactive arthropathy after *Salmonella*, *Yersinia* or *Shigella* enteritis than a B27-negative individual. This encouraged Ebringer *et al.* (*257, 258*) to search for Gram-negative organisms in patients – organisms that might cross-react with B27 as a form of molecular mimicry. They found cross-reactivity with *Klebsiella pneumoniae* and showed that the load of this organism in the stool of patients was higher when the disease was active.

A further significant finding was made by Seager *et al.* (*259*): lymphocytes from spondylitic patients reacted feebly to the organism *in vitro*, and a rabbit antiserum against a particular subspecies of *Klebsiella* lysed the lymphocytes of B27-positive patients but not of B27-positive normal individuals. Furthermore, according to Geczy *et al.* (*260*) *Klebsiella* culture supernatants possessed a factor that rendered B27-positive cells from normal individuals susceptible to lysis by anti-*Klebsiella* antibody. These findings strongly suggested cross-reactivity as a mechanism, but they were not universally accepted. McMichael and Bell (*261*) have recently reviewed the four possible mechanisms underlying the B27 association with several diseases in the light of modern notions of MHC molecule structure and peptide presentation. The mechanisms include the possibility of cross-reactivity and a complex "arthritogenic peptide model". It is at present far from clear which, singly or in combination, is primarily responsible.

H-2 restriction phenomena and antigen presentation

Thanks to the observation that many immune responses (e.g. against the minor histocompatibility antigens and against viruses) can occur only in the context of the appropriate MHC alleles (H-2 restriction), and that MHC molecules are specially adapted to bind and present self and foreign peptides, it has become apparent that the functions of histocompatibility antigens are fundamental to the workings of the immune response. This has already been considered in Chapter 3 as well as above in connection with the structure of class I and II molecules. At the same time MHC molecules provide a basis for the distinction between self and non-self. The evolution of these basic molecules and that of their relatives in the supergene family (immunoglobulins, the mouse Thy-1 antigen, CD4 and CD8 molecules, and the T cell receptor) have been the cause of much speculation. Klein (see *11*) has studied the frequency of H-2 alleles in wild mouse populations and has discussed the speed and mechanisms of their evolution at some length. He has speculated that as speciation occurred, each species must start with 15–20 alleles at the polymorphic loci and that to generate about 100 alleles would take substantially longer than one million years. Evolution would come about by natural selection and/or genetic drift.

Bodmer (*262*) has considered the evolution of the HLA system and has argued that early on there must have occurred "fusion of the gene for an Ig domain, possibly derived from a cellular adhesion molecular function, with a gene for a peptide binding domain ... This event, which must have taken place at least 5–7 hundred million years ago in early Cambrian or even pre-Cambrian organisms, was followed by a series of duplications and divergence, leading eventually to the present set of genes". He believes that the first HLA molecule was probably "a homodimer of a fused immunoglobulin and peptide binding domain analogous to the HLA class II molecules", and that class I molecules then arose by duplication of the N-terminal peptide binding domain of the primitive molecule or by "an independent fusion event between the genes for an immunoglobulin domain and an already duplicated peptide binding domain", followed by association with β-microglobulin.

An up-to-date picture of the complexity of the HLA system can be found in the recent review by Campbell (263) and the map compiled by Campbell and Trowsdale (264).

The "Minor" Histocompatibility Antigens: Minor but Important?

Although MHC antigens vary in strength they generally incite strong allograft responses; that is, of course, why they were designated as 'major' antigens. There are, however, a large number of genetic loci quite separate from the MHC region and often located on different chromosomes that code for 'weak' histocompatibility antigens – weak in the sense that their sole presence in an allograft will bring about an immune response so feeble that the graft is rejected very slowly or, in some cases, not at all. They are nonetheless important because certain multiple minor differences can be additive and produce between them a strong response, and because they provide a target for chronic graft-versus-host reactions. They may also play a role in the response of patients to HLA-identical organs, especially when they are siblings, although proof of this has been hard to come by.

The antigen determined by the Y chromosome (H-Y)

In the mouse
The first minor antigen to be discovered, and one that has continued to arouse great interest, is the H-Y antigen – so-called because its allele is located on the Y chromosome. It is present on the nucleated cells of males, but not females, in experimental animals as well as in humans. It was discovered in 1955 by E.J. Eichwald and C.R. Silmser (265) by serendipity. In a very brief paper in *Transplantation Bulletin*, of which Eichwald was an editor and which was to be the forerunner of *Transplantation*, they explained that their observation that male skin grafts are rejected by females of the same inbred strain had arisen from experiments designed to determine "the number and types of genes influencing the fate of skin homografts", using unrelated backcross mice. If Klein (11) is to be believed, it all came about because Eichwald had given his new technician, Silmser, the task of perfecting his skin grafting technique and found to his dismay that some intrastrain grafts were rejected, albeit rather slowly. Both accounts could, of course, be right, but if Klein's story is correct it is an interesting example of Medawar's (266) claim that most scientific papers, including his own, were fraudulent because they misrepresent "the processes of thought that accompanied or gave rise to the work that is described . . .". According

to Eichwald (personal communication) both explanations are in fact correct, the one leading to the other. At any rate, on careful analysis of the skin graft data the unsuccessful grafts were almost invariably male grafts transplanted to females of the same strain or to F1 hybrids. Having ruled out faulty technique Eichwald and Silmser wrote disarmingly that "We are unable to explain the results satisfactorily".

A possible explanation was quickly forthcoming, for in the same number of the journal T.S. Hauschka (267) discussed Eichwald and Silmser's data. After considering and dismissing several possibilities he suggested that the most probable explanation was a gene determining a transplantation antigen linked to the Y chromosome, though he could not exclude androgen dependence. A few months later Snell (268) considered the question in great detail and, having quoted a previous publication by Eichwald, Silmser and Christensen (269) that skin grafts are a far more sensitive indicator of alloreactivity than tumors, concluded that "It is not therefore implausible to postulate a Y chromosome histocompatibility gene in the mouse". Snell pointed out that some H-2 antigens are weaker than others, the genes having "low penetrance", and quoted unpublished data by one of his collaborators, Sheila Counce, who had encountered very slow rejection of skin grafts exchanged between two coisogenic strains (i.e. strains with the same H-2 complex, but differing in the rest of their genome). Survival times were 31 and 24 days respectively and "here donor and host differ at the H-3 locus. We already had evidence from tumor grafting that H-3 was a 'weaker' locus than H-2." Thus the concept of a weak or minor histoincompatibility was established and many more minor loci, of the order of at least 40, were to be identified.

Eichwald is a man of many parts and an affectionate biographic sketch of him was published by J.E. Murray (270) in 1984. He was one of the editors of both journals that were to play an important role in the development of transplantation and an account of how these journals were formed has been given by N. Kaliss (271).

Before mentioning some of the other minor antigens it may be appropriate to follow the history of H-Y. It was soon shown that H-Y was operative in a number of mouse strains (272) although Prehn and Main (273) could not detect it in two strains. Feldman (272) reported experiments from which he deduced that male tissues incited some kind of cytotoxic response in females. On the other side of the coin, Billingham and Silvers (274, 275) had no difficulty in inducing tolerance for the H-Y antigen by inoculating male spleen cells intravenously into female neonatal mice, and Mariani et al. (276) succeeded in inducing tolerance in fully adult mice by giving larger numbers of cells, again intravenously. The H-Y antigen was clearly carried on spermatozoa of the mouse as Katsh, Talmage and Katsh (277) observed accelerated or delayed responses to intrastrain male skin grafts by females, depending on the number of sperms inoculated. The H-Y antigen was thus clearly established as a transplantation antigen, though a minor one in view of its relative weakness compared with H-2 antigens.

Billingham and Silvers, whose neonatal tolerance experiments have been mentioned above, made the biology of H-Y one of their special interests. They showed, for example, that the H-Y antigen was identical in different strains (278), that the basis of the variable results in different strains – females of some strains rejecting all male grafts, females of other strains none at all – was caused by the genotype of the female, which influenced her reactivity to react, as well as by the genetic background of the male, which influenced the expression of H-Y (279). "Thus the complete penetrance of the Y factor in C57 mice is due to the females of this strain being relatively strong reactors against male skin isografts, and not because the antigen is strongest in this strain", they wrote in *Nature* in 1968 together with Barbara Sandford (280) when they considered whether H-Y was Y-linked or sex-influenced. They concluded that "While our observations are consistent with the fact that the male antigen is determined by a histocompatibility locus associated with the Y chromosome, they certainly do not prove this to be the case". And they quoted some work by Poláčková and Vojtíšková (281) showing that a significant proportion of male C57 skin grafts from mice that had been castrated at birth were accepted by adult females of the same strain.

The literature on H-Y became so extensive that it is impossible to trace the development of this fascinating antigen in detail. E. Simpson (282) wrote a comprehensive review in 1982 of the role of H-Y as a minor transplantation antigen. A few issues of special interest will, however, be highlighted here.

First, the same H-Y antigen is expressed in the males of all strains of mice, even in those in which the females do not appear to respond to it. The most persuasive evidence for this was the fact that females of a responder strain could be made tolerant neonatally by the inoculation of male cells from a non-responder strain (275). Second, Gasser and Silvers (283, 284) and Bailey and Hoste (285) found that the ability of female mice to reject male skin isografts was largely determined by the H-2 genotype of the female. For example, out of ten strains tested, six possessed the H-2b allele and were all good responders to H-Y, whereas the other four, which lacked this allele, were poor responders (284). The conclusion that the H-2 locus largely controlled reactivity against H-Y was supported by other studies of this group (286, 287) and in retrospect it seems to have been a clear pointer to the phenomenon of H-2 restriction, which affects both minor histocompatibility and many other antigens, such as those of viruses. A further important step was the demonstration that the H-Y antigen of rats and mice is homologous: thus male lymphoid cells of some rat strains sensitized female mice against male mouse skin grafts (288).

Third, the nature of the response provoked by H-Y needs to be considered. Simpson, in her review (282), pointed out that like other minor histocompatibility antigens, H-Y elicits good cellular (see below) but poor antibody responses. The first group to uncover a cellular cytotoxic response to H-Y were Goldberg, Shen and Tokuda (289) when they showed, in a preliminary communication, that mouse spleen cells taken from females previously sensitized against male skin grafts caused low level lysis of radiolabeled lymph node cells from normal males after incubation for 2–3 days. The assay used by them was that of Canty and Wunderlich (290). "Thus we have in our hands a workable *in vitro* technique for the demonstration of cellular immunity against a minor histocompatibility cell surface antigen." It was E. Simpson and her colleagues at the Clinical Research Center, Harrow, who developed this test and used it to dissect the anti-H-Y cytotoxic response.

In their 1975 contribution, Gordon, Simpson and Samuelson (291) showed conclusively that:

(1) Partially purified primed female spleen cells gave strong cytotoxic responses when cultured for five days with irradiated radiolabeled male spleen cells.

(2) The cytotoxic cells were T lymphocytes.

(3) No response developed in non-responder strains.

(4) The cytotoxic activity was restricted to male target cells histocompatible with the responder strain "over at least a portion of the major (H-2) histocompatibility complex".

They concluded that "the H-Y target cell antigen may be specified by the H-2 complex". They invoked the demonstration by Shearer and by Zinkernagel and Doherty (see Chapters 1, p. 31, and 2, p. 82) of H-2-restricted responses to trinitrophenyl-modified syngeneic cell antigens and to viral antigens, and accepted that either of the two hypotheses put forward by Zinkernagel and Doherty (292) – based on "altered self" or "intimacy" – could be applicable to the H-Y model. A year later Simpson's group pooled their data with those of an American group (293) and showed that "at least some component of H-Y is detected on allogeneic cells *in vivo* during primary sensitization, and that the second set cell-mediated response to H-Y is not necessarily restricted by the H-2 haplotype of the sensitizing strain". In 1977 Simpson's group (294) demonstrated that the H-2 restriction of H-Y required sharing of the K and/or D end of H-2 between the cytotoxic female cell and the male target cell. Their finding that F1 hybrid mice produced from two non-responder strains could be responders led them to think that there was Ir gene complementation, probably in the I-C region. H-2 restriction of minor antigens was thus clearly established.

Fourth, Simpson *et al.* (295) took up the hypothesis proposed by Wachtel *et al.* (296) a decade earlier that H-Y might play a role in primary sex determination. They studied sxr5-carrying female mice obtained from crossing females carrying the T(16;X)16H translocation with sxr-carrying males. The female progeny was both H-Y positive and fertile, demonstrating clearly that H-Y does not impair reproduction in adult females.

Finally, to bring the story of H-Y into the era of molecular biology and right up to date, Rötzschke *et al.* (297) identified a naturally occurring endogenous peptide that can be eluted from class I antigens, giving substance to the notion that the H-Y antigen can be reprocessed *in vivo* by antigen-presenting cells of host origin and presented in the context of H-2 (293). Scott *et al.* (298) have now succeeded in identifying a ubiquitously expressed gene on the short arm of the Y chromosome of the mouse, Smcy, and have established that it encodes an H-YKk epitope (defined as the octamer peptide TENSGKDI) that is not found on the X chromosome, which in turn carries the homologous gene smcx. "These findings provide a genetic basis for the antigenic difference between males and females that contributes towards a tissue transplant rejection response", they wrote. It is a fitting climax to a story that began exactly 40 years before with Eichwald and Silmser's unexplained observations.

In humans

The H-Y antigen has its homolog in other species such as the rat, in which the cytotoxic response to H-Y has likewise been found to be restricted by class I antigens (299, 300). It is therefore hardly surprising that in the mid-1970s a Dutch group provided evidence for its existence in humans. Thus Goulmy *et al.* (301, 302) demonstrated HLA-A2 restricted cytotoxicity of a woman's lymphocytes after she had rejected a male bone marrow transplant, the cytotoxic response being directed mainly at H-Y. Although the biologic function of the H-Y chromosome remains unknown, its existence in man appears to play an adverse role in clinical bone marrow transplantation (303). In kidney transplantation the situation is less clear, although Thoenes, Urban and Doering (304) found that the presence of minor antigens in rat kidneys, additional to MHC antigens, adversely affected the induction of immunologic enhancement.

Other minor histocompatibility antigens

In the mouse

Minor antigens other than H-Y were first discovered in the mid-1950s in Snell's laboratory in Bar Harbor, thanks to the production of coisogenic mouse strains by a series of crosses that introduced on to the background of an inbred strain a gene for graft resistance originally present in the other parent of the initial cross. These weak loci, which were unrelated to H-2 and present on a variety of chromosomes, were designated H-1, H-3 and so on. By 1955 H-3 had been provisionally identified (305) and H-1 by the following year, and they were to be the avant-garde of more than 40 such loci. Counce et al. (306) tested mice differing at the H-3 locus not only with tumors, but also with skin grafts, which gave more quantitative results thanks to their greater sensitivity to weak immune responses. Mean survival times were 31 and 25 days in two different strain combinations differing for H-3, compared with a time of nine days for skin transplanted to H-2-incompatible mice. It was in this paper that the terms 'strong' and 'weak' loci were introduced.

J.H. Berrian and C.F. McKhann, two American workers, made it their business to find out the precise effects minor antigens had on the development of immunity and tolerance, and they published a series of papers in the first half of the 1960s. Transplantation of skin allografts to donor mice differing from the recipients only by the H-3 antigen produced very variable survival times, from 16 to more than 60 days (307), though second-set grafts were rejected more uniformly (8–11 days). Among the possible explanations they considered were prolongation of survival due to tolerance or enhancement, and graft adaptation as suggested by Woodruff (308). Whereas the route by which mice received sensitizing doses of lymphoid cells did not matter greatly for H-2 antigens (309), it affected the outcome very critically when the difference was confined to H-3, the intravenous route establishing tolerance rather than immunity (310). Lymph nodes draining the graft site showed an onset of weight gain at the same time, regardless of whether the difference was strong or weak (311), although the peak response was always near the time of rejection, and this suggested to McKhann that the development of transplantation immunity was biphasic. This and other parameters were further explored by McKhann and Berrian (312) in the same year, when they concluded from skin transplantation and adoptive transfer of immunity studies that:

(1) The longer survival of H-3 disparate grafts was not due to limited antigen release.
(2) Although the transfer of immunizing capacity from graft to host occurred in four days, as for H-2 grafts, a further four days at least were required before a second-set response could be demonstrated.

(3) The regional lymph nodes played a lesser role than in the destruction of H-2 incompatible grafts, as described by Billingham, Brent and Medawar (*313*).

Finally, McKhann published several papers showing that:

(1) The effects of H-1 and H-3 could be additive (*314*).
(2) The effects of immunization with spleen cells were slower in onset but of longer duration for H-3 than for H-2, and immunity could be more easily interfered with for H-3 by, for example, the removal of the regional lymph node at an early stage (*315*).
(3) The intravenous inoculation of spleen cells into adult mice established a longlasting tolerance when the donor differed only for H-3 (*316*), a result that was obtained only with the greatest difficulty and by the use of repeated doses of viable cells in strains differing for H-2 (*317*).

By 1966, 15 minor histocompatibility loci had been identified in the mouse (*318*), 13 of them autosomal and two associated with the sex chromosomes, Y and X. Skin graft survival times differed widely, from 15 to more than 300 days. The H-X antigen was discovered by Bailey (*319, 320*), again by serendipity, when he was grafting mice for an entirely different purpose. In the event he found that skin allografts exchanged between reciprocal male hybrids of several strains were unexpectedly rejected, a result that could have been caused by an antigen carried on either the Y or the X chromosome. He was able to decide that the antigen was associated with the X chromosome when he discovered that it was the skin of the paternal strain – the carrier of the contrasting X chromosome – that was rejected by the hybrid male. Rejection was very slow and usually took 5–9 weeks. Bailey went on to identify a number of other minor loci (*321*).

The additive effect of minor antigens had already been hinted at by McKhann for H-1 and H-3, and Graff *et al.* (*322*) showed very clearly that the effect of multiple antigens could have a cumulative effect on skin graft survival – a point of interest in bone marrow transplantation. Hildemann (*323*) provided evidence for the notion that it was the interallelic combination rather than the H-locus as such that determined the intensity of responsiveness, and he confirmed that graft dose was an important factor, a large dose tending to prolong survival. It was M.J. Bevan (*324*) who showed beyond doubt that the cytotoxic T cell response to minor antigens is MHC-restricted, and Groves and Singer (*325*) later established the same mechanism for tolerance induction to minor self antigens.

In humans

Large numbers of minor loci have been discovered in the mouse and in other animal species thanks to intricate breeding protocols and analysis by tumor and skin grafting. This is clearly not possible in the search for human minor loci and it is hardly surprising that their existence has been demonstrated only in the last two decades. In 1976–1977 Goulmy *et al.* (*326, 327*) provided the first indication of the existence of a human H-Y antigen: a female patient with aplastic anemia who had been given a bone marrow graft from her brother rejected the graft and, subsequently, her lymphocytes could be shown to mount an *in vitro* HLA-A2 restricted cytotoxic response against a panel of male cells. The existence of an HLA-A2 (and B7) restricted human H-Y antigen was confirmed by Pfeffer and Thorsby (328) in the context of kidney transplantation from an HLA-identical brother, and it was concluded that in this case the self-HLA-restricted cytotoxicity against H-Y was "a major cause of rejection". This may, however, have been exceptional, for Ellison et al. (329) were unable to detect an adverse H-Y effect when analyzing the data from a large number of zero-mismatched living donor renal transplants.

Other human minor loci have been identified (330, 331). Remarkably, the HLA-2.1-bound peptide representing one of these (HA-2) was identified in the same year as the mouse H-Y peptide. This became possible after an HLA-A2.1-restricted cytotoxic T cell clone recognizing HA-2 was established from a patient with severe graft-versus-host disease after an HLA-identical bone marrow transplantation. Den Haan et al. (332) were able to conclude that it probably originated "from a member of the non-filament-forming class I myosin family", and that "Because HA-2 has a phenotype frequency of 95% in the HLA-2.1-positive population, it is a candidate for immunotherapeutic intervention in bone marrow transplantation".

Other antigens that could be considered to be minor antigens are the tissue-restricted Sk antigens present in mouse skin and first described by Boyse et al. (333) and the H-2 restricted epa antigens of epidermal cells defined by Steinmuller, Tyler and David (334). Steinmuller's review (335) covers the whole range of tissue-specific/restricted histocompatibility antigens.

Thus it would appear that minor antigens may be of considerable clinical importance, although their biologic role is not completely understood. It is of great interest that a viral origin has been suggested for them, and some persuasive evidence for this has been presented by Colombo, Jarnisch and Wettstein (336) for endogenous retroviruses introduced into mouse embryos. The skin of such mice was rejected by normal coisogenic recipients and cytotoxic responses could be generated to the antigen, which they designated H-43. If their observation has general validity – and it may not – it would explain why both minor and viral antigens should operate via the same mechanism (i.e. MHC restriction).

The puzzle of minor histocompatibility antigens has been freshly considered by Roopenian (337) in the light of contemporary knowledge of allograft rejection and histocompatibility antigens.

An Apology and a Comment

It may well appear that I have painted a far too detailed picture in this chapter. I have done this for several reasons, foremost among them that the story of histo-incompatibility illustrates that the history of biology is often made not by quantum leaps but by a plethora of small steps involving an army of participants; and at the risk of tedium I have tried to do justice to those involved. The other reason is that the story shows how unpredictable the pathways of science can be. What began with some seemingly esoteric observations on red cell antigens in the mouse grew into one of the central features of the immune responsive mechanism.

The story of the histocompatibility antigens is one of compelling interest. The earliest pioneers – Gorer and Snell – were driven along this path because they hoped that it would lead to a better understanding of the pathogenesis of tumors. When it turned out that the antigens involved were of importance in the transplantation of normal tissues and organs the enthusiasm that sustained workers in this field was based on the hope that a detailed knowledge of the transplantation antigens, as they were then called, would greatly facilitate clinical transplantation. Along the way came the realization that the molecules that were being studied were of the greatest importance to the functioning of the immune system, and this provided a spur for the molecular immunologists to discover the detailed structure of these molecules. There can be no doubt that with its unique record of international cooperation and collaboration, which helped to uncover a crock of gold at the end of the rainbow, this story has been one of the greatest triumphs of twentieth-century immunology even though it has not solved the problem of tissue and organ transplantation.

References

1. Irwin, M.R. & Cole, L.J. (1936) *J. Exp. Zool.* **73**, 85.
2. Owen, R.D. (1945) *Science* **102**, 400.
3. Bittner, J.J. (1935) *J. Genet.* **31**, 471.
4. Little, C.C. (1941) In *Biology of the Laboratory Mouse*, ed. G.D. Snell, p. 279, Dover Publ., N.Y..
5. Hauschka, T.S. (1952) *Cancer Res.* **12**, 615.
6. Snell, G.D. (1953) *J. Natl. Cancer Inst.* **14**, 691.
7. Little, C.C. (1914) *Science* **40**, 904.
8. Little, C.C. & Tyzzer, E.E. (1916) *J. Med. Res.* **33**, 393.
9. Gorer, P.A. (1936) *J. Genet.* **32**, 17.
10. Gorer, P.A. (1936) *Brit. J. Exp. Path.* **17**, 42.
11. Klein, J. (1986) *Natural History of the Major Histocompatibility Complex*, John Wiley, N.Y..
12. Klein, J. (1975) *Biology of the Mouse Histocompatibility-2 Complex*, Springer–Verlag, Berlin.
13. Snell, G.D. (1948) *J. Genet.* **49**, 87.
14. Snell, G.D. (1941) *Biology of the Laboratory Mouse*, Dover Publ., New York.
15. Gorer, P.A., Lyman, S. & Snell, G.D. (1948) *Proc. Roy. Soc. B.* **135**, 499.
16. Dunn, L.C. & Caspari, E. (1945) *Genetics* **30**, 543.
17. Snell, G.D. (1991) In *History of Transplantation: Thirty-five Recollections*, ed. P.I. Terasaki, p. 19, U.C.L.A. Typing Lab., Los Angeles.
18. G.E.W. Wolstenholme & M.P. Cameron (eds) (1954) *Preservation and Transplantation of Normal Tissues*, Ciba Found. Symp., J. & A. Churchill Ltd., London.
19. Medawar, P.B. (1957) In *The Harvey Lectures 1956–7*, p. 144, Academic Press, N.Y..
20. Medawar, P.B. (1962) In *Transplantation*, Ciba Found. Symp., eds, G.E.W. Wolstenholme & M.P. Cameron, p. 1, J. &. A. Churchill, London.
21. Medawar, P.B. (1961) *Biogr. Mem. Roy. Soc.* **7**, 95.
22. Gorer, P.A. (1950) *Brit. J. Cancer* **4**, 372.
23. Gorer, P.A. & Mikulska, Z.B. (1954) *Cancer Res.* **14**, 651.
24. Gorer, P.A. & O'Gorman, P. (1956) *Transpl. Bull.* **3**, 142.
25. Amos, D.B. (1953) *Brit. J. Exp. Path.* **34**, 414.
26. Snell, G.D. (1951) *J. Natl. Cancer Inst.* **11**, 1299.
27. Hoecker, G.F., Counce, S.J. & Smith, P. (1954) *Proc. Natl. Acad. Sci. U.S.A.* **40**, 1040.
28. Amos, D.B., Gorer, P.A. & Mikulska, Z.B. (1955) *Proc. Roy. Soc. B.* **144**, 369.
29. Snell, G.D., Smith, P. & Gabrielson, F. (1953) *J. Natl. Cancer Inst.* **14**, 457.
30. Allen, S.A. (1955) *Cancer Res.* **15**, 315.
31. Gorer, P.A. (1956) *Adv. Cancer Res.* **4**, 149.
32. Shreffler, D.C. & Owen, R.D. (1963) *Genetics* **48**, 9.
33. Passmore, H.C. & Shreffler, D.C. (1970) *Biochem. Genetics* **4**, 351.
34. Shreffler, D.C. (1965) In *Isoantigens and Cell Interactions*, ed. J. Palm, p. 11, Wistar Institute Press, Philadelphia.

35. Démant, P., Capková, J., Hinzová, E. *et al.* (1973) *Proc. Natl. Acad. Sci. U.S.A.* **70**, 863.
36. Snell, G.D. (1968) *Folia Biol. (Prague)* **14**, 335.
37. Ivanyi, P. (1970) *Curr. Topics Microbiol. Immunol.* **53**, 1.
38. Meo, T., Krasteff, T. & Shreffler, D.C. (1975) *Proc. Natl. Acad. Sci. U.S.A.* **72**, 4536.
39. Fu, S.M., Kunkel, H.G., Brusman, H.P. *et al.* (1974) *J. Exp. Med.* **140**, 1108.
40. Meo, T., Atkinson, J.P., Bernoco, M. *et al.* (1977) *Proc. Natl. Acad. Sci. U.S.A.* **74**, 1672.
41. Powis, S.H. & Geraghty, D.E. (1995) *Immunology Today* **16**, 466.
42. Lilly, F., Boyse, E.A. & Old, L.J. (1964) *Lancet* **2**, 1207.
43. McDevitt, H.O. & Tyan, M.L. (1968) *J. Exp. Med.* **128**, 1.
44. McDevitt, H.O. & Chinitz, A. (1969) *Science* **163**, 1207.
45. Benacerraf, B. & McDevitt, H.O. (1972) *Science* **175**, 273.
46. McDevitt, H.O., Deak, B.D., Shreffler, D.C. *et al.* (1972) *J. Exp. Med.* **135**, 1259.
47. McDevitt, H.O. & Benacerraf, B. (1969) *Adv. Immunol.* **11**, 31.
48. Thorsby, E. (1971) *Eur. J. Immunol.* **1**, 57.
49. Thorsby, E. (1971) *Tissue Antigens* **1**, 294.
50. Davies, D.A.L., Manstone, A.J., Viza, D.C. *et al.* (1968) *Transplantation* **6**, 571.
51. Woodruff, M.F.A. (1969) *Transplantation* **7**, 290.
52. Davies, D.A.L., Viza, D.C., Colombani, J. *et al.* (1969) *Transplantation* **8**, 740.
53. Klein, J. & Shreffler, D.C. (1972) *Tissue Antigens* **2**, 78.
54. Hirschfeld, J. (1965) *Science* **148**, 968.
55. Snell, G.D., Cherry, M. & Demant, P. (1971) *Transpl. Proc.* **3**, 183.
56. Klein, J. & Shreffler, D.C. (1972) *J. Exp. Med.* **135**, 924.
57. Amos, D.B. (1990) In *Clinical Transplantation 1989*, ed. P.I. Terasaki, p. 61, U.C.L.A. Typing Lab., Los Angeles.
58. *Histocompatibility Testing* (1965) Nat. Acad. Sci. – Nat. Res. Council, Washington D.C.
59. Dausset, J. & Nenna, A. (1952) *Compt. Rend. Soc. Biol. (Paris)* **146**, 1539.
60. Payne, R. (1957) *Vox Sang.* **2**, 233.
61. Dausset, J., Nenna, A. & Brecy, H. (1954) *Blood* **9**, 969.
62. Whyte, H.M. & Yee, I.L. (1956) *Austr. Ann. Med.* **5**, 214.
63. Killmann, S-A. (1957) *Acta Rheumat. Scand.* **3**, 209.
64. Dausset, J. (1958) *Acta Haematol. (Basel)* **20**, 156.
65. Payne, R. & Rolfs, M.R. (1958) *J. Clin. Invest.* **37**, 1756.
66. Van Rood, J.J., Van Leeuwen, A. & Eernisse, J.G. (1958) *Vox Sang.* **4**, 427.
67. Van Rood, J.J., Eernisse, J.G. & Van Leeuwen, A. (1958) *Nature* **181**, 1735.
68. Spielman, W. (1955) *Bibl. Haematol.* **3**, 7.
69. Rogers, B.O. (1963) In *Diseases of the Nervous System*, Monogr. Suppl., **24**, 3.
70. Amos, D.B., Gorer, P.A., Mikulska, Z.B. *et al.* (1954) *Brit. J. Exp. Path.* **35**, 203.
71. Dausset, J., Ivanyi, P. & Ivanyi, D. (1965) In *Histocompatibility Testing*, p. 51, Munksgaard, Copenhagen.
72. *Histocompatibility Testing* (1967), eds E.S. Curtoni, P.L. Mattiuz & R.M. Tosi, Munksgaard, Copenhagen.
73. Walford, R.L. (1990) In *History of HLA. Ten Recollections*, ed. P.I. Terasaki, p. 123, U.C.L.A. Tissue Typing Lab., Los Angeles.
74. Van Rood, J.J. (1962) In *Leucocyte Groupng. A Method and its Application*, Thesis, Leiden.
75. Van Rood, J.J., D'Amaro, DJ., Doetjes, R.S. *et al.* (1972) *Tissue Antigens* **2**, 196.
76. Terasaki, P.I. & McClelland, J.D. (1964) *Nature* **204**, 998.
77. Mittal, K.K., Mickey, M.R., Singal, D.P. *et al.* (1968) *Transplantation* **6**, 913.
78. Mittal, K.K., Mickey, M.R. & Terasaki, P.I. (1969) *Transplantation* **8**, 801.
79. Terasaki, P.I. (1965) In *Histocompatibility Testing*, p. 171, Nat. Acad. Sci. – Nat. Res. Council, Washington, D.C.
80. Terasaki, P.I. (1991) In *History of Transplantation: Thirty-five Recollections*, ed. P.I. Terasaki, p. 511, U.C.L.A. Tissue Typing Lab., Los Angeles.
81. Sanderson, A.R. & Batchelor, J.R. (1967) In *Histocompatibility Testing 1967*, ed. E.S. Curtoni, P.L. Mattiuz & R.M. Tosi, p. 367, Munksgaard, Copenhagen.
82. Van Rood, J.J. & Van Leeuwen, A. (1963) *J. Clin. Invest.* **42**, 1382.
83. Payne, R., Tripp, M., Weigle, J. *et al.* (1964) *Cold Spring Harbor Symp. Quant. Biol.* **29**, 285.

84. Kissmeyer-Nielsen, F., Svejgaard, A. & Hauge, M. (1968) *Nature* **219**, 1116.
85. Terasaki, P.I. (ed.) *History of HLA. Ten Recollections*, U.C.L.A. Tissue Typing Lab., Los Angeles.
86. Dausset, J., Colombani, J., Legrand, L. *et al.* (1969) *Presse Méd.* **77**, 859.
87. Dausset, J., Walford, R.L., Colombani, J. *et al.* (1969) *Transpl. Proc.* **1**, 331.
88. Mickey, M.R., Singal, D.P. & Terasaki, P.I. (1969) *Transpl. Proc.* **1**, 347.
89. Walford, R.L., Finkelstein, S., Hanna, C. *et al.* (1969) *Nature* **224**, 74.
90. Thorsby, E., Sandberg, L. Lindholm, A. *et al.* (1970) *Scand. J. Haemat.* **7**, 195.
91. Solheim, B.G., Bratlie, A., Sandberg, L. *et al.* (1973) *Tissue Antigens* **3**, 439.
92. Taylor, R.B., Duffus, P.H., Raff, M.C. *et al.* (1971) *Nature New Biol.* **233**, 225.
93. Bach, F.H. & Voynow, N.K. (1966) *Science* **153**, 545.
94. Amos, B.D. & Bach, F.H. (1968) *J. Exp. Med.* **153**, 545.
95. Bach, F.H., Widmer, B., Segall, M. *et al.* (1972) *J. Exp. Med.* **136**, 1430.
96. Bach, F.H., Widmer, B., Segall, M. *et al.* (1972) *Science* **176**, 1024.
97. Klein, J., Widmer, B., Segall, M. *et al.* (1972) *Cell. Immunol.* **4**, 442.
98. Sachs, D.H. & Cone, J.L. (1973) *J. Exp. Med.* **138**, 1289.
99. Sachs, D.H., Winn, H.J. & Russell, P.S. (1971) *J. Immunol.* **107**, 481.
100. Hämmerling, G.J., Mauve, G., Goldberg, E. *et al.* (1975) *Immunogenetics* **1**, 428.
101. Hauptfeld, V., Klein, D. & Klein, J. (1973) *Science* **181**, 167.
102. David, C.S., Shreffler, D.C. & Frelinger, J.A. (1973) *Proc. Natl. Acad. Sci. U.S.A.* **70**, 2509.
103. Klein, J., Hauptfeld, M. & Hauptfeld, V. (1974) *Immunogenetics* **1**, 45.
104. Shreffler, D., David, C.S., Götze, D. *et al.* (1974) *Immunogenetics* **1**, 188.
105. Van Rood, J.J. & Eijsvoogel, V.P. (1970) *Lancet* **1**, 698.
106. Eijsvoogel, V.P., Schellekens, P. Th. A., Breur-Vriesendorp, B. *et al.* (1970) *Transpl. Proc.* **3**, 85.
107. Sorensen, F.S. & Nielsen, L.S. (1970) *Acta Path. Microbiol. Scand.* **78B**, 719.
108. Sengar, D.P., Mickey, M.R., Myhere, B.A. *et al.* (1971) *Transfusion* **11**, 251.
109. Mempel, W., Albert, E. & Burger, A. (1972) *Tissue Antigens* **2**, 250.
110. *Histocompatibility Testing 1975*, Munksgaard, Copenhagen.
111. *Histocompatibility Testing 1977*, Munksgaard, Copenhagen.
112. Du Pasquier, L. Chardonnens, X. & Miggiano, V.C. (1975) *Immunogenetics* **1**, 482.
113. Klein, J. (1970) *Science* **168**, 1362.
114. Klein, J. (1971) *Nature* **229**, 635.
115. Klein, J. (1973) *Transplantation* **13**, 291.
116. Zaleska-Rutczynská, Z. & Klein, J (1977) *J. Immunol.* **119**, 1903.
117. Klein, J. & Rutczynská, Z. (1977) *J. Immunol.* **119**, 1912.
118. Festenstein, H. (1966) *Ann. N.Y. Acad. Sci.* **129**, 567.
119. Festenstein, H., Abbasi, K., Sachs, J.A. *et al.* (1972) *Transpl. Proc.* **4**, 219.
120. Festenstein, H. (1974) *Transplantation* **18**, 555.
121. Abbasi, K. & Festenstein, H. (1973) *Eur. J. Immunol.* **3**, 430.
122. Röllinghoff, M., Pfizenmeier, K. Trostmann, H. *et al.* (1975) *Eur. J. Immunol.* **5**, 560.
123. Sachs, J.A., Huber, B. & Festenstein, H. (1973) *Transpl. Proc.* **5**, 1373.
124. Huber, B., Démant, P. & Festenstein, (1973) *Transpl. Proc.* **5**, 1377.
125. Nisbet, N.W. & Edwards, J. (1973) *Transpl. Proc.* **5**, 1411.
126. Huber, B., Peña-Martinez, J. & Festenstein, H. (1973) *Transpl. Proc.* **5**, 1373.
127. Salaman, M.H., Wedderburn, N., Festenstein, H. *et al.* (1973) *Transplantation* **16**, 29.
128. Marrack, P. & Kappler, J. (1990) *Science* **248**, 705.
129. Herman, A., Kappler, J., Marrack, P. *et al.* (1991) *Ann. Rev. Immunol.* **9**, 745.
130. Kappler, J., Pullen, A.M., Callahan, J. *et al.* (1989) *Cold Spring Harbor Symp. Quant. Biol.* **54**, 401.
131. Pullen, A.M., Potts, W., Wakeland, E.K. *et al.* (1990) *J. Exp. Med.* **171**, 49.
132. Marrack, P., Blackman, M., Kushnir, M. *et al.* (1990) *Nature* **332**, 840.
133. Klein, J. (1977) In *The Major Histocompatibility System in Man and Animals*, ed. D. Götze, p. 339, Springer–Verlag, Berlin.
134. Klein, J. (1979) *Science* **203**, 516.
135. Kahan, B.D. & Reisfeld, R.A. (1969) *Science* **164**, 514.
136. Davies, D.A.L. (1969) *Transplantation* **8**, 51.
137. Colombani, J., Colombani, M., Viza, D.C. *et al.* (1970) *Transplantation* **9**, 228.

138. Sanderson, A.R. (1968) *Nature* **220**, 192.
139. Shimada, A. & Nathenson, S.G. (1967) *Biochem. Biophys. Res. Commun.* **29**, 828.
140. Summerell, J.M. & Davies, D.A.L. (1969) *Transpl. Proc.* **1**, 479.
141. Hämmerling, U., Davies, D.A.L. & Manstone, A.J. (1971) *Immunochem.* **8**, 7.
142. Sanderson, A.R., Cresswell, P. & Welsh, K.I. (1971) *Proc. Symp. Immunogenet. of the Mouse H-2 System*, p. 238, Karger, Basel.
143. Sanderson, A.R. & Welsh, K.I. (1974) *Transplantation* **18**, 197.
144. Sanderson, A.R. & Welsh, K.I. (1974) *Transplantation* **17**, 281.
145. Terhorst, C., Robb, R., Jones, C. *et al.* (1977) *Proc. Natl. Acad. Sci. U.S.A.* **74**, 4002.
146. Peterson, P.A., Rask, L., Sege, K. *et al.* (1975) *Proc. Natl. Acad. Sci. U.S.A.* **72**, 1612.
147. Vitetta, E.S., Uhr, J.W., Klein, J. *et al.* (1977) *Nature* **270**, 535.
148. Silver, J. & Hood, L. (1976) *Nature* **73**, 599.
149. Blankenhorn, E.P., Cecka, J.M., Goetze, D. *et al.* (1978) *Nature* **274**, 90.
150. Orr, H.T., López de Castro, J.L., Lancet, D. *et al.* (1979) *Biochem.* **18**, 5711.
151. Orr, H.T., López de Castro, J.L., Parham, P. *et al.* (1979) *Proc. Natl. Acad. Sci. U.S.A.* **76**, 4395.
152. Rothbard, J.B., Hopp, T.P., Edelman, G.N. *et al.* (1980) *Proc. Natl. Acad. Sci. U.S.A.* **77**, 4239.
153. Trägårdh, L., Rask, L., Wiman, K. *et al.* (1980) *Proc. Natl. Acad. Sci. U.S.A.* **77**, 1129.
154. Coligan, J.E., Kindt, T.J., Uehara, H. *et al.* (1981) *Nature* **291**, 35.
155. Bjorkman, P.J., Strominger, J.L. & Wiley, D.C. (1985) *J. Mol. Biol.* **186**, 205.
156. Reyes, A.A., Schöld, M. & Wallace, R.B. (1982) *Immunogenetics* **16**, 1.
157. Maloy, W.L. & Coligan, J.E. (1982) *Immunogenetics* **16**, 11.
158. Springer, T.A., Kaufman, J.F., Terhorst, C. *et al.* (1977) *Nature* **268**, 213.
159. McMillan, A., Cecka, J.M., Murphy, D.B. *et al.* (1977) *Proc. Natl. Acad. Sci. U.S.A.* **74**, 5135.
160. Silver, J., Russell, W.A., Reis, B.L. *et al.* (1977) *Proc. Natl. Acad. Sci. U.S.A.* **74**, 5135.
161. Cook, R., Vitetta, E.S., Capra, J.D. *et al.* (1977) *Immunogenetics* **4**, 437.
162. Silver, J., Walker, L.E., Reisfeld, R.A. *et al.* (1979) *Mol. Immunol.* **16**, 37.
163. Kaufman, J.F. & Strominger, J.L. (1982) *Nature* **297**, 694.
164. Gotz, H., Kratzin, H., Thinnes, F.P. *et al.* (1983) *Hoppe-Seyler's Z. Physiol. Chem.* **364**, 749.
165. Walker, L.E., Hewick, R., Hunkapiller, M.W. *et al.* (1983) *Biochem.* **22**, 185.
166. Bjorkman, P.J., Saper, M.A., Samraoui, B. *et al.* (1987) *Nature* **329**, 506.
167. Bjorkman, P.J., Saper, M.A., Samraoui, B. *et al.* (1987) *Nature* **329**, 512.
168. Brown, J.H., Jardetzky, T., Saper, M.A. *et al.* (1988) *Nature* **332**, 845.
169. Brown, J.H., Jardetzky, T.S., Gorga, J.C. *et al.* (1993) *Nature* **364**, 33.
170. Snell, G.D., Russell, E., Fekete, E. *et al.* (1953) *J. Natl. Cancer Inst.* **14**, 485.
171. Billingham, R.E., Brent, L. & Medawar, P.B. (1954) *Proc. Roy. Soc. B.* **143**, 43.
172. Klein, J. (1986) *Natural History of the Major Histocompatibility Complex*, p. 394, John Wiley, N.Y.
173. Rychliková, M. Démant, P. & Ivanyi, P. (1971) *Nature New Biol.* **230**, 271.
174. Démant, P. (1970) *Folia Biol. (Praha)* **16**, 373.
175. Klein, J. (1972) *Tissue Antigens* **2**, 262.
176. Rapaport, F.T. & Converse, J.M. (1968) In *Human Transplantation*, eds F.T. Rapaport & J. Daussset, p. 304, Grune & Stratton, N.Y.
177. Rapaport, F.T., Dausset, J., Converse, J.M. *et al.* (1965) In *Histocompatibility Testing*, p. 97, Munksgaard, Copenhagen.
178. Dausset, J., Rapaport, F.T., Colombani, J. *et al.* (1965) *Transplantation* **6**, 701.
179. Dausset, J., Rapaport, F.T., Ivanyi, P. *et al.* (1965) In *Histocompatibility Testing 1965*, p. 63, Munksgaard, Copenhagen.
180. Medawar, P.B. (1946) *Brit. J. Exp. Path.* **27**, 15.
181. Rapaport, F.T., Dausset, J., Converse, J.M. *et al.* (1965) *Transplantation* **3**, 490.
182. Van Rood, J.J., Van Leeuwen, A., Schippers, A. *et al.* (1965) In *Histocompatibility Testing*, p. 37, Munksgaard, Copenhagen.
183. Amos, D.B., Ward, F.E., Zmijewski, C.M. *et al.* (1967) *Transplantation* **6**, 524.
184. Ceppellini, R. (1968) In *Human Transplantation*, eds F.T. Rapaport & J. Dausset, p. 21, Munksgaard, Copenhagen.
185. Amos, D.B., Seigler, H.F., Southworth, J.G. *et al.* (1969) *Transpl. Proc.* **1**, 342.
186. Dausset, J. & Rapaport, F.T. (1969) *Transpl. Proc.* **1**, 649.

187. Dausset, J., Rapaport, F.T., Legrand, J. *et al.* (1969) *Nouv. Rev. Franc. d'Hématol.* **9**, 215.
188. Thorsby, E. & Kissmeyer-Nielsen, F. (1968) *Vox Sang.* **14**, 417.
189. Brent, L. (1965) In *Histocompatibility Testing*, p. 3, Munksgaard, Copenhagen.
190. Murray, J.E. (1964) *Transplantation* **2**, 14.
191. Good, I.J. (1952) *Lancet* **2**, 289.
192. Newth, D.R. (1961) *Transpl. Bull.* **27**, 452.
193. Brent, L. & Medawar, P.B. (1963) *Brit. Med. J.* **2**, 269.
194. Gray, J.G. & Russell, P.S. (1965) In *Histocompatibility Testing*, p. 105, Munksgaard, Copenhagen.
195. Gray, J.G. & Russell, P.S. (1963) *Lancet* **2**, 863.
196. Starzl, T.E., Marchioro, T.L., Terasaki, P.I. *et al.* (1965) *Ann. Surg.* **162**, 749.
197. Vredevoe, D.L., Terasaki, P.I., Mickey, M.R. *et al.* (1965) In *Histocompatibility Testing*, p. 25, Munksgaard, Copenhagen.
198. Terasaki, P.I., Vredevoe, D.L., Porter, K.A. *et al.* (1966) *Transplantation* **4**, 688.
199. Vredevoe, D.L., Mickey, M.R., Goyette, D.R. *et al.* (1966) *Ann. N.Y. Acad. Sci.* **129**, 521.
200. Van Rood, J.J., Van Leeuwen, A. & Bruning, J.W. (1967) *J. Clin. Pathol.* **20** (suppl. *Symp. Tissue Org. Transplant.*), 504.
201. Singal, D.P., Mickey, M.R. & Terasaki, P.I. (1969) *Transplantation* **7**, 246.
202. Patel, R. & Terasaki, P.I. (1969) *New Engl. J. Med.* **280**, 735.
203. Batchelor, J.R. & Joysey, V.C. (1969) *Lancet* **1**, 790.
204. Batchelor, J.R. & Hackett, M. (1970) *Lancet* **1**, 581.
205. Terasaki, P.I. & Mickey, M.R. (1971) *Transpl. Proc.* **3**, 1057.
206. Mickey, M.R., Kreisler, M., Albert, E.D. *et al.* (1971) *Tissue Antigens* **1**, 57.
207. Terasaki, P.I. (1990) In *History of HLA: Ten Recollections*, ed. P.I. Terasaki, p. 213, U.C.L.A. Tissue Typing Lab., Los Angeles.
208. Dausset, J. & Rapaport, F.T. (1971) *Transpl. Proc.* **3**, 979.
209. Dausset, J. & Rapaport, F.T. (eds) (1971) *Transpl. Proc.* **3**, 979–1131.
210. Opelz, G., Mickey, M.R. & Terasaki, P.I. (1974) *Transplantation* **17**, 371.
211. Oliver, R.T.D., Sachs, J.A., Festenstein, H. *et al.* (1972) *Lancet* **2**, 1381.
212. Van Hooff, J.P., Schippers, H.M.A., Van der Steen, G.J. *et al.* (1972) *Lancet* **2**, 1385.
213. Eijsvoogel, V.P., Van Rood, J.J., Du Toit, E.D. *et al.* (1972) *Eur. J. Immunol.* **2**, 413.
214. Bildsoe, P., Freiesleben-Sorensen, S., Pettirossi, O. *et al.* (1970) *Transpl. Rev.* **3**, 36.
215. Ceppellini, R., Curtoni, S., Leigheb, G. *et al.* (1965) In *Histocompatibility Testing*, p. 13, Munksgaard, Copenhagen.
216. Russell, P.S., Nelson, S.D. & Johnson, G.J. (1966) *Ann. N.Y. Acad. Sci.* **129**, 368.
217. Bach, F.H. & Kisken, W.A. (1967) *Transplantation* **5**, 1046.
218. Van Rood, J.J. & Eijsvoogel, V.P. (1970) *Lancet* **1**, 698.
219. Bach, F.H., Day, E. & Bach, M.L. (1971) *Tissue Antigens* **1**, 39.
220. Van Rood, J.J., Van Leeuwen, A., Keuning, J.J. *et al.* (1975) *Tissue Antigens* **5**, 72.
221. Solheim, B.G., Bratlie, A., Winther, N. *et al.* (1975) In *Histocompatibility Testing*, p. 713, Munksgaard, Copenhagen.
222. Albrechtsen, D., Bratlie, A., Nousiainen, H. *et al.* (1978) *Immunogenetics* **6**, 91.
223. Ting, A. & Morris, P.J. (1978) *Lancet* **1**, 575.
224. Albrechtsen, D., Flatmark, A., Jervell, J. *et al.* (1978) *Lancet* **2**, 1126.
225. Persijn, G.G., Gabb, B.W., Van Leeuwen, A. *et al.* (1978) *Lancet* **1**, 1278.
226. Moen, T., Albrechtsen, D., Flatmark, A. *et al.* (1980) *New Engl. J. Med.* **303**, 850.
227. Svejgaard, A. (1982) *Transplantation* **33**, 1.
228. Lundgren, G., Groth, C.G., Albrechtsen, D. *et al.* (1986) *Lancet* **2**, 66.
229. Dick, H.M., Briggs, J.D., Wood, R.F.M. *et al.* (1972) *Tissue Antigens* **2**, 345, 480.
230. Van Rood, J.J. (1987) *Transpl. Proc.* **19**, 139.
231. Hardy, M.A. (1987) *Transpl. Proc.* **19**, 144.
232. Persijn, G.G., D'Amaro, J., Lange, G.M. *et al.* (1989) *Transpl. Proc.* **21**, 656.
233. Opelz, G. (1990) *Transpl. Proc.* **23**, 46.
234. Möller, E. (1990) *Transpl. Proc.* **23**, 63.
235. Carlsson, B., Wallin, J., Bohme, J. *et al.* (1987) *Hum. Immunol.* **20**, 95.
236. Opelz, G., Mytilineos, J., Scherer, S. *et al.* (1991) *Lancet* **383**, 461.
237. Middleton, D., Scherer, S., Dunckley, H. *et al.* (1988) *Transpl. Int.* **1**, 161.

238. Brodsky, F.M., Parham, P., Barnstable, C.J. *et al.* (1979) *Immunol. Rev.* **47**, 3.
239. Lilly, F., Boyse, E.A. & Old., L.J. (1964) *Lancet* **2**, 1207.
240. Nandi, S. (1967) *Proc. Nat. Acad. Sci. U.S.A.* **58**, 485.
241. Amiel, J.L. (1967) In *Histocompatibility Testing 1967*, p. 79, Munksgaard, Copenhagen.
242. Van Rood, J.J., Van Leeuwen, A. & Schippers, A. (1968) *Cancer Res.* **28**, 1415.
243. Van Rood, J.J. (1973) *Neth. J. Med.* **16**, 65.
244. Forbes, J.F. & Morris, P.J. (1970) *Lancet* **2**, 849.
245. Van Rood, J.J., Van Hoof, J.P. & Keuning, J.J. (1975) *Transpl. Rev.* **22**, 75.
246. McDevitt, H.O. & Bodmer, W.F. (1974) *Lancet* **1**, 1269.
247. Dausset, J. & Svejgaard, A. (eds) (1976) *HLA and Disease*, Inserm, Paris.
248. Van Rood, J.J. (1975) *Genetics* **79** (suppl.), 277.
249. Ryder, L.P., Anderson, E. & Svejgaard, A. (eds) (1979) *HLA and Disease Registry; Third Report*, Munksgaard, Copenhagen.
250. Bodmer, W.F. (1980) *J. Exp. Med.* **152**, 3535.
251. Batchelor, J.R. & Welsh, K.I. (1982) In *Clinical Aspects of Immunology*, 4th edn, eds P.J. Lachmann & D.K. Peters, p. 283, Blackwell, Oxford.
252. Tiwari, J.L. & Terasaki, P.I. (1985) *HLA and Disease Associations*, Springer-Verlag, N.Y.
253. Batchelor, J.R. & McMichael, A.J. (1987) *Brit. Med. Bull.* **43**, 156.
254. Brewerton, D.A., Caffrey, M., Hart, F.D. *et al.* (1973) *Lancet* **1**, 904.
255. Schlosstein, L., Terasaki, P.I., Bluestone, R. *et al.* (1973) *New Engl. J. Med.* **288**, 704.
256. Brewerton, D.A. (1978) *J. Roy. Soc. Med.* **71**, 331.
257. Ebringer, A., Cowling, P., Ngwa Suh, N. *et al.* (1976) In *HLA and Disease*, eds J. Dausset & A. Svejgaard, p. 27, Inserm, Paris.
258. Ebringer, A., Cawdell, D.R., Cowling, P. *et al.* (1978) *Ann. Rheumat. Dis.* **37**, 146.
259. Seager, K., Bashir, H.V., Geczy, A. *et al.* (1979) *Nature* **277**, 68.
260. Geczy, A.F., Alexander, K., Bashir, H.V. *et al.* (1983) *Immunol. Rev.* **70**, 23.
261. McMichael, A. & Bell, J. (1991) *Res. Immunol.* **141**, 475.
262. Bodmer, W.F. (1995) In *Cancer Surveys: Molecular Mechanisms of the Immune Response* **22**, 5.
263. Cambell, R.D. (1993) In *Genome Analysis* **5**, 1, Springharbor Lab. Press.
264. Campbell, R.D. & Trowsdale, J. (1993) *Immunol. Today* **14**, 349.
265. Eichwald, E.J. & Silmser, C.R. (1955) *Transpl. Bull.* **2**, 148.
266. Medawar, P.B. (1963) *The Listener* **70**, Sept. 12, 1963; reprinted in *The Power and the Glory* (1990), ed. D. Pyke, p. 228, Oxford Univ. Press, Oxford.
267. Hauschka, T.S. (1955) *Transpl. Bull.* **2**, 154.
268. Snell, G.D. (1956) *Transpl. Bull.* **3**, 29.
269. Eichwald, E.J., Silmser, C.R. & Christensen, P.E. (1955) *Transpl. Bull.* **2**, 57.
270. Murray, J.E. (1984) *Transplantation* **37**, 1.
271. Kaliss, N. (1984) *Transplantation* **37**, 3.
272. Feldman, M. (1958) *Transplantation* **5**, 15.
273. Prehn, R.T. & Main, S. (1956) *J. Nat. Cancer. Inst.* **17**, 35.
274. Billingham, R.E. & Silvers, W.K. (1958) *Science* **128**, 780.
275. Billingham, R.E. & Silvers, W.K. (1960) *J. Immunol.* **85**, 14.
276. Mariani, T., Martinez, C., Smith, J.M. *et al.* (1959) *Proc. Soc. Exp. Biol. Med.* **101**, 596.
277. Katsh, G.F., Talmage, D.W. & Katsh, S. (1964) *Science* **143**, 41.
278. Billingham, R.E. & Silvers, W.K. (1963) *Ann. Rev. Microbiol.* **17**, 531.
279. Silvers, W.K. & Billingham, R.E. (1967) *Science* **158**, 118.
280. Silvers, W.K., Billingham, R.E. & Sandford, B.H. (1968) *Nature* **220**, 401.
281. Polačková, M. & Vojtišková, M. (1968) *Folia Biol. (Praha)* **14**, 93.
282. Simpson, E. (1982) *Immunol. Today* **3**, 97.
283. Gasser, D.L. & Silvers, W.K. (1971) *J. Immunol.* **106**, 875.
284. Gasser, D.L. & Silvers, W.K. (1971) *Translantation* **12**, 412.
285. Bailey, D.W. & Hoste, J. (1971) *Translantation* **11**, 404.
286. Gasser, D.L. & Silvers, W.K. (1971) *J. Immunol.* **106**, 875.
287. Wachtel, S.S., Gasser, D.L. & Silvers, W.K. (1973) *Science* **181**, 570.
288. Silver, W.K. & Yang, S-L. (1973) *Science* **181**, 570.
289. Goldberg, E.H. Shen, F.W. & Tokuda, S. (1973) *Transplantation* **15**, 334.

290. Canty, R.J. & Wunderlich, J.R. (1970) *J. Natl. Cancer Inst.* **45**, 761.
291. Gordon, R.D., Simpson, E. & Samuelson, L.E. (1975) *J. Exp. Med.* **142**, 1108.
292. Zinkernagel, R.M. & Doherty, P.C. (1975) *Lancet* **1**, 1406.
293. Gordon, R.D., Mathieson, B.J., Samuelson, L.E. *et al.* (1976) *J. Exp. Med.* **144**, 810.
294. Hurme, M., Hetherington, P.R., Chandler, P. *et al.* (1977) *Immunogenetics* **5**, 453.
295. Simpson, E., Maclaren, A., Chandler, P. *et al.* (1984) *Transplantation* **37**, 17.
296. Wachtel, S.S., Ohno, S., Koo, G.C. *et al.* (1975) *Nature* **257**, 235.
297. Rötzschke, O. Falk, K. Wallny, H-J. *et al.* (1990) *Science* **249**, 283.
298. Scott, D.M., Ehrmann, I.E., Ellis, P.S. *et al.* (1995) *Nature* **376**, 695.
299. Gunther, E. & Wurst, W. (1984) *Immunogenetics* **20**, 1.
300. Gunther, E. (1985) *Transpl. Proc.* **17**, 1849.
301. Goulmy, E., Termijtelen, A., Bradley, B.A. *et al.* (1976) *Lancet* **2**, 1206.
302. Goulmy, E., Termijtelen, A., Bradley, B.A. *et al.* (1977) *Nature* **266**, 544.
303. Storb, R., Prentice, D.L. & Thomas, E.J. (1977) *J. Clin Invest.* **59**, 625.
304. Thoenes, G.H., Urban, G. & Doering, I. (1974) *Immunogenetics* **3**, 239.
305. Snell, G.D., Counce, S., Smith, P. *et al.* (1955) *Proc. Am. Ass. Cancer Res.* **2**, 46.
306. Counce, S., Smith, P., Barth, R. *et al.* (1960) *Ann. Surg.* **144**, 198.
307. Berrian, J.H. & McKhann, C.F. (1960) *J. Natl. Cancer Inst.* **25**, 111.
308. Woodruff, M.F.A. (1959) In *Biological Problems of Grafting*, Congr. Coll. d'Univers. Liège, **12**, 80.
309. Billingham, R.E., Brent, L. & Mitchison (1957) *Brit. J. Exp. Path.* **38**, 467.
310. Berrian, J.H. & McKhann, C.F. (1960) *Ann. N.Y. Acad. Sci.* **87**, 106.
311. McKhann, C.F. (1961) *J. Surg. Res.* **1**, 294.
312. McKhann, C.F. (1961) *J. Immunol.* **86**, 170.
313. Billingham, R.E., Brent, L. & Medawar, P.B. (1955) *Proc. Roy. Soc. B.* **143**, 58.
314. McKhann, C.F. (1964) *Nature* **201**, 937.
315. McKhann, C.F. (1964) *Transplantation* **2**, 613.
316. McKhann, C.F. (1964) *Transplantation* **2**, 620.
317. Brent, L. & Gowland, G. (1963) *Nature* **192**, 1265.
318. Graff, R.J., Hildemannn, W.H. & Snell, G.D. (1966) *Transplantation* **4**, 425.
319. Bailey, D.W. (1963) *Transplantation* **1**, 70.
320. Bailey, D.W. (1964) *Transplantation* **2**, 203.
321. Bailey, D.W. (1972) *Mouse Newsletter* **45**, 15.
322. Graff, R.J., Silvers, W.K., Billingham, R.E. *et al.* (1966) *Transplantation* **4**, 605.
323. Hildemann, W.H. (1970) *Transpl. Proc.* **2**, 24.
324. Bevan, M.J. (1975) *J. Exp. Med.* **142**, 1349.
325. Groves, E.S. & Singer, A. (1983) *J. Exp. Med.* **158**, 1483.
326. Goulmy, E., Termijtelen, A., Bradley, B.A. *et al.* (1976) *Lancet* **2**, 1206.
327. Goulmy, E., Termijtelen, A., Bradley, B.A. *et al.* (1977) *Nature* **266**, 544.
328. Pfeffer, P.F. & Thorsby, E. (1982) *Transplantation* **33**, 52.
329. Ellison, M.D., Norman, D.J., Breen, T.J. *et al.* (1994) *Transplantation* **58**, 818.
330. Goulmy, E. (1988) *Transpl. Rev.* **2**, 29.
331. De Bueger, M. & Goulmy, E. (1993) *Transpl. Immunol.* **1**, 28.
332. Den Haan, J.M.M., Sherman, N.E., Blokland, E. *et al.* (1995) *Science* **268**, 1476.
333. Boyse, E.A., Lance, E.M., Carswell, E.A. *et al.* (1970) *Nature* **227**, 901.
334. Steinmuller, D. Tyler, J.D. & David, C.S. (1981) *J. Immunol.* **126**, 1747.
335. Steinmuller, D. (1984) *Immunol. Today* **5**, 234.
336. Colombo, M.P., Jarnisch, R. & Wettstein, P.J. (1987) *Proc. Nat. Acad. Sci. U.S.A.* **84**, 189.
337. Roopenian, D.C. (1992) *Immunol. Today* **13**, 7.

Biographies

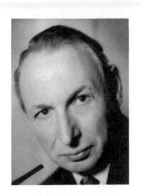

PETER ALFRED GORER
(1907–1961)

Peter Gorer was born in London, the son of Edgar Gorer, a well-known collector of oriental art, and Rachel Alice Cohen. He received a public school education (in the English sense) and showed little promise as a scholar. From an early age he developed a love of natural history and this may explain why he transferred from dentistry to medicine after becoming a student at Guy's Hospital, London. This interest became a lifelong passion and he was a keen lepidopterist and fisherman, and an active member and President of the British (Fly) Casting Association. In the 1950s he was a close friend of T. Edwards, the English Champion Caster, and his second wife, Elizabeth Bruce Keucher, whom he married in 1947, also became an enthusiastic angler. (His first wife had died of tuberculosis a few years after their wedding.)

Gorer's interest in natural history led him away from clinical medicine into pathology. After completing his medical studies he joined J.B.S. Haldane, the distinguished geneticist, at University College, London, and there the ground was prepared for his later work on the histocompatibility antigens of the mouse. On moving to the Lister Institute he began his life's work – the study of the genetic and antigenic basis of tumor transplantation, and this continued unabated when he returned to Guy's Hospital as a morbid histologist and hematologist in 1940. Apart from a year spent in Bar Harbor, where he developed a close collaboration and friendship with G.D. Snell, he remained at Guy's for the remainder of his relatively short life. (Snell recalls that, thanks to "another bit of fortune", Gorer left Bar Harbor just before the Laboratory was destroyed by fire; the other (bit of good fortune) had been to meet the librarian and secretary to the Director, who was to become his wife.)

Gorer published his first papers on the antigen(s) that were later to become the H-2 antigens – antigens present on mouse red blood and tumor cells – some ten years before he went to Bar Harbor with the aid of crude antisera, and he devised a complex agglutination technique that enabled him to identify several antigens. The most prominent of these was called antigen II, and this later became H-2. He subsequently combined his serologic expertise with Snell's knowledge of and interest in tumor transplantation, and it was this collaborative venture that allowed the story of H-2 to unfold in all its glory.

Gorer was an original, creative thinker, something of an eccentric, often some-what carelessly dressed and a heavy smoker, even when lecturing. Perhaps it is not altogether surprising that he was underestimated at Guy's Hospital, where he was Reader in Experimental Pathology and where his promotion to a Professorship was not considered until after he had been elected to Fellowship of the Royal Society in 1960, shortly before his death from lung cancer.

Gorer had a succession of very bright students and collaborators, among them D.B. Amos, J.R. Batchelor, A.E. Boyse and G. Hoecker, all of whom have made their mark in immunogenetics and transplantation immunology. He was greatly admired by them and several of them have published their affectionate recollections of him in volume 24 of *Immunogenetics*, 1986, as has J. Klein.

Gorer was undoubtedly the father of histocompatibility antigens and must be ranked among the most influential workers in the field of immunology this century. He was also a combative proponent of humoral antibodies as mediators of allograft reactions, a subject on which he and Medawar agreed to differ until a resolution came about when a role for both antibodies and lymphocytes was defined. Barbara Mikulska was his trusted assistant who helped him to refine the agglutination assay. There was something faintly patrician about Peter Gorer; according to A.E. Boyse, he "kept gentleman's hours, seldom appearing before lunch and often not at all". He excelled in conversation, being amusing, witty and full of laughter. Tragically, this great pioneer died at the height of his powers.

GEORGE D. SNELL
(1903–1996)

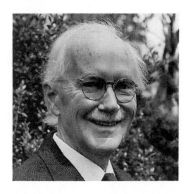

George Snell (his middle-name is unknown to most people, but I understand that it is Davis, after his grandfather) is without doubt one of the fathers of modern immuno-genetics although he himself, in his *Recollections* (1), pays tribute to the earlier pioneers like W. Castle ("the father of mammalian genetics in this country") and C.C. Little, who was instrumental in founding the Jackson Laboratory in 1929 in Bar Harbor, Maine. Having spent his childhood in Brookline, Massachusetts, he graduated from Dartmouth College and took his Ph.D. at Harvard, his main interest having been in mouse genetics. It was therefore a natural development for him to join the Jackson Laboratory in 1935 – the beginning of an astonishingly creative association that lasted until his retirement in 1973. (Indeed, George continued to live close to the Laboratory. His wife Rhoda died in 1995 and he in June 1996.)

Snell's achievements are towering and they have provided the basis of our modern understanding of transplantation genetics. The creation of large numbers of highly inbred mouse strains and their congenic lines alone constituted a major advance, but Snell and his colleagues used these tools to unravel the complexities of the H-2 histo-compatibility system of the mouse and its function in terms of tumor and skin transplantation. It was Snell who coined the term "histocompatibility" genes (H genes for short). His studies using tumors were complemented brilliantly by those of P.A. Gorer in London, who had identified mouse red cell antigens that were to become H-2. The two pioneers collaborated closely for several years at a time when few others were interested in the genetics of transplantation.

Snell became immensely influential for the next generation of histocompatibility geneticists by providing them with both intellectual leadership and the sophisticated array of inbred lines with which to dissect H-2 and discover non-H-2 loci. Snell and his colleagues did much to identify and study the properties of the antigens expressed by these genes. Apart from Gorer his many colleagues included at one time or another C.C. Little, A. Cloudman, N. Kaliss, G. Hoecker, S. Counce, J.H. Stimpfling, R.J. Graff, W.H. Hildemann, D.W. Bailey, I.F.C. McKenzie, P. Démant and I. Hilgert, the latter two visiting Research Fellows from Prague. Together with Kaliss, Snell also published some seminal papers shedding light on the phenomenon of immunologic enhancement of tumors and in 1938 he edited *The Biology of the Laboratory Mouse*, a book that has since been through several editions and has remained the standard work for anyone working with mice. In 1988, long after his retirement, Snell published a sociophilosophical book *Search for a Rational Ethic* in which he raised his sights to problems such as biologic and evolutionary ethics and the genetic basis of human behavior.

Snell had always been a modest man who preferred to shun the limelight and that personal trait, together with great singlemindedness and his preoccupation with scientific problems, the significance of which was not always readily understood by his contemporaries, led some people to undervalue him. Though a great personal friend of Peter Gorer's his relationship with Peter Medawar was apparently somewhat fragile, a state of affairs probably engendered by the very different personalities of these two great scientists.

The academic world has showered Snell with honors, from honorary degrees and membership of national societies to a multiplicity of prizes and medals, culminating in the award of the Nobel Prize in Physiology and Medicine, which he shared with J. Dausset and B. Benacerraf in 1980.

1. G.D. Snell (1991) In *History of Transplantation: Thirty-five Recollections*, ed. P.I. Terasaki, p. 19, U.C.L.A. Tissue Typing Laboratory, Los Angeles.

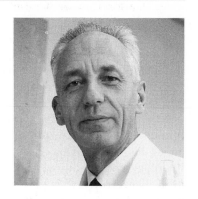

**JEAN BAPTISTE GABRIEL
JOACHIM DAUSSET
(1916–)**

Jean Dausset was born in Toulouse in the south of France although he spent most of his life in Paris, where he completed his medical studies and subsequently carried out most of his research. In 1948 he spent a year on an internship and residency at Harvard Medical School before he became Director of the Laboratory of the French National Blood Transfusion Center at the tender age of 34. He wrote to me: "My interest in leucocytes came naturally from my background studying erythrocyte groups since 1952. I was accustomed to red cell agglutination either direct or indirect (Coombs' test). I tried to apply this technique to leucocytes. It was as simple as that!". Simple or not, it was Dausset who was the first to identify a human major histocompatibility antigen, which he called MAC, though he was very closely followed by Rose Payne and Jon Van Rood, both of whom independently published papers in the same year – 1958 – describing the existence of histocompatibility antigens on human blood white cells. At that time many transplantation immunologists like P.B. Medawar were skeptical of the usefulness and importance of antibodies such as the iso-agglutinins, believing that it was the cellular response against allografts that really mattered, and I recall Dausset visiting Medawar's laboratory full of enthusiasm but receiving a polite but somewhat puzzled response. Evidently even Medawar did not appreciate the importance of Dausset's findings. Dausset cannot recall Medawar's reaction, "which was thus probably neutral".

Although many others took part in unraveling the human leukocyte antigen (HLA) story – Payne, Van Rood, Bodmer, Amos, Ceppellini, Terasaki, Bach, and Batchelor, to name but a few – it was MAC that set the ball rolling. Dausset became a regular participant at the Histocompatibility Conferences and Workshops and it was thanks to his flexibility and that of others that MAC eventually became HLA-A2, appropriately the very molecule that was the first to be crystallized and to have its three-dimensional structure elucidated 30 years after its discovery. Dausset continued to play an important role in the dissection of the HLA system and one of his special contributions, in collaboration with Felix Rapaport, was to demonstrate its importance in determining the fate of human skin allografts. The effect of HLA incompatibilities versus matching was never very great in non-immunosuppressed individuals, but it was sufficiently significant to encourage many workers to study the HLA system and to apply typing methods to the selection of living related or cadaveric kidney donors. Dausset would be the first to admit that the discovery of HLA was greatly aided and abetted by the previous work on the mouse H-2 system. The combined work of those working on experimental animals and with human material was to expose the true functions of the major histocompatibility molecules as vital signals to the cells of the immune system. "Looking back at this saga," he wrote in 1990, "which continues to unfold at present, the HLA adventurers may be justified in feeling a certain sense of achievement" (1)

Dausset was and is a shy and modest man and he has remained so despite receiving all kinds of honors, awards and decorations, both in his own country and abroad. Among his many prizes the most coveted will undoubtedly be the Nobel Prize for Physiology and Medicine, which he was awarded jointly in 1980 with G.D. Snell and B. Benacerraf. He is married to Rose, originally a Spaniard, and they have two children. During the war he was a Captain in the French Medical Corps and he took part in the French, Tunisian and Normandy campaigns. Dausset has published numerous scientific papers and written or co-edited a number of books. Having founded the Centre d'Étude du Polymorphisme Humain in Paris he is continuing to take an intense interest in all aspects of human individuality, especially the predictive value of HLA genotypes.

1. J. Dausset (1990) In *History of HLA: Ten Recollections*, ed. P.I. Terasaki, p. 3, U.C.L.A. Laboratory, Los Angeles.

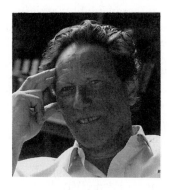

JOHANNES JOSEPH VAN ROOD
(1926–)

Jon Van Rood was born in The Hague, The Netherlands, in 1926. His father had been an engineer and his mother a musician; his stepfather a portrait painter. In "HLA and I" (1) he recalls the turbulent times of his late adolescence during the German occupation. Having been imprisoned twice he finished up in hiding with others in a cold, ill-lit cellar where he had to resort to eating daffodil bulbs (personal communication) in order to survive, and where he nonetheless managed to study science subjects in preparation for his medical studies at the University of Leiden. There he was greatly influenced by some of his teachers, especially Professor J. Mulder and Professor Van Loghem.

Apart from a sabbatical year at the Public Health Research Institute of the City of New York (1962) Van Rood's working life was spent in Leiden in various capacities, first as head of the Department of Hematology, of which he became Chairman in 1976, and later as Chairman of the Leiden Institute for Immunology. He married Sacha, Baronesse van Tuyll van Serooskerken, in 1956 and they had three children.

A paper published by P.B. Medawar in 1946 showing that skin and blood leukocytes shared the same transplantation antigens "formed the basis of my scientific life". He wrote to me recently "My entry in transplantation immunology was a beautiful case of serendipity" when, as a young resident in medicine, he was confronted with a patient who developed a severe non-hemolytic transfusion reaction due to leukocyte antibodies. It turned out that the antibodies had been formed as a result of pregnancy and Van Rood analyzed this problem with the help of a computer, the first time that this had been done in Europe. This stood him in good stead when he analyzed his early, very complex human leukocyte antigen (HLA) data, and others soon followed suit. The use of computers was a great innovation that allowed the appraisal and comparison of wordwide HLA antibody data to advance at a gallop rather than at a snail's pace. Van Rood and two colleagues published their first paper on the identification of histocompatibility antigens using the sera of multiparous women in 1958 – the same year in which J. Dausset and R. Payne published similar results. Van Rood's family studies were of the greatest importance in unraveling the genetics of HLA. It is unfortunate that the Nobel Committee did not see fit to include him among the recipients of the 1980 Prize in Physiology and Medicine, for not only was he a co-discoverer of HLA but he has continued to the present day to make many significant contributions to the HLA story.

Van Rood is an ebullient participant at congresses and smaller meetings and has been a key member of the series of Histocompatibility Workshops, always willing to take on those who disagree with his often strongly held convictions. He is a stout proponent of tissue typing in organ transplantation, despite some skepticism from transplant surgeons. A keen sailor, he has conducted memorable summer schools in immunology on a two-masted schooner in the Zuider See. He is also a keen and stately skier and a regular attender of the W. Brendel "ski-conferences" in Austria. Van Rood was Founder and Chairman of the European Foundation of Immunogenetics and of Eurotransplant (1967), and co-founder of the European Bone Marrow Transplantation Group. He has been a member of numerous editorial boards and research institutes and an editor of several journals. He has been showered with honors and prizes, including the Karl Landsteiner Memorial Award, the Robert Koch Medal and the James Blundell Award of the British Blood Transfusion Society. His honorary degrees come from universities in The Netherlands, Belgium, Italy, France, Chile, and Germany, and he is a Fellow of the Royal College of Physicians and the Royal College of Pathologists, London. In 1985 he received the order of Knighthood of the Dutch Lion, and in 1991 he became Commander of the Order of Oranje Nassau.

1. J.J. van Rood (1993) *Ann. Rev. Immunol.* 11, 1.

5 Fetally and Neonatally Induced Immunologic Tolerance

"Tolerance, like the secondary response and the nature of immunological 'memory', has become something of a testing ground for theories of the immune response."

P.B. Medawar, 1961

Having evolved as an all-embracing defense against pathogens and parasites, the mammalian immune system is a highly sophisticated, complex and integrated network (see Chapter 1). Although its complexity could only be guessed at half a century ago, it was clear then that it provided a formidable barrier to the transplantation of foreign tissues and organs. Earlier attempts to transplant allogeneic skin or kidneys had usually either failed or claims for their survival had later been shown to be spurious. There were, nonetheless, some straws in the wind that suggested that tissue transplantation might one day become a reality.

Evidence from Embryology

For embryologists working in the first half of the twentieth century, one of the most challenging problems was posed by the differentiation of the embryo and its component parts. To what extent is the differentiation of a limb bud, for example, already programmed – or is it influenced by factors emanating from its local environment? In which cells reside the power to determine pattern and color formation in birds? These and other questions were studied to some degree *in vitro*, but one of the most popular approaches was to transplant embryonic tissues to another individual. Because there was already some understanding that the transplantation of tissues to genetically different adults was doomed to failure, and because it was thought important for the tissue to develop in a developmentally similar environment, the hosts were either amphibian larvae or, most commonly, chick embryos at about the same level of development as the graft. Although the importance of the immune system in graft rejection was not appreciated at that time, with hindsight these studies clearly demonstrated the immunologic immaturity of both amphibian embryos and larvae and avian embryos and suggested that a small proportion of such grafts could survive into adulthood.

This is a large field in its own right and although of interest in the context of immunologic tolerance, it is not directly relevant to this history. However, it does seem appropriate to consider some of the most important examples.

In amphibia, the first successfully if temporarily established xenogeneic grafts were by Born in 1897 (*1*), when he created chimeras by transplanting frog tissues into toad embryos or larvae. Lewis (2), a decade later, used this kind of model, albeit frog into newt, to study the differentiation of optic vesicles, and found that they completed their differentiation successfully. A similar approach was followed by Hewitt (3) in 1934; he too observed more or less normal differentiation of xeno-geneic optic vesicles in frog or axolotl embryos, but described gradual atrophy of the grafts. Because a lowering of the ambient temperature not only reduced the growth rate differences between graft and host, but also lengthened graft survival, he concluded that the different growth rates probably accounted for the eventual atrophy of the grafts – clearly a fallacious argument. Geinitz (4) carried out extensive studies, this time between newt and frog embryos, likewise highlighting the near-normal differentiation of embryonic grafts in their larval hosts.

Evidence from the transplantation of embryonic chick tissues to chick embryos is equally compelling; it was a widely used method for studying limb and feather differ-entiation, the migration of pigment cells from the neural crest, and the formation of feather color patterns. Others were bold enough to transplant xenogeneic tissues to chick embryos, again with remarkable success.

The first to explore the chick embryo as a host for foreign tissues were Rous and Murphy (5), who inoculated embryos with rat sarcoma cells a few years before World War I and found that these survived well during the incubation period of the eggs. In a series of elegant and incisive studies published in 1912–1914, Murphy took this early observation a great deal further. He showed that the chick embryo has no defense against rat sarcoma cells (6), that few small round lymphoid cells infiltrate the grafted tissue in the embryo and that a defense develops at the time of hatching, accompanied by the appearance of small lymphoid cells around the grafts (7). Of greatest consequence was his finding that the *in vitro* growth of rat sarcoma tissue was inhibited by the concomitant presence of adult chicken spleen fragments or bone marrow cells, whereas other adult tissues had no such effect (8). *In vivo*, the concomitant transplantation of rat sarcoma and adult chicken spleen or bone marrow caused the sarcoma cells to degenerate and die, even when they were not directly in contact, accompanied by "massive collections of lymphocytes around the edges and in clumps associated with the blood vessels of the tumor" (8,9). Murphy thus showed with the utmost clarity that the avian embryo is immunoincompetent and that this immature state can be reversed by the provision of adult immunologi-cally competent cells. It seems surprising that workers who followed him did not make more of these important discoveries, though it is probable that World War I, the start of which coincided with the publication of these important papers, diverted attention from them.

Transplantation of limb buds and other tissues became a much used approach of experimental embryologists following the description by Hamburger in 1933 of a relatively simple transplantation technique (10). Apart from Hamburger himself (11), the workers who made the greatest impact were Eastlick, Willier and Rawles. Eastlick (12–14) transplanted embryonic tissues of other avian species to the chick embryo; many grafts survived and differentiated well, though not in every combination. He noted that the time of appearance and severity of "incompatibility reactions" depended on the donor species (14). One duck graft survived for as long as 13 months, but most failed to survive the reaction that developed close to or after hatching. "The reaction seems to affect seriously the vascular system of the graft as indicated by stasis and edema. . . . Although it has not been demonstrated experimentally, it seems logical to assume that the foreign proteins of the heteroplastic grafts sensitize the hosts so that defense mechanisms are brought into play." He went on to speculate that in the embryo the graft and host tissues "may have become more or less 'adjusted' to one another during the embryonic period, and that this *tolerance* (my italics) may not be lost at once". This is as near as the experimental embryologists ever got to understanding the basis of their successful transplants and to the notion that the presence of foreign tissue in the developing embryo could bring about a long-lasting change in host reactivity, and it was the first time that the term 'tolerance' had been applied. Willier (*15*), Willier and Rawles (*16*) and Rawles (*17–20*) tended to take survival in embryos for granted and merely used the transplantation technique to pursue their own objectives in the study of embryonic differentiation.

It is appropriate to mention here the experiments of Danforth and Foster, who in 1929 showed that skin allografts transplanted to newly hatched chicks generally failed to survive after the initial take, but that a small proportion survived for more than a year, fully integrated into the host to the extent that the host acquired muscular control over the graft hair follicles (*21*). Their goal was to study genetic and endocrine factors in the fowl and they were not interested in the possible immunologic implications of their observations. They cited Loeb's 'individuality differentials' (*22*), inadequate vascularization or sex differences between the donor and host as possible causes for the lack of survival of the majority of grafts.

In all probability the early experimental embryologists could have developed the notion of tolerance long before Owen's discovery of red cell chimerism in cattle (*23*), had they been less committed to their own objectives and more inquisitive about the basis of the successful transplants in chick and amphibian embryos and the reasons for their destruction in early adult life.

The Cattle Story: Vital Landmarks and the Concept of Self/Non-self

In the early 1940s R.D. Owen was an Associate Professor of Genetics and Zoology at the University of Wisconsin, where together with C. Stormont he was studying the genetics of red blood cell antigens of cattle. In the course of this work Owen made the extraordinary discovery that the red cells of dizygotic twins carried not only their own genetic antigens but also possessed red cells displaying the antigens of their partner. This work was published in 1945 (*23*, see also *24*). The cellular chimerism was variable in degree but long lasting.

Owen was quick to link his profoundly important discovery to the anatomic findings of Lillie earlier in the century, who had shown that bovine dizygotic twins invariably develop a fusion of their placentae early in embryonic life (*25–27*). The resulting passage of sex hormones from the genetic male to the genetic female embryo severely disturbs the sexual development in the female, causing it to be a sterile "freemartin". Lillie was clearly excited by "this natural experiment enabling us to draw far-reaching conclusions as to the origin and the differentiation of sex-characters in mammals", but he would have been astonished to know that his findings also provided an explanation for one of the seminal discoveries of modern immunology a quarter of a century later.

Owen realized that placental fusion was at the root of his findings, red cell chimerism having been established as a consequence of the exchange of hemopoietic stem cells during embryonic life. Although he wrote that "Several interesting problems in the fields of genetics, immunology and development are suggested by these observations", he chose to focus the application of his finding on the identification of the sterik freemartin twin, as it is outwardly indistinguishable from a normal twin in the first few years of life. Quite apart from any biological implications the discovery may have held at the time it was clearly of some importance to cattle farmers.

A year later Owen, Davis and Morgan published a further paper, in which they described "the strange case of 'Old Glory', a cow who was turned out to pasture ...". Old Glory proceeded to have quintuplets over a period of 24 hours and they were given the names of the 'Big Five' superpowers at that time. All proved to be chimeric for the red cells of the other partners (28).

Red cell chimerism in cattle twins was highlighted a few years later, when Burnet and Fenner published the second edition of their monograph on *The Production of Antibodies* (29). This was a perceptive and prescient discussion of every aspect of antibody formation, with sections on the immunologic behavior of young animals, the 'self-marker' concept, the development of 'marker' recognition in embryonic life, and tissue transplantation immunity in relation to immunologic theory. They speculated that as fetal mammals and chick embryos are incapable of antibody production and the full capacity to do so develops only slowly in the young animal, "the process by which self-pattern becomes recognizable takes place during the embryonic or immediately post-embryonic stages" (30). The detailed reasoning for the self-marker hypothesis was at the time, and still is, hard to follow and they made one error in postulating that their hypothesis encompassed only "expendable" cells. Thus, Burnet and Fenner wrote that "If in embryonic life expendable cells from a genetically distinct race are implanted and established, no antibody response should develop against the foreign cell antigen when the animal takes on independent existence" (31). It is in this context that they quoted Owen's cattle studies, and they concluded: "A very interesting field for direct experimentation is opened up by this finding, particularly if the same type of phenomenon can be induced by intravenous inoculation of foreign embryonic cells in chick embryos" (31).

The second speculation Burnet and Fenner made in this context was that "following a generalized non-fatal infection by a pathogenic microorganism of the embryo *in utero*, the animal after birth would be incapable of responding with antibody production to injection or infection with the same microorganism" (32). In support of this they quoted the work of Traub (33–35). He had studied the natural history of strains of mice infected with lymphocytic choriomeningitis virus, in which the infected colony appeared to have reached a state of symbiosis with the non-lethal virus. The adults were carriers and the young, though infected *in utero*, showed no clinical evidence of illness. Of greatest consequence was the finding that mice exposed *in utero* to the virus were resistant to subsequent intracerebral challenge, and that no neutralizing or complement-fixing antibody was detectable in their blood. Following a discussion of various aspects of Traub's studies, Burnet and Fenner went on to say with great aplomb: "These phenomena are clearly complex but there is the development of a tolerance to the foreign microorganism during embryonic life which is in line with the present hypothesis" (32). Because Fox and Laemmert (36), working with yellow fever virus introduced into chick embryos, were unsuccessful in bringing about a state of tolerance, Burnet and Fenner considered that "more than mere casual presence of the antigen in the embryo is necessary if subsequent immunological reactivity is to be modified in the way we have suggested" (37). This point was confirmed by Burnet's laboratory a year later when they failed to induce tolerance to the influenza virus (38).

A year after publication of Burnet and Fenner's monograph, G.V. Lopashov and O.G. Stroyeva (39) produced a lengthy, discursive and speculative paper in a Russian journal on "The development of immunological reactions and the problem of incompatibility of transplanted tissues" (title translated). In it they discussed how the organism might distinguish between self proteins and foreign proteins, and in a groping way they conclude that unresponsiveness to self had its origins in adaptive changes during embryonic life. They associated this process with the reticuloendothelial system (RES), to which they attributed a nutritional function as well as the source of "proteins, antibodies and phagocytes". In translation it is far from easy to follow their speculations, and the linking of the supposed nutritional functions of the RES with recognition of non-self is misleading. However, the germ of an independent self–non-self theory seems to be there. To quote one or two of their remarks: "During the process of ontogenesis a tissue system capable of immunological reaction must first come into contact with proteins (and protein complexes) belonging to the same organism, products of its organs and cells. Its universal reactivity gives us no reason to suppose that the immune system possesses a predetermined ability to react only to foreign proteins and not to its own, that it has an inborn capability to distinguish between them, nor that this capability first appears outside the process of ontogenetic development. Therefore one may suppose with greater certainty that the immune system's encounter with the products of the rest of the body are anything but inconsequential. Later on the immune system will not produce antibodies to the tissues of the self, and the phagocytes it produces will not destroy those tissues . . . At some point a state of compatibility is achieved that allows the immune system and self proteins to tolerate one another in coexistence" (40). They undermined the thrust of their argument by assuming that the cause of the compatibility thus achieved is that the "developing blood cells, coming into contact with proteins circulating in the blood, themselves begin to produce proteins that correspond more closely to the cells already formed than could have been determined by one initial group of proteins in the ovum" (40). They seem to imply here that the expression of proteins expressed by cells (cellular histocompatibility antigens?) can be fundamentally altered by antibodies produced by the embryo and that this accounts for the failure of the adult immune system to respond to self antigens. The point is not wholly clear but seems to be borne out by their subsequent statement that "It is probable that the formation of the individual, specific composition of blood proteins thus achieved is, one way or another, dependent upon the changing metabolic conditions, particularly with regard to nutrition, which exist during the organism's development, in each case creating protein compositions which are unique to the individual" (40).

This self–non-self recognition hypothesis is so problematic that it cannot be equated with Burnet and Fenner's, as Hašek's group have done in some of their earlier publications (*41, 42*). However, it is of some interest that ideas of this kind should have preoccupied a distinguished Soviet embryologist (G.V. Lopashov) in the scientific ambience prevailing in the Soviet Union at that time.

Within two years of the publication of Burnet and Fenner's monograph (*29*) further important evidence was to emerge from the study of cattle dizygotic twins. P.B. Medawar became Professor of Zoology at Birmingham University, England, in 1947 and R.E. Billingham was a postdoctoral Fellow working with him on problems of tissue transplantation. From their separate recollections (*43, 44*) it would appear that they embarked on a series of skin grafting experiments in cattle because of a chance meeting at the Eighth International Congress of Genetics in Stockholm in July, 1948 between Medawar and a Scottish geneticist, H.P. Donald, who was Director of the Agricultural Research Council's Animal Breeding and Genetics Research Organization in Edinburgh. Donald was studying genetic and environmental differences in cattle, using identical and fraternal twins, and central to his study was the problem of distinguishing with certainty between these two kinds of twins. Medawar declared, apparently over cocktails, that "in principle the solution is extremely easy: just exchange skin grafts between the twins and see how long they last. If they last indefinitely you can be sure these are identical twins, but if they are thrown off after a week or two you can classify them with equal certainty as fraternal twins" (*43*). His offer to demonstrate the technique of skin grafting led to a joint venture carried out at an experimental farm about 40 miles from Birmingham, where Medawar and Billingham soon mastered the art of exchanging skin grafts between young calves, despite a total lack of surgical facilities. Their results astounded them: not only identical twins but also fraternal twins, including twins of opposite sex, usually accepted their grafts, though they rejected grafts from their parents or from siblings of separate birth (*45, 46*), as would be expected. Gross inspection of the grafts at regular intervals was backed up by careful histologic information, and the evidence that dizygotic cattle twins, despite their quite different genetic constitution, accepted each other's skin grafts, though not always permanently, was absolutely conclusive. Several decades later it was shown that there can indeed be a very wide range in the survival times of such skin grafts (*47, 48*) and the possibility was raised that this might be caused by the presence of skin-specific (SK) antigens described in some strains of mice (*49*).

In their first (1951) paper (*45*) Billingham *et al.* referred to Owen's earlier discovery of red cell chimerism and explained that their own experiments provided direct confirmation of his hypothesis that cell precursors must have been exchanged *in utero*, and they suggested that the mechanism might be akin to "desensitisation". However, they pointed out that "In one important respect the mechanism of acquired tolerance to tissue homografts in twin cattle differs from desensitisation in the ordinary sense. The embryo is immunologically inactive: it does not manufacture antibodies and cannot therefore be said to become 'desensitised' to an antigen to which it is not in any case sensitive" (*45*); and they went on to speculate that the critical issue might be that antigen confronts "the embryo's gradually awakening faculty of immunological response".

It is of interest that Medawar and Billingham did not become aware of Owen's vital discovery until they were well into their skin grafting study, which began early in 1949. According to Medawar (*50*), "We came upon the answer not through any exertion of our own but by browsing in an exciting-looking book newly published by Frank Macfarlane Burnet and Frank Fenner – *The Production of Antibodies* (1949)." Billingham's memory is more precise. "One day, as we were leaving the farm, troubled by confirmation of the mutual acceptance of each other's grafts by unequivocal dizygotic twins, i.e. those of dissimilar sex, which we were completely at a loss to explain, we met Dr Donald and briefed him on the status of the project. He advised us to go home and read 'Immunogenetic consequences of vascular anastomoses established between bovine twins', a 1945 paper by Ray D. Owen published in *Science* which he felt might help resolve our problem" (*44*). Yet Medawar had undoubtedly read the monograph as a reviewer some time after its publication in 1949, for he published an unsigned review of the book in *Nature* in August, 1950 (*51*). I am in possession of his review copy, which he had annotated liberally, though curiously not in relation to Owen's discovery and its implications. The review was undoubtedly written by Medawar because a cutting was attached to his copy of the book, the style is unmistakably his, and in summarizing matters that were new to the second edition he wrote "Another is the chapter on transplantation immunity, containing the suggestion (which this reviewer is looking forward to trying out) that the response to the grafting of foreign homologous cells has something in common with the type of sensitivity provoked by tuberculin." Such a project was not, in fact, attempted by him and L. Brent until the late 1950s, whereas the study on acquired tolerance commenced within 18 months of the publication of his review article, after at least six months of planning and preparation. But in any case, the initiation of the cattle skin grafting project was early in 1949, well before the publication of the Burnet and Fenner book, the English edition of which did not appear until March 1950 and long before Medawar had written his review. (Consultation with the editor of *Nature* has confirmed that Medawar had indeed been its author.) It is perhaps idle to speculate whether Medawar and his group would have embarked on the mouse tolerance study had they been put off the cattle skin grafting project by an earlier awareness of Owen's red cell chimerism story.

Owen's 1945 paper and the Burnet and Fenner monograph greatly influenced Medawar's subsequent thinking. Combined with the cattle skin graft data of his own team, it led directly to the formulation of a strategy designed to prove that tolerance could be induced experimentally and that it had a significance well beyond that of 'nature's experiment' in cattle.

Experimental Verification of the Tolerance Concept

The Medawar School: early studies

The strategy discussed above to prove that tolerance could be induced experimentally was conceived during the course of 1951, and its execution coincided with Medawar's move to the Department of Zoology at University College, London. He was accompanied by R.E. Billingham and by L. Brent, whose Ph.D. thesis was to be largely devoted to the topic of acquired immunologic tolerance. Medawar had wisely decided to use inbred mice, which had become available thanks to the pioneering work of G.D. Snell in Bar Harbor. Quite apart from their far less heterogeneous response to skin grafts, these mice had the great advantage that the cell and skin graft donors did not have to be one and the same animal. The strains that became available were CBA (agouti), provided by N.A. Mitchison and A/Jax (white), obtained directly from Bar Harbor. A third strain (AU and later C57Bl; black) was used as a third party control for experiments testing the specificity of tolerance. The choice of strains was fortuitous and it emerged only later that the two main strains differed only for class I histocompatibility antigens, for which tolerance is achieved relatively easily and by mechanisms involving clonal deletion rather than suppression.

The work was begun early in 1952. Although the techniques were simple, the project turned out to be frustratingly difficult, for pregnant mice did not take very kindly to a radical laparotomy and the inoculation of their embryos with a mixture of allogeneic tissue fragments and cells of adult spleen, testis and kidney. Many litters were aborted or born dead. Matters were improved by abandoning laparotomy in favor of incision into and mobilization of the abdominal skin and injection through the semitransparent body wall, though accuracy was inevitably sacrificed. The aim was to inject the allogeneic cells directly into the embryonic abdominal cavity, but this was by no means always achieved. Attempts were also made to inject allogeneic cells into newborn recipients. Despite all manner of setbacks, which included the accidental use of one F1 hybrid litter of recipients (thus guaranteeing the survival of the skin test grafts!), an error that was fortunately discovered by the suspicious investigators by appropriate skin graft tests, sufficient data had been accumulated by the middle of 1953 for the first paper to be published in *Nature* (52). Surviving mice that had received foreign cells were given a skin graft from the donor strain about eight weeks after birth. Although not every mouse proved to be tolerant, grafts on some of them showed either prolonged or permanent survival. The 'actively acquired tolerance' was entirely specific for grafts of the cell donor strain, and because tolerated grafts that were retransplanted to mice syngeneic with the host animals were rejected it was concluded that tolerance was due to a specific failure of the host's immunologic response rather than to graft adaptation. The mouse data were reinforced by some preliminary experiments in chick embryos, which were inoculated intravenously (via one of the chorioallantoic veins) with blood taken from an allogeneic embryo of about the same age. Here strict pairing of Rhode Island Red blood and skin donors with their White Leghorn recipients was essential as no inbred strains of chickens were available. Again, some grafts had survival times well in excess of the grafts transplanted to normal chicks two weeks after hatching, and two showed permanent survival, with normal growth of red feathers showing up dramatically against the white feathers of the surrounding skin.

In their discussion Billingham, Brent and Medawar (52) referred to Burnet and Fenner's prediction that "the exposure of animals to antigens before the development of the faculty of immunologic response should lead to tolerance rather than to heightened resistance", and they went on to say that "our experiments do not yet bear upon the fundamental problem of whether the production of antibodies represents an *inherited* derangement of protein synthesis, that is, a transformation which can persist through repeated cell divisions after the disappearance of the antigen originally responsible for it . . . In our experiments there is no reason to doubt that at least some of the cells of the foetal inoculum survived as long as the tolerant state which they were responsible for creating", a prediction that turned out to be correct.

Apart from noting that tolerant females injected with male cells were fertile, Billingham, Brent and Medawar referred to Owen's previous findings in cattle, to the first case of human red cell chimerism in dizygotic twins (53), and to the demonstration by Cannon and Longmire (54) that although 5–10% of allogeneic skin grafts from newly hatched donors were accepted by newly hatched chicks, this was no longer the case when grafts were transplanted two weeks after hatching. Finally, they discussed the concept of tolerance in relation to other phenomena that occur in adult life, namely Felton's immunologic paralysis (55), oral desensitization to certain drug allergies (56), and the enhancement of tumor growth following pretreatment of the recipients with lyophilized tissue preparations from the donor strain (57) (see also Chapter 6).

It is worth pausing to consider the extraordinary state of immunologic ignorance prevailing in 1951, when this study was begun. The function of lymphocytes was still highly controversial and essentially unknown, their subpopulations had not been identified, the role of the thymus was mysterious, the study of the histocompatibility antigens of the mouse was in its infancy, and inbred strains of mice, now the basic tool of immunologists, were only just becoming readily available. True, the phenomenon of immunologic enhancement (57) (see Chapter 6) was already being studied, but was ill-understood. Cellular immunology had yet to be invented (except in the Metchnikoff sense) and it is striking that the *Nature* paper by Billingham, Brent and Medawar (52) refers exclusively to how their data might bear on the problem of antibody formation, despite Medawar's earlier demonstration that rabbit skin allografts are heavily infiltrated with host lymphocytes (58).

The concept of tolerance and its implications created a stir in the biologic world, its first public airing having taken place at a meeting of the British Society for Experimental Biology in London in 1953. With characteristic generosity Medawar and Billingham had asked the most junior member of the team (L. Brent) to address the packed meeting.

Although this team of workers published a number of papers in the years following the *Nature* publication (52), their next most significant contribution was the description of their by now extensive data in 1956 (59). This paper, published with numerous color photographs, established immunologic tolerance as a universal phenomenon of fundamental importance, not only in the context of tissue transplantation but also in normal development. The specificity of tolerance was confirmed, and it was shown that a variety of nucleated cells, but not red cells, could elicit it. It was not an "all or nothing" phenomenon in that all degrees of tolerance were observed, from permanent to transient acceptance of skin grafts. A "null period" in which neither tolerance nor immunity were induced by the intraperitoneal and subcutaneous introduction of allogeneic cells was postulated – a concept that was later abandoned when it was shown that the induction of tolerance after birth depended upon the number of cells in the inoculum and the route used (60, 61) (see also page 197), the intravenous route being by far the most efficient (62). Both Koprowski (63) and Bollag (64) had already shown that tolerance to allogeneic or xenogeneic tumors could be induced by cells introduced into murine embryos, and Simonsen (65) had found that susceptibility to the Rous sarcoma virus was increased in young turkeys by their previous inoculation *in ovo* with adult chicken blood. Billingham, Brent and Medawar (59) extended these findings by demonstrating that allogeneic mammary tumor tissue implanted into newborn mice could elicit tolerance for skin grafts. Of great theoretic importance was their finding that well-established skin allografts on tolerant mice could be destroyed adoptively by the introduction of lymphoid cells syngeneic with the hosts: the fact that this could be done not only by cells presensitized against donor strain antigens but also by normal cells led Billingham *et al.* to conclude that tolerance was caused by a 'central failure' of the immune response and not, like immunologic enhancement (see below), by intercession at a peripheral level. Once the clonal selection theory of antibody formation had become accepted (66–68) tolerance was seen as a prime example of clonal inactivation or deletion.

The *Philosophical Transactions of the Royal Society* paper by Billingham, Brent and Medawar (59) also described experiments with chick embryos and with fetal rats and rabbits. Intravenous injection of embryonic or adult blood into ten-day-old chick embryos induced skin graft tolerance in some of the recipients, but it was noted that "experiments with *adult* blood . . . met with about 95% mortality. . . . Deaths occurred towards the end of incubation, i.e. 4 to 5 days after inoculation; the fact that the blood of adult ducks was usually inoffensive, and that not all chicken donors were guilty, suggests an infective cause of death". This is the only reference to the mortality encountered in this tolerance study and, with the benefit of hindsight, its cause was clearly graft-versus-host disease; a condition that was recognized by Simonsen (69) and by Billingham and Brent (62) a year later (see Chapter 8). There is little doubt that a heavy mortality was encountered in the rodent experiments, but there was a tendency to dismiss this as being due to technical problems. It is strange that Medawar's group, which was so creative in other respects, did not at that time suspect that there might have been another cause of death and that they did not discover graft-versus-host disease several years earlier than proved to be the case.

The placement of "a miscellany of adult tissues (kidney, spleen, heart and lung)" on to the chorioallantoic membrane of 8–11-day-old chick embryos was sufficient to prolong the survival of subsequently transplanted skin grafts from the cell donors, but no experiments were carried out to ascertain whether donor cells had migrated into the embryos. The intravenous inoculation of allogeneic whole blood or leukocytes into newly hatched chicks met with partial success, and it was clearly established that tolerance induction was a function of properties residing in viable nucleated cells; red cells, plasma or leukocytes that had been killed by a variety of methods failed to induce tolerance.

Of some significance was the discovery that fertile double-yolked eggs produced two embryos which, like cattle twin embryos, were found to have a free anastomosis of their circulations. Owen's findings of red cell chimerism in cattle twins were confirmed in these natural chick twins as well as in chick embryos of different breeds that had been parabiosed by an ingenious technique developed by Hašek (70) (see p. 192): both proved to be red cell chimeras and tolerant of each other's skin grafts, though some asymmetry was noted in the duration of graft survival in the experimental twin partners.

Billingham, Brent and Medawar included in their *Philosophical Transactions of the Royal Society* paper (59) a discussion of tolerance in normal development, based on Burnet and Fenner's prediction of tolerance on the grounds that "antibody-forming cells, characteristic scavengers (*sic*), must 'learn' to distinguish between substances which are proper to the individual and those which may later gain entry from outside." They distinguished between "the specialized and complex substances that are formed in the later stages of cellular differentiation" and the isoantigens responsible for transplantation immunity. Were it not for the phenomenon of tolerance, it was argued, isoantigens might lead to the formation of autoantibodies. The exceptional examples of casein and spermatozoal antigens were cited as molecules that develop too late in life to induce tolerance and which therefore, when injected into adults, will provoke the formation of antibodies. Lens protein, on the other hand, was potentially antigenic because it is sequestered from the immune system during the critical embryonic period and thus cannot induce tolerance. The isoantigens (alloantigens) that incite rejection responses were different because they were represented in every living nucleated cell, including the cells of the immune system: "a future antibody-forming cell does not learn not to react against substances which are part of its own fabric". In the 1956 paper this was the extent of the discussion concerning the relationship between tolerance and autoimmunity, but the subject was fully aired by Brent and Medawar two years later at the Seventh International Congress of Microbiology (71).

The contribution of the Hašek School

I have already alluded to the fact that Milan Hašek, working in Prague, published his first observations on the effects of parabiosis of chick embryos (70) in the same year in which Billingham, Brent and Medawar published their *Nature* paper (52). They appeared in a Czech journal that was at that time not readily accessible to, and certainly not read by, most biologists in the West. The paper was written in Russian but had a German summary. Fortunately one of Medawar's departmental colleagues, Dr A. Comfort, brought it to the notice of the Medawar group and managed to translate parts of it.

Although Hašek had used certain immunologic markers to establish the degree of protein exchange between duck and chicken parabionts by the presence of antibodies against duck serum, this was not primarily an immunologic paper. Spurred on by the Lysenko and Michurin doctrine of the inheritance of acquired characteristics, Hašek was at that time interested in whether the exchange of blood elements between chick embryos of different breeds or embryos of different species would lead to "vegetative hybridisation", a state in which the parabionts were expected to display some of the characteristics of their partners. The use of embryos semed to him to be particularly favorable because of their inability to make antibodies.

Hašek's early papers (70, 72) provide an interesting example of scientific work conceived on misguided scientific principles that resulted in erroneous interpretations, but led to the establishment of a valid and sophisticated technique, which he and his colleagues (and later others, too) put to good use. In these papers, homage was paid to the studies of I.V. Michurin, T.D. Lysenko and their collaborators, "who have demonstrated vegetative hybridization on a vast scale in plants", and the "non-scientific, idealistic theory of genes invented by the disciples of Weissman and Morgan" were berated (70). In the befogged and, for dissenters, dangerous climate prevailing in Eastern Europe at the time it is perhaps not surprising that Hašek should have found it necessary to conform and to interpret his data in a politically

acceptable way. What he did establish clearly was that the technique of *in ovo* parabiosis led to the exchange of blood elements and that antibodies against serum
proteins were not formed by the parabiont partners; and that even active immunization after hatching failed to induce the formation of antibodies. More dubiously,
he claimed to have found differences in body weight as a result of parabiosis, so
that the chick partner of a duck embryo would later in life have a body weight
halfway between that of a normal chicken and a duck. Further, Hašek claimed to
have found long-lasting changes in feather coloration, thanks to "an increase in
biological vigor and immunological changes". He concluded that his study confirmed
his group's earlier observations involving the exchange of egg-white between chick
embryos (*41, 73*), and that the concept of vegetative hybridization had an important
place in Michurian biology, providing the key to an understanding of non-sexual
changes in the life of organisms. "Vegetative hybridization can clearly be brought
about in animals and this opens up a far broader path to the solution of those questions concentrating on the guided alteration in heredity of (somatic) characteristics."
It is of more than passing interest that Hašek had previously published a paper
purporting to show that following the inoculation of duck egg-white into chick
embryos, the number of chromosomes in the embryos was significantly increased
(*74*).

Medawar and L. Brent met Hašek at an international conference in 1954. Hašek
proved to be an engaging and highly intelligent man who responded with enthusiasm
to the suggestion that his published work on vegetative hybridization could very well
be interpreted in terms of acquired immunologic tolerance, and he was presented
with a copy of the 1953 *Nature* paper (*52*). Thereafter the publications from Hašek's
laboratory struck a very different note: the western literature on tolerance was fully
acknowledged, the political references disappeared, and the experimental studies of
the Prague group were interpreted in immunologic terms. This completed a process
that had already begun in 1954 in a paper that was still written in Russian (with a
German summary), describing the fate of allo- and heterografts after embryonic parabiosis – success was recorded with the former and some prolongation of survival
with the latter (*75*). "Vegetative hybridization" had become "vegetative approximation" (Annäherung), and many of the western references from Billingham, Brent and
Medawar's 1953 paper were cited.

Although much of the subsequent work continued to be published in Russian,
though now with summaries in English, two papers by Hašek and T. Hraba appeared
in the newly formed *Folia Biologica* in 1955 (*76*) and in the following year (*77*),
both written in fluent English, this time with summaries in Russian. They were,
respectively, concerned with the importance of phylogenetic relationships between
donor and recipient in the induction of "immunologic approximation", and the
immunologic consequences following parabiosis between turkey and hen embryos.
As far as I can ascertain it was J. Grozdanovič, working in Hašek's laboratory, who
was the first of the Czech workers to use the term "immunologic tolerance" (*78*) in
describing the induction of tolerance to a xenogeneic tumor.

The first paper published by Hašek in a western journal was in *Nature* in 1955
(*79*), when he and T. Hraba briefly summarized their data on the immunologic
consequences of parabiosis between avian embryos. The capacity for hemagglutinin
production was specifically impaired in chicken parabionts, but red cell chimerism

could not be demonstrated. The authors pointed out that in this respect, as in the matter of fertility, their data differed from those of Owen's natural cattle twins, which showed lasting red cell chimerism and infertility in the female (23, 24, 28). Billingham, Brent and Medawar (59) confirmed the fertility of tolerant animals in both chickens and mice a year later, and demonstrated variable red cell chimerism in fully adult parabionts with the aid of a battery of specific antisera provided by R.D. Owen. They concluded that "Hašek's inference, from his failure to demonstrate chimerism, that chimerism and the inhibition of antibody formation are essentially different phenomena, cannot therefore be upheld". Hašek and Hraba went on to show that in xenogeneic parabiosis (duck and chicken) neither natural antibodies nor acquired antibodies could be suppressed and they suggested that the Burnet and Fenner hypothesis (29) needed to take into account the nature of the antigen. In this paper the Czech authors restricted themselves to the use of "inhibition of antibody production", leaving vegetative "hybridization" and "approximation" in limbo, but evidently not yet ready to adopt the term "tolerance".

I have considered the early Czech transplantation history in some detail for more than one reason. First and foremost, Milan Hašek entered the field of unresponsiveness induced in embryos at a very early stage – his first relevant paper appeared in the same year (1953) in which Billingham, Brent and Medawar published their first data on actively acquired tolerance – and his role therefore deserves to be carefully assessed and acknowledged. Second, his story is a salutary lesson in the destructive effect a repressive regime can have on the development of science. Third, it was to Hašek's great credit to have had the courage to move away from the prescribed theories once his eyes had been opened, for it certainly continued to be hazardous in Czechoslovakia and the Eastern block generally to subscribe to what would have been considered to be subversive and western-inspired ideas. Indeed, in the long run he had to pay a heavy price (see p. 228). Finally, it bears on the question of how fundamental a debt the discovery of tolerance owes Hašek and his school. I have formed the impression that Hašek and his colleagues made numerous valuable contributions, particularly in opening up the study of xenogeneic transplantation and tolerance and in the provision of the technique of parabiosis of avian embryos. However, the phenomenon was discovered independently by Medawar's group by 1953, preceded as it had been by the cattle twin skin transplantation studies (45, 46), and had generated such an impetus of its own and such widespread interest among biologists and immunologists in the West that its further development was well assured. In view of the unfortunate misinterpretation by Hašek of his own early data the sentiments expressed by J. Dausset that Hašek "ought to have at least shared the Nobel Prize with F. Macfarlane Burnet and Peter Medawar" (80) must, I think, be regarded as controversial. It could, indeed, be argued that a far weightier claim could have been made for R.D. Owen's inclusion.

Hašek proceeded to build up a sizeable team of workers at the Institute of Experimental Biology and Genetics in Prague (now the Institute of Molecular Genetics). Under his and J. Šterzl's leadership it became the most advanced center of immunology in Eastern Europe and remained so until his removal as Director following the collapse of the Dubcek revolution in 1968. He influenced a large number of Czech scientists, from T. Hraba, J. Chutná, I. Hilgert, A. Lengerová, V. Hašková, K. Nouza, V. Holáň and J. and P. Ivanyi to M. Holub (who has since become a well known poet), J. Klein, and P. Démant, and because of the adverse political climate prevailing in Czechoslovakia many of these emigrated to the West and especially to the United States. The scientific memoirs and personal recollections of Milan Hašek, published in a recent monograph (81), form a fitting tribute to Hašek's powers of leadership, influence and personality (see also p. 228). Since his untimely death some of his later collaborators, prominent among them V. Holáň, have been continuing the Prague tradition of studying various aspects of neonatal tolerance.

Further Development of the Concept of Neonatal Tolerance

By 1956 the principle of tolerance, seen as an acquired and highly specific abrogation of responsiveness to histocompatibility (transplantation) antigens following their inoculation into immunologically incompetent animals, was well established. The early observations had shown that the ubiquitous allograft reaction, which with few exceptions was known to lead to the downfall of allografts transplanted to adults (see Chapter 2), could be circumvented by purely biologic means, and this provoked a flood of further investigations.

The state of the art in 1956 was summarized at a historic meeting held in March at the Royal Society, London, and published later that year (82). It was organized by P.B. Medawar, who also made the introductory remarks, and F.M. Burnet was in the Chair. Contributions came from some of the leaders in the field. R.D. Owen discussed erythrocyte antigens in relation to tolerance induction (83) and B. Cinader and J.M. Dubert (84) outlined their data on tolerance induction in neonatal rabbits to human albumin – a study that confirmed previously published investigations with alum-precipitated bovine albumin (85), human albumin (86) and bovine albumin and human plasma (87) – and they suggested that tolerance was due to "some functional modification of the antibody-forming mechanism . . . that may not require the continued presence of antigen". There followed a highly pertinent discussion on the fate of protein antigens inoculated into experimental animals by J.H. Humphrey, summarizing evidence suggesting that protein antigens can survive in the liver long after they have been eliminated from the circulation, and postulating that tolerance depended on "an acquired ability to break down the particular foreign antigenic substance fast enough to prevent it acting as an antigen" – a hypothesis that lost its plausibility when it was shown that the maintenance of tolerance depended upon continued cellular chimerism or, in the case of soluble proteins, repeated inoculation of the antigen. H. Koprowski (88) gave an account of his group's tumor transplantation study, coming to the conclusion that the growth of allogeneic and xenogeneic tumors in mice inoculated *in utero* with normal donor strain cells was due to an adaptation of the host rather than a change in the antigenic nature of the tumors. R.J.C. Harris (89) described experiments on the induction of tolerance in turkeys to the Rous sarcoma "agent". M. Hašek (90) discussed his group's extensive data on the induction of tolerance in birds to xenogeneic (heterologous) red cell antigens following either intravenous inoculation of blood in the last quarter of incubation or after parabiosis: success depended on the taxonomic relationship between the donor and recipient, and in the duck it was possible to induce tolerance even after hatching. R.E. Billingham and L. Brent (91) described for the first time their method of injecting neonatal mice intravenously and showed that it could be an effective method of making mice at least partially tolerant to skin allografts. Both mice and chickens were made tolerant to the skin of two different strains by the concomitant inoculation at birth of blood from the two strains, but the survival time of the grafts was not necessarily symmetric. They concluded that "our interpretation of the experiments on heterologous tolerance is in accord with this taxonomic classification", and they stated that, in contradiction to Hašek and Hraba's earlier claim (76, 79), "we are therefore disinclined to believe that Burnet and Fenner's 1949 'self-marker' concept requires modification in order for it to uphold a distinction between homologous and heterologous antigens". In his concluding remarks, F.M. Burnet (92) made two points worth noting. First, "At a theoretical level I believe that the recent work provides general support for the self-marker concept that Fenner and I proposed in 1949. The differentiation between self and non-self must not, however, be taken too literally. The important division may be between the components of expendable cells and all other materials. As Medawar pointed out, there are subtle distinctions to be made between various tissues according to their time of maturing and their relation to the scavenging cells of the body". Second, in his concluding sentence he stated: "Immunology seems to be ready for a new phase of activity that may be even more fruitful than its first flowering in the hands of Ehrlich and Bordet half a century ago". This big claim has been at least partially justified by subsequent events, even though the world continues to await the dramatic impact of immunology on medicine comparable to that following the discoveries of the early pioneers.

This meeting provided an important landmark in the development of the tolerance concept, and it encouraged activity in many laboratories throughout the world and on the part of many hundreds of investigators. Other conferences, too, reflected this steep rise in interest and excitement, among them the biannual Tissue Homotransplantation Conferences sponsored by the New York Academy of Sciences and organized by the energetic surgeons J.M. Converse and B.O. Rogers. (The latter was also the co-editor of *Transplantation Bulletin*, the only journal specializing in transplantation and the forerunner of the journal *Transplantation*.) This series began in 1954 (93) and concluded with the Seventh Conference in 1966 (94), its role thereafter having been taken over by the International Congresses of The Transplantation Society. This society was formed at the end of the 1964 meeting in New York with the adoption of a constitution and the election of its first President, P.B. Medawar. Its First International Congress in 1968 in Paris and all subsequent biannual congresses have been published in *Transplantation Proceedings*, edited by the indefatigable F.T. Rapaport. Surprisingly, the first of the New York meetings in 1954 contained only one paper on neonatal tolerance (from the Medawar stable) and the input of papers devoted to tolerance in subsequent meetings did not increase nearly as rapidly as that from other areas of tissue transplantation. (The overall interest in transplantation was quantitatively revealed by the ever increasing length of the Conference Proceedings: from the First in 1954, which was a mere 89 pages, to the Seventh in 1966 (884 pages) to the massive multi-volume tomes of the Transplantation Society Congresses.) Yet it is clear from the Symposium held in Liblice in 1961 under the auspices of the Czechoslovak Academy of Sciences (95) that there was a huge ground swell of interest in the phenomenon of tolerance in all its manifestations and in its putative mechanisms, and this was further emphasized by a later and more specialized conference in New York, this time on *Immunological Tolerance to Microbial Antigens* (96). Other international meetings followed.

The development of the concept of neonatally induced tolerance – ignoring for the time being the induction of tolerance in adult animals (see Chapter 6) – was given impetus by attempts to resolve a number of problems: the precise period of an animal's life in which tolerance can be readily induced; the question of its specificity, which was challenged by several groups; the role played by antigen in its maintenance; the establishment of its universality in relation to self-antigens and non-histocompatibilty antigens; above all, the problem of the mechanism(s) underlying its induction; and the role played by the different regions of the major histocompatibility complex (MHC). The rest of this chapter is devoted to these questions.

The "null" (or "neutral") period

Some indication that the induction of unresponsiveness is possible in only very young animals was provided by the transplantation of allografts to chicks in the first fortnight after hatching. Thus, Cannon and Longmire (54) found that grafts placed within three days of hatching had a survival rate of 5–10%, a figure that declined to 1% at 4–6 days and zero at 14 days. Their attempt to boost these figures by administering cortisone was successful in that a higher proportion of chicks (20%) that received their transplants within the first three days now failed to reject them. Woodruff (97) attempted a similar strategy in rats: having shown with Simpson using skin allografts that newborn rats are susceptible to tolerance induction (98), he tried to lengthen the postnatal period in which tolerance could be induced by treating the recipients with cortisone. Unlike Billingham, Brent and Medawar (59) working with mice, he was partially successful.

The concept of a null period, in which the immunologic development of an animal is such that the introduction of antigens will incite neither tolerance nor immunity, was developed by Billingham, Brent and Medawar in 1956 (59). It was based on their finding that out of a large number of newborn mice inoculated intraperitoneally soon after birth with crude suspensions of fragments and cells from several adult donor strain organs, relatively few became tolerant and the remainder were neither tolerant nor immune. "So far as homografts are concerned the epoch of birth represents, for the great majority of mice, a *null period* during which exposure to an antigenic stimulus confers neither tolerance nor immunity to any appreciable degree."

This concept soon required revision. For example:

(1) Within a year Billingham and Brent (62, 99) had shown that cleaned up suspensions of adult spleen cells inoculated into newborn mice *intravenously* were remarkably effective in inducing long-lasting tolerance in some strain combinations. This observation was soon confirmed by R.A. Good's group in Minneapolis (100) after L. Brent had demonstrated the intravenous route of inoculation to them on a visit in the summer of 1956.

(2) The proportion of tolerant mice injected at birth could be increased, and the period in which tolerance to skin grafts could be induced was extended, by using larger doses of donor cells (101, 102). Even adult mice were rendered unresponsive by multiple doses of H-2 incompatible donor strain cells (103) or by a single large dose of H-2 compatible cells (104).

(3) Inoculation of very small numbers of viable or large numbers of irradiated donor cells into newborn mice sensitized the animals sufficiently for them to become invulnerable to the graft-versus-host disease that would normally be expected from the inoculation of larger numbers of parental strain donor cells on the second day (*105*). The same pre-treatment prevented tolerance induction to skin allografts by the inoculation of a tolerance-inducing inoculum on the fourth day (*106*).

(4) In species with long gestation periods, such as the sheep, the fetus was found to be capable of skin allograft rejection at 117 days when grafts were implanted subcutaneously (*107*), and this was later found to apply to orthotopic skin allografts transplanted as early as the eightieth day (*108*) (i.e. close to the end of the third trimester). In the rhesus monkey fetus a roughly similar situation was shown to prevail, in that orthotopic skin allografts transplanted on the fifty-eighth day (gestation period 165 days) were rejected normally (*109*), the histologic picture being virtually indistinguishable from that of rejection in the adult. Antigens such as sheep red blood cells were also shown to induce antibody formation in the fetuses of these large animal species and Uhr (*110*) demonstrated that guinea pigs presented with antigens such as diphtheria toxoid, bovine serum albumin or ovalbumin one or two weeks before birth gave typical delayed-type hypersentivity skin reactions when tested on the first day following birth. For a detailed survey of the early and extensive work on the development of immunity the reader is referred to Šterzl and Silverstein's exhaustive review (*111*).

(5) Finally, studies on the male-specific minor histocompatibility antigen, H-Y, provided the final nail in the coffin for the notion that there is a null period closely associated with the immediate postnatal period of animals. Following on the heels of Billingham and Brent's demonstration that it is far from difficult to inject newborn mice intravenously (*62*) there came a clutch of papers, many of them from R.A. Good's laboratory in Minneapolis, not only pointing to the ease with which neonatal female mice can be rendered tolerant to male skin grafts by the intravenous inoculation of syngeneic male cells (*112, 113*) – even in very small numbers (*114, 115*) – but showing that the tolerance-inducing or adaptive period extends well into postnatal life for this relatively weak antigen (*112, 116*). This point was further emphasized by the demonstration (*117*) that even adult females become tolerant to syngeneic male skin following parabiosis, the time taken (two weeks) being far shorter than for strains differing at the H-2 locus (seven weeks). Others showed at roughly the same time the feasibility of creating tolerance in adult parabionts joined together with mice of totally different strains, both H-2 compatible and non-compatible (*118, 119*), or by multiple intravenous inoculation of cells into adult recipients (*102, 120*).

It is clear, then, that insofar as a null or neutral period exists it is essentially movable, depending on the strength of the antigen, the dose at which it is administered and the route by which it is presented.

Where does this leave the human neonate then? By analogy with other species with long gestation periods one could reasonably expect it to be past the adaptive period in which the induction of tolerance is still possible. Although the human newborn is by no means immunologically fully mature – it depends for its protection from infectious organisms to some degree on maternal antibodies transmitted in the milk – it is capable of certain responses soon after birth (see below).

Encouraged by the work of Puza and Gombos (121), who claimed to have observed some degree of tolerance to skin allografts taken from adult dogs whose blood had been used in total transfusions of puppies 3–4 days after birth, Albert et al. (122) drew attention in 1959 to a single human case illustrating, they thought, the same phenomenon. A baby with erythroblastosis had been transfused with Rh-negative blood 40 hours after birth, followed by two subsequent transfusions from different adult donors. This boy was given a skin graft from the blood donor seven years later and the authors claimed that this graft, though undergoing all kinds of trials and tribulations, survived for at least 81 days: "Two black hairs had disappeared, one remained alive"! Bearing in mind the great difficulties of assessing skin graft rejection when it is subacute there must be some considerable doubt concerning the survival of this graft, and the doubt is sharpened by an extraordinary postscript appearing in the paper though not in the oral presentation. Evidently it had later emerged that, thanks to an administrative error, the skin donor had not been one of the blood donors; if tolerance had indeed developed to his graft this must have been brought about by wholly nonspecific mechanisms. On balance one is inclined to dismiss this anecdotal case as invalid.

A year later Fowler, Schubert and West (123) described the fate of skin allografts from donors whose blood had been used in exchange transfusions in 12 newborn infants who were being treated for jaundice. Transfusions were given in the first few days of life and the skin grafts were applied a day or two later. Six of them had been treated with stored blood and the skin grafts had come from either the two blood donors or from the father or mother: all grafts were rejected acutely. The other six had received skin from their specific blood donors, and here rejection was considerably delayed though the grafts were eventually rejected or were undergoing rejection at the time of biopsy. The authors did not overinterpret their data and concluded that "The newborn human infant already displays a highly developed homograft rejection mechanism". It is, in any case, quite possible that the clinical condition of the babies was partly responsible for the limited prolongation of survival.

This and subsequent studies indicated that the human neonate is immunologically sufficiently well developed to banish all thought of tolerance induction – a conclusion that is well supported by evidence (124–126) showing that the human neonate is capable of antibody production and the development of delayed-type hypersensitivity reactions. Although it is theoretically not impossible that tolerance to a given donor such as the father or the mother could be induced by intrafetal inoculation of viable cells the complexities of such a procedure, with the overriding need to avoid graft-versus-host disease, would probably be too great, yet experiments in the fetal sheep (127), baboon (128) and rhesus (129) and cynomolgus (130) monkey have been attempted with human application in mind. Such an approach is likely to be over-taken by gene transfer to individuals with single gene disorders. The answer P.B. Medawar is said to have given to a question after one of his lectures on tolerance, that the phenomenon had absolutely no clinical applicability (131), was entirely realistic for at that time (1957) Medawar could not have foreseen the great impact the concept of tolerance would have on the initiation of a helter-skelter search for methods to induce specific unresponsiveness in adult animals, including man.

It is of interest that Van Rood and his colleagues have found (*132*) that, when tissue typing human organ graft recipients and their potential donors, there are some "permissible mismatches" of certain HLA antigens (usually A or B) against which the graft recipient does not make antibodies. They claimed that such antigens are non-inherited maternal antigens (NIMA) towards which tolerance had been induced during fetal life by the accidental passage of maternal cells into the fetal circulation. There are at present some difficulties with this interpretation, not least among them the lack of persuasive evidence for cellular chimerism in such individuals; yet in the mouse (*133*) (but not in the rat (*134*)) supporting evidence has been provided, in that young mice have been shown to have maternal lymphocytes in their lymphoid tissue associated with prolonged survival of maternal skin.

The question of specificity

In their 1956 monograph Billingham, Brent and Medawar (*59*) considered the tissue and individual (or strain) specificity of acquired tolerance. They presented cogent evidence against tissue specificity, for whole blood, blood leukocytes, and a mixture of adult tissues, and even a mammary carcinoma, induced tolerance to skin allografts from the same donor strain. It was later shown that a wide variety of tissues such as spleen, bone marrow, lymph nodes and thymus are effective inducers of tolerance of skin or kidney allografts, and this lack of tissue specificity in tolerance induction has never been challenged. (The exceptions are non-nucleated mammalian and nucleated avian red blood cells, the latter lacking histocompatibility antigens and both having a finite lifespan.) Billingham, Brent and Medawar concluded that ". . . this leads to an inference of a much more radical kind – that skin epithelium contains no antigens not also present in the leukocytes." Many years later it was shown that although class I histocompatibility antigens are ubiquitously represented on tissues, red cells excepted, class II antigens have a more restricted distribution (see Chapter 2).

By contrast, these authors found that tolerance was rigorously individual or strain specific in both mice and chickens and it is therefore surprising that doubts about this arose later. According to them, "tissues from one donor should confer *tolerance* of tissues taken from another only when the second donor contains *no* antigens not also present in the first . . . therefore, tolerance was strictly specific to donors isogenic with those that provided the cells for the foetal inoculation, and the power of tolerant mice to react upon homografts from unrelated donors was not perceptibly impaired." A previous finding "that a tolerated homograft underwent a temporary setback during the rejection of a homograft from a new and different donor" (*52*) was "corrected" in a 1955 paper (*135*): "The mistake was due to using partially tolerant animals. . . . When tolerance is complete, a homograft from a new donor is destroyed without a perceptible reaction upon the homograft already present."

Doubts about the stringency of individual specificity were first expressed by Terasaki, Cannon and Longmire (*136*), who induced a low-level tolerance in embryonic chicks by the intravenous inoculation of embryonic blood that had come from a donor of the same breed or from one of a different breed. When the recipients were challenged with skin grafts from chicks other than the blood donor there was a small, but apparently significant, overall improvement in graft survival compared with normal controls. These authors were at a loss to explain their findings though they discounted antigenic similarity between the blood and the skin donors. Interpretation of these data is complicated by the fact that the breeds used were not inbred. Among other examples of tolerance that were not fully individual were the following.

(1) Hašek's group (137) described a single turkey that had been parabiosed in embryonic life with a chicken. It failed to reject xenogeneic skin grafts taken from two "third-party" chickens as well as an allograft, although a skin graft from another xenogeneic species (guinea fowl) was promptly rejected. It would appear that tolerance to xenoantigens had overridden the recognition of alloantigens of the donor as well as the host species – a finding that has never been adequately explained.

(2) In a model of tolerance to allogeneic skin grafts, Zeiss (138) noticed some non-specific manifestations in tolerant rats, though she found this to be the exception rather than the rule; she excluded graft-versus-host disease as a possible cause, but was unable to discriminate between an innate ability to respond and genuine cross-tolerance.

(3) Holáň et al. (139) found that the suppressor lymphocytes generated in their mouse model of neonatally induced tolerance were nonspecifically suppressive in one strain combination when spleen cells were transferred to syngeneic recipients, but not in the reciprocal combination.

However, these ill-explained exceptions – and interestingly they seem to have their counterpart in tolerance induced in adult animals (see Chapter 6) – do not overthrow the overall concept of individual specificity in neonatal tolerance, for this has frequently been confirmed in neonatally induced allogeneic tolerance. The problem has more recently been reinvestigated in two laboratories with the aid of a battery of inbred strains and their recombinants. Thus, Streilein and Klein (140) showed that tolerant mice vigorously reject third-party skin allografts expressing strong class I antigens foreign to both donor and recipient. They found, surprisingly, that third-party grafts expressing the tolerated class I antigens plus weak class II antigens were rejected with special dispatch, and this was true also for third-party grafts carrying the host's own class II and the tolerated donor class I antigens. In interpreting these findings these workers suggested that tolerant animals possess precursors of cytotoxic T lymphocytes with the capacity to recognize and react against the tolerated donor K and D antigens, and that this potential, suppressed in some way (probably by suppressor T cells), can be "brushed aside when the same strong antigens are presented in an inappropriate genetic context". Such an explanation would probably also account for the data of Holáň et al. (139) referred to above.

Holáň (141) returned to this problem recently and carried out some careful experiments in which he looked for confirmation that tolerance in mice had a nonspecific element. He was quite unable to do so and concluded that "neonatally induced tolerance to skin allografts in mice is absolutely specific", thus vindicating the original claims made by Billingham, Brent and Medawar (51). Those cases of nonspecificity described in the literature are probably exceptional and are likely to owe their existence to special features of the experimental model.

Some reflections on the issue of specificity are in order here. As tolerance is an immunologic event it undoubtedly makes sense that it should be restricted to the antigens that were used to incite it in any one individual. So far as clinical transplantation is concerned, specificity is something of a double-edged weapon. Its great attraction is that it leaves the tolerant subject fully responsive to other and potentially harmful antigens, such as those carried by infectious organisms. This consideration makes the induction of some form of tolerance in man so attractive when compared with the blunderbuss approach inherent in the use of chemical immunosuppressive agents. On the other hand, the induction of specific unresponsiveness in patients would be a great deal simpler if its specificity were less stringent (see Chapter 6). That it is possible, in some instances, to induce tolerance in adult animals with only some of the antigens expressed on an organ allograft is of great interest and possibly holds some clinical potential (see Chapter 6).

The concept of split tolerance

The notion that a mouse might become tolerant to some of the histocompatibility antigens present in tolerance-inducing cells, but not to others, stems from the observation that the inoculation of allogeneic hybrid cells into neonatal mice may induce tolerance of skin grafts for one of the parental strains of the hybrid but not for the other. This finding was described by Billingham and Brent (99) as 'split tolerance'. They proposed two hypotheses: selection by the neonatal recipient against donor cells carrying the least favored antigens, and transformation by some host cells, leading to the acquisition by some host cells of the more favored antigens. Both hypotheses seem extremely far-fetched in retrospect, and Brent and Courtenay, a few years later, provided evidence against them (142). They did, however, confirm the original data and they also showed the continued chimerism of hybrid cells carrying both sets of antigens in mice that had rejected skin grafts from one of the parental strains. The alternative hypotheses put forward by them to explain their findings were not much more plausible than those they replaced and they were later made redundant by the demonstration that some mouse strains carry a skin-specific (SK) antigen not present in the lymphoreticular cells normally used for tolerance induction (49, 143). The observation that a human recipient fully accepted a fraternal twin kidney following whole body irradiation without subsequent immunosuppression, but rejected the donor's skin graft (144), suggests that an SK antigen might have been involved. The demonstration that newly hatched chicks made tolerant to skin allografts can nonetheless produce antidonor antibodies has also been ascribed to split tolerance (145) though it might well have been a case of incomplete tolerance.

Does maintenance of tolerance depend on the continuous presence of the antigen?

In their 1956 monograph Billingham, Brent and Medawar (59) had drawn attention not only to the long-lasting red cell mosaicism described by Owen in cattle dizygotic twins, but also to their finding that natural chicken twins have, and artificial synchorial twinning of chicken embryos brings about, a state of red cell chimerism. Further, they found that skin graft tolerance was firmly linked to red cell chimerism: when the latter disappeared in one pair of parabionts later in life, the skin grafts that had been tolerated well until then underwent chronic rejection. The emphasis here was on red cell chimerism because, thanks to the work of R.D. Owen, a number of specific antibodies had become available for identifying chicken red cells. Thus, ". . . it is virtually certain that red-cell chimerism must entail a tolerance of skin homografts, for red-cell chimerism comes about when blood cells are exchanged in foetal life. . . . There is, of course, no reason why a tolerance of skin homografts produced by the inoculation of tissues lacking red-cell precursors (e.g. tumour fragments) should lead to red-cell chimerism". Although donor cell chimerism was therefore firmly linked to tolerance, there was at that time no evidence for the presence of donor cells other than those of hemopoietic origin. They made one other point in relation to Hašek and Hraba's inability to demonstrate red cell chimerism in chicken parabionts (79) despite depressed antibody responses against their partner's red cells: "An existing state of red-cell chimerism must of necessity imply a failure to form the appropriate iso-agglutinins, but the disappearance of chimerism does not imply that iso-agglutinins will thereupon be formed". In the study of Billingham, Brent and Medawar parabionts that had lost their red cell chimerism were nonetheless deficient in their antibody responses against their partner's red cells. It is not at all clear whether they thought that the partial tolerance displayed by a shortfall in antibody production after the termination of red cell chimerism was brought about by the continued presence of other kinds of donor cells. At any rate, they went on to say that "Hašek's inference, from his failure to demonstrate chimerism, that chimerism and the inhibition of antibody formation are essentially different phenomena, cannot therefore be upheld".

Evidence for the maintenance of the tolerant state by donor antigen came from studies of cellular chimerism on the one hand, and from the use of soluble protein antigens in the induction of tolerance on the other. Billingham, Brent and Medawar (59) had shown that viable cells were essential: nucleated and replicating cells lost their ability to induce tolerance after they had been killed by methods that preserved their physical integrity, and even nucleated chicken red cells were of no use. This was an issue analyzed fastidiously by Mitchison: the tolerance induced in embryonic or newly hatched chicks with purified allogeneic red blood cells continued for as long as regular transfusions were administered, but tolerance was lost 25–29 days after the transfusions were terminated (146). Mitchison had used the elimination rates of chromium-labeled red cells from the donor as a test for tolerance, and his results were decisive in showing that the presence of the antigen is essential for maintaining the tolerant state. His demonstration had been preceded by Simonsen's finding that the maintenance of a partial tolerance induced in chicken embryos by human blood depended on repeated weekly transfusions (147).

Other evidence came hard and fast, not least the finding that graft-versus-host disease, often chronic in nature, ensues when fully allogeneic immunocompetent cells are injected into fetal or neonatal rodents (see below). Billingham and Brent (99) studied the question of donor cell chimerism using a variant of Mitchison's design (148): they discovered donor cells in significant numbers in all tissues (spleen, lymph nodes, bone marrow, kidney, liver, thymus, blood) tested, but failed to find such cells in partially tolerant mice that had rejected their skin grafts after a period of time. With perhaps undue caution they stated, nonetheless, that "The question of whether a lasting tolerance of homologous tissues depends upon the persistence in the hosts of donor strain cells must for the time being remain unanswered", for although a clear association had been established, proof was lacking, they felt, that tolerance could not continue without donor cells. The persistence of donor cell chimerism was later established quantitatively by Silobrčić, using the T6T6 chromosomal marker in CBA mice: a level of 12–15% was found in the spleen and lymph nodes of tolerant mice and, though declining with age, the donor cells never disappeared altogether, even in old mice (149).

Convincing proof came from two laboratories. Silvers (150) removed long-tolerated skin grafts from adult females that had been made tolerant at birth to syngeneic male skin carrying the minor H-Y histocompatibility antigen. The skin grafts had been transplanted soon after birth and the mice had never received a cellular inoculum. On removal of the grafts the mice regained immunologic competence to H-Y – clear evidence that the continued presence of the H-Y molecule had been directly responsible for tolerance maintenance. An ingenious variant of this approach was followed by Lubaroff and Silvers a few years later (151). They worked with mice that had been made tolerant to allogeneic skin grafts by the classic method, and they destroyed the donor chimeric cells as well as the skin grafts by transferring sensitized C3H-anti-A cells into tolerant CBA mice carrying healthy A strain grafts. The C3H cells adoptively transferred differed from their CBA hosts for minor antigens and would eventually be rejected, though evidently not before they had effectively undermined the tolerant state of the hosts. When fresh A strain skin grafts were subsequently transplanted to the same animals they were rejected, presumably by host lymphocytes that had regenerated in the absence of donor antigen. However, inoculation of F1 hybrid cells following the adoptive transfer of sensitized cells ensured acceptance of fresh skin grafts. The same workers (152) had previously destroyed donor cell chimerism in rats with specific antisera directed against donor strain antigens, a procedure that would not be expected to harm the skin grafts directly (see Chapter 2); yet the skin grafts did undergo rejection, presumably because of the previous removal of donor cells by antibodies. Harris, Harris and Farber subsequently confirmed in mice that tolerance could be broken by alloantibodies, though persuaded by the kinetics of skin graft rejection they were inclined to believe that graft destruction was mainly brought about by a direct effect of the antibodies on the graft (153).

These immunogenetic studies received powerful backing from investigations involving tolerance induction to soluble protein antigens. Following pioneering work (85–87) showing that tolerance to a variety of proteins such as bovine serum albumin can be induced in neonatal rodents followed by multiple doses of the tolerogen, the question soon arose of whether the maintenance of tolerance required further and regular inoculations of the tolerogen. According to Cinader and Dubert (154), rabbits that had received a large dose of bovine serum albumin soon after birth remained unresponsive for as long as 600 days, but although this received some support (155) it was challenged by others who found that repeated doses of the tolerogen were essential if the unresponsiveness was to be prevented from decaying. Thus, Wolfe et al. showed that the unresponsiveness induced by a single large dose of bovine serum albumin given intraperitoneally to 50-hour-old chicks declined significantly by 12 weeks (156), and the same was found to be true when chick embryos were inoculated intravenously on the fifteenth day of incubation (157). Smith and Bridges (158) subjected the hypothesis that antigen persistence is essential to the most rigorous quantitative examination, again in rabbits. In their hands a single large intraperitoneal dose of one of several proteins given to neonatal rabbits induced a specific unresponsiveness for 90–120 days, but this time-limited unresponsiveness could be indefinitely prolonged by repeated injections of the tolerogen. They also showed that the initial dose given to the neonatal rabbit was of considerable importance. It would appear that repeated challenge with the tolerogen to test the immune status of the rabbits could itself have prolonged the tolerant state – a point that may well explain the earlier data of Cinader and Dubert (154). Smith and Bridges concluded that "The data ... appear to be consistent with an hypothesis that the persistence of the originally injected antigen in critical tissues is directly or indirectly responsible for inhibition of the immune response to this antigen at subsequent challenge ... The data presented would suggest that the critical antigen may be located intracellularly ... ".

It would therefore seem that the persistence of the tolerogenic stimulus is vital for the maintenance of tolerance. Evidently the constantly turning-over population of lymphocytes must be exposed to the tolerogen to reacquire unresponsiveness, which is clearly not a property passed on to the cellular progeny of tolerant cells. Whether the tolerogen has a direct effect on antigen-specific T and B lymphocytes or on cells with the capacity for specific suppression is a question that will be examined below, as will the possibility that in adult animals tolerance can be maintained by signals emanating only from the test graft in the absence of detectable chimerism.

Very recently the question of donor cell chimerism has been raised by T.E. Starzl in relation to human liver allograft recipients – a possibility that, surprisingly, had not previously received attention. According to Starzl's group, donor cells migrate from the transplanted organ to the tissues of the recipient (159–161), and they have pointed to a possible analogy between this drug-induced unresponsiveness and neonatally induced tolerance – a question that will be discussed further in Chapter 7.

The universality of the tolerance phenomenon

Medawar had begun his activities in allotransplantation in the mid-1940s by studying human and rabbit skin allografts (see Chapter 2). It was therefore natural that he and his colleagues should continue to use skin grafts as their analytic tool. Not only is the surgical procedure of skin transplantation extremely simple, especially in small rodents, but it is also relatively non-traumatic to the animals. Furthermore, the monitoring of graft survival can be carried out by naked eye inspection on a day to day basis once the bandage has been removed after the grafts have firmly healed in – in practice from the sixth or seventh day after the operation; and small biopsies or whole grafts can be readily removed for histologic examination. Renewed hair growth in the graft is a sure sign of the health of the graft, and there can be little doubt that the early photographs of white-haired grafts on agouti murine recipients, of brown or black-haired grafts on albino hosts, and perhaps most strikingly, of brown feathers growing profusely from a Rhode Island Red graft on a White Leghorn chicken (59) made a deep impression on the biologic and immunologic communities. Kidney transplantation in rats did not become possible until the late 1960s and it is therefore hardly surprising that most workers entering the field of tolerance readily followed the example of the University College group.

The mouse remained the favored species, primarily because, thanks to the work of Snell and his colleagues at Bar Harbor, numerous highly inbred strains and their congenic lines became increasingly available, facilitating analysis of the phenomenon. Thus, the influence of different parts of the H-2 histocompatibility locus, the intricacies of which were rapidly being revealed in terms of subregions and individual antigenic determinants, could be examined (see below). In addition mechanisms could be studied by the adoptive transfer of viable lymphocytes from one mouse to another of the same inbred strain – not to mention the determination of both tissue and individual specificity and exploration of the question of graft as opposed to host adaptation. Hašek and his colleagues had successfully used the chicken and other avian species, in which the embryo is accessible to manipulation either by parabiosis (70) or by inoculation of cell suspensions via one of the chorioallantoic veins (59); but even they turned increasingly to the mouse in their later studies.

However, it soon became evident that other species, usually outbred, were amenable to tolerance induction immediately or soon after birth, provided that the neonates were still relatively immature immunologically. The work of Woodruff and Simpson (98) pointed to the rat as an excellent species from this point of view, and despite the almost uniformly unsuccessful attempts by Billingham and Brent (99) – conceivably but improbably explained by their use of skin grafts that had been frozen in 15% glycerol at −79° C – the neonatal rat was soon used by others. Those working with soluble protein antigens (see above) turned to the neonatal rabbit even before publication of Woodruff and Simpson's paper (98), mainly because the rabbit, unlike the mouse, was known to be a good producer of antibodies and because it was assumed that the neonate would be immunologically sufficiently immature. As we have seen above, this expectation was largely justified.

As the larger mammalian neonates have been shown to be well past the adaptive period for tolerance induction (107–111) it is puzzling that at least one claim has been made for the induction of tolerance to human albumin in the neonatal goat (162). Other species more akin in their immunologic development to the mouse, in which tolerance has been successfully induced after birth, include the Syrian hamster (163); and LaPlante et al. showed that the pouch young of the North American opossum not only accepted maternal skin grafts for very long periods, but that 60% with long-surviving grafts also accepted a second maternal graft, while rejecting a third-party graft normally (164). Gengozian et al. revealed that fraternal twins of the marmoset, a small New World primate in which there is a high incidence of placental vascular anastomosis, were invariably chimeric in their lymphoreticular tissues (165) and tolerant of each other's skin when tested in adult life (166), thus further corroborating the earlier work of Owen in another species.

It has therefore been firmly established that any species whose neonates are immunologically still immature is suitable for the induction of tolerance after birth. It will be seen in Chapter 6 that even immunologically competent adults can be rendered tolerant provided other strategies are used to reduce their immunologic status to that of a newborn mouse.

In view of the fact that tolerance lacks tissue specificity except where tissue-specific antigens can operate as alloantigens, as for the SK antigen, it follows that the use of spleen cells or whole blood can induce tolerance not only to skin, but to other tissues and organs. This was demonstrated strikingly by Simonsen and his colleagues (167) when they transplanted a kidney from one dizygotic cattle twin to another (in which the tolerogenic signal must have come from blood cell precursors), and it has been amply confirmed in the rat with kidneys and other organs (168) and in the mouse for the ovary (169) and the adrenal gland (170). However, as will be seen in Chapter 6, some organs and tissues have more stringent requirements than others and that for the long-term survival of skin grafts nothing but the most complete form of unresponsiveness suffices. Patterson (171) was one of the first to show that inoculation of allogeneic spinal cord into newborn rats prevented the recipients from producing a paralytogenic response when challenged later in life with adjuvant-incorporated spinal cord. Tolerance has been induced for many microbial organisms including the Rous sarcoma virus (172) and *Shigella paradysenteriae* (173).

The concept of tolerance was thus established as having validity in many species, for a variety of tissues and organs, and for antigens other than histocompatibility antigens. Although restricted to immunologically incompetent animals it triggered a vast field of research devoted to the induction of tolerance in adult animals and ultimately in man, and it set the 'gold standard' for a form of unresponsiveness that was specific, independent of continuous immunosuppression and essentially harmless to the tolerant individual. It threw a ray of light on the known unresponsiveness to 'self' and it was instrumental in the development of theories seeking to explain the mechanisms underlying immunologic unresponsiveness.

Mechanisms of Tolerance

Clonal deletion

In their 1953 *Nature* paper Billingham, Brent and Medawar (52) did not express any view as to the mechanism of tolerance, except to speculate that it might owe something to the action of "tissue haptens" that were themselves non-antigenic but contained the determinant groupings conferring specific activity on complete antigens. They quoted the work from several laboratories that had already induced some form of unresponsiveness in adult animals – Felton's 'immunologic paralysis' with pneumococcal polysaccharide (55), Chase's orally induced desensitization to simple chemical compounds (56) and the work by Casey, Snell and Kaliss and their colleagues on the enhancement of tumor growth with the aid of lyophilized allogeneic tissue preparations (see 57 and Chapter 6). In their 1956 paper (59) Billingham, Brent and Medawar developed the notion that unlike tumor enhancement, tolerance represented "a primary central failure of the mechanism of the immunologic reaction", the critical evidence having come from experiments in which tolerance was abolished by the introduction into tolerant mice of not only presensitized but also normal syngeneic lymph node cells. It was argued that this proved that tolerance could not have been peripheral, for example through the intervention of antibodies or antigen–antibody complexes, because the normal lymphoid cells would have been expected to come under the influence of any prevailing peripheral suppressive mechanism and the tolerant state should have continued unabated. It was not until several years later – once it had been shown that lymphocytes bring about the rejection of allografts (174), that individual antibody-producing cells can respond to only one antigen or a very restricted range (175–177) and Burnet had fully developed his clonal selection hypothesis (68) – that tolerance as well as self-tolerance was interpreted as being due to the elimination of a clone or clones of antigen-reactive lymphocytes. The breaking of tolerance by normal syngeneic lymphoid cells was a cornerstone of this theory.

In his Nobel Prize lecture, given on December 12th 1960 (*178*), Medawar did not develop the theory of tolerance a great deal further, being content to leave the more theoretic speculations to Burnet on the same occasion (*179*). The latter, in discussing the immunologic recognition of self, suggested some variants of his clonal selection hypothesis and stated that "circulating globulin (as postulated by Jerne, *180*) can be categorically eliminated in view of the phenomena of graft-versus-host reactions and any attempt to give an observable basis to the concept must be concerned with the immunologically competent cell (as envisaged by Talmage, *66* and Burnet, *68*) . . . The elimination of self-reactive patterns would . . . result when prenatal contact with self-components occurred. The residue would be available to react with and 'recognize' foreign configurations entering during the period of independent life". In support of his ideas he referred to graft-versus-host lesions in the chorioallantoic membrane of chick embryos to which limited numbers of blood leukocytes had been added, the difference between negative and positive membranes (multiple lesions) having been attributed to a single antigenic determinant in the host (*181*). Overall, Burnet reiterated his belief that both self-recognition and tolerance develop on a cellular, "and probably on a clonal", basis.

Preceding the Nobel Lectures by about a year, Medawar had published a closely argued analysis of theories of tolerance (*182*). The argument was based on two major assumptions:

(1) That the maintenance of tolerance depends on the persistence of the antigen(s).
(2) That any one antibody-forming cell or its lineage responds to only one antigen at a time (*175–177*).

He eventually arrived at two "self-consistent" theories:

(1) The Burnet–Lederberg hypothesis that cells preadapted to react upon particular antigens are eliminated from the organism, and persisting antigen is needed to induce tolerance in stem cells that differentiate throughout life. Accordingly, tolerance was a property of the organism rather than of the cell, a question first posed by Woodruff (*183*).
(2) A theory that is based on the assumption that an antibody-forming cell can respond to any antigen with which it comes first into contact, and that tolerance "involves some change in the immature antibody-forming cell other than death and elimination". He pointed out that the latter "has one interesting logical consequence, namely that whereas the effect of antigen upon embryos is to induce immunologic tolerance, the effect of antigen upon adults is twofold: to evoke an immune response from some cells and tolerance from others" (*184*), as was postulated by Loutit (*185*).

Considering the overall state of knowledge at the time – for example, this was before the distinction between T and B lymphocytes was appreciated – this is a remarkably clear statement encapsulating the two possibilities that continue to exercise the minds of immunologists even now, and the probability is that these two theories do in fact account for the different forms of tolerance that are known to exist. However, the concept of clonal deletion of antigen-reactive T lymphocytes held sway after it had been shown experimentally that the immune response is indeed clonal. It is of some interest that Medawar, who with Burnet may be thought of as the founder of cellular immunology, was at this time still thinking exlusively in terms of antibody-producing cells. Some ambivalence remained, for Medawar concluded that "The somewhat scholastic exercise ... cannot distract attention from the fact that we still have no idea of the nature of the change that occurs *within* cells when they become tolerant – supposing that there is such a thing as a tolerant cell".

The concept of clonal deletion received support from a variety of quite different experimental observations, which seem to have stood the test of time. Thus, tolerant mice were shown to lack cells able to respond in graft-versus-host assays against donor antigens (186–189) or to suppress such reactions (190); and antidonor reactivity was likewise absent when tested by the *in vitro* mixed lymphocyte reaction (MLR) or cell-mediated lympholysis (CML) assays (189, 191–194). This was found to correlate with the absence or virtual absence of cytotoxic T cell precursors (195), which the limiting dilution technique made particularly persuasive (196–200) when it became available in the 1980s. It soon became apparent, however, that this was true mainly for class I histocompatibility antigens (198, 201), tolerance to class II having a different explanation (202) (see below). There was also a hint that selection might be against high affinity B cells (203, 204) and that it occurs within the thymus (205).

Other evidence adding weight to the clonal deletion hypothesis came from the confirmation that tolerance is broken by the adoptive transfer of normal cells, in this case small lymphocytes (174), although it later transpired that this did not apply to tolerance to class II molecules (206), thus explaining the difficulty some workers had in repeating the experiments of Billingham, Brent and Medawar (59). As already noted, the latter had fortuitously chosen strains of mice for these experiments that differed from their donors only for class I molecules. Further, Nossal and his colleagues were the first to show that tolerance to minor (but not major) histocompatibility antigens (207) and to soluble proteins (208) can be abrogated by giving tolerant mice a sublethal dose of X-irradiation, suggesting to them that radiation had selected a residual non-tolerant subpopulation of host cells. However, other workers (209, 210) were unable to break tolerance to soluble proteins in this way and it is in any case possible to interpret the findings in other ways. Finally, in a decade in which it became fashionable to explain tolerance in terms of blocking antibodies (see below) the role of such antibodies was nonetheless questioned by some workers after rigorous investigations (211).

Not long after the discovery in 1961 of the role of the thymus gland in the development of the immune system (212) (see Chapter 1) Waksman and his colleagues went a long way towards linking the thymus gland with the events leading to the induction of tolerance. This was done initially in experiments in which the thymus of tolerant animals was transplanted to thymectomized irradiated adult rats. This resulted in specific tolerance to bovine gamma globulin (213, 214) as measured by antibody formation and delayed type skin reactions. Later, similar results were obtained by the inoculation of bovine gamma globulin directly into the thymus of irradiated adult rats (215–217) (see also Chapter 6). The intrathymic route proved to be significantly more efficient than intravenous administration of the antigen, suggesting that the thymus played a special role in tolerance induction. This point was strongly reinforced by the later demonstration by Robinson and Owen (*218*) that *in vitro* culture of embryonic thymus tissue from 14-day-old fetuses, together with adult mitomycin-treated allogeneic spleen fragments, prevented the development of specific mixed lymphocyte reaction reactivity, and this was interpreted as the *in vitro* induction of tolerance in thymic tissue. When the thymic explants were first cultured on their own for three days, tolerance was no longer induced.

By the end of the 1960s evidence began to accrue that neonatally induced tolerance, and indeed specific unresponsiveness induced in adult animals, could have very different explanations, for first antigen–antibody complexes and later suppressor cells came into vogue (see below). Interest in clonal deletion waned correspondingly and revived only when the availability of monoclonal antibodies reacting with T cell receptors using specific V-β segments made it possible to pin down the fate of cells in the thymus and the periphery in a very precise way. The laboratory of J.W. Kappler and P. Marrack played a decisive role here: the paper these workers published with N. Roehm in 1987 (*219*) showed beyond reasonable doubt that potentially self-reacting T cells expressing V-β 17α are present in the immature thymocyte population but are selectively eliminated from both the peripheral T cell population and the mature thymocyte pool of mice expressing IE (class II MHC antigens of the mouse). Despite earlier demonstrations (*220–222*) that in some experimental systems potentially self-reacting clones are present in the mature lymphocyte population – suggesting that some unknown mechanism (anergy?) was preventing them from responding to self-antigens – this finding established that clonal elimination is probably the foremost mechanism securing self-tolerance, which can be supplemented when necessary by anergy or active suppression in order to obviate the danger of autoimmune responses. This principle was soon extended to tolerance towards Mls (mixed lymphocyte stimulation) antigens (see Chapter 4) in adult mice (*223–226*) as well as to neonatal tolerance to Mls antigens. Marrack *et al.* (*224*) showed that clonal deletion can come about as a result of an interaction between thymic T cells major histocompatibility complex (MHC) molecules expressed on bone marrow-derived cells.

That two modalities of tolerance can come about in the thymus – clonal deletion and clonal inactivation (anergy) – was demonstrated by Roberts, Sharrow and Singer (*227*), though in a radiation chimera model. (The development of the concept of anergy will be discussed in Chapter 6.) Although the precise details of what happens in these intrathymic interactions remain to be elucidated, these investigations, using molecular technology, have restored the concept of clonal deletion as a critically important mechanism in self-tolerance and, by implication, also in tolerance to allogeneic antigens. The wheel has turned full circle: what was surmised from relatively crude biologic experiments in the 1950s has been vindicated by precise molecular techniques some three decades later.

Suppressive mechanisms

Antibodies and antigen–antibody complexes
Antibodies can be instrumental in enhancing allogeneic tumor growth – a form of specific inhibition of the immunologic response. This has been known since Kaliss demonstrated in the mid-1950s that the phenomenon of enhancement, originally induced by the pretreatment of adult animals with lyophilized preparations of the

donor's tumor or normal tissue, can be brought about by alloantisera containing antibodies directed against the donor's histocompatibility antigens (228). Indeed, feedback inhibition with specific antibody is a well-established phenomenon (229–231). It is therefore not surprising that investigators began to look for antibodies or antigen–antibody complexes in models of neonatally induced tolerance.

The idea that 'blocking' antibodies or antigen–antibody complexes might be responsible for a wide variety of experimentally induced models of specific unresponsiveness was strongly promoted by the work of K.E and I. Hellström (232) (see Chapter 6), who conducted their early work at the Karolinska Institute, where they had been graduate students of Professor George Klein, the reknowned tumor biologist; they later moved to the United States. The assays they used were originally the colony inhibition test and later cytotoxicity inhibition. When turning their attention to mice that had been made tolerant in neonatal life, they and their collaborators found in the serum of mice (233) and rats (234) 'blocking factors,' thought to be antigen–antibody complexes, that inhibited normal host cells *in vitro* from responding to the donor strain's histocompatibility antigens; when 'tolerant' lymphoid cells were cultured in normal serum, MLR-reactive or cytotoxic cells were uncovered. In view of the earlier work of Billingham, Brent and Medawar (59) and the then prevailing view that tolerance was not mediated by active suppression their data caused something of a sensation and not a little controversy. They received support from Chutná *et al.* (235), G.A. Voisin and his colleagues in Paris, who described at roughly the same time the occurrence of "facilitation-enhancing antibodies" in the sera of tolerant mice (236, 237), and T.G. Wegmann's laboratory, which found serum blocking factors in tetraparental mice (238), animals resulting from the fusion of early embryos and thus exposed to the allogeneic antigens from a very early stage (239). Such mice had been shown by Mintz and Silvers (240) to be strongly chimeric, to accept skin grafts from the strains that had contributed to their formation and not to suffer from graft-versus-host disease after inoculation of their lymphocytes, and to have normal responses to third-party antigens (i.e. to be a good model for self-tolerance).

Brent *et al.* (241) reviewed the evidence for and against active suppression in neonatal tolerance as well as in other forms of tolerance, and concluded that serum factors (and suppressor cells) can be involved in "partial tolerance", (i.e. where tolerance had not been induced fully as evidenced by the permanent survival of skin allografts and by the survival of a second graft from the same donor). For example, serum from fully tolerant mice had not been found to inhibit cytotoxicity of sensitized cells in the mixed lymphocyte reaction (242) or cytotoxic chromium release (243) assays and it did not interfere with the mixed lymphocyte reaction of normal cells (243). The controversy seemed, then, to center on the methods used to induce tolerance, especially the route of injection and the number of cells used, as well as on the strain combinations involved, for some strains are less amenable to tolerance induction than others. There was also a tendency to draw generalized conclusions from data that showed statistical significance but which were nonetheless less than overwhelmingly conclusive, either in terms of the degree of inhibition or the proportion of animals exhibiting it.

The concept of blocking factors gradually faded away as a tenable explanation for neonatal tolerance, partly because of the conflicting evidence, and partly because they were superseded by the notion of suppressor cells. In 1972 Rouse and Warner dealt a mortal blow to the notion that antibodies were an essential component of tolerance by showing that tolerance could be readily induced in bursectomized chicks that were incapable of antibody production (244).

A comment on 'fashion' in immunologic research

I have already referred to 'vogues in immunologic' research, and it is perhaps appropriate to comment on this interesting phenomenon. The wave of papers describing blocking factors in the first half of the 1970s was replaced by yet another wave of papers – a giant wave – which explained experimental systems that had previously been thought to be driven by clonal detection/inactivation and then (at least by some) by blocking factors exclusively in terms of suppressor or, more specifically, T suppressor cells. It is not easy to account for this, though the lack of precision of the biologic techniques used, the bewildering array of models, and the particular preference of the investigators may well have had something to do with it.

Despite a vast amount of evidence that suppressive T cell populations are demonstrable in both neonatal tolerance and in adult models of specific tolerance, many molecular immunologists even now question the existence of such a mechanism and prefer to interpret their data exclusively in terms of anergy. This is mainly because a tolerant cell has yet to be identified, no phenotypic markers distinguishing suppressor cells from cytotoxic cells having been found, and no gene rearrangement having been demonstrated in T suppressor cells. This skepticism is compounded by the fact that molecular immunologists have often seemed to be unaware of the work of cellular immunologists, thus creating an artificial gulf that has been detrimental to the development of the field in the last ten years. Although it may be unrealistic to suggest it, progress in immunology might well have been faster and with fewer contradictions if investigators had applied not only their own pet assays to their experimental models but also those used by others, and even directly compared one model with another. But that may be advancing a too perfectionist view of the conduct of science!

Suppressor cells

Although the name Richard K. Gerson tends to be associated with the discovery of suppressor cells, and in particular suppressor T lymphocytes, several other strands can be discerned, primarily through the work of Bertie F. Argyris, Peter J. McCullagh and Wulf Dröge. It was Argyris, working as a postdoctoral fellow at the Carnegie Institution of Washington, who first described a phenomenon that she called "adoptive tolerance" (245). She made C3H mice tolerant of CBA minor histocompatibility antigens and several months later transferred large numbers of spleen, lymph node and bone marrow cells to lethally irradiated adult C3H mice; the majority of these cell recipients proved to be tolerant to CBA skin grafts, and they were found to be chimeric for donor strain (CBA) antigens. The study included several controls but unfortunately did not preclude the possibility that in this 'weak' H-2 compatible strain combination, chimeric cells in the tolerant cell donors may have been responsible for inducing actively acquired tolerance in the irradiated recipients. The claim that "lymphoid tissue from a tolerant mouse can be transferred to a new environment without prejudicing its 'tolerant' behavior" cannot therefore be sustained, a criticism that can be applied to some later studies involving the transfer of cells from tolerant animals. Although Argyris in later years described the occurrence of T suppressor cells and macrophages with suppressive activity in animals sensitized to allogeneic tumors and in neonatal spleens, this issue was never clarified by her.

The discovery of specific suppressor lymphocytes stems from experiments conducted in adult animals. Thus, Gershon and his assistant K. Kondo described some complex experiments in 1970 in which thymectomized and lethally irradiated mice were reconstituted with bone marrow cells and made tolerant to sheep red blood cells. The reactivity of these animals was studied with or without the addition of thymic cells or T lymphocytes (246). Although the mechanisms were far from clear they concluded that the induction of tolerance and immunity in bone marrow-derived cells "seems to require the cooperation of T lymphocytes". This work was conducted in the late 1960s in the Chester Beatty Laboratories of the Institute of Cancer Research, London, where Gershon had spent a year.

In 1971 Gershon and Kondo published studies that took the story a step further; they now felt able to describe the transfer of tolerance with T lymphocytes as "infectious tolerance" (247), and in 1972 Gershon et al. discussed the possibility that suppressor T lymphocytes could be responsible (248). Dröge likewise published data in 1971 showing that thymus cells in young chickens can cooperate with bursa-dependent cells, not only in the production of anti-*Brucella abortus* antibodies, but also in mediating a suppressive effect (249). The implications of these discoveries and the contributions of McCullagh, Dröge and others working with adult systems will be discussed in Chapter 6. As far as neonatally induced tolerance is concerned these researchers were highly influential in alerting other workers to the possibility that suppressor T lymphocytes might be underpinning at least some aspects of this phenomenon.

That suppressive mechanisms may be involved in maintaining neonatally induced tolerance had been foreshadowed by:

(1) Experiments indicating that tolerance cannot always be broken by the adoptive transfer of normal syngeneic lymphocytes, even when administered in large numbers (250–252).

(2) The observation that *in vitro* culture of lymphocytes from tolerant animals led to a break in tolerance (253) – at the time interpreted as evidence favoring the existence of tolerant cells, but with the benefit of hindsight more likely to have been brought about by the loss of suppressor cells. This was later confirmed by the finding that the spleens of tolerant animals can possess activated CD4, CD8 and B lymphocytes (254).

(3) Silvers' observation that the surgical removal of certain lymph nodes from mice demonstrably tolerant of skin allografts caused graft destruction in some animals, especially if they were freshly transplanted grafts from the donor strain (255).

(4) Stockinger's demonstration, again later in 1984, that the frequency of precursor cytotoxic cells with specificity for the donor's histocompatibility antigens rose steeply in tolerant cell populations after 'absorption' on monolayers of syngeneic blast cells with receptors for the tolerogen (256) – a strong argument against clonal deletion in Stockinger's experimental system and suggestive of the presence of anti-idiotypic regulatory T lymphocytes.

More direct proof of immunoregulation by suppressor cell populations in neo-natally induced tolerance soon became available. The papers dealing with this are numerous and I shall restrict my discussion to a few. Elkins (257) was among the first to demonstrate specific suppressor cell populations capable of extenuating graft-versus-host reactions, but paradoxically he found these were demonstrable only after the termination of tolerance. At about the same time suppressor cells were described in tetraparental mice (258), curiously by the same authors who had previously found blocking antibodies in such animals. McCullagh worked with a model of tolerance to sheep red blood cells in which rats repeatedly received the red cells, starting on day one: not only did normal syngeneic lymphoid cells inoculated into tolerant rats become tolerant themselves within three days rather than break the tolerant state (259), but thoracic duct lymphocytes taken from tolerant animals could not only decrease but also augment the immune responses of normal cells, depending on the ratio of cell mixtures used (260). McCullagh therefore envisaged that cells could act as suppressor cells in certain circumstances and that this was a factor in the maintenance of tolerance. He subsequently implicated cells of host rather than of donor origin in experiments with rats that had been tolerized to histocompatibility antigens (261).

Two other laboratories were to leave little doubt that specific suppressor lympho-cytes could play a role in maintaining neonatal tolerance. Dorsch and Roser, working at that time in Sydney, Australia, described T suppressor cells in DA rats tolerant of PVG histocompatibility antigens that were capable of transferring the tolerant state to irradiated adult recipients (262). They concluded that "It is therefore clear that the injected syngeneic T cells alone must have been responsible for the specific suppression which induced tolerance in the irradiated recipients of tolerant T-cell inocula. This result implies that true transplantation tolerance is a positive response mediated by T cells which belong to the recirculating pool of small lymphocytes." This paper followed close on the heels of another published in 1974 showing that the transfer of tolerance was due to humoral or cellular suppressor mechanisms (263), a finding that Dorsch and Roser understandably found to be inconsistent with the clonal deletion hypothesis. They subsequently confirmed their findings with highly purified populations of T lymphocytes (264), but went on to advance the hypoth-esis that the suppressor lymphocytes were of *donor* origin (i.e. that they belonged to the F1 donor chimeric cell population, bringing about suppression by anti-idio-typic mechanisms) (265). Such a mechanism had gained credence through the early work of Ramseier (266) and Binz and Wigzell (267) in the induction of specific unre-sponsiveness in adult animals. However, the work of the latter – involving the raising of anti-idiotypic responses for prolonging skin allograft survival – was never substantiated in more than a limited number of strain combinations in the rat, and even then led to only limited prolongation of skin allograft survival (see Chapter 6).

The other group providing evidence for suppressor cells in tolerant mice was Hašek's. Although they seemed to be unaware of the earlier work of Argyris (245), Hilgert, Kristofová and Rieger, studying tolerance in a restricted H-2 combination, essentially followed her experimental approach and felt able to argue that tolerance might be an active process (268). In 1977 Rieger and Hilgert (269) and Holáň, Chutná and Hašek (270) showed that some degree of prolongation could be achieved by the adoptive transfer of cells from tolerant mice or rats across wider genetic disparities, though no attempt was made at this stage to identify the suppressor cells as T lymphocytes, and the prolongation was observed in only a relatively small proportion of animals. On the contrary, a year later Holáň, Chutná and Hašek presented evidence suggesting that the suppressor cells were nylon wool-adherent (*271*), a characteristic not normally associated with T lymphocytes. However, numerous other investigations following in the wake of the earlier work identified the suppressor cells in animals made tolerant at birth as T lymphocytes (see, for example, *272*).

In the 1980s it became clear that whether clonal deletion or regulation by suppressor cells is responsible for tolerance largely depends on the nature of the histocompatibility differences between the donor and the recipient. Streilein and Klein, in a study published in 1980 using H-2 congenic strains of mice and their recombinants, found that class I molecules function rather poorly as tolerogens in neonatal animals, whereas class II molecules induced tolerance with relative ease (*273*). Indeed, they showed that class I antigens can become effective tolerogens if conjoined with class II in the same inoculum, and they suggested that I-J alloantigens were perhaps capable of inducing suppressor mechanisms. A year later Streilein and Gruchella published data involving the adoptive transfer of cells from tolerant mice supporting this notion, when they showed that class I differences can trigger clonal deletion but that tolerance to class II molecules depends on some kind of suppressor mechanism (*274*). Their data were backed up by Streilein's laboratory in 1987: tolerogen-reactive lymphocytes were only slightly depleted in mice tolerant of class II molecules and yet there was a total absence of mixed lymphocyte reaction-reactivity (*275*). These data are not easy to reconcile with the original observation of Billingham, Brent and Medawar (*59*) that tolerance to what were later shown to be class I molecules was readily induced in the newborn mouse. More or less concomitantly with Streilein's group, Holáň and Hašek found that the D end of the H-2 region was considerably more tolerogenic than the K end, and that animals injected at birth with cells bearing the full H-2 differences became tolerant easily to grafts disparate at the D, but not the K end (*276, 277*). These workers concluded that there was no dependence on I-J. Perhaps the last word on these complex problems has not yet been uttered. The reader may wish to consult the review by Wood and Streilein (*278*).

Nonspecific suppressor cells in neonatal rodents

The earlier work relating to the immunologic status of fetal and neonatal animals has been well reviewed by Šterzl and Silverstein (*111*) and by Solomon (*279*). The immunologic immaturity of fetal and neonatal rodents is solidly documented (*280, 281*) but there has been some divergence of opinion as to the cause. Although some believe they have found evidence for a shortfall in the number of T lymphocytes or their precursors (*281–284*), possibly due to a thymosin deficiency in the neonate (*285*), others have suggested a dearth of antigen-presenting cells. Thus Argyris (*286*) was the first to suggest that there was a deficit of antigen-processing macrophages in the murine neonate: the provision of syngeneic adult macrophages significantly enhanced the antibody response to sheep red blood cells, and her hypothesis later received strong support from others (*287, 288*).

An alternative explanation, for which there is a considerable amount of support, is that nonspecific suppressor mechanisms are operative at certain developmental stages, thereby interfering with the development of immunologic responses. For example, it has been shown that neonatal lymphoid tissues can possess cells that have all the functional hallmarks of suppressor cells. Olding and Oldstone (*289*) were the first to show that human neonatal blood lymphocytes can interfere with *in vitro* proliferation of maternal or unrelated adult lymphocytes, and others found much the same suppressive phenomenon when studying lymphoid cells from the neonatal mouse (*290–293*). The work of Medawar and Malkovský suggested that one of the critical features of the neonatal mouse's immune system is a lack of the lymphokine interleukin-2 (IL-2): mice given recombinant IL-2 at birth failed to become tolerant to allogeneic cells injected concomitantly (*294*). This finding has, however, not been confirmed in the chicken (*295*), and it has recently been reinterpreted by Desquenne-Clark, Kimura and Silvers as being due to the loss of tolerance in donor chimeric cells of the SK antigen of the skin (*296*). The observation by Lipoldová, Zajičová and Holáň (*297*) that suppressor mechanisms in neonatal mice do not inhibit the proliferation of adult spleen cells stimulated with IL-2, and that the inability of newborn mice to produce IL-2 and to synthesize IL-2 receptors contributes to their immunologic immaturity, is relevant. As neonatal spleen cells do not synthesize messenger ribonucleic acid for 55 kDa IL-2 receptor it is probable that an important defect is the lack of IL-2 receptors (*298*).

Another group studying natural suppressor cells in the neonatal mouse spleen is S. Strober's; they have compared such cells with suppressor cells found in mice subjected to total lymphoid irradiation and found them to be closely similar, with the same 'null' phenotype (*299*). These nonspecific natural suppressor cells have been cloned and shown to be capable of suppressing the mixed lymphocyte reaction (*300*) and the *in vitro* generation of cytotoxic lymphocytes (*301*), and to have a unique cell surface phenotype (*301*). The significance of these cells following TLI will be considered in Chapter 6. If they are indeed indistinguishable from neonatal suppressor cells it would lend support to the notion that total lymphoid irradiation and perhaps other forms of immunosuppression reduce the adult lymphoid system to its neonatal equivalent, thus facilitating tolerance induction.

What the function of such nonspecific suppressive mechanisms might be is open to debate, but they could ensure that at a time when potentially self-reactive lymphocytes are still being eliminated there cannot be self-destructive immune responses. It is of interest in this connection that it has been claimed that the repertoire of antigen-specific cells is almost identical in neonatal and adult mice (*302*).

Allogeneic tolerance and self-tolerance

The concept of "horror autotoxicus", embodying the paradigm that the body's immune system does not and cannot react against its own cellular components, stemmed from the finding by Ehrlich and Morgenroth (*303*) that goats inoculated with allogeneic red cells produced antibodies against them, but failed to do so when inoculated with their own blood, and it was they who coined this dramatic term (*304*). Since these early experiments a number of exceptions have been noted, mainly for tissues that are normally sequestered from the developing and the mature lymphoid system (e.g. the lens proteins of the eye) or for sequestered cells that are not fully differentiated until the lymphoid system has attained maturity (e.g. spermatozoal antigens).

Although the early workers were quick to see the link between tolerance to allo-geneic antigens and tolerance to self-components – the latter providing the *raison d'être* for the former – it was E.L. Triplett (*305*), a biologist working at Santa Barbara University, who produced highly persuasive evidence in favor of this hypothesis. He removed the buccal component of the pituitary gland of larvae of the tree frog *Hyla regilla* before the gland had differentiated and produced adult-type proteins. The extirpated gland was 'parked' in somewhat older larvae and eventually transplanted back into the original donor larvae after they had reached immunologic maturity, in practice during the metamorphosis stage. A significant number of such animals rejected their own pituitary, a point that was easily observed by the effect a surviving graft had on the pigmentation of the recipient. The study was well controlled and Triplett concluded that "these experiments indicate that the immune system does not possess the genetic information necessary to discriminate between 'self' and 'foreign' antigenic determinants. Ability to recognize antigens as self is a property acquired by contacting these antigens during the period before immunologic compe-tence is acquired". This paper, which has been rather neglected in the onward march of immunology, demonstrated vividly that tolerance to foreign antigens and self-tolerance owe their existence to essentially the same mechanisms. It is therefore not surprising that both self-tolerance (*306–309*) and tolerance to allogeneic minor histo-compatibility antigens have been shown to be MHC-restricted (*310, 311*).

Is tolerance inherited?

Billingham, Brent and Medawar (*59*) had satisfied themselves at a very early stage that tolerance was not inherited. They had done this by mating tolerant males and females and showing that their progeny rejected skin grafts of the donor strain quite normally. Hašek *et al.* (*312*) later confirmed this in a xenogeneic system. It is there-fore surprising that this issue, which hinges on the possible Lamarckian transmis-sion of tolerance, was revived in the late 1970s, initially with the publication of a theoretic monograph by E.J. Steele (*313*) and subsequently by experimental findings by Steele and R.M. Gorczynski claiming that the progeny of tolerant parents displayed hyporesponsiveness to donor strain antigens in a microcytotoxic assay (*314, 315*). These data could not be confirmed by Brent *et al.* (*316, 317*). This controversy has been well and dispassionately reviewed by Hašek, Lodin and Holáň (*318*) and the curious reader is encouraged to consult this paper, in which the evidence for and against the Lamarckian inheritance of tolerance is evaluated. The authors were, however, unaware of yet another set of negative findings published by Smith several years before (*319*).

As one of the participants in this controversy I can add that it generated some heat at the time. This was partly because Steele spent a year in Medawar's department at the Clinical Research Center in Northwick Park while some of Medawar's colleagues, in collaboration with the writer, were unsuccessfully (as it turned out) attempting to repeat Steele and Gorczynski's findings, and partly because the *New Scientist* (the foremost popular British science magazine), several prestigious British newspapers and the British Broadcasting Corporation gave the controversy a great deal of publicity. In the 1981–1982 period a number of articles were published in the *New Scientist*, one by Steele ("Lamarck and immunity: the tables turned") criticizing the data published by Brent *et al.* in *Nature*, followed by a response by Brent *et al.* (". . . the tables unturned") and yet a further response from Steele (". . . a conflict resolved"), criticizing and reworking each other's statistical analyses! The last word should, I think, belongs to Hašek, Lodin and Holáň (*318*), written in 1985: "In conclusion, there is as yet no good evidence from experimental results to support the theory of genetic transmission of immunological tolerance". This confirms Medawar's more general critique of Lamarckian inheritance when, long before this immunologic controversy, he rigorously reviewed the biologic and genetic evidence for and against the theory. Thus he concluded his "A Commentary on Lamarckism" (*320*) by stating that "I am not aware of any experiments that have a greater claim upon our attention than these four (examples), though of many which have far less. It is therefore the generally held view that the case for Lamarckian inheritance in metazoa is unproven".

Conclusions

Some prominence has been given here to the phenomenon of tolerance in immunologically immature animals for several reasons.

(1) Tolerance has unquestionably had a profound influence on the development of modern immunology, especially on the theories concerning the induction of immune responses. It has affected our understanding of self-tolerance and, hence, of autoimmunity; and it has led to the realization that some successful allografts, especially bone marrow and other tissues possessing significant numbers of mature lymphocytes, can complicate matters disastrously for the host by generating a graft-versus-host response, a problem of great significance in bone marrow transplantation to this day (see Chapter 8).

(2) Tolerance studies have provided immunology with many techniques and assays that have been valuable in other contexts.

(3) Of great importance is the explosive effect tolerance has had on the search for an experimental solution to the problem of inducing specific unresponsiveness in adult animals and in man. The discovery of tolerance in the 1950s not only made it permissible to engage in the search for the "Holy Grail" (see Chapter 6) but provided a powerful incentive to do so; and it provided the gold standard by which such approaches needed to be judged.

(4) The phenomenon is of particular interest from a strictly historical point of view because it is possible to chart its progress from the early vital discoveries with their rather simplistic explanations to the present time, when the subtleties and complexities of tolerance, and its multifaceted nature, are more fully appreciated.

(5) It has taught us that, however important certain single experiments or observations may be, they usually have antecedents that scientists as well as historians ignore at their peril.

Addendum to Chapter 5

Just before this manuscript was taken to the publishers a paper was published in *Science* by J.P. Ridge, E.J. Fuchs and P. Matzinger (*321*), accompanied and supposedly supported by two others (*322, 323*) as well a by an introductory *Research News* article by a scientific journalist (*324*). Ridge, Fuchs and Matzinger re-examined neonatally induced tolerance in mice to the H-Y antigen. Because they were able to prevent tolerance induction to H-Y and to bring about priming to that minor histocompatibility antigen by using cell inocula enriched for dendritic cells, and because tolerance could be induced in adult mice by very large doses of male B lymphocytes, the authors concluded that:

(1) There is nothing very special about the neonatal period.
(2) "Tolerance is not determined by the self or nonself origin of the antigen but rather by the conditions under which it is introduced."

They tied their conclusions to P. Matzinger's 'danger' model (*325*) of cell activation, "which suggests that the immune system does not discriminate between self and nonself but between dangerous and harmless entities, and that the primary distinction is made by antigen-presenting cells, which are activated to up-regulate costimulatory molecules only when induced by alarm signals from their enviroment . . ."

There are all kinds of problems with the 'danger' notion, and in some respects Ridge, Fuchs and Matzinger would seem to be reinventing the wheel in that it has long been known that tolerance induction can be frustrated in neonatal mice by the introduction of exogenous interleukin (IL)-2 (*326*) and that tolerance to H-Y can be established in adult mice with large doses of cells (see p. 198 and Chapter 4). Such findings can be accommodated without abandoning the self–nonself theory on which much of modern immunology is founded. That there is indeed something special about the neonatal period is clear from numerous investigations (see above). It would be wise to suspend judgement on both the "danger" hypothesis and the interpretation of their recent experiments by Ridge, Fuchs and Matzinger.

References

1. Born, B. (1987) *Arch. f. Entwmech.* **4**, 349, 518.
2. Lewis, W.H. (1907) *Amer. J. Anat.* **7**, 146.
3. Hewitt, D.C. (1934) *J. Exp. Zool.* **69**, 235.
4. Geinitz, B. (1925) *Entwmech.* **5**, 419.
5. Rous, P. & Murphy, J.B. (1911) *J. Amer. Med. Ass.* **56**, 741.
6. Murphy, J.B. (1912) *J. Amer. Med. Ass.* **59**, 874.
7. Murphy, J.B. (1914) *J. Exp. Med.* **19**, 181.
8. Murphy, J.B. (1914) *J. Exp. Med.* **19**, 513.
9. Murphy, J.B. (1914) *J. Amer. Med. Ass.* **62**, 199.
10. Hamburger, V. (1933) *Anat. Rec.* (suppl.) **55**, 58.
11. Hamburger, V. (1938) *J. Exp. Zool.* **77**, 379.
12. Eastlick, H.L. (1939) *Nature* **144**, 380.
13. Eastlick, H.L. (1939) *Proc. Natl. Acad. Sci.* **25**, 551.
14. Eastlick, H.L. (1941) *Physiol. Rev.* **14**, 136.
15. Willier, B.H. (1941) *Amer. Nat.* **75**, 136.

16. Willier B.H. & Rawles, M.E. (1941) *Physiol. Zool.* **13**, 177.
17. Rawles, M.E. (1938) *Anat. Rec.* (suppl.) **72**, 68.
18. Rawles, M.E. (1944) *Physiol. Zool.* **17**, 167.
19. Rawles, M.E. (1945) *Physiol. Rev.* **20**, 248.
20. Rawles, M.E. (1952) *N.Y. Acad. Sci.* **55**, 302.
21. Danforth, C.H. & Foster, F. (1929) *J. Exp. Zool.* **52**, 443.
22. Loeb, L. (1921) *Biol. Bull.* **15**, 143.
23. Owen, R.D. (1945) *Science* **102**, 400.
24. Owen, R.D. (1946) *Genetics* **31**, 227.
25. Lillie, F.R. (1916) *Science* **43**, 611.
26. Lillie, F.R. (1917) *J. Exp. Zool.* **23**, 371.
27. Lillie, F.R. (1923) *Biol. Bull.* **44**, 47.
28. Owen, R.D., Davis, H.P. & Morgan, R.F. (1946) *J. Hered.* **37**, 290.
29. Burnet, F.M. & Fenner, F. (1949) *The Production of Antibodies*, 2nd ed. Macmillan, Melbourne, London.
30. Burnet, F.M. & Fenner, F. (1949) *The Production of Antibodies*, 2nd ed. p. 102 Macmillan, Melbourne, London.
31. Burnet, F.M. & Fenner, F. (1949) *The Production of Antibodies*, 2nd ed. p. 103 Macmillan, Melbourne, London.
32. Burnet, F.M. & Fenner, F. (1949) *The Production of Antibodies*, 2nd ed. p. 104 Macmillan, Melbourne, London.
33. Traub, E. (1936) *J. Exp. Med.* **64**, 183.
34. Traub, E. (1938) *J. Exp. Med.* **68**, 229.
35. Traub, E. (1939) *J. Exp. Med.* **69**, 801.
36. Fox J.P. and Laemmert, H.L. (1947) *Amer. J. Hyg.* **46**, 21.
37. Burnet, F.M. & Fenner, F. (1949) *The Production of Antibodies*, 2nd ed. p. 105 Macmillan, Melbourne, London.
38. Burnet, F.M., Stone, J.D. and Edney, M. (1950) *Austr. J. Exp. Biol. Med. Sci.* **18**, 291.
39. Lopashov, G.V. and Stroyeva, O.G. (1950) *Usp. Sov. Biol.* **30**, 234.
40. Lopashov, G.V. and Stroyeva, O.G. (1950) *Usp. Sov. Biol.* **30**, p. 253.
41. Hašková, V. (1953) *Czechosl. Biol.* **2**, 167.
42. Hašek, M. & Hraba, T. (1955) *Folia Biol.* **1**, 1.
43. Medawar, P.B. (1986) *Memoirs of a Thinking Radish.* p. 111, Oxford Univ. Press, Oxford.
44. Billingham, R.E. (1991) In *History of Transplantation: Thirty-five Recollections*, ed. P.I. Terasaki, p. 80, U.C.L.A. Tissue Typing Laboratory, Los Angeles.
45. Anderson, D., Billingham, R.E., Lampkin, G.H. *et al.* (1951) *Heredity* **5**, 379.
46. Billingham, R.E., Lampkin, G.H., Medawar P.B. *et al.* (1952) *Heredity* **6**, 201.
47. Stone, W.H., Cragle, R.G., Swanson, E.W. *et al.* (1965) *Science* **148**, 1335.
48. Stone, W.H., Cragle, R.G. & Johnson, D.F. (1971) *Transplantation* **12**, 421.
49. Boyse, E.A. & Old, L.J. (1968) *Transplantation* **6**, 619.
50. Medawar, P.B. (1986) *Memoirs of a Thinking Radish.* p. 112, Oxford Univ. Press, Oxford.
51. Medawar P.B. (unsigned book review) *Nature* **166**, 204.
52. Billingham, R.E., Brent L. & Medawar, P.B. (1953) *Nature* **172**, 603.
53. Dunsford, I., Bowley, C.C., Hutchison, A.M. *et al.* (1953) *Brit. Med. J.* **2**, 81.
54. Cannon, J.A. & Longmire, W.P. (1952) *Ann. Surg.* **135**, 60.
55. Felton, L.D. (1949) *J. Immunol.* **61**, 107.
56. Chase, M.W. (1946) *Proc. Soc. Exp. Biol. Med. N.Y.* **61**, 257.
57. Snell, G.D. (1952) *Cancer Res.* **12**, 543.
58. Medawar, P.B. (1944) *J. Anat. (London)* **78**, 176.
59 Billingham, R.E., Brent, L. & Medawar, P.B. (1956) *Phil. Trans. Roy. Soc. London, Ser. B.* **239**, 357.
60. Howard, J.G. & Michie, D. (1962) *Transpl. Bull.* **29**, 1.
61a. Brent, L. & Gowland, G. (1961) *Nature* **192**, 1265.
61b. Brent, L. & Gowland G. (1962) In *Mechanisms of Immunological Tolerance*, p. 237, Czech. Acad. Sci. Prague.
62. Billingham, R.E. & Brent, L. (1957) *Transpl. Bull.* **4**, 67.
63. Koprowski, H. (1955) *Nature* **175**, 1087.

64. Bollag, W. (1955) *Experientia* **11**, 227.
65. Simonsen, M. (1955) *Nature* **175**, 764.
66. Talmage, D.D. (1957) *Annu. Rev. Med.* **8**, 239.
67. Burnet, F.M. (1957) *Austr. J. Sci.* **20**, 67.
68. Burnet, F.M. (1959) *The Clonal Selection Theory of Acquired Immunity*, Cambridge Univ. Press, Cambridge.
69. Simonsen, M. (1957) *Path. Microbiol. Scand.* **40**, 480.
70. Hašek, M. (1953) *Czechosl. Biol.* **2**, 265.
71. Brent, L. & Medawar, P.B. (1959) In *Recent Progress in Microbiology*, p. 181, Almqvist & Wiksell, Stockholm.
72. Hašek, M. (1953) *Czechosl. Biol.* **2**, 25.
73. Vojtisková, M. & Hašek, M. (1953) *Czechosl. Biol.* **2**, 220.
74. Hašek, M. (1952) *Czechosl. Biol.* **1**, 144.
75. Hašek, M. (1954) *Czechosl. Biol.* **3**, 344.
76. Hašek, M. & Hraba, T. (1955) *Folia Biol.* **1**, 1.
77. Hraba, T. (1956) *Folia Biol.* **2**, 165.
78. Grozdanovič, J. (1956) *Folia Biol.* **2**, 296.
79. Hašek, M. & Hraba, T. (1955) *Nature* **175**, 764.
80. Dausset, J. (1989) In *Realm of Tolerance*, ed. P. Ivanyi, p. 3, Springer–Verlag, Berlin, Heidelberg.
81. Ivanyi P (ed.) (1989) *Realm of Tolerance*, pp. 314, Springer–Verlag, Berlin, Heidelberg.
82. A discussion meeting on immunological tolerance (1956) *Proc. Roy. Soc. B.* **146**, p. 1092.
83. Owen, R.D. (1956) *Proc. Roy. Soc. B.* **146**, p. 146.
84. Cinader, B.P. & Dubert, J.M. (1956) *Proc. Roy. Soc. B.* **146**, p. 146.
85. Hanan, R.Q. & Oyama, J. (1954) *J. Immunol.* **73**, 49.
86. Cinader, B. & Dubert, J.M. (1955) *Brit. J. Exp. Path.* **36**, 515.
87. Dixon, F.J. & Maurer, P.H. (1955) *J. Exp. Med.* **101**, 245.
88. Koprowski, H., Gail, T. & Love, R. (1956) *Proc. Roy. Soc. B.* **146**, p. 37.
89. Harris, R.J.C. (1956) *Proc. Roy. Soc. B* **146**, p. 59.
90. Hašek, M. (1956) *Proc. Roy. Soc. B.* **146**, p. 67.
91. Billingham, R.E. & Brent, L. (1956) *Proc. Roy. Soc. B.* **146**, p. 78.
92. Burnet, F.M. (1956) *Proc. Roy. Soc. B.* **146**, p. 90.
93. *Ann. N.Y. Acad. Sci.* (1955) **59** (3), p. 277.
94. *Ann. N.Y. Acad. Sci.* (1966) **129** (1), p. 884.
95. Hašek, M., Lengerová, M. & Vojtisková, M. (eds) (1962) *Mechanisms of Immunological Tolerance*, p. 544, Publ. House of the Czech. Acad. Sci. **181**.
96. Friedman, H. (ed.) (1971) *Ann. N.Y. Acad. Sci.* **181**, p. 315.
97. Woodruff, M.F.A. (1957) *Ann. N.Y. Acad. Sci.* **64** (5), 792.
98. Woodruff, M.F.A. & Simpson, L.O. (1955) *Brit. J. Exp. Path.* **36**, 494.
99. Billingham, R.E. & Brent, L. (1959) *Phil. Trans. Roy. Soc. London*, ser. B, **242**, 439.
100. Martinez, C., Aust, J.B., Smith, J.M. & *et al.* (1958) *Proc. Soc. Biol. Med.* **97**, 736.
101. Brent, L. & Gowland, G. (1961) *Nature* **192**, 1265.
102. Brent, L. & Gowland, G. (1962) *Nature* **196**, 1298.
103. Shapiro, F., Martinez, C., Smith, J.H. *et al.* (1961) *Proc. Soc. Exp. Biol. Med.* **106**, 472.
104. McKhann, C.F. (1962) *J. Immunol.* **88**, 500.
105. Michie, D. & Howard, J.G. (1962) *Transpl. Bull.* **29**, 1.
106. Brent, L. & Gowland, G. (1963) *Transplantation* **1**, 372.
107. Schinkel, O.G. & Ferguson, K.A. (1953) *Austr. J. Biol. Sci.* **6**, 533.
108. Silverstein, A.M., Prendergast, R.A. & Kraner, K.L. (1964) *J. Exp. Med.* **119**, 955.
109. Silverstein, A.M. & Kraner, K.L. (1964) In *Molecular and Cellular Basis of Antibody Formation*, eds J. Šterzl *et al.*, p. 341, Publ. House Czech. Acad. Sci., Prague.
110. Uhr, J.W. (1960) *Nature* **187**, 957.
111. Šterzl J. & Silverstein, A.M. (1967) *Adv. Immunol.* **6**, 337.
112. Billingham, R.E. & Silvers, W.K. (1958) *Science* **128**, 780.
113. Mariani, T., Martinez, C., Smith, J.M. *et al.* (1958) *Proc. Soc. Exp. Biol. Med.* **99**, 287.
114. Billingham, R.E. & Silvers, W.K. (1960) *J. Immunol.* **85**, 14.
115. Mariani, T., Martinez, C., Smith, J.M. *et al.* (1959) *Proc. Soc. Exp. Biol. Med.* **101**, 596.

116. Lustgraaf, E.C., Fuson, R.B. & Eichwald, E.J. (1960) *Transpl. Bull.* **26**, 145.
117. Skowron-Cendrzak, A. & Konieczná-Marcynská, B. (1959) *Nature* **184**, 1590.
118. Rubin, B.A. (1959) *Nature* **184**, 205.
119. Martinez, C., Smith, J.M., Shapiro, F. *et al.* (1959) *Proc. Soc. Exp. Biol. Med*, **102**, 413.
120. Shapiro, F., Martinez, C., Smith, J.M. *et al.* (1961) *Proc. Soc. Exp. Biol. Med* **106**, 472.
121. Puza, A. & Gombos, A. (1958) *Transpl. Bull.* **5**, 30.
122. Albert, F., Lejeune-Ledant, G., Moureau, P. *et al.* (1959) In *Biological Problems of Grafting*, eds F. Albert & P.B. Medawar, p. 369, Blackwell Sci. Publ., Oxford.
123. Fowler, R., Schubert, W.K. & West, C.D. (1960) *Ann. N.Y. Acad. Sci.* **87** (1), 403.
124. Osborn, J.J., Dancis, J. & Julia, J.F. (1952) *Pediatrics* **9**, 736.
125. Uhr, J.W., Dancis, J. Finkelstein, M.S. *et al.* (1962) *J. Clin. Invest.* **41**, 1509.
126. Uhr, J.W., Dancis, J. & Newmann, C.G. (1960) *Nature* **187**, 1130.
127. Flake, E.D., Harrison, M.R., Adzick, N.S. *et al.* (1986) *Science* **233**, 776.
128. Roodman, G.D., Vandeberg, H.L. & Kuehl, T.J. (1988) *Bone Marrow Transpl.* **3**, 141
129. Bond, S.J., Harrison, M.R., Crombleholme, T.M. *et al.* (1980) *Blood* **70** (suppl. 1), 1017.
130. Brent, L., Linch, D.C., Rodeck, C.H. *et al.* (1989) *Immunol. Letters* **21**, 55.
131. Calne, R.Y. (1989) In panel discussion on the role of immunology in the development of clinical transplantation, *Immunol. Letters* **21**, 82.
132. Claas, F.J.J., Gijbels, Y., Van der Velden-de Munck J. *et al.* (1988) *Science* **241**, 1815.
133. Zhang, L. & Miller, R.G. (1993) *Transplantation* **56**, 918.
134. Propper, D.J., Woo, J., Stewart, K.N. *et al.* (1992) *Transplantation* **52**, 331.
135. Billingham, R.E., Brent, L. & Medawar, P.B. (1955) *Ann. N.Y. Acad, Sci.* **59**, 409.
136. Terasaki, P.I., Cannon, J.A. & Longmire, W.P. (1958) *J. Immunol.* **81**, 246.
137. Hašek, M., Hraba, T. & Hort, J. (1959) *Nature* **183**, 1199.
138. Zeiss, I.M. (1966) *Immunology* **11**, 597.
139. Holáň, V., Hašek, M., Hilgert, I. *et al. Transpl. Proc.* **13**, 608.
140. Streilein, J.W. & Klein, J. (1980) *Proc. Roy. Soc. B.* **107**, 475.
141. Holáň, V. (1990) *Transplantation* **50**, 1027.
142. Brent, L. & Courtenay, T.H. (1962) In *Mechanisms of Immunological Tolerance*, eds. M. Hašek, A. Lengerová & M. Vojtisková, p. 113, Publ. House Czech. Acad. Sci., Prague.
143. Boyse, E.A., Lance, E.M., Carswell, E.A. *et al.* (1970) *Nature* **227**, 901.
144. Murray, J.E., Merrill, J.P., Dammin, G.J. *et al.* (1960) *Surgery* **48**, 272.
145. Štark, O., Křen, V., Frenzl, B. *et al.* (1962) In *Mechanisms of Tolerance*, eds M. Hašek, A. Lengerová & M. Vojtisková p. 123, Publ. House Czech. Acad. Sci., Prague.
146. Mitchison, N.A. (1959) In *Biological Problems of Grafting*, eds F. Albert & G. Lejeune-Ledant, p. 239, Blackwell Scientific Publ., Oxford.
147. Simonsen, M. (1959) *Acta Path. Microbiol. Scand.* **39**, 21.
148. Mitchison, N.A. (1956) *Brit. J. Exp. Path.* **37**, 239.
149. Silobrčić, V. (1971) *Eur. J. Immunol.* **1**, 313.
150. Silvers, W.K. (1968) *J. Exp. Med.* **128**, 69.
151. Lubaroff, D.M. & Silvers, W.K. (1973) *J. Immunol.* **111**, 65.
152. Lubaroff D.M. & Silvers, W.K. (1968) *J. Immunol.* **104**, 1236.
153. Harris, T.N., Harris, S. & Farber, M.B. (1973) *Transplantation* **15**, 383.
154. Cinader, B. & Dubert, J.M. (1956) *Proc. Roy. Soc. B.* **146**, 18.
155. Weigle, W.O. & Dixon, F.J. (1958) *Proc. Soc. Exp. Biol. Med.* **98**, 213.
156. Wolfe, H.R., Temelis, C., Mueller, A. *et al.* (1957) *J. Immunol.* **79**, 147.
157. Tempelis, C.J., Wolfe, H.R. & Mueller, A.P. (1958) *Brit. J. Exp. Path.* **39**, 328.
158. Smith, R.T. & Bridges, R.A. (1958) *J. Exp. Med.* **108**, 227.
159. Starzl, T.E., Demetris, A.J., Trucco, M. *et al.* (1992) *Lancet* **340**, 876.
160. Starzl, T.E., Demetris, A.J., Trucco, M. *et al.* (1992) *New Engl. J. Med.* **328**, 745.
161. Starzl, T.E., Demetris, A.J., Murase N. *et al.* (1992) *Lancet* **339**, 1579.
162. Carter, B.G. & Cinader, B. (1960) *Ann. N.Y. Acad. Sci.* **87** (1), 363.
163. Billingham, R.E., Sawchuck, G.H. & Silvers, W.K. (1960) *Transpl. Bull.* **26**, 446.
164. LaPlante, E.S., Burrell, R., Watne, A.L. *et al.* (1969) *Transplantation* **7**, 67.
165. Gengozian, N., Batson, J.S., Greene, C.T. *et al.* (1969) *Transplantation* **8**, 633.
166. Porter, R.P. & Gengozian, N. (1969) *Transplantation* **8**, 653.

167. Simonsen, M. (1955) *Ann. N.Y. Acad. Sci.* **59**, 448.
168. Mullen, Y. & Hildemann, W.H. (1975) *Transplantation* **20**, 281.
169. Martinez, C., Aust, J.B. & Good, R.A. (1956) *Transpl. Bull.* **3**, 128.
170. Medawar, P.B. & Russell, P.S. (1959) *Immunology* **1**, 1.
171. Patterson, P.Y. (1958) *Ann. N.Y. Acad. Sci.* **73** (3), 811.
172. Simonsen, M. (1955) *Nature* **175**, 763.
173. Friedman, H. & Gaby, W.L. (1960) *J. Immunol.* **85**, 478.
174. Gowans, J.L., McGregor, P.D. & Cowen, D.M. (1963) In *The Immunologically Competent Cell*, eds. G.E.W. Wolstenholme & J. Knight p. 20. J.A. Churchill, London.
175. Coons, A.H. (1958) *J. Cell. Comp. Physiol.* **52** (suppl. 1), 55.
176. Nossal, G.J.V. & Lederberg, J. (1958) *Nature* **181**, 1419.
177. White, R.G. (1958) *Nature* **182**, 1383.
178. Medawar, P.B. (1961) *Science* **133**, 303.
179. Burnet, F.M. (1961) *Science* **133**, 307.
180. Jerne, N.K. (1960) *Ann. Rev. Microbiol.* **14**, 341.
181. Burnet, F.M. & Burnet, D. (1960) *Nature* **188**, 376.
182. Medawar, P.B. (1960) In *Cellular Aspects of Immunity*, Ciba Found. Sym., p. 134. Churchill, London.
183. Woodruff, M.F.A. (1959) In *Biological Problems of Grafting, A Symposium*, eds F. Albert & P.B. Medawar p. 258, Blackwell, Oxford.
184. Medawar, P.B. (1960) In *Cellular Aspects of Immunity*, Ciba Found. Sym., p. 145 Churchill, London.
185. Loutit, J.F. (1956) In *Lectures on the Scientific Basis of Medicine* **5**, 439, Athlone Press, London.
186. Billingham, R.E., Defendi, V., Silvers, W.K. *et al.* (1962) *J. Natl. Cancer Inst.* **28**, 365.
187. Wilson, D.B., Silvers, W.K. & Nowell, P.C. (1967) *J. Exp. Med.* **126**, 655.
188. Gorczynski, R.M., Macrae, S. & Till, J.E. (1978) *Scand. J. Immunol.* **7**, 453.
189. Gruchella, R.S. & Streilein, J.W. (1982) *Immunogenetics* **15**, 111.
190. Elkins, W.L. (1972) *Cell. Immunol.* **4**, 192.
191. Brooks, C.G. (1975) *Eur. J. Immunol.* **5**, 741.
192. Silvers, W.K., Elkins, W.L. & Quimby, F.W. (1975) *J. Exp. Med.* **142**, 2312.
193. Von Boehmer, H., Sprent, J. & Nabholz, M. (1975) *J. Exp. Med.* **141**, 322.
194. Wood, P.J. & Streilein, J.W. (1982) *Eur. J. Immunol.* **12**, 188.
195. Elkins, W.L. (1973) *J. Exp. Med.* **137**, 1097.
196. Nossal, G.J.V. & Pike, B.L. (1981) *Proc. Natl. Acad. Sci. U.S.A.* **48**, 3844.
197. McCarthy, S.A. & Bach, F.H. (1981) *J. Immunol.* **131**, 1676.
198. Feng, H.M., Glasebrook, A.L., Engers, H.D. *et al.* (1983) *J. Immunol.* **131**, 2165.
199. Carnaud, C., Ishazaka, S.T. & Stutman, O.J. (1984) *J. Immunol.* **133**, 45.
200. Wood, P.J., Strome, P.G. & Streilein, J.W. (1985) *Transpl. Proc.* **17**, 1137.
201. Wood, P.J., Strome, P.G. & Streilein, J.W. (1987) *J. Immunol.* **138**, 3661.
202. Mohler, K.M. & Streilein, J.W. (1987) *J. Immunol.* **139**, 2211.
203. Tite, J.P. & Playfair, J.H.L. (1978) *Immunology* **34**, 1089.
204. Wood, P.J., Socarras, S. & Streilein, J.W. (1987) *J. Immunol.* **139**, 3236.
205. Macphail, S. & Stutman, O. (1989) *J. Immunol.* **143**, 1795.
206. Gruchella, R.S., Strome, P.G. & Streilein, J.W. (1983) *Transplantation* **36**, 318.
207. Fefer, A. & Nossal, G.J.V. (1962) *Transpl. Bull.* **29**, 447.
208. Mäkelä O. & Nossal, G.J.V. (1961) *J. Immunol.* **88**, 613.
209. Denhardt, D.T. & Owen, R.D. (1960) *Transpl. Bull.* **7**, 394.
210. Boyden, S.V. & Sorkin, E. (1962) *Immunology* **5**, 370.
211. Brent, L., Brooks, C. & Lubling, N. (1972) *Transplantation* **14**, 382.
212. Miller, J.F.A.P. (1961) *Lancet* **2**, 748.
213. Isaković, K., Smith, S.B. & Waksman, B.H. (1965) *J. Exp. Med.* **122**, 1103.
214. Smith, S.B., Isaković, K. & Waksman, B.H. (1966) *Proc. Soc. Exp. Biol. Med.* **121**, 1005.
215. Staples, P.J., Gery, I. & Waksman, B.H. (1966) *J. Exp. Med.* **124**, 127.
216. Horiuchi, A. & Waksman, B.H. (1968) *J. Immunol.* **100**, 947.
217. Horiuchi, A. & Waksman, B.H. (1968) *J. Immunol.* **101**, 1322.
218. Robinson, H.H. & Owen, J.J.T. (1977) *Clin. Exp. Immunol.* **27**, 322.
219. Kappler, J.W., Roehm, N. & Marrack, P. (1987) *Cell* **49**, 273.
220. Smith, J.B. & Pasternak, R.D. (1989) *J. Immunol.* **121**, 1889.

221. Battisto, J.R. & Pouzio, N.M. (1981) *Prog. Allerg.* **28**, 169.
222. Glimcher, L. & Shevach, E. (1982) *J. Exp. Med.* **156**, 640.
223. Kappler, J.W., Staerz, U., White, J. *et al.* (1988) *Nature* **332**, 35.
224. Marrack, P., Lo, D., Brinster, R., *et al.* (1988) *Cell* **53**, 627.
225. MacDonald, H.R., Schneider, R., Lees, R.K. *et al.* (1988) *Nature* **332**, 40.
226. Speiser, D.E., Schneider, R., Hengartner, H. *et al.* (1989) *J. Exp. Med.* **170**, 595.
227. Roberts, J.L., Sharrow, S.O. & Singer, A. (1990) *J. Exp. Med.* **171**, 935.
228. Kaliss, N. (1957) *Ann. N.Y. Acad. Sci.* **64**, 977.
229. Uhr, J.W. & Möller, G. (1968) *Adv. Immunol.* **8**, 81.
230. Cinader, B. (ed.) (1971) *Regulation of the Antibody Response*, 2nd edn. Charles Thomas, Springfield, Ill.
231. Dwyer, J.M. & Kantor, F.S. (1973) *J. Exp. Med.* **137**, 32.
332. Hellström, K.E. & Hellström, I. (1970) *Ann. Rev. Microbiol.* **24**, 373.
233. Hellström, I., Hellström, K.E. & Allison, A.C. *Nature* **230**, 49.
234. Bansal, S.C., Hellström, K.E., Hellström, I. *et al.* (1973) *J. Exp. Med.* **137**, 590.
235. Chutná, J., Hašek, M., Sládeček, M. *et al.* (1973) *Folia Biol.* **19**, 252.
236. Voisin, G.A. (1971) *Cell. Immunol.* **2**, 670.
237. Voisin, G.A., Kinsky, R.G. & Duc, H.T. (1971) *J. Exp. Med.* **135**, 1185.
238. Phillips, M, Martin, W.J., Shaw, A.R. *et al.* *Nature* **234**, 146.
239. Mintz, B. (1962) *Science* **138**, 594.
240. Mintz, B. & Silvers, W.K. (1971) *Science* **158**, 1484.
241. Brent, L., Brooks, C.G., Medawar, P.B. *et al.* (1976) *Brit. Med. Bull.* **32**, 101.
242. Beverley, P.C.L., Brent, L., Brooks, C. & *et al.* (1973) *Transpl. Proc.* **5**, 679.
243. Brooks, C.G. (1975) *Eur. J. Immunol.* **5**, 741.
244. Rouse, B.F. & Warner, N.L. (1972) *Eur. J. Immunol.* **2**, 102.
245. Argyris, B.F. (1963) *J. Immunol.* **90**, 29.
246. Gershon, R.K. & Kondo, K. (1970) *Immunology* **18**, 723.
247. Gershon, R.K. & Kondo, K. (1971) *Immunology* **21**, 903.
248. Gershon, R.K., Cohen, P., Hencin, R. *et al.* (1972) *J. Immunol.* **108**, 586.
249. Droege, W. (1971) *Nature* **234**, 549.
250. Billingham, R.E., Silvers, W.K. & Wilson, D.B. (1963) *J. Exp. Med.* **118**, 397.
251. Tong, J.L. & Boose, D. (1970) *J. Immunol.* **105**, 426.
252. Terman, D.S., Minden, P. & Crowle, A.J. (1973) *Cell. Immunol.* **6**, 273.
253. McGregor, D.D., McCullagh, P.J. & Gowans, J.L. (1967) *Proc. Roy. Soc. B.* **168**, 229.
254. Bandeira, A., Coutinho, A., Carnaud, C. *et al.* (1980) *Proc. Acad. Sci. U.S.A.* **86**, 272.
255. Silvers, W.K. (1974) *J. Immunol.* **113**, 804.
256. Stockinger, B. (1984) *Proc. Natl. Acad. Sci. U.S.A.* **81**, 220.
257. Elkins, W.L. (1972) *Cell. Immunol.* **4**, 192.
258. Phillips, S.M. & Wegmann, T.G. (1973) *J. Exp. Med.* **137**, 291.
259. McCullagh, P. (1970) *Aust. J. Exp. Biol. Med. Sci.* **48**, 369.
260. McCullagh, P. (1974) *Eur. J. Immunol.* **4**, 540.
261. McCullagh, P. (1975) *Aust. J. Exp. Biol. Med. Sci.* **53**, 431.
262. Dorsch, S. & Roser, B. (1975) *Nature* **258**, 233.
263. Dorsch, S. & Roser, B. (1974) *Aust. J. Exp. Biol. Med. Sci.* **52**, 33 and 45.
264. Dorsch, S. & Roser, B. (1982) *Transplantation* **33**, 518.
265. Dorsch, S. & Roser, B. (1982) *Transplantation* **33**, 525.
266. Ramseier, H. (1973) *Eur. J. Immunol.* **3**, 156.
267. Binz, H. & Wigzell, H. (1976) *J. Exp. Med.* **144**, 1438.
268. Hilgert, I. Kristofová, H. & Rieger, M. (1975) *Folia Biol. (Praha)* **21**, 409.
269. Rieger, M. & Hilgert, I. (1977) *J. Immunogenet.* **4**, 61.
270. Holáň, V., Chutná, J. & Hašek, M. (1977) *Folia Biol. (Praha)* **23**, 66.
271. Holáň, V., Chutná, J. & Hašek, M. (1978) *Nature* **274**, 897.
272. Gorczynski, R.M. & Macrae, S. (1979) *J. Immunol.* **122**, 737, 747.
273. Streilein, J.W. & Klein, J. (1980) *Proc. Roy. Soc. B.* **207**, 461.
274. Streilein, J.W. & Gruchella, R.S. (1981) *Immunogenetics* **12**, 161.
275. Mohler, K.M. & Streilein, J.W. (1987) *J. Immunol.* **139**, 221.

276. Holáň, V. & Hašek, M. (1981) *Immunogenetics* **12**, 465.
277. Hašek, M. & Holáň, V. (1981) *Scand. J. Immunol.* **14**, 669.
278. Wood, P.J. & Streilein, J.W. (1984) *Transplantation* **37**, 223.
279. Solomon, J.B. (1971) *Foetal and Neonatal Immunology*, p. 234, American Elsevier Publ. Co., New York.
280. Bortin, M.M., Rimm, A.A. & Goldstein, E.C. (1969) *J. Immunol.* **103**, 683.
281. Chiscon, M.O. & Golub, E.S. (1972) *J. Immunol.* **108**, 1379.
282. Spear, P.G., Wang, A-L., Rutishauer, U. *et al.* (1973) *J. Exp. Med.* **138**, 557.
283. Mosier, D.E. (1974) *J. Immunol.* **112**, 305.
284. Pilarski, L.M. (1977) *J. Exp. Med.* **146**, 887.
285. Goldstein, A.L., Guha, A., Howe, M.L. *et al.* (1971) *J. Immunol.* **106**, 773.
286. Argyris, B.F. (1968) *J. Exp. Med.* **128**, 451.
287. Landahl, C.A. (1976) *Eur. J. Immunol.* **6**, 130.
288. Lu, C.Y., Calamai, E.G. & Unanue, E.R. (1979) *Nature* **282**, 327.
289. Olding, L.B. & Oldstone, M.B.A. (1974) *Nature* **249**, 161.
290. Mosier, D.E. & Johnson, B.M. (1975) *J. Exp. Med.* **141**, 216.
291. Skowron-Cendrzac, A. & Ptak, W. (1976) *Eur. J. Immunol.* **6**, 451.
292. Ptak, W. & Skowron-Cendrzac, A. (1977) *Transplantation* **24**, 45.
293. Argyris, B.F. (1978) *Cell. Immunol.* **34**, 354.
294. Malkovský, M., Medawar, P.B., Hunt, R. *et al.* (1984) *Proc. Roy. Soc. B.* **220**, 439.
295. Tempelis, C.H., Hala, K., Kromer, G. *et al.* (1988) *Transplantation* **45**, 449.
296. Desquenne-Clark, L., Kimura, H. & Silvers, W.K. (1988) *Transplantation* **46**, 774.
297. Lipoldová, M., Zajičová, A. & Holáň, (1990) *Immunology* **71**, 497.
298. Holáň, H., Lipoldová, M. & Zajičová, A. (1991) *Cell. Immunol.* **137**, 216.
299. Oseroff, A., Okada, S. & Strober, S. (1984) *J. Immunol.* **132**, 101.
300. Schwadron, R., Gandour, D.M. & Strober, S. (1985) *J. Exp. Med.* **162**, 297.
301. Schwadron, R. & Strober, S. (1987) *Transpl. Proc.* **19**, 354.
302. Dwyer, J.M. & Mackay, I.R. (1972) *Immunology* **23**, 871.
303. Ehrlich, P. & Morgenroth, J. (1900) *Berl. Klin. Wschr.* **37**, 453. (English translation in *The Collected Papers of Paul Ehrlich* (1957), vol. 2, ed. F. Himmelweit, p. 205, Pergamon, London.)
304. Ehrlich, P. & Morgenroth, J. (1901) *Berl. Klin. Wschr.* **38**, 251. (English translation as for ref. 303, p. 246.)
305. Triplett, E.L. (1962) *J. Immunol.* **89**, 505.
306. Matzinger, P. & Waterfield, D.J. (1980) *Nature* **285**, 492.
307. Groves, E.S. & Singer, A. (1983) *J. Exp. Med.* **158**, 1483.
308. Matzinger, P., Zamoyska, R. & Waldmann, H. (1984) *Nature* **308**, 738.
309. Rammensee, H-G. & Bevan, M.J. (1984) *Nature* **308**, 741.
310. Kimura, H., Desquenne-Clark, L., Miyamato, M. *et al.* (1986) *J. Exp. Med.* **164**, 2031.
311. Waite, D.J., Miller, R.A. & Sunshine, G.H. (1989) *Cell. Immunol.* **117**, 70.
312. Hašek, M., Hort, J., Lengerová, A. *et al.* (1963) *Folia Biol. (Praha)* **9**, 1.
313. Steele, E.J. (1979) *Somatic Selection and Adaptive Evolution; On the Inheritance of Acquired Characters*, Williams & Wallace, Toronto.
314. Gorczynski, R.M. & Steeles, E.J. (1980) *Proc. Natl. Acad. Sci. U.S.A.* **77**, 2871.
315. Gorczynski, R.M. & Steele, E.J. (1981) *Nature* **289**, 678.
316. Brent, L., Rayfield, L.S., Chandler, P. *et al.* (1981) *Nature* **290**, 508.
317. Brent, L., Chandler, P., Fierz, W. *et al.* (1982) *Nature* **295**, 242.
318. Hašek, M., Lodin, Z. & Holáň, V. (1985) *Surv. Immunol. Res.* **4**, 35.
319. Smith, R.N. (1981) *Nature* **292**, 767.
320. Medawar, P.B. (1981) In *The Uniqueness of the Individual*, 2nd revised edn, pp. 82–83, Dover Publ., N.Y.
321. Ridge, J.P., Fuchs, E.J. & Matzinger, P. (1996) *Science* **271**, 1723.
322. Sarzotti, M., Robbins, D. & Hoffman, P.M. (1996) *Science* **271**, 1726.
323. Forsthuber, T., Yip, H.C. & Lehmann, P.V. (1996) *Science* **271**, 1728.
324. Pennisi, E. (1996) *Science* **271**, 1665.
325. Matzinger, P. (1994) *Annu. Rev. Immunol.* **12**, 991.
326. Malkovský, M. & Medawar, P.B. (1984) *Immunol. Today* **5**, 340.

Biographies

RAY DAVID OWEN (1915–)

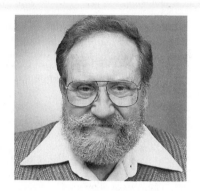

It is rare that a single paper, a briefly written one at that like the one Ray Owen published in *Science* in 1945, has a decisive impact on the course of science. In discovering the red cell mosaicism of cattle dizygotic twins and explaining it in terms of Lillie's much earlier description of the shared placentation of such twins, Owen exerted a profound influence on the thinking of F.M. Burnet and the subsequent studies of P.B. Medawar and his colleagues. Although Owen was co-author of a number of subsequent publications, ranging from genetics, tolerance, bone marrow transplantation and blood groups, none could match this *Science* paper in overriding importance. Medawar wrote to him on October 24th, 1960: "Of the five or six hundred letters I have had about this Nobel prize, yours is the one I most wanted to receive. I think it is *very wrong* that you are not sharing in this prize; the only consolation is that all your professional colleagues have a perfectly clear under-standing of the fact that you started it all. . . I was very much touched by your characteristically generous and modest letter".

Owen was brought up on a dairy farm in Wisconsin and his father, who was also a cattle fancier, aroused his interest in genetics. His Ph.D. studies at the University of Wisconsin were largely concerned with the biochemical and developmental genetics of birds. Influenced by M.R. Irwin, who is reputed to have coined the term 'immuno-genetics', and in collaboration with C. Stormont, he then worked on the genetics of red cell antigens in cattle, and this led to his germinal discovery. In 1947 he became Associate Professor of Biology at the California Institute of Technology, where he remained as a senior and highly respected faculty member until his retirement. He had a succession of postgraduate students who made names for themselves – among them I. Rapaport, W.H. Hildemann, H. Gershowitz, J. Berrian, D. Shreffler – and by influencing a succession of graduate students and postdoctoral fellows (including this author) and working as Dean of Students he remained a potent influence until his retirement. He became Professor Emeritus in 1983 and he and his wife June continue to be associated with Caltech. He selflessly spent a significant part of his life serving national and international scientific institutions, reviewing grant applications and scientific papers, and recruiting students, as well as ensuring their welfare once they had commenced their studies.

All who came within Owen's orbit will remember him as an intellectually sharp, stimulating, highly knowledgeable and at the same time modest man who was always willing to help other scientists, whether young or old. His interests outside his professional life were his family, home and garden, and his many friends. He received numerous honors including in 1966 the Gregor Mendel Medal of the Czechoslovak Academy of Sciences to mark the Mendel Centenary. In June 1996, the University of Wisconsin, Madison, held a Symposium in Ray Owen's honor to mark the 50th anniversary of the publication of his paper in *Science*.

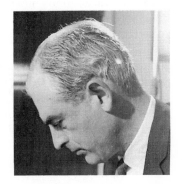

**PETER BRIAN MEDAWAR
(1915–1987)**

Peter Medawar was born in Brazil, his father having been Lebanese and his mother English. He was educated at a prestigious English public (=private!) school, Marlborough College, and took a degree in Zoology at Oxford University, followed by a Phil.D. It was in Oxford that he met his wife Jean, a student at the time, who became his lifelong companion and his chief support during his lengthy illness.

Medawar was one the foremost biologists of his generation and once he had turned his powerful mind to the subject of transplantation, he stamped his authority and creativity on a rapidly developing field. Modern transplantation immunology can be said to have begun with his demonstration, in the mid-1940s, of the immunologic basis of skin allograft rejection, and the development of cellular immunology received a great impetus from his studies. The discovery of acquired tolerance, made with Billingham and Brent, was probably his greatest achievement, for which he shared the Nobel Prize with Macfarlane Burnet in 1960. However, he made numerous other contributions to the study of graft rejection and he played an important role in demonstrating the activity of anti-lymphocyte serum and the mechanism of its action. In the 1950s he and his two research associates (Billingham and Brent) were playfully known in the United States as 'The Holy Trinity'! As if all this was not enough, he left his Chair of Zoology at University College, London, in 1962 to become the Director of Britain's foremost center of medical research, the National Institute for Medical Research, a post to which he brought great distinction and which he had to relinquish after his first catastrophic cerebral hemorrhage in 1969. He bore his physical disablement with heroic courage and good humor: not only did he continue to enjoy life (although his sporting hobbies of playing squash and cricket had come to an end), but he added to his list of books seven others, all written in his inimitably witty, stylistically elegant and intellectually probing manner. He was no mean philosopher of science, as is clear from some of his essays, and he was a great admirer and close friend of Karl Popper. His last book, written after several further and increasingly disabling strokes, was the autobiographic: *Memoirs of a Thinking Radish* (1986). All his books were read with enjoyment by scientists and laymen alike.

Medawar was a charismatic man and had a wide circle of admirers. He was showered with honors – from becoming one of the youngest Fellows of the Royal Society and the recipient of the Royal Society's Copley Medal to his knighthood in 1965 and the Queen's Order of Merit in 1981. Numerous national scientific societies made him an honorary member and he collected honorary degrees as others collect stamps. Appropriately, he was elected to be the first President of The Transplantation Society. Although he appreciated these honors he bore them lightly and he retained a sense of proportion and a mischievous sense of humor. His friends and colleagues (and there were many, from all over the world) and all who encountered him will remember him as a brilliant, genial, generous, and approachable man whose conversational ability, lectures and writings were never less than inspiring and always to the point. One of his passionate and lifelong interests was opera, and listening to his favorites helped to sustain him until the end.

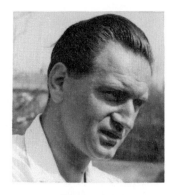

MILAN HAŠEK (1925–1984)

Like Medawar, Milan Hašek had the physical stature of a giant. He had a keen intellect and despite his earlier belief in communism he communicated an overwhelming *joie de vivre*, which he was only too happy to share with his friends and colleagues at the end of a day's work or conferencing. He delighted in drinking unsuspecting friends 'under the table' and engaging them (while still relatively sober) in such physical contests as chair lifting and arm wrestling. He had a knack of making visitors welcome and shared his scientific and political thoughts and enthusiasms with them without reserve.

Hašek was born in Prague, where he spent virtually all his life. Having taken a medical degree at Charles University he joined the Institute of Biology as a research scientist in 1950 and then became head of the Department of Experimental Biology and Genetics. In 1962 he was promoted to Director of the Institute. His wife Vera was a transplantation immunologist too who managed to reconcile her professional life with bringing up three children. He remarried in the 1970s. The contribution Hašek and his colleagues made to the development of tolerance has already been described (p.192). He entered the field developing and applying the technique of parabiosis of avian chick embryos and studying the biologic consequences of such a union. His first publication on this came in the same year (1953) in which Billingham, Brent and Medawar. published their first tolerance paper. Hašek, whose powers of leadership were considerable, built up a large research group in Prague and under his direction his Institute became the most advanced, prestigious and productive in Eastern Europe. At that time the latest equipment was not always available in Czechoslovakia and it is a great tribute to the Czech workers that they contributed so handsomely to immunology despite this handicap. Hašek organized a number of international symposia in Liblice castle, near Prague, and these played an important role in forging close links between the Czech school and western immunologists, as well as advancing the field generally. Those who were present will remember these meetings with much pleasure, even though they were somewhat overshadowed by the repressive political climate of the time. Hašek's brutal removal from the Institute Directorship in 1970 followed his signing of the Dubcek Declaration in 1968 and the Soviet invasion of his country and, though eventually rehabilitated as a scientist, these events may well have played a role in his premature death.

Hašek and his colleagues published a huge number of papers, many of them in their 'house' journal, *Folia Biologica*. With Holáň he published a textbook on immunity (in Czech). He was made an honorary member of many national societies, was a member of editorial boards and international committees (including those of The Transplantation Society, of which he was a founding member), and received several prizes, including the Emil von Behring Preis of the Philipps Universität, Marburg (1968). His sudden, unexpected and inadequately explained death in 1984 was a blow not only to his family, friends and colleagues but to the whole immunologic community. It is an indication of the affection and esteem in which he was held that those of his former students and colleagues who had emigrated published an impressive memorial volume in 1989 – *Realm of Tolerance* – describing their studies, and many poignant recollections of Milan Hašek may be found in this book.

6 Immunoregulation: The Search for the Holy Grail

*"Good scientists study the most important problems they think
they can solve. It is, after all, their professional business to solve
problems, not merely to grapple with them. The spectacle of a scientist
locked in combat with the forces of ignorance is not an inspiring
one if, in the outcome, the scientist is routed."*

P.B. Medawar, 1961

In Chapter 5 I have dealt with the phenomenon of fetally or neonatally induced tolerance at length because it created the intellectual climate for the development of a vast new immunologic field of research – that of immunoregulation. It was certainly not intended to set neonatal tolerance apart from immunoregulation; indeed, most models of specific immunoregulation achieved in adult animals, and sometimes even in man, are considered to be examples of tolerance, in keeping with its wider definition of an acquired state of specific unresponsiveness regardless of the model used or the mechanism responsible. Thus R.H. Schwartz, in his recently published review on immunoregulation, called his chapter "Immunological Tolerance" (1). For an up-to-date account of this complex and important field, especially of its molecular basis, the reader is advised to consult this excellent review.

Schwartz very reasonably chose to discuss tolerance by referring to mechanisms rather than to the models used. From a historian's viewpoint this approach, though logical, introduces a level of complexity that might well interfere with the reader's ability to follow the historic thread. I have therefore decided to use the other approach, with all its other disadvantages.

A search for the Holy Grail? The ability to modulate an animal's and by analogy a patient's immunologic responses at will, with minimal or no side-effects, has undoubtedly become the prime objective in immunology. It is hardly necessary to point to the huge benefits this would confer, not only in tissue and organ transplantation but in a wide range of medical areas, including the autoimmune diseases, the allergies, some forms of cancer and the immunodeficiency syndromes. It would be no exaggeration to say that the practice of medicine would be utterly transformed. However, while numerous animal models have more or less successfully shown that it is possible to induce specific tolerance in adult animals, though usually not without the aid of nonspecific adjuncts, there is still a long way to go before this knowledge can be applied clinically, despite previous optimistic forecasts, including one from the present author (2)! The search for the Holy Grail is nevertheless being actively pursued by many laboratories throughout the world and one would have to be a congenital pessimist, and one lacking in imagination to boot, to claim that these efforts will not, in due course, bear fruit.

Although it could be argued that vaccination and immunotherapy are part of immunoregulation, they are excluded from this history because they are concerned with the induction of immunity rather than with its prevention. Those interested in the history of immunization may wish to consult references 3–5.

The Phenomenon of Immunologic Enhancement

The roots of this phenomenon, arguably the first example of specific immuno-regulation, may be found in the attempts by the early tumor biologists to elicit immunity by the previous inoculation of live or dead tumor cells – a branch of the biologic sciences that developed explosively in the late nineteenth and the early part of the twentieth centuries (see Chapter 2) and that has been comprehensively reviewed by Schöne (6), Tyzzer (7) and Woglom (8). Critical was the observation by Flexner and Jobling that the resistance of rats to the growth of a transplantable rat sarcoma could be lowered by the inoculation of an emulsion of the tumor tissue, heated to 56°C, 10–30 days before challenging the recipients with live sarcoma cells (9). This finding, which they described as the "promotion" of tumor growth, was soon confirmed by Bashford, Murray and Haaland (10). It more or less coincided with obervations that enzymatically degraded or mechanically disintegrated tumor cells, far from immunizing the recipients against the tumor, as had been expected, accelerated its growth. Thus Haaland (11), who concluded that the immunizing property of transplantable mouse tumors was dependent on the living cell and associated with a certain period of *in vivo* growth, observed that "far from inducing any increased resistance, inoculation of disintegrated cells only seems to manure the soil for a subsequent growth of tumours". This was corroborated by others – by Leitch in the same year with a saline extract of a mouse carcinoma (12), by Bisceglie (13) with a cell-free tumor filtrate and by Bertolotto (14) with multiple doses of nucleoproteins prepared from mouse carcinomas. Surprisingly, Favilli (15) was able to stimulate growth of Ehrlich's mouse carcinoma by multiple previous inoculations of sodium caseinate. More than a decade later Chambers and Scott, having failed to extract an immunizing factor from irradiated or untreated rat tumor cells, studied the results of tumor autolysis and found evidence for two factors, one stimulating tumor growth and the other inhibiting it (16). These workers went on to use a supernatant extracted from Jensen's rat sarcoma to enhance the growth of the tumor (17).

It was with this background that Casey published his first paper in 1932 (18) describing the experimental enhancement of growth of the Brown–Pearce rabbit tumor, though he seemed to be less than well acquainted with the literature. He used an autolytic approach for the preparation of tumor extracts, one of such crudity as to make a contemporary biologist's hair stand on end! For example, rabbits bearing the tumor were left "in the ice-box (26–32° F)" for two weeks (in some cases for two months), whereupon a saline emulsion of the tumor was prepared and inoculated into the right testicles of normal adult rabbits. This was followed by the inoculation of fresh tumor cells into the left testicles. Compared with a control group that had not been pretreated the tumors grew more rapidly and to a larger size, caused the death of a greater proportion of recipients, and resulted in a higher incidence of metastases. The effect could be observed using an intracutaneous site (19) and obtained with dessicated tissue or with material that had been filtered.

Attempts by Casey and his colleagues to analyze the nature of enhanced tumor growth were not particularly successful, even though by 1949, encouraged by the experiments of Snell's group (see below), they had begun to use inbred C57BL mice (20). They used mammary mouse carcinoma tissue from a number of tumor lines, minced and ground in a mortar with saline after storage at 0°C for many months. Their main finding was to confirm the work of Snell's group and to show that enhanced tumor growth was specific. Unfortunately by this time they had chosen to call the unknown growth-promoting material the XYZ factor and the phenomenon the XYZ effect, which they defined as "the decreased incidence and more rapid increment of local and metastatic transplanted tumors following the prior injection in the same or distant sites of an extract from the homologous tumor" (20). Because the factor had been shown to be filtrable and thermolabile they flirted with the idea that it was "an inert contaminating virus" in the tumor cells. They persisted with the XYZ terminology until 1952 (21), and it was left for G.D. Snell, N. Kaliss and their colleagues at Bar Harbor, working with inbred strains of mice and with allogeneic tumors, to uncover its immunologic basis.

The observation by Snell's group that pretreatment with lyophilized mammary carcinoma tissue enhanced the tumor's growth in allogeneic hosts provided a valuable tool for the analysis of the phenomenon of immunologic enhancement, as it now became known. In their 1946 paper (22) they describe, for several inbred strains of mice, what happened when frozen and dried (lyophilized) preparations of an allogeneic A strain carcinoma were inoculated into the hosts over a seven week period preceding transplantation of the live tumor. There was usually uncontrolled tumor growth resulting in the death of the host mice, whereas the tumor grew only transiently in untreated animals before rejection occurred. In one strain combination they found the opposite effect – protection against the tumor. These authors provided a good review of the previous literature on immunization and growth promotion, and suggested that "The diversity of the results just noted is probably to be explained by the complexity of the genetic basis of tissue specificity". They went on to estimate the number of "loci" (the first use of this term in place of "genes"?): it "certainly exceeds 10 and is probably less than 30, and the most probable estimate would appear to be in the neighbourhood of 16 or 20" – an underestimate as it later transpired, but in the light of knowledge at that time a good prediction of the complexity of the histocompatibility system of the mouse. They went on to say that some of the genes might be "minor genes", that the loci "act to induce an immune reaction to a transplanted tumor by producing some substance not produced by the particular allele carried by the host", and that "There is no reason to suppose that the number of such substances exceeds the number of genes concerned", though it could be less. Finally, they drew attention to the difficulty of unraveling the complexities of the phenomenon of tissue specificity with non-inbred animal stocks and explained that "With this in mind, methods have been developed for producing special inbred stocks identical with standard stocks now available except that each stock will be differentiated by carrying a recessive allele of some one of the loci concerned with tissue specificity" (i.e. the congenic lines that later proved so fundamentally important in the dissection of the H-2 system).

This paper put the XYZ effect and tumor enhancement in general on a scientific basis, and two years later a further paper from Snell's laboratory (23) analyzed the phenomenon in seven inbred strains using nine different tumors: both inhibition and enhancement were observed, and "some specificity" was found when the lyophilized tumor donors and the fresh tumor donors came from different strains. However, tumors originating from the same strain gave strong cross-reactions.

Progress now became very rapid. It was shown that the enhancing material was present in filtered tissue extracts prepared by digestion with hyaluronidase (24), that inoculation of tissue preparations was effective only if made at least one day before tumor transplantation but that the effect of treatment with lyophilized tissue can be very long-lasting (25), and – very significantly – that enhancement can also be brought about by pretreatment with normal tissue preparations from the strain from which the tumor had come (26). This effect was species-specific (27). The enhancing substances were thus firmly nailed to the flag of the H-2 histocompatibility system, as argued persuasively in 1954 by Snell (28), who showed in mouse strains with known D and K genotypes that enhancement occurred only if the tumor and the normal enhancing tissues shared a factor lacking in the host. Snell therefore concluded that the enhancing substance "must be a product of the H-2 locus", and he cited convincing evidence that the effect was due to an immunologic response. Having recently become aware of the tolerance studies by Billingham, Brent and Medawar (see Chapter 5) he suggested, erroneously as it turned out, that the phenomenon should be named "actively acquired tolerance" and he added, speculatively, that it may owe its existence to the incorporation in the host's cells of the foreign H-2 molecules. This speculation was nipped in the bud by the observation by Kaliss that enhancement is antibody-mediated (see below) although, curiously, it was echoed by Kaliss himself as late as 1955 (29). Kandutsch and Reinert-Wenck (30) later studied the chemical nature of the enhancing substances – they were found in tumor and spleen tissue, but in lower concentrations in the liver, kidney and stomach – and concluded that they were mucoproteins.

The first indication that immunologic enhancement could be antibody-mediated came in 1952 with the demonstration by Kaliss and Molomut (31) that allo-antisera produced in rabbits or mice by immunization with a mixture of tumor and spleen and kidney from the tumor strain led to "marked growth, and some takes" of two allogeneic tumors that would normally be expected to regress in all hosts. While drawing attention to the parallel between this outcome and that previously obtained with lyophilized tissues, the authors were wary not to draw general conclusions from this finding, though they saw a rough correlation between the sera's hemagglutinating titers and their biologic activity. This paper was soon followed up by the demonstration (32) that resistance to sarcoma I could be broken down by previous treatment of the hosts with one or other of two allo-antisera raised in mice by immunization with spleen cells only, despite the fact that one of the sera had no detectable complement-fixing antibodies – a result that mirrored pretreatment with lyophilized tumor preparations.

Kaliss published a number of other papers (33–35) cementing the link between allo-antibodies and enhancement, though attempts to appraise the possible mechanisms came rather later (35, 36). By showing that the active fraction of the enhancing antisera was associated with the globulin and probably the gammaglobulin fraction,

Kaliss and Kandutsch (37) had laid the basis for a plausible immunologic explanation, though this still left open the question of whether enhancement was brought about by an effect on the immune system or by selection of cells within the tumor. Gorer (38) had earlier found an association between enhancing procedures and the formation of high titers of hemagglutinating allo-antibodies. Of considerable relevance was the finding by Mitchison and Dube (39) that the enhanced state could be abrogated by treatment of the hosts with lymph node cells of immunized mice, whereas normal lymph node cells were ineffective. Their study therefore seemed to distinguish functionally between enhancement and tolerance, for the latter could be abolished by both normal and presensitized cells (40).

Until Billingham, Brent and Medawar (41) attempted to enhance the survival of skin allografts little was known about whether tumors were unique in this respect; indeed, this had generally been assumed to be the case because of the finding by Billingham and Sparrow (42) that trypsinized epidermal cells inoculated intravenously into allogeneic rabbits substantially prolonged skin graft survival. Little was known of the mechanism underlying this observation and it was shown to be a peculiarity of the intravenous route. The attempt by Billingham, Brent and Medawar (41) to prolong skin allograft survival in mice by pretreatment with lyophilized kidney, liver or spleen preparations showed that the conditions that ensured the uncontrollable growth of a tumor led to only a few days of prolonged skin graft survival. Because they used inbred strains for which precise median survival times of graft survival were known they nevertheless believed "that even a few days' postponement of graft breakdown represents an impairment of immunity which is quite great enough to allow a tumor homograft to get out of immunological control", especially as they had previously shown in experiments on tolerance "that a tumor allograft may grow and kill its host in the face of a residual immunity strong enough to destroy a skin homograft completely". It therefore seemed that the growth rate characteristic of tumors provided the key, but later studies on the long-term survival of vascularized organ allografts following enhancement regimens showed that this was not the case (see below). Instead, the exquisite sensitivity of skin to even feeble immune responses was almost certainly responsible for the unimpressive results obtained by Billingham, Brent and Medawar and this was confirmed by G. Möller's demonstration (43) that the same pretreatment that prolonged skin allograft survival only minimally procured substantial survival of ovarian grafts.

Two other lines of evidence need to be mentioned. First, the finding by Voisin and Kinsky that enhancing antisera raised by the inoculation of lyophilized preparations into adult mice had the power to inhibit graft-versus-host reactions (runting) in newborn mice following the introduction of immunologically competent allogeneic cells (44). Further, sera obtained from mice made conventionally tolerant at birth had the power to enhance tumor growth in the appropriate strain combination, despite the absence of conventionally identifiable antibodies (45, 46), though antibodies thought to belong to the IgA class were uncovered by the synergic hemagglutination technique. Voisin's contributions to the field of enhancement and tolerance, which began with a speculative paper in 1962 (47) and included a careful review of the phenomenon of enhancement (48) a year later, were probably underrated. The reasons for this are not clear, but the fact that some of them were published in French (which, if true, would suggest a somewhat insular outlook by the Anglo-

Saxon scientific community) and some in Symposia volumes in which economy with words was not always of the essence may have had something to do with it. An additional factor, perhaps, was Voisin's introduction of the term "facilitation" in place of enhancement – a term that had resonance in both French and English and to which he clung despite the reluctance of other immunologists to adopt it. Thus Medawar, in bringing the very informative and successful 1962 *Ciba Symposium on Transplantation* to a close stated that although a neutral word that could also encompass normal tissues might be desirable and he was attracted by the term facilitation "it is too late to persuade anybody to use that now" (49).

The other line of evidence came from Brent and Medawar (50), who continued their earlier exploration with Billingham (41) of the effects enhancing antisera have on skin allografts. They confirmed that graft prolongation was minimal and far outweighed by the use of multiple doses of the vital dye trypan blue, and they showed that the immunogenicity of crude cell-free allogeneic extracts inoculated into mice could be largely prevented by sera with anti-donor strain antibodies. They argued that because direct mixing of antiserum and tissue extract before inoculation did not lead to loss of immunogenicity, their data could not be interpreted in terms of an afferent inhibition of the immune response. They thus reversed their previous conclusion (41), which had been based on the erroneous assumption of nuclear (= graft sensitizing – "T") and cytoplasmic (= antibody-inducing – "H") antigens. Because antisera were unable to counteract even the feeblest pre-existing immunity, efferent inhibition (i.e. at the level of the target tissue – the skin grafts) was thought to be equally improbable. Like Snell *et al.* (51) before them they thought that their data could best be accommodated by a form of central inhibition (i.e. at the level of the immunocompetent cell), though by means "at present unknown".

Snell *et al.* (51) had arrived at their conclusion after ruling out a suggestion originally made by Kaliss (35) that tumor enhancement was brought about by some physiologic alteration of the tumor. This they were able to do by showing that tumors transplanted directly from the donor strain had the same growth rate and power to overwhelm their allogeneic hosts as tumors that had been grown in mice of the host strain following enhancing pretreatment. On the other hand, they found that enhancing antisera greatly inhibited the immunity that would normally be conferred on mice by the inoculation of immune lymph node cells, thus allowing tumor implants of the appropriate type to grow out of control. Further, the administration of allogeneic cells together with antiserum suppressed antibody formation. They concluded that "These results provide an adequate explanation of the phenomenon of immunological enhancement". Indeed, several years earlier Pikovski and Schlesinger (52) had pretty well ruled out tumor alteration when in their hands tumors that had been maintained in passively enhanced rats for a number of generations were readily accepted by normal recipients of the original donor strain. For their part, Brent and Medawar (50) went on to speculate that because hyperimmunization with repeated doses of allogeneic spleen cells led to high antibody titers but a lowering of cellular sensitivity, an early sensitive phase is superseded by a phase in which cells "are preoccupied by the manufacture of humoral antibodies". They quoted several papers based on other systems in support of this notion, which in modern terms might conceivably be accounted for by the existence of T1 and T2 CD4-positive lymphocytes, the one concerned with providing "help" in the induction of delayed-type hypersensitivity effectors and the other with help for B lymphocytes in antibody formation (53).

All the mechanisms put forward at this time to account for the phenomenon of enhancement had to accommodate the fact that alloantibodies were capable of mediating its development and that an immune response to the alloantigens of the donor strain – present on tumor as well as normal tissues – was clearly involved. Four other hypotheses were put forward.

(1) First, that antibody might bring about some cell selection within the transplanted tumor, favoring cells able to escape from the cellular sensitivity aroused; but this notion was dismissed almost as quickly as it had been formed (54, 55).

(2) The second, proposed by Snell (56, 57), involved the "walling-off" by specific antibody of the antigenic sites on the tumor cells, thus preventing them from sensitizing the host (i.e. another form of afferent inhibition). This was dismissed by Kaliss on the grounds that in some cases he was able to bring about enhanced growth by giving the antiserum as late as day 7–10 after tumor transplantation (34), and by Gorer when he drew attention to the fact that exceedingly small amounts of antibody could cause enhancement (58, 59). (Bearing in mind that Kaliss was working in Snell's institute at Bar Harbor and that they collaborated extensively it seems a little odd to see this cut and thrust in their published work!)

(3) Third, Feldman and Globerson believed that tumor survival in the face of an evident allograft response was due to an increased antibody-induced expression of alloantigens on the cell surface, thus making the cells less vulnerable (60).

(4) Finally, Gorer (58) saw a similarity between desensitizing antibodies in certain depressed states of allergy and enhancing antibodies, and suggested that this "anergy", as it "is sometimes described", might account for Mitchison and Dube's suggestion (39) that pretreatment blocks the defensive cellular response while leaving antibody production intact.

Many years later anergy was to be invoked to account for many forms of specific inhibition of the immune response (see below).

Further evidence for the notion that antibodies can block the immune response ('blocking antibodies') came in a flood of papers from the laboratory of K.E. and I. Hellström, who demonstrated such antibodies not only in animals (61–65) and human tumor patients (66, 67) with growing tumors, but also in other biologic situations involving the transplantation of allogeneic tissues and cells, as in tolerant mice (68) or rats (69, 70), tetraparental mice (71), bone marrow chimeras (72) and human long-term kidney transplant patients (73). The factors involved were variously described as blocking antibodies or antigen–antibody complexes (74), but their mode of action was not fully elucidated. Nonetheless, despite objections raised against the conclusions drawn from tolerant mice (see Chapter 5), blocking factors of one kind or another seemed to sweep everything before them in the early 1970s and appeared to offer a plausible explanation for the phenomenon of enhancement and many other forms of specific unresponsiveness (75).

In an attempt to create some order from this welter of often contradictory information and interpretation Batchelor stated in 1968 that "Much of the earlier argument about enhancement was due to a reluctance to accept the fact that more than one mechanism might operate" (76), and this probably hit the nail on the head. As so often in biologic research, there were indeed a great many models! G. Möller, in an elegant earlier series of publications designed to elucidate the mechanism of passively induced tumor enhancement, found that:

(1) Inhibition of the immune response was directly related to the number or strength of the antigenic sites that were not coated with antibody (77).
(2) Enhancement was obtained with tumor cells that were coated with antibodies in the absence of circulating antibodies in the hosts (78).
(3) Antibodies antagonized the neutralizing effect exerted by presensitized lymphoid cells on tumor growth when all three elements were mixed together before inoculation into adult mice (79).

His overall conclusion was that efferent inhibition had occurred (80). While confirming that the survival of skin allografts was only barely prolonged by enhancing antisera he nevertheless found that ovarian allografts were more amenable in this respect (43), thus drawing attention to the importance of the target tissue. By demonstrating that antibody-coated tumor cells survived in allogeneic hosts, but non-coated cells inoculated concomitantly did not, Möller satisfied himself that an efferent rather than a central influence was paramount. In reviewing some of the literature, Batchelor (76) wrote that "It seems likely, therefore, that one of the critical factors which decides whether a graft is destroyed by antibody *in vivo* or whether it survives and shows enhanced growth is the amount of complement fixed by the reaction", and he cited the work of Chard (81) and Chard, French and Batchelor (82), making use of Fab and F(ab')2 fragments from H-2 antibodies, to support his contention: although these fragments could bind to cells they were not cytotoxic, but were nonetheless able to suppress the *in vivo* growth of the appropriate tumor.

The enhanced growth of tumors is thus probably brought about by more than one mechanism involving efferent and central pathways. However, the phenomenon was largely removed from the realm of tumor biology when in the late 1960s it became possible to transplant kidneys in the rat and it became apparent that allogeneic kidneys were highly susceptible to the action of enhancing protocols involving treatment with both antigen and antibody (83) or antibody alone (84). Enhancement therefore became subsumed into the more general category of specific immunosuppression/immunoregulation/tolerance and this will be dealt with in the next section. Interest in the enhancement of tumors waned correspondingly; the early work has, however, been well reviewed (85–87).

Enter Microvascular Surgery and the Rat Kidney Allograft

S. Lee's technical advance in transplanting kidneys from one rat to another (88, 89) opened up new vistas, for at last transplantation immunologists working with inbred rodents were freed from the constraints of having to use mainly tumors (a special case?) or skin grafts (easy to perform, but perhaps too vulnerable?). It facilitated the study of kidney allograft rejection in inbred strains and at the same time put transplantation immunology more closely in touch with clinical kidney transplantation, which by then had already taken off though – despite the use of immunosuppressive drugs – it still yielded relatively poor results (see Chapter 7). Clearly, an immuno-regulatory protocol for kidney transplant recipients was highly desirable, and at last it became possible to pursue this objective. It should be said that this development occurred against a backdrop of great surgical advances in the experimental trans-plantation of organs, mainly in dogs, commencing with the early attempts at kidney transplantation by Ullmann (90) and Carrel (91) at the turn of the century. This was followed by a wave of renewed interest and an armory of refined techniques after World War II in the transplantation of both kidneys and livers. (For references see the excellent historic accounts of organ transplantation by Woodruff (92) and Moore (93) and Chapter 2.) It was Moore and his colleagues at the Peter Bent Brigham Hospital in Boston who first described a workable one-stage transplantation technique for the canine liver (94). Feldman et al. later went on to use Lee's kidney transplantation technique to study the mechanism of allograft rejection in inbred rats made tolerant at birth (95), showing that the animals were tolerant to both skin and kidney grafts from the same donor strain, that the tolerance could be broken adoptively though sometimes with difficulty, and that grafts could be injured by humoral factors as well as by lymphoid cells. Lee and Edgington in the same year described a technique for heterotopic liver transplantation in the rat with which they studied the process of liver allograft rejection (96).

It was Stuart, Saitoh and Fitch (83), however, who in 1968 were the first to apply Lee's surgical innovation to the study of renal allograft enhancement by transplanting (Lewis x BN) F1 kidneys into Lewis recipients, which were given donor strain spleen cells one day before and hyperimmune Lewis-anti-BN serum immediately before and after the operation, both intravenously. They thus combined both active and passive immunization. All ten kidneys in the experimental group, which was bilaterally nephrectomized, showed long-term survival with near-normal blood urea nitrogen. Kidney graft survival was shown to be specific for the donor strain, and although treatment with either spleen cells alone or hyperimmune serum alone produced some prolonged survival it was the combined treatment that was most effective. Here at last was a clear demonstration that protocols known to induce tumor enhancement were equally effective in prolonging the life of organ allografts. The paper was published in the same volume number of *Science* as a paper by Axelrad and Rowley (97) showing that the induction of delayed-type hypersensitivity to sheep red blood cells (SRBC), induced by red cells administered intradermally in Freund's adjuvant, could be specifically suppressed by either passively administered anti-SRBC or by intravenous inoculation of SRBC given shortly before sensitization. These authors speculated that the effect of the antibody might have been through interaction with antigen or with antigen-reactive cells, thus limiting the proliferation of cells mediating delayed-type hypersensitivity; and that the antibody might have committed such cells to proliferation of antibody-producing cells, so reducing the number of cells available to develop a hypersensitivity response. "The combined treatment presumably summates these two effects", they wrote. Hence treatment protocols were equally effective for delayed-type hypersensitivity and for allograft rejection, a finding that supported the link that had been established earlier between these two immunologic events (see Chapter 2).

The use of passively administered antisera to bring about the permanent survival of rat kidney allografts was given a great boost by the work of French and Batchelor one year later, when they showed that using inbred strains different from those used by

Stuart, Saitoh and Fitch, rats given F1 hybrid kidneys and several doses of hyperimmune anti-donor antiserum administered repeatedly in the first 4 days following renal transplantation sustained their grafts indefinitely (84). The effect was again highly strain-specific and the animals bearing the enhanced allografts produced some cytotoxic anti-donor antibody in the early stages, though titers had declined greatly or were down to zero by ten weeks. These workers found that when parental strain kidneys were transplanted using the same enhancing protocol, prolongation of survival, though substantial, was limited. They were inclined to attribute this to the greater antigenic load carried by homozygous tissues, thus either increasing the requirement for antibody or making the kidneys more vulnerable to antibody-mediated damage. French and Batchelor pointed to the potential clinical interest of these data, either as a prophylactic treatment where there were known human leukocyte antigen (HLA) incompatibilities or in the treatment of rejection crises.

Enhancement/Tolerance of Rat Kidneys

The reports by Stuart and his colleagues and by French and Batchelor triggered an explosion of research in which the rat kidney became the chief object of attention; indeed, it can be said that, just as tolerance had dominated the 1950s and 1960s, so the enhancement of kidneys and other organs became a dominant preoccupation of the 1970s and 1980s. Some of the earlier work has been well reviewed (98, 99) (see especially the comprehensive review by Morris; 100). Here I will restrict myself to the main advances and to the hypotheses put forward to account for the long-term and highly specific survival of kidney allografts in the rat. It must, however, be said that the enhancement procedures:

(1) Did not work equally well in all strain combinations tested (101).
(2) Were often dependent on the use of F1 hybrid kidneys (102).
(3) Tended to be less successful in large animals such as primates (103, 104) and dogs (105, 106). (Mybergh and Smit's results in baboons (104) were, however, obtained with liver allografts, using a polyspecific antiserum; substantially improved survival was obtained when the recipients were also treated with donor bone marrow cells.)

This prompted J.W. Fabre (107), who has contributed substantially to the analysis of the phenomenon, to publish an article in 1982 entitled "Rat kidney allograft model: was it all too good to be true?". He argued that virtually any form of temporary immunosuppression, even in "difficult" rat strain combinations, tended to lead to the long-term acceptance of kidney allografts, and he suggested that this was probably true because unlike the human kidney (108), that of the rat has an endothelium lacking Ia (i.e. class II) antigens (109, 110). He linked this fact with the known antigen-presenting role of interstitial dendritic cells (111) and the high probability that in the rat they represent the chief "passenger leukocyte" of the kidney (112) and act as the major target for enhancing antibodies (110); and he argued that whereas human vascular endothelial cells can stimulate in the mixed lymphocyte reaction (MLR) and present antigens (113), this additional facility was not available to the rat. As dendritic cells were capable of migration (114) a freshly transplanted rat kidney would lose them within a few days, leaving it without a significant antigen-presenting capacity, in contrast to the human kidney. Donor dendritic cells that had migrated to other tissues of the recipient might be expected, he argued, to be opsonized by the enhancing antibodies and hence eliminated. (The whole question of passenger leukocytes is considered in Chapter 2.) This explanation for the relative ease with which passive enhancement can be brought about for rat kidneys does not, of course, explain how the enhancement mechanism operates, and others have addressed this question (see below); nor does it invalidate the use of the rat as an experimental species, though it emphasizes the importance of verifying experimental protocols in other, and especially in larger, species.

Before describing mechanisms that have been proposed it is necessary to consider what kind of antibodies play a role in enhancement.

Class of antibody involved

It has been confirmed many times over that an enhanced state can be established by either active sensitization before transplantation or by the passive administration of anti-donor alloantibody at the time of grafting. The class of antibody responsible has been the source of some disagreement though the evidence has, on the whole, favored immunoglobulin (IgG) or its subclasses. The first to address this question comprehensively were Mullen and Hildemann and their colleagues (*115–118*), who concluded that the effective antibodies were to be found primarily in the IgG but not the IgM fraction, and that IgG2 was active. Indeed, they showed that IgM administered in a weak strain combination curtailed graft survival (*118*). Their conclusion received support from others (*119*) and was consistent with studies on the enhancement of tumor allografts (*120–125*), but a role for IgM, if less marked and predictable, was suggested by data from certain protocols relating to both kidney (*126–128*) and tumor (*129, 130*) enhancement. Claims for the involvement of anti-Ia (i.e. anti-class II) antibodies in heart (*131*) or kidney (*132, 133*) enhancement have been made but have also been disputed (*134, 135*), an important point that has already been alluded to and that will be further considered under mechanisms (below).

Specificity

Like neonatally induced tolerance, enhancement is a specific event – a point well established for tumors by G. Möller (*77*) and for mouse skin allografts by Jeekel, McKenzie and Winn (*136*), who used a battery of congenic strains differing at a single well-defined locus. Nevertheless, some cross-reactivity has been encountered for kidney allografts (*137, 138*) and for skin allografts (*139*), but McKenzie, Fabre and Morris (*140*) established that this was not a common event and that when it happened the sera were usually weak. In general it would seem that enhancement is a donor-specific phenomenon.

The Mechanism of Enhancement in Kidney Allograft Survival

Batchelor and Welsh (*98*) distinguished between two distinct phases in the induction of enhancement: induction, in which the host's response is delayed or suppressed, and maintenance, when a graft is firmly established and may survive indefinitely without further treatment. These two stages are characterized by properties that are most readily explained by different mechanisms, and most workers have since accepted this distinction as useful and informative. I will therefore deal with possible mechanisms under these two headings.

Inductive stage

This stage immediately follows the administration of antibodies or, in the case of active enhancement, pretreatment with antigenic preparations of some kind or another, that leads to the formation of anti-donor antibodies by the graft recipient. Among the possible mechanisms proposed to account for the inductive phase are:

(1) Walling off (or coating) of the antigenic sites on the target tissue by antibody (56, 57).
(2) Interference with immunogenic passenger cells.
(3) A central suppression of the immune system by interaction between antigen or antigen–antibody complexes and antigen-reactive lymphocytes (50, 52) (see below).

The first of these hypotheses was found to be untenable not only in tumor studies (34, 58, 59) (see above), but also in the transplantation of rat kidneys, for Fabre and Morris were able to induce enhancement with extremely small doses (10–50 μl) of antibody (141) – not nearly enough to cover all the antigenic sites of the kidney. The same is true for the maintenance stage, in that it has been shown by Fine et al., using a labeled anti-donor antibody that kidneys in enhanced and non-enhanced rats take up the same amount of antibody,, that there is a continuous turnover of bound antibody, and that long-surviving kidneys have plenty of free antigenic sites (142). Although it cannot be ruled out that antibody coating plays some role, especially in view of the favorable F_1 hybrid effect, it is necessary to examine the evidence for alternative explanations, in the first place in the inductive phase.

The early evidence favoring some form of central inhibition of the immune response has already been dealt with above; it was based entirely on tumor and skin allograft transplantation. In rats with passively enhanced kidneys it has likewise been found that there is a marked early inhibition of the humoral response (143, 144) and that this can be especially true for early IgM production (144).

Some form of central inhibition is attractive in view of the finding that passively administered antibody interferes with the production of the recipient's antibody response, both after tumor (51) and kidney (143, 144) transplantation, with the effect being especially marked for the early IgM response (144). Indeed, Snell et al. (51) had shown that there was both a delay and impairment of the cellular response in mice soon after treatment and tumor transplantation. Interestingly enough, Uhr and Möller, in reviewing in 1968 the topic of immunoregulation by antibody to a variety of antigens (121), were unable to suggest any plausible mechanism other than that antibody interacts specifically with antigenic determinants. They thought that the simplest explanation was that antigenic determinants on the antigen molecule were rendered sterically unavailable to the immune system – a possibility that, as stated above, has been rendered improbable so far as enhancement is concerned.

Their alternative suggestion – that the metabolism of antigen is altered by binding with antibody – is clearly equally inapplicable to the prolonged survival of tissue and organ grafts.

We are left then with the notion – advocated extensively by the Hellströms and their colleagues – that once antibody has bound to antigen in the graft and the resulting complexes are shed into the circulation, they can interact with antigen-specific receptors of lymphocytes both in the periphery and the central lymphoid organs, thus inhibiting their ability to respond. This notion continued to receive support in experimental models – for skin (145, 146), hearts (147), kidneys (119) and cells (148) – as well as in clinical renal transplantation (149, 150) though not always necessarily in the early stages. A plausible mechanism that has been put forward for the action of complexes is that following interaction between complexes and specific antigen-reactive lymphocytes, the lymphocytes are removed from the circulation and catabolized by macrophages, thus leaving the animal with a deficiency of potentially reactive cells. This phenomenon, known as ARCO (antigen-reactive cell opsonization) will now be considered.

The idea that an antibody directed against the Rh (D) antigen of red blood cells can clear such cells from the circulation of an Rh-negative individual, and therefore prevent sensitization, we owe to the work of Clarke et al. (151) (see also 152), who showed that Rh-positive cells inoculated into Rh-negative men were cleared from the circulation within 24 hours if an incomplete antibody was administered within 30 minutes, and that this interfered with the induction of antibodies against them. Others subsequently applied this protocol to the prevention of hemolytic disease of the newborn (see Chapter 3). This is the classic example of the abortion of an immune response by the removal of the antigen before it is able to activate the immune system, in this case possibly by lysis but more probably by opsonization and removal of the cells by the reticuloendothelial system. By depleting the body of lymphocytes that would be critically involved in the induction of a specific immune response, ARCO works at the other end of the immune arc.

ARCO depends on the formation of antigen–antibody complexes that form a bridge between antigen-reactive cells (ARC) and macrophages by virtue of being concomitantly bound to ARC via free sites on the antigen and to macrophages via the Fc portion of the antibody molecule. When both occur, the ARC are avidly phagocytosed and thus not only removed, but destroyed. The phenomenon was first demonstrated in 1977 by Hutchinson and Zola (153) when they showed that rabbit-anti-rat antilymphocyte sera, strenuously absorbed with purified rat red cells, were strongly opsonic in that they were instrumental in diverting radiolabeled antibody-coated splenocytes to the liver of rat recipients. These sera had anti-Ia-like specificity (153) and were capable of prolonging kidney allograft survival (154), in keeping with the observation that Ia (i.e. class II) antibodies can be effective mediators of enhancement (see above). These observations arose from the notion that the prime action of enhancing antisera is on ARC (98) and that macrophages are involved in some form in antibody-mediated suppression (155–157). The term ARCO was not formally proposed in the paper by Hutchinson and Zola referred to above (153) but it was used by the same authors in another publication that same year (158).

ARCO is a relatively simple and elegant way of modulating immune responses. It has been successfully employed to modulate responses to sheep red blood cells (159), kidney allografts (*154, 158*), tumors (*160*) and skin allografts (*161*). It is prevented if animals are depleted of macrophages (*159*), unaffected by decomplementation of mice (*162*) and is not operative in mice made tolerant neonatally (*161*), thus emphasizing the distinction between tolerance and enhancement. Interestingly, it could be brought about by the use of an antibody with a specificity that has nothing to do with histocompatibility antigens. Thus, following the demonstration by Sinclair and Law (*163*) that antibody against the hapten trinitrophenol (TNP) coupled to stimulator cells used in a cytotoxicity assay suppressed the response to the relevant alloantigens, Hutchinson and Brent (*164*) went on to show that TNP coupled to soluble histocompatibility antigens of the graft donor strain, injected into mice together with anti-TNP antibody, prolonged the life of unmodified tumor allografts – a principle that was soon extended to skin and kidney allografts (*165, 166*). They therefore raised the possibility that passive enhancement procedures might be applied to clinical transplantation without the problems inherent in the production of enhancing alloantibodies and the danger of causing hyperacute rejection. It seems surprising that no attempts seem to have been made to exploit this approach in larger animals and clinically.

Maintenance phase

Mechanisms that have at one time or another been proposed to account for the maintenance phase of enhancement, in which the graft is fully established and no longer subject to the direct influence of the passively administered antibody, include:

(1) The release of tolerogenic antigen from the graft leading to clonal deletion or other forms of tolerance.
(2) Formation of antigen–antibody complexes involving antibodies actively produced by the graft recipient.
(3) Development of anti-idiotypic antibodies.
(4) The generation of suppressor cells.
(5) Graft adaptation.

Although some of these could be operative at the same time and reinforce each other, others are mutually incompatible. These possibilities will now be briefly considered in their historic context, but first it is necessary to examine what is known of the immunologic status of enhanced rats towards the antigens of the donor strain.

The immunologic status of enhanced kidneys in rats

There was a general consensus that the lymphoid organs (i.e. the spleen and lymph nodes) of enhanced rats carrying healthy allografts can react normally against donor strain antigens when tested *in vitro* by a variety of tests. This was true for graft-versus-host reactivity (GVHR) (*116, 167–170*), fully confirmed with the aid of T lymphocytes some two decades later (*171*), mixed lymphocyte culture reactivity (MLR) (*168, 172–174*) and cell-mediated lympholysis (CML) (*143, 144*) – features that again distinguish at least some forms of neonatally induced tolerance from enhancement. Likewise, donor strain cells inoculated into kidney-bearing enhanced rats elicited strong cell-mediated responses as measured *in vitro*, with the grafts continuing to function normally (*144*). Nonetheless, the demonstration that there was a shortfall of cells with GVHR potential in the blood of enhanced rats, but not in the spleen and lymph nodes (175) – a finding that was in agreement with earlier work (115, 116) – still left open the possibility that ARCO or other modulating influences were brought to bear on the recipient's lymphocytes in the circulation rather than in the lymphoid organs, producing a specific lymphocyte deficiency where it matters most. It is, however, clear that neither clonal deletion nor anergy applies to these animals.

Antigen–antibody complexes
Apart from the data of Tilney and Bell (176), attempts to transfer enhancement passively with serum from enhanced rats have generally been negative (see for example 177), and this is a strong argument against the participation of blocking factors. On the other hand, the phenomenon of ARCO undoubtedly operates, not only in recently enhanced rats but also in animals well into their maintenance phase (154), thus leaving open the possibility that this mechanism plays an important role in preventing the host from destroying the graft.

Anti-idiotypic antibodies
The concept that an animal can make antibodies or other immune responses against the receptor or a portion thereof of its own antibodies (the receptor being by definition unique to its own body and therefore potentially immunogenic) is owed to a great extent to the early work of Ramseier and Lindenmann (178), who built on the observation by Oudin and Michel (179) that antibody receptor sites bear antigenic ("idiotypic") determinants that can evoke antibodies in animals belonging to the same species. Ramseier and Lindenmann postulated that it should therefore be possible to elicit antibodies in F_1 hybrid mice against cells from mice of either parental inbred strain, and they showed this to be the case using an indirect, cumbersome and not easily quantifiable test that measured the "product of antigenic recognition" (PAR) (180). Thus, supernatants of cultures of parental and F_1 hybrid cells, containing shed PAR, were injected into the skin of Syrian hamsters, where they set up a lesion containing variable numbers of polymorphonuclear cells. These cells were counted and compared with appropriate controls. The demonstration that anti-idiotypic antibodies can suppress responses to histocompatibility antigens is of particular relevance here, especially as it was also shown that auto-anti-idiotypic antibodies can be detected in inbred rats sensitized against the tissues of an allogeneic strain (181), the rise in titer taking place as the alloantibody response waned. A possible physiologic role in the control of antibody production and of cellular immunity in the maintenance stage of enhancement was therefore given considerable credence.

That anti-idiotypic antibodies have the power to inhibit GVHR *in vivo* was first shown by Joller (182), who studied the mortality of F1 newborn mice given parental spleen cells that had been treated *in vitro* with the appropriate antibody. Binz, Lindenmann and Wigzell (183) as well as McKearn (184) observed this to be true also for the local GVHR measured by enlargement of the popliteal lymph nodes following inoculation of lymphoid cells into the footpads of rats. Other *in vitro* effects claimed for anti-idiotypic sera were on the generation of murine cell-mediated cytotoxicity (185) and on the MLR in the mouse (186), though this worked only when the responder cells were precultured with the antiserum as well as with complement – a finding that was later confirmed by Binz and Wigzell (*187*). The latter (see also *188*) made use of a previous observation of theirs that normal (Lewis) rats have idiotypic receptor molecules with specificity for other Ag-B (rat) histo-compatibility antigens (in this case DA) in their sera and urine: they isolated these molecules, cross-linked them with glutaraldehyde and injected them with Freund's adjuvant into normal Lewis rats. They claimed that such rats lacked *in vitro* MLC reactivity, that the sera together with complement specifically inhibited the normal MLC reaction, and that DA skin grafts transplanted to the rats had significantly longer survival times than grafts transplanted to control animals (*187, 188*). They speculated on the possible application of their techniques to the manipulation of the immune system in transplantation, allergic disorders, and certain autoimmune diseases. The possible application of the anti-idiotypic strategy to clinical problems was further discussed by the same workers a year later (*189*). Significantly, the same group (*190*) showed that MLC reactivity and the local GVHR could be impaired when lymphoid cells from rats had been sensitized with purified T lymphoblasts (i.e. cells expected to possess a high density of antigen-binding idiotypic receptors as well as alloantigens).

It should be noted that at least two dissenting voices were raised at the time by workers who had been unsuccessful in verifying the claims made by the Swedish group. The first was K. Fischer Lindahl, working in M. Simonsen's laboratory, who at quite an early stage studied the interaction of anti-receptor antibodies in MLR, rather than place reliance on the clumsy PAR assay previously used by Ramseier and Lindenmann. She was unable to show that the MLR was either impaired or delayed although the sera she used were active in the PAR assay, and she found that skin allografts were rejected normally by treated rats (*191*). Fischer Lindahl suggested that the results in the PAR assay might have been due to contaminating B lympho-cytes and she doubted – rightly as it turned out – that the T cell receptor (the structure of which was at that time quite unknown) was an immunoglobulin. It may be of significance that she used a different strain combination than that habitually used by Binz and Wigzell's group, and indeed one of the criticisms leveled against that group's work was that their data were obtained in the main with one particular strain combination and that the universality of the effects had therefore not been satisfactorily established (*192*).

The other negative paper came from Fitch and Ramseier (*193*) – the latter having been one of the workers who originally described anti-idiotypic phenomena with the aid of the PAR assay. Treatment of responder lymphocytes with anti-idiotypic antisera and complement failed to inhibit the generation of cytotoxic T lymphocytes in MLR, and potentially cytolytic cells once generated could not be inhibited although the sera produced the expected and specific depression of PAR reactivity. In discussing their results, Fitch and Ramseier suggested that their discordant data might be explicable if different subsets of T lymphocytes were involved in PAR and cytolytic activities, and that in the study of Binz and Askonas (*186*) only a few of a large number of batches of antisera had proved to be active.

What evidence has been put forward then to show that the anti-idiotypic approach can bring about the survival of allografts? It must be said that it is rather limited. In a paper published in *Nature* in 1976 Binz and Wigzell (*187*) showed, again in the DA to Lewis rat strain combination, that the mean survival of DA skin grafts was prolonged to 30 days (or, in a larger group, 24 days) in Lewis rats that had been subjected to two treatments with Lewis-anti-DA idiotypes obtained from normal sera, cross-linked with gluteraldehyde, and presented in Freund's adjuvant. This prolongation of survival was strain-specific and the lymphocytes from some of the rats were non-reactive to DA antigens in an MLC assay. Strangely enough, there was evidence for the presence of anti-idiotypic antibodies some time after the rats had rejected their grafts.

The other evidence rested on the demonstration that a strictly limited prolongation of adult cardiac allografts was brought about by auto-immunization of rats with syngeneic anti-donor T lymphocyte blasts (one of five grafts surviving for more than 100 days), although better results were achieved when neonatal hearts were transplanted to the pinna of the ear (194). Batchelor and French were even less successful when testing AS rats that had been immunized against AS anti-August idiotype (using Freund's adjuvant) with F_1 hybrid kidneys: only one of ten survived indefinitely, almost all the others being rejected more or less normally (195) (note that their paper is a useful review of enhancement of kidney allografts). In the same year, Stuart, McKearn and Fitch (196) published data showing that rats immunized with both donor strain spleen cells and alloantibody directed against them displayed a peak of anti-idiotypic antibody ten days later, that the titer declined rapidly, and that F_1 kidneys transplanted at the height of this antibody response survived indefinitely. This was highly circumstantial evidence for the notion that survival of the grafts was mediated either partially or exclusively by anti-idiotypic antibodies, and the authors went on to provide some evidence implicating the involvement of suppressor cells in the maintenance phase (see below). Investigations in outbred primates, predominantly by Mybergh's South African group (104, 197, 198), showed that although enhancement of allogeneic livers could be achieved the results were not nearly as good as in the rat, and to secure prolonged survival in a high proportion of experimental subjects other strategies had to be resorted to, such as the use of cyclophosphamide or other immunosuppressive drugs or the inoculation of donor bone marrow cells.

Although great hopes were thus raised in the 1970s that anti-idiotypic responses could be harnessed in the cause of clinical transplantation and in many other spheres of medicine requiring modulation of the immune response, these have not yet been realized. When reviewing the clinical potential of this approach, Brent and Kilshaw (192) sounded a note of caution in the mid-1970s, based on:

(1) The fact that most of the data on the prolongation of graft survival – in fact most of the data on the induction of anti-idiotypic antibodies – had been generated from a single rat strain combination.
(2) The complexity of the manipulations required.
(3) The dependence on the clinically unacceptable Freund's adjuvant.
(4) The impermanence of allograft survival achieved.
(5) The puzzling presence of antibodies well after graft rejection had occurred.

Nonetheless, anti-idiotypic antibody responses are undoubtedly generated in many animals and human subjects sensitized against a variety of antigens (199–202) other than histocompatibility antigens, and they may well play a role, though almost certainly not the only one, in damping down normal immune responses. Their occurrence following blood transfusions in experimental animals and in man has also been noted and it is possible that there might be a positive correlation with good graft survival (see Chapter 7). Indeed, as the anti-idiotype is the mirror image of the specific antigen the hope continues to be entertained that anti-idiotypic vaccines might become feasible, especially in conditions such as human immunodeficiency virus (HIV) infection; and anti-idiotypes play a central role in Jerne's network theory of antibody production and its control (see Chapter 1).

Anti-Lymphocyte Serum (ALS)

Anti-lymphocyte serum (ALS) may be defined as a serum containing antibodies against the lymphocytes of another species, the antibodies having been raised by inoculating xenogeneic lymphocytes (e.g. those of mice or human beings) into animals that are known to be good producers of antibody, such as rabbits or horses. When injected into animals of the species that provided the sensitizing lymphocytes it brings about a sharp drop in the number of circulating lymphocytes and consequently immunologic impairment. Although the potential of ALS, experimental as well as clinical, was highlighted by the pioneering studies of M.F.A. Woodruff and his colleagues in the 1960s (see below), this approach had clearly exercised the minds of earlier workers.

Early studies

Chew, Stephens and Lawrence, in their publication of 1936 (203), rightly acknowledge the first furrows ploughed in this field at the turn of the century by E. Metchnikoff, M. Funck, S. Flexner and C.H. Bunting, all of whom raised anti-leukocytic sera by inoculating xenogeneic cells into adult animals. In this they were way ahead of their time, even though they did not appreciate the profound immuno-suppressive effects that the treatment of animals with such sera could have. It is ironic that Metchnikoff, the cogent and even partisan advocate of the role of phago-cytic cells as opposed to antibodies in the body's defense against infections and other foreign intruders could, with a little imagination, be regarded as the "grandfather" of ALS. In his lengthy and indeed rather wordy paper published in 1899 on "Études sur la resorption des cellules" (204) he described experiments in which the inoculation of bull spermatozoa into guinea pigs brought about not only a state of active phago-cytosis, but also the appearance of a "serum substance" that immmobilized the spermatozoa, a process that came about more quickly when a second inoculum was applied. He confirmed this result *in vitro* and found that immobilization did not depend on agglutination or cellular destruction. The same idea was applied to the "resorption" of leukocytes: splenic fragments from rats injected into guinea pigs produced a serum that agglutinated and destroyed rat leukocytes. Mononuclear cells were the first to disappear, followed by polynuclear cells, and later by mast cells. He encountered a lack of tissue specificity in that a serum induced by "lymphatic ganglia" comprising, it was thought, predominantly mononuclear cells, was equally effective against polynuclear cells.

The other three workers published their studies in the next few years and they corroborated Metchnikoff's findings and extended them. Funck's considerable achievement was to show that the *in vivo* effect was mirrored *in vitro*: a guinea pig anti-rabbit spleen serum, obtained by six intraperitoneal inoculations of a cellular emulsion, caused cellular abnormalities and the total destruction of rabbit peritoneal exudate cells within 24 hours when used undiluted, whereas normal serum proved to be harmless (205). This antiserum was again not specific for mononuclear cells, and lack of specificity was also shown by an anti-bone marrow serum, though it destroyed the polynuclear cells of the exudate more quickly than mononuclear cells. In the same year (1900) Besredka described leukocytotoxins prepared in the rabbit and guinea pig against each other's lymph glands, and showed that at a 1:20 dilution they completely destroyed peritoneal lymphoid cells (206). The sera appeared to be labile in that they lost their lytic activity when heated to 55° C for 30 minutes – Buchner (207, see also Chapter 1) had discovered complement (alexin) the year before – and they were distinctly toxic, leading to illness or even death of the animals. Flexner (208) found that he lost too many of his rabbits from infection and settled for the goose as the producer of antisera against guinea pig cells. The sera were injected subcutaneously into guinea pigs, sometimes after heating to 56°C in order to make them non-hemolytic, and he autopsied the recipients to study the manifold changes in the lymphoid tissues and in the bone marrow. Flexner concluded that ". . . in the cytotoxins we possess agents which act with great energy upon the lymphoid tissues" and stated that "The absence of specificity of reaction of the organs to the several cytotoxins is undeniable". He also made one perspicacious if tentative prediction: "It is, indeed, possible that the primary changes are in the circulating white blood cells. I must confess to some skepticism regarding such a probability".

It was Bunting, a year later, who provided evidence for this prediction in the same American journal (209). He followed Flexner closely in producing goose-anti-rabbit sera and studied the effect of the sera on the peripheral white blood cells of the rabbit recipients. A myelotoxic serum given intraperitoneally caused a drop in the total number of white cells followed by hyperleukocytosis by 32 hours, and the lymphocytes likewise showed an early, but not very marked decline, with recovery by 32 hours. When testing a lymphocytotoxic serum, the total number of white cells fell somewhat, followed by a rebound, whereas lymphocyte numbers were halved by four hours, with subsequent recovery and rebound. Although normal serum also had some effect, this was not nearly as marked as for the experimental sera, and Bunting thought he had detected some specificity. In discussing the decline in the number of cells, he stated that "This leucopenia may be due to the withdrawal of leukocytes from the circulation or to their destruction within the circulation. Of the finer mechanism of the process the experiments allow no speculation". Other early workers who raised cytotoxic sera in rabbits against rat lymphoid tissues were Christian and Leen (210), who measured cytotoxicity by observing the cessation of the ameboid movement of rat leukocytes; and Pappenheimer (211), whose rabbit anti-rat thymus or anti-human tonsil sera were cytotoxic and agglutinating, activities that absorption with red blood cells did not reduce. Heating of these sera removed cytotoxicity but not their agglutinating powers.

Thus the scene had been set for further investigation of a potentially important experimental approach to immunosuppression, but interest in these antisera subsided and the next significant development did not occur until 1936, when Chew, Stephens and Lawrence published their first paper in the *Journal of Immunology* (*203*). They prepared rabbit-anti-guinea pig sera against carefully isolated peritoneal exudate cells, which they claimed were predominantly polymorphonuclear neutrophils (lymphocytes amounted to 1–4%), and they studied the effect of these antisera on the peripheral blood and on a variety of organs of the recipient guinea pigs. Circulating neutrophils were depressed, with little effect on lymphocytes, and monocytes, eosinophils, basophils, platelets and red cells were essentially unaffected compared with animals that had been treated with normal serum. When the antiserum was administered by the intracardiac route the drop in neutrophil numbers was extremely rapid and the authors concluded that destruction must have occurred on contact with antibody. Interestingly, Chew, Stephens and Lawrence found that when antiserum was administered repeatedly a marked "tolerance" developed (i.e. the effect became less marked). They considered that this might have been caused by antibodies against rabbit serum proteins, but dismissed the idea (probably prematurely) because a "desensitizing" dose of normal rabbit serum did not reverse the "tolerance". Finally, they showed that the antiserum was not injurious to other tissues, that the period of neutropenia could be prolonged by daily injections of increasing amounts of antiserum, and that in such animals neutrophils were not available for the mediation of local tissue reactions.

This paper by Chew, Stephens and Lawrence was designed to study an anti-neutrophil antiserum but it raised, nonetheless, some interesting points that also pertain to ALS. A year later Chew and Lawrence published a further paper, this time describing the preparation of an anti-lymphocytic antiserum (*212*). The serum was decomplemented by heating and absorbed with washed guinea pig and sheep red cells – the latter to remove anti-Forssman antibodies. It was sterilized by filtration and stored in ampoules in the refrigerator where it remained potent for at least a month. Their method of preparation provided the basis of more recent studies. On inoculation into guinea pigs the serum caused considerable lymphopenia in the circulation (with only a very transient neutropenia) that lasted for at least 40 hours following a single dose, and which could be prolonged for at least ten days by repeated doses. Overall the effect was remarkably specific for lymphocytes. When the animals were autopsied the only pathologic change found was hyperplasia of the lymphoid tissues and "a peculiar appearance of the liver cells", without necrosis, in animals that had received multiple doses.

The work of the American group described above was taken up in Great Britain by Cruickshank (*213*), who briefly reviewed both the old and the more recent literature and concluded that the reduction in circulating lymphocytes after ALS treatment had been achieved only by Chew's group. The ALS Cruickshank prepared in rabbits was against rat lymph node cells; the hemolysins having been absorbed, it was highly effective in reducing the number of circulating rat lymphocytes. Cruickshank showed that exposure of a boiled suspension of lymph node cells to the antiserum led to an antigen–antibody reaction in which complement was used up – the first proof that at least some of the effects of ALS are mediated by cytotoxic antibodies – and that splenectomy of the serum recipients had no apparent effect on ALS action. Lymphocytes in the nodes and in the spleen were left undamaged by the limited treatment used in his experiments. Finally, he showed that the antibodies were species-specific in that their action on mouse and rabbit lymphocytes was minimal.

The strange case of "anti-reticular cytotoxic serum"

At this point I will digress momentarily. Perusal of the *American Review of Soviet Medicine* shows that some Soviet workers were greatly preoccupied by the therapeutic activity of certain "anti-reticular cytotoxic sera" (i.e. antisera prepared against cells of the recticuloendothelial system), and this subject was reviewed in a paper by A.A. Bogomolets that was first published in Russian in 1942 and which was adapted and translated for the above journal by S.H. Fisher (*214*). It is all rather mind-boggling! Fired by Metchnikoff's hypothesis that small doses of cytotoxic serum can "strengthen the function of the most valuable elements in the body and to cause a weakening of the agressive tendencies of the phagocytes", Bogomolets and others carried out "a great number of experiments" summarized in this article, which in the main consists of rather vague and naive speculations. I shall not attempt more than a superficial synopsis here. In studying the effect of such sera on "carcinogenic transplants" (details of the sera and the experimental animals are lacking), both blocking and prophylactic doses were encountered. Others showed, apparently, that "stimulation of the connective tissue with anti-reticular serum in many cases leads to complete disappearance of large carcinogeneous tumors in mice and decreases in the number of metastases . . . ."; that although large doses inhibited the growth of osteoblasts, "stimulating doses greatly accelerate the healing of fractures"; and that these sera could be used to treat "a number of human diseases where it seemed necessary to stimulate the trophic, plastic, or protective functions of the physiologic system of the connective tissue". These diseases included not only a variety of human tumors, but surgical infections, postpartum infections, sepsis, acute rheumatism, lung abscesses, osteomyelitis of the jaw, bone fractures and the formation of calluses! The sera had to be used in very small doses if an opposing effect was to be avoided.

Bogomolets believed that the serum acted by "stimulating the plastic, protective, and trophic functions of the system of connective tissue", which does not leave us much the wiser. "I would compare the action of our serum, though I wish to stress that this is merely a comparison, with the action of a match causing a conflagration", he wrote. It would seem that this paper was delivered at a conference in the Soviet Union in 1942 on "*The Therapeutic Action of Anti-Reticular Cytotoxic Serum*", at which some 40 reports were made. Bogomolets concluded that ". . .it is possible to hope . . . that this new means of pathogenetic therapy, anti-reticular cytotoxic serum, may prove to be highly useful for the restoration of the health and strength of the heroic protectors of our great motherland". At the same conference B.E. Linberg reported on the efficacious treatment in a rear evacuation hospital of gunshot fractures, frostbite, slow healing wounds and chronic pulmonary empyema resulting from gunshot wounds (*215*). The conference formally stamped its seal of approval on anti-reticular cytotoxic serotherapy with sera prepared in animals and, from the 2500 clinical observations presented, accepted a clear therapeutic effect for frostbite and wounds, infectious diseases (from spotted typhus to tonsillitis), and "diseases of the nervous system" (e.g. duodenal and gastric ulcers and eczema).

Anti-reticular cytotoxic serum, which never entered the mainstream of immunology and medicine, was clearly something of a black box, and its early widespread clinical application in the Soviet Union seems to be yet another manifestation of the uncritical pursuit of biomedical science in that period of the Soviet Union's history. Marchuk's method of preparing the serum (*216*) was generally adopted. A few years later R. Straus and his colleagues in the United States published several papers in the *Journal of Immunology*:

(1) Reviewing the literature (*217*), from which they concluded that, despite a feeling of skepticism, "the rationale and the claims for the effect of ACS (anti-reticular cytotoxic serum) seem worthy of independent study".
(2) Describing in detail the preparation of such sera in rabbits and goats against splenic tissue and bone marrow from human cadavers, their titration for antibodies and complement, their species specificity and their storage at 4° C (*218*).
(3) Confirming that small ("stimulating") doses of serum accelerated the healing of bone fractures in rabbits, whereas large ("depressing") doses slowed down the healing process (*219*).

I have attempted to discover the fate of what became known as "Bogomolet's serum"; although numerous papers were published over the next 15 years or so, they appeared largely in Soviet or unknown western journals. However, at least four American groups studied the therapeutic efficacy of the serum: Rogoff *et al.* (*220*) found that it did not ameliorate experimentally induced polyarthritis in guinea pigs or rheumatoid arthritis in patients; Anigstein, Whitney and Beninson (*221*) observed that it was protective in guinea pigs against typhus and spotted fever, but noted that normal serum likewise attenuated both conditions; and Kling failed to find any benefit in the treatment of osteoarthritis (*222*). Kling wrote: "The sensational press notices omitted the word acute (i.e. from rheumatism, author) and both the public and physicians were fired with expectation that a cure for all forms of rheumatism was discovered. A great clamour was raised ... and in this country (the United States, author) it was immediately introduced into the therapy of various forms of arthritis. ... On the basis of our material and a review of the literature it is concluded that there is no indication for anti-reticular cytotoxic serum in the treatment of osteoarthritis and fibrositis". Finally, Rifkinson (*223*) failed to detect any influence of the serum on the healing of incised cerebral wounds in rats.

Despite these negative reports, Bogomolet's serum was later written about with considerable enthusiasm in German and Austrian medical journals (*224–226*), though Leger (*227*) warned that it furthered the healing of bone fractures in only a minority of cases. Loiseleur attempted a rather naive analysis of its mode of action in one experimental model (*228*). However, although to my knowledge a formal "obituary" for Bogomolet's serum was never written (not unusual for biologic phenomena that have failed to withstand the test of time) interest in it faded away in the early 1960s, having been overtaken by the development of highly specific antisera of various kinds and by the study of the immunosuppressive properties of ALS. What actions it did exert, especially in the treatment of infectious conditions, may have been brought about by a hit-and-miss activation of the reticuloendothelial system, though the likely presence of immunosuppressive antibodies would make even that rather charitable speculation improbable. Anti-lymphocyte antibodies might, however, have been responsible for the amelioration of conditions with an autoimmune component; thus, Currey and Ziff (*229*) later demonstrated the efficacy of ALS in the prevention of experimentally induced polyarthritis in the rat.

The modern study of anti-lymphocyte serum

It was a letter published by *Nature* in 1951 by Woodruff and Forman (*230*), in which they described their attempt to reveal an *in vitro* action of ALS, that drew attention to the earlier work of Chew and Lawrence (*212*) and Cruickshank (*213*). Although Woodruff and Forman confirmed that a rabbit-anti-rat ALS that had been decomplemented brought about a rapid and severe lymphopenia *in vivo* they could not demonstrate a cytotoxic effect when rat lymph node cells were incubated with the antiserum in the presence of guinea pig complement. They concluded that "This suggests that the action of the serum *in vivo* is probably not due to direct destruction of lymphocytes in the bloodstream", though their data seem to suggest that they may have been misled by very high background levels of cytotoxicity in an assay that depended on the uptake of a vital dye by dead cells.

Inderbitzen kept the subject alive by showing that inoculation into guinea pigs of an antiserum prepared in rabbits against guinea pig lymph node cells not only depleted the animals of lymphocytes but suppressed delayed cutaneous allergic reactions such as the tuberculin reaction (*231*), which was already then known to be associated with a heavy infiltration of the reaction site with lymphocytes. On the other hand, a serum directed against polymorphonuclear cells did not have such an effect. These data were confirmed some years later by Waksman and Arbouys (*232*), who went on to demonstrate that contact sensitivity could likewise be suppresssed but that the action of ALS did not extend to passive cutaneous anaphylaxis, an antibody-mediated phenomenon. They were able to delay the onset of experimental allergic encephalomyelitis as well as the onset of rejection when skin allografts were transplanted to serum-treated recipients. Strikingly, there was some effect even in presensitized guinea pigs in that second-set skin grafts did not undergo the same degree of ischemia as in controls, and in some grafts vascularization occurred, followed by a tempo of rejection characteristic of a first-set response. Waksman's laboratory followed this up by showing that anti-lymph node sera produced a marked blood lymphopenia if administered repeatedly (though the effect became less marked with continued treatment), that this was accompanied by the depletion of small lymphocytes in the nodes, that the suppression of delayed hypersensitivity reactions (though not allergic encephalomyelitis) closely correlated with the degree of lymphopenia achieved, and that absorption of sera with normal blood white cells led to the loss of both the lymphopenic and the suppressive effects (*233*). They concluded "tentatively" that "a circulating mononuclear cell, probably the small lymphocyte, is the primary reactant in the various types of delayed hypersensitive reactions" – a conclusion that proved to be correct.

Although Waksman's group in Boston were the first to show that ALS could weaken the response to skin allografts, it was left to Woodruff and Anderson working in Edinburgh to draw the attention of transplantation immunologists to the fact that the life of skin allografts could be *substantially* prolonged. This they did in a letter to *Nature* in 1963 (*234*), in which they reported on experiments involving *in vivo* lymphocyte depletion by thoracic duct cannulation and/or treatment with ALS in inbred rats. Either of these treatments (ALS was given daily for 14 days from the day after skin grafting, and cannulation was conducted for five days before grafting) more or less doubled the median survival time (MST) of allografts, but administered in tandem the MST went up dramatically to 35 days. There followed an avalanche of publications confirming and extending the immunosuppressive activity of ALS in a variety of species and analyzing its mode of action.

It is not possible or indeed necessary to give a blow by blow account of subsequent developments, though it is of interest to note the contributions of some of the early workers – a few of them still active in the field. A year after the appearance of their vital *Nature* paper, Woodruff and Anderson (235) enlarged on their findings by showing that preoperative thoracic duct drainage and postoperative treatment with ALS for 89 days permitted rat skin allografts to survive for long if variable periods, with a mean survival time of over 100 days. (Two of five rats died with intact grafts, presumably from infection.) Because this long-term survival was achieved despite the fact that lymphocyte levels returned to near normal after about three weeks and that cessation of treatment did not necessarily result in graft rejection, these workers concluded that "it seems unlikely that the effect can be completely accounted for by lymphocyte destruction". Indeed, one animal seemed to have become permanently tolerant. Nonetheless, cell death was clearly an important component of ALS action because the histologic picture in spleens and lymph nodes displayed "widespread death of lymphocytes". They concluded that "From the point of view of the surgery of replacement, the results are encouraging" and they announced that similar experiments were being conducted in dogs, as a preliminary to human application. "There are, however, obvious dangers in administering heterospecific sera and great caution will be required in any clinical trial." A paper published by D. Hume's group in the same year described the power of ALS to destroy rat lymphocytes *in vitro* and to bring about a sustained lymphopenia *in vivo* if administered daily for three weeks (236), a result in conflict with the work of Woodruff's laboratory. They postulated that Woodruff and Anderson's serum may not have been powerful enough to eliminate enough lymphocytes to prevent the production of anti-ALS antibodies.

Gray, Monaco and Russell, working in Boston, published a brief report in 1964 in *Surgical Forum* which extended the study of ALS to inbred mice (237). Daily inoculations of mice with an ALS raised in rabbits brought about skin allograft survival for more than 30 days, though some recipients died during the course of the treatment – a problem avoided by administering the serum only three times a week for two weeks. The primary, but not the secondary response to *Salmonella* II antigen was depressed and the antiserum showed species, but not strain, specificity. Curiously, these authors referred to the 1964 paper of Woodruff and Anderson as "in press", but seemed to be unaware of the Edinburgh workers' earlier *Nature* paper. Gray's coworkers were P.S. Russell, who like Woodruff had already made his mark in the field of transplantation and who likewise went on to become a distinguished transplant surgeon/immunologist, and A.P. Monaco, who made the application of ALS to the solution of graft rejection his major interest in the years to come and who has made manifold scientific and surgical contributions to the field.

The same group, with M. Wood, published extensive data on the production, properties and immunosuppressive powers of ALS in inbred mice. Apart from confirming previous findings, such as the presence of agglutinins and cytotoxins and the lymphopenia induced in mice, they found precipitins to mouse serum proteins, were able to bring about sustained lymphopenia by continuing the treatment without the morbidity reported by others and, significantly, found that ALS was less immunogenic than normal rabbit serum (238), a finding that was correctly attributed to the immunosuppressive action of ALS. Absorption of ALS with non-lymphoid mouse cells left its activity unimpaired, and chronic low dose or acute high dose treatment led to extensive lymphocyte depletion in the lymphoid organs. In an accompanying paper (239) these workers reported that:

(1) Their ALS was effective in prolonging skin allograft survival across a strong H-2 barrier (they published the first picture of an ALS-treated mouse carrying a healthy skin allograft).
(2) Prolonged treatment of mice to maintain allografts indefinitely resulted in a wasting syndrome and death associated with lymphoid atrophy.
(3) Seven daily doses of ALS were most effective when given just before skin transplantation and not at all if treatment was delayed until one week after transplantation.
(4) The ALS was effective even in presensitized animals and when xenografts (rat) were transplanted.
(5) Crude gammaglobulin extracted from ALS was as immunosuppressive as the whole serum.
(6) ALS absorbed with normal mouse serum did not show any impairment of immunosuppressive function, ruling out the possibility that its action in prolonging graft survival was primarily on mouse antibodies against the skin grafts and thus providing "evidence against a significant role of humoral antibody in allograft rejection".

These workers concluded that the action of ALS was intimately associated with its ability to deplete the recipients of lymphocytes (i.e. it had a 'central' effect, and that this provided further evidence for the significant participation of lymphocytes in skin allograft rejection).

Although P.B. Medawar has sometimes been seen as the 'high priest' of ALS – an accolade that is perhaps more appropriate to M.F.A. Woodruff – it is only at this point that he and his colleagues entered the arena. However, it was an area of research that suited Medawar's analytical style, and he, together with several bright and committed American postdoctoral Fellows working with him at the National Institute for Medical Research, soon made some signal contributions to the literature. Levey and Medawar (the latter rigorously following the rule of publishing in alphabetic order) published two papers in 1966 in which they pushed the state of knowledge considerably further and discussed the mode of action of ALS. In the first of these (240) they described their method of preparing the antiserum by the intravenous inoculation of weanling mouse thymus and lymph node cells into rabbits, and showed that:

(1) Treatment of mice with the ALS on days two and five after skin grafting was the most effective way of prolonging graft survival.
(2) The recipients' lymphoid cells, especially those of the thymus, were coated with antibody – a point already made by Dumonde et al. (241).
(3) More prolonged survival could be achieved by treatment for up to four weeks but that, once treatment ceased, rejection occurred rapidly.
(4) ALS could overcome a state of presensitization.

(5) Normal and immune lymphocyte transfer reactions in guinea pigs were totally abolished by a rabbit-anti-guinea pig serum, thus setting ALS apart from other immunosuppressive agents.

Finally, they concluded that the antiserum induced tolerance for the foreign serum proteins – erroneously, as it turned out, for the mouse is notoriously inefficient at generating antibody responses. In considering the mechanisms that might be responsible for these findings, they concluded that while the lymphocytolytic effect probably played a role it could not provide a full explanation, more or less ruled out antigen competition as an important factor, and felt unable to exclude the possibility that the antiserum acted by neutralizing a humoral thymus factor (242). They expressed some doubts about the "attractive" "blind-folding" hypothesis (i.e. the coating of the potentially reactive lymphocytes with xenogeneic antibody, thus rendering them unable to recognize foreign antigen) because the theory "does not account for the power of antisera to institute a state of specific tolerance, if indeed they do". They concluded that, whatever the mechanism, "heterologous antilymphoid antisera are the most powerful immunosuppressive agents yet described".

In their second publication Levey and Medawar (243) extended these data by showing that abolition of a pre-existing state of sensitivity with ALS caused the mice to revert to a state of "virgin" reactivity – soon to be confirmed by Medawar's colleague E.M. Lance (244) – and that agents that interfered with cellular turnover (such as hydrocortisone or sublethal irradiation) enhanced the action of ALS. Strangely, ALS proved to be effective in mice that had been strongly sensitized against rabbit immunoglobulin although no long-term surviving grafts were found in such animals: "The fact that ALS seems to abolish or prevent the inception of a reaction against itself is of some clinical importance". (Later reports, especially in large animals and in man, showed that ALS does indeed incite the formation of antibodies, thus limiting its use – see below.) Potent ALS could be prepared in rabbits with pure epidermal cells and fibroblastic L cells, thus indicating that ALS "is not specific in any histological sense", and by the use of crude thymocyte subcellular fractions. Unlike Jeejeebhoy (245) they found that thymectomy did not potentiate the effect of ALS, though Jeejeebhoy's observation was later vindicated. The non-reactivity produced by ALS was not antigen-dependent, and they concluded that graft prolongation could not be classified as immunologic tolerance. Finally, they added one further hypothesis to explain the action of ALS: "sterile inactivation" of lymphoid cells (analogous to that produced by phytohemagglutinin), which "forestalls or supplants all other immunological commitments". "Though it may not stand up to closer scrutiny, this hypothesis accounts adequately for the properties of ALS described so far. . . There seems little room for a theory that attributes the effect of ALS to lymphocytolysis or lymphocytic depletion." And they concluded by stating that "ALS appears to be devoid of intrinsic or acute toxicity, and its clinical possibilities therefore deserve close attention".

Although all the early work was carried out in mice and rats – the existence of inbred strains greatly facilitating reliable experimentation and analysis – the years 1966–1967 witnessed a great spurt in the application of ALG (antilymphocyte globulin) to larger mammals, primarily the dog, as this was seen as an essential prerequisite for its clinical application. The first groups to publish highly encouraging data in 1966 came from the United States, United Kingdom and Germany (246–251) and they were soon followed up by others, thus establishing that ALG was without question an immunosuppressive agent potent not only in rodents. This conclusion was greatly fortified by the demonstration by Balner, Van Bekkum and their colleagues that both skin allograft rejection and GVHRs in rhesus monkeys could be severely impaired by ALS or anti-thymocyte serum (ATS) (252–254).

The immunogenicity of anti-lymphocyte serum

Once it had been demonstrated that the immunosuppressive powers of ALS reside in the gammaglobulin fraction (255–258), Lance and Dresser set out to study the immunogenicity of rabbit gamma-IgG in mice (259). They were motivated by the possibility that the mode of action of ALS was essentially one of antigen competition. They found that although normal rabbit gammaglobulin was poorly immunogenic in mice and readily induced a state of paralysis or tolerance (260), gammaglobulin from ALS was highly immunogenic, repeated doses leading to the rapid elimination of radiolabeled molecules. However, a state of non-reactivity could be induced by the previous exposure of the recipient mice to a high dose of normal serum gammaglobulin or by closely spaced doses of ALS, and they concluded that the hypothesis of antigenic competition could therefore not be excluded. Nonetheless, because the prior induction of paralysis with normal serum gammaglobulin did not diminish the potency of ALS in prolonging skin allograft survival (256), Lance and Dresser felt that "the immuno-genicity of ALS is irrelevant to its mode of action in the promotion of homograft survival", a view that was confirmed by Woodruff's Edinburgh group in the same year (261). Nonetheless, this demonstration of the production of antibodies against ALS gammaglobulin, though explaining some of the toxic consequences of ALS treatment such as nephritis (262–264) makes the outcome of the continuous administration of ALS to mice every four days from birth and for many months all the more remark-able: the response to skin allografts and other manifestations of cellular immmunity were almost completely suppressed for as long as the treatment continued (265), with-out any significant pathologic changes in the recipients (266). Presumably tolerance to the serum proteins must have been successfully induced, though Nehlsen and Simpson, both members of Medawar's research group at the National Institute for Medical Research, Mill Hill, did not examine the mice for anti-rabbit serum antibodies. (However, some of the recipients developed polyomas, the virus probably having been introduced with the ALS.) Previously, Lance (267), another member of Medawar's team, had treated mice with two different regimens of ALS for six months: mice that received weekly rather than more widely spaced doses accepted skin allografts far more readily and developed tolerance to the rabbit gammaglobulin. It was left to Dalton, Anderson and Sanders (268) to draw attention to the fact that, at least in the rat, sensitization to an ALS prepared in one species (rat) could be circumvented by the subsequent use of a serum prepared in another (horse).

As early workers had drawn attention to the probability that the production of anti-ALS antibodies could be a vital limiting factor in the clinical use of ALS, a number of workers set out to prevent anti-ALS antibodies by tolerizing (or para-lyzing) the recipients with normal serum or gammaglobulin from the ALS-producing species. Denman and Frenkel (269) found that rats tolerant to rabbit gammaglobulin

(RGG) were more prone to develop a wasting disease produced by ALS, and Howard, Dougherty and Mergenhagen (270) not only confirmed this in mice but showed that skin allograft survival was more prolonged in such animals when treated with ALS as did Hardy, Quint and Monaco (271), who also found that previous sensitization of mice to ALG had an adverse effect on its immunosuppressive action. Raju and Grogan (272) confirmed in rats that tolerance induction potentiated the effect of ALS, but found it to be immunosuppressive even in the presence of anti-rabbit serum protein antibodies. Tolerance induction to ALS was successfully accomplished in dogs (273, 274) too, but rhesus monkeys tended towards sensitization rather than tolerance when normal horse globulin was inoculated (275). Svehag et al. were, however, successful in macaque monkeys (276). Perhaps these conflicting data are not too surprising, considering that Golub and Weigle, using inbred strains of mice and carefully controlled conditions, found considerable variability in tolerance induction to human gammaglobulin, depending to some degree on the strain, the level of residual aggregates in the protein solutions and the timing (277).

In patients, the question of tolerance to the serum proteins of the ALG-producing species was not answered unequivocally. That in part explains why ALG has been and is still being used largely as a potent weapon against rejection crises rather than as a primary immunosuppressant, despite the fact that an early report on kidney transplantation was favorable (278), as was a later report on its use in human cardiac transplantation (279). (ALG was in any case used less frequently when monoclonal antibodies against T lymphocytes became available; see below.) Although Taub et al. (280) showed in a single patient with aplastic anemia that one large dose of equine gammaglobulin induced tolerance to a subsequent course of ATG, and Butler et al. (281) in the same year confirmed in transplant recipients that previous treatment with aggregate-free normal horse immunoglobulin prevented antibody formation to subsequently administered therapeutic ALG, others were either unsuccessful in inducing tolerance (282) or even found that some patients were sensitized (283). Nonetheless Hanto et al. (284) recently showed ALG to be as effective as the monoclonal anti-lymphocytic antibody OKT3 but the higher proportion of patients in the ALG group who developed cytomegalovirus infections gave the monoclonal antibody a clear edge, yet the problem of sensitization remains (see below).

The mechanism of action of anti-lymphocyte serum/anti-thymocyte serum

ALS was thus shown to have a profound effect on cell-mediated responses, including the allograft reaction, and its efficacy clearly extended not only to skin grafts but also to organs such as the kidney and to a variety of species. As GVHR (see Chapter 8) is, likewise, a cell-mediated response it was not long before it was demonstrated that ALS is equally effective in subduing or altogether preventing GVHR as measured by the spleen weight gain assay (285) or the death of the recipients (286), and this was subsequently amply confirmed by other workers. In the same year (1967) Van Bekkum's group in the Netherlands (287) found the same to be true for secondary disease, following whole body irradiation of mice and the transfer of allogeneic bone marrow cells. However, here treatment of the cell *donors* was found to be more effective than treatment of the recipients. These workers found, too, that although ALS produced in cynomolgus monkeys prevented secondary disease in rhesus monkeys, it did so only when inoculated into the recipients, and all animals developed fatal virus infections and thrombocytopenia. However, although most attention was paid to cell-mediated responses it soon became clear that humoral responses could also be affected. Thus, Woodruff and his colleague K. James showed that antibody responses to both bovine serum albumin (288) and sheep red blood cells (289) could be suppressed, though the target was almost certainly the then unknown T helper lymphocyte required for the production of some antibodies. The same group confirmed the finding of Harris and Harris (290) that the *in vitro* treatment of presensitized cells prevents such cells from transferring sensitivity adoptively (291), a finding that agreed with Levey and Medawar's *in vivo* abolition of the presensitized state (243).

I have already indicated that a variety of hypotheses have been put forward to account for the dramatic immunosuppressive action of ALS. There are several early reviews on ALS in which these hypotheses have been evaluated (292–295; see also the earlier discussion by Levey and Medawar, 296) and I will confine myself to the most salient points.

Selective depletion of circulating lymphocytes

First advanced by Lance on mainly functional and morphologic grounds (267), this hypothesis has remained the most persuasive even though it may not be the only mechanism. Among evidence already mentioned was Levey and Medawar's demonstration that although ALS is highly effective in preventing sensitization by skin allografts, it cannot oppose sensitization by the intravenous injection of as few as five million spleen cells (296), presumed to be due to the fact that such cells "home" to the less affected lymphoid organs, whereas the destruction of skin grafts is brought about by circulating lymphocytes. Also relevant are the findings that the residual cells in ALS-treated animals are mainly short-lived (293) and that ALS has a selective effect on thymus-derived antigen-sensitive cells (297, 298) and on the cellular, but not the humoral, response to histocompatibility antigens (299).

The removal of lymphocytes from the circulation soon after ALS treatment is well documented; it is in part brought about by complement-mediated destruction (300) and largely by opsonization and phagocytosis in the liver (301–302). One consequence of the elimination of peripheral lymphocytes is that with repeated doses of ALS, the central lymphoid organs become depleted of lymphocytes, despite some early observations to the contrary. For example, Russell and Monaco (303) found that although lymph nodes underwent enlargement the number of recoverable cells was greatly diminished; and, like Jeejeebhoy (245), they showed that adult thymectomy prior to ALS treatment "dramatically augmented" immunosuppression. Clearly, interference with the production of T lymphocytes by the thymus gravely prejudiced the recovery of T cell function in ALS-treated animals, as might indeed be expected if the T lymphocytes are mainly affected.

Blindfolding

This concept, which involved the coating of lymphocytes with the foreign serum proteins, thus preventing them from interacting with target cells, was proposed by Levey and Medawar (240) but quickly abandoned by them when they discovered that cells can remain immunoincompetent after repeated cell divisions (304). The idea seemed to receive support when Brent, Courtenay and Gowland showed that reactivity in a GVHR system could be restored to ALS-treated lymphocytes by *in vitro* trypsinization (286), but lost credence following the unsuccessful attempt by Lance to confirm their data (305).

Enhancement

The possibility that antibodies present in ALS act specifically on antigens of the graft was considered by Levey and Medawar (240), but rejected by them because ALS raised against the murine donor strain was as effective, but not more so, than sera raised against the recipient strain; and the later finding that ALS, though species-specific, prolonged the survival of xenografts seemed to justify their dismissal of this hypothesis. There was, nonetheless, some circumstantial evidence favoring it, principally the finding that rabbit-anti-mouse epidermal cell antibodies (306) as well as ALS (307) produced some prolongation of skin allograft survival when the grafts were preincubated in the sera, and the even earlier observation by Guttmann *et al.* (308, 309) that treatment of rat kidney donors with ATS improved kidney allograft function and morphology. (The *Journal of Experimental Medicine* paper by Guttmann's group is the third in a long and admirable series, published mainly in *Transplantation*, in which they systematically studied the mechanisms responsible for kidney allograft rejection in rats and ways of modulating the allograft response.) Furthermore, treatment of rats given skin allografts with anti-epidermal sera raised in rabbits prolonged skin allograft survival (310, 311). However, little further support has since been registered for this hypothesis, and the demonstration by Guttmann, Lindquist and Ockner that the passive transfer of serum from rats with greatly prolonged kidney allograft survival after ATG treatment did not transfer the unresponsiveness (312) further argued against the enhancement hypothesis. It is more than likely that some of the reported effects pointing to an enhancement mechanism were brought about by the action of the antisera on passenger leukocytes in the grafts, causing the grafts to be less immunogenic – a possibility raised by Callender *et al.* (313).

Sterile activation

This notion was put forward by the ever inventive Levey and Medawar team (243), namely that ALS might bring about a generalized activation of the immune system that "forestalls or supplants all other immunological commitments", perhaps analogous to the activation triggered by phytohemagglutinin. Accordingly, blast formation and cell division would occur but without "specific immunological performance", and, according to Levey and Medawar, such a hypothesis would account (in 1966) for all findings relating to ALS "so far". It does not, however, receive a mention in their review of mechanisms a year later (296), and in the 1973 review of Medawar's group (295) they listed the objections to it, including the observation by Denman, Denman and Holborow (314) that a massive drop in the number of circulating lymphocytes can occur soon after ALS administration without detectable blast cell formation.

Tolerance induction

Whilst ALS can undoubtedly assist very powerfully in the induction of tolerance to skin and kidney allografts (see later), Levey and Medawar (296) ruled out tolerance induction as an explanation of its primary action, mainly because it normally operates nonspecifically and irrespective of the strength of the antigenic stimulus. Such an explanation would also be in conflict with an observation made by numerous workers that there is usually a return to full reactivity within a relatively short time after cessation of ALS treatment (240, 246). Nonetheless, grafts have sometimes been retained for considerable periods after cessation (305).

In their review, Lance, Medawar and Taub (295) also ruled out antigenic competition, interference with a thymic hormone, and action via a non-immunologic pathway. They conclude that "the alternative proposals to the hypothesis of selective depletion of recirculating lymphocytes are found wanting in one respect or another, yet the possibility of dual or multiple mechanisms cannot be completely excluded".

A very recent study concerning the specificity of antibodies in ATG (anti lymphocyte globulin) goes a long way towards explaining why ALG/ATG is so extraordinarily potent. Although this question had previously been investigated, the study of Rebellato et al. (315) has revealed antibody specificities in much finer detail by analyzing batches of rabbit-anti-human ATG in rhesus monkeys. Present in these preparations were as many as 23 specificities, including seven that were T cell-specific and seven (at high titer) binding to non-T cell antigens. Many of these antibodies were directed against signal transduction and adhesion molecules, were detectable at the time when recovery of reactivity takes place, and persisted for long periods. The authors therefore postulated that these antibodies contribute to the hyporesponsiveness induced by ATG and that the multiple specificities of ATG help to explain why it can be more effective in suppressing the cell-mediated response than specific anti-T cell monoclonal antibodies.

Although Medawar and his colleagues entered in the field relatively late it is clear that they made massive experimental contributions and formulated a number of useful working hypotheses concerning the mode of action of ALS.

Anti-lymphocyte serum as an adjunct in the induction of specific tolerance

It is clear, then, that the presence of a skin or kidney allograft in a mouse treated with ALS does not necessarily lead to the induction of specific tolerance to that graft; to achieve tolerance another strategy, involving the inoculation of lymphoid cells from the graft donor, is needed. Such a strategy was first devised by Monaco et al. (246), who were able to convert the nonspecific though longlasting unresponsiveness induced in mice by a combination of adult thymectomy and ALS treatment into a state of specific unresponsiveness by the intravenous infusion of a single high dose of F_1 hybrid donor strain lymphoid cells. Though their first experiments, in which they used an H-2 incompatible strain combination that was strongly disparate, were largely unsuccessful they nevertheless showed that cellular chimerism had been created (246). However, they soon discovered that specific tolerance could be induced in this way in a high proportion of mice if the immunogenetic disparity was less marked (i.e. differences confined to H-2 class I), that mice with long-lived skin allografts accepted a second graft from the donor strain but rejected third-party grafts, and that the tolerance could be abolished by the adoptive transfer of normal syngeneic lymphoid cells (316).

Enter Lance and Medawar with a massive paper devoted to tolerance induction in ALS-treated mice, published in 1969 (317). Working mainly with a class-1 disparate strain combination and with potent ALS preparations given in a few pulses in the first week after skin transplantation, they showed that long-term tolerance could be induced, albeit in a minority of the experimental subjects, without the aid of thymectomy and with far smaller numbers of F_1 hybrid lymphoid cells than those used by Monaco *et al.* They established the optimal time for the administration of the cells and the intravenous route as superior to others, showed that there was a positive correlation between cell dose and efficacy, demonstrated the specificity of the tolerance, and found it possible to overcome to some degree a pre-existing immunity. Tolerance induction "obeyed the conventional rule that it is more difficult in proportion to the antigenic disparity between donor and host" and it could be potentiated by low doses of irradiation or cyclophosphamide. Tolerance extended to the formation of humoral anti-donor strain antibodies, and although cellular chimerism was present it faded with time. Lymphoid cells from tolerant animals retained their ability to react against donor strain and third-party antigens in a GVHR assay. A single dose of cell-free extracted antigen was ineffective, but repeated doses every two weeks brought about some limited prolongation of graft survival. Lance and Medawar argued that the differences between conventional and ALS-induced tolerance could be explained in terms of cellular population dynamics, the cells inoculated in the latter being at a selective disadvantage *vis-à-vis* the regenerating lymphoid system of the host, thus explaining the relatively short-lived tolerance.

This study opened up the possibility of inducing long-lasting tolerance without previous thymectomy and the essential finding was soon confirmed by others (*318*; these workers showed additionally that the skin grafts themselves provide an important source of antigen maintaining the tolerance); and it encouraged many other workers to establish experimental models using ALS as the prime immunosuppressant. One of these was Nisbet, who found that pretreatment of parental strain mice with ALS before undergoing parabiosis with F_1 hybrids greatly facilitated the induction of tolerance (*319*). I shall confine myself in the main to two approaches designed for possible clinical application by employing antigens that, like the F_1 hybrid cells inoculated by Monaco *et al.* and Lance and Medawar, would not complicate matters by causing GVHR's: the addition of adult bone marrow cells or the use of extracted cell-free antigen. Both experimental designs were among the first to reveal that suppressor T lymphocytes (Ts) can be involved in this form of tolerance.

The use of bone marrow cells

Monaco and Wood's group, working in Boston, described a mouse model in 1971 which was based on Lance and Medawar's but made use of donor strain bone marrow rather than F_1 hybrid lymphoid cells (*320*). Skin allograft survival was prolonged though only a few grafts survived for long periods, and there was no graft-versus-host disease (GVHD). The group has worked on this model ever since. Although previous thymectomy markedly improved skin allograft survival the tolerance was not accompanied by chimerism (*321*) and Ts could not be demonstrated (*322*), whereas the same treatment without thymectomy led to the formation of Ts, demonstrable in adoptive transfer assays (*323*). The non-specificity of the suppressor cells found in ALS-treated mice (*324*) was converted into donor specificity by the presence of antigen (in the form of cells and skin grafts) (*325*) and, interestingly, the majority of Ts, which were detected *in vitro*, were derived from the donor cell inoculum (326). This finding was analogous to the description by Muraoka and Miller (327) of bone marrow derived Ts that can suppress, *in vitro*, the cytotoxicity against stimulator cells syngeneic with them – a finding that was to lead to the concept of "veto cells" (328–330) (see below). While others, using a cell-free system, have uncovered the existence in skin graft-tolerant mice of host-derived Ts that suppress the response against donor antigens (see below), Wood *et al*. have recently described, in their model, a marked reduction in the number of antigen-specific host cytotoxic T lymphocytes, a finding which they have attributed to veto cells of donor origin (331). (Suppressor cells that act nonspecifically after ALG treatment have been described not only in mice, but also in rhesus monkeys (332).) It is possible that in this model, as in others, more than one mechanism was operative, for Monaco and his colleagues had earlier also found evidence implicating blocking factors, reminiscent of immunologic enhancement (333).

In the Wood/Monaco mouse model long-term prolongation of graft survival was often confined to a minority of experimental subjects unless thymectomy was also carried out, and the group has in the main used one particular strain of F_1 hybrid recipients or strain combinations disparate for relatively weak H-2 or non-H-2 antigens. It is, nonetheless, of particular interest because the treatment with both ALS and bone marrow cells was entirely postoperative and because J. Thomas and her colleagues have applied the model very successfully to rhesus monkeys (334) whose unresponsiveness – as that of mice – seems to depend on the appearance of veto cells of donor origin (335).

Quite independently and predating the study by Thomas *et al*. by a decade, Mybergh's group in Johannesburg had also used ALG in combination with a low dose of donor bone marrow cells in baboons to induce long-term tolerance to liver allografts – a treatment that did not depend on continuous immunosuppression and that was superior to regimens involving the long-term administration of prednisolone and azathioprine (336). Indeed, the inoculation of donor bone marrow cells has been applied to clinical transplantation (albeit with drug-based immunosuppression) in an attempt to induce specific tolerance, and whilst it is too early to say whether this has been beneficial it has certainly not led to any harmful consequences (see Chapter 7). The case for doing so has beeen cogently argued by Monaco *et al*. (337).

Like Liegeois, Charreire and Brennan before them (338), Monaco and Wood's group found that animals treated with ALS and bone marrow cells became cellular chimeras (333), a phenomenon that both groups described as "microchimerism" because of the relatively low level of detectable donor cells. In the study of Liegeois, Charreire and Brennan, this amounted to 3.6%; this might well have been an underestimate as their method of detection was confined to dividing cells carrying the distinctive chromosomal T6 marker. Despite the introduction of the prefix "micro" the chimerism does not appear to differ quantitatively very greatly from that described in mice made tolerant *in utero* or at birth with F_1 hybrid cells (see Chapter 5), though it is sometimes hard to demonstrate. Chimerism, which has also been demonstrated in the rhesus monkey model of Thomas *et al*. (335), has been given a direct clinical interest by the recent demonstration in Pittsburgh that human liver allograft recipients develop donor cell chimerism in their tissues (339, 340), a matter that is discussed further in Chapter 7. One critical question is whether the chimeric state is responsible for the maintenance of the unresponsiveness or whether it is merely its consequence. The fact that specific tolerance has been induced in experimental animals that, by definition, cannot be chimeras in the accepted sense suggests that, when it does occur, it is an effect rather than a cause, though it may depend on the underlying mechanisms and the allograft involved.

Mention should be made here of the work of Floersheim, who made a substantial contribution to the experimental application of ALS in conjunction with immuno-suppressive drugs and who showed, early on, that the addition of donor spleen cells can greatly enhance the durability of the tolerant state. Thus, he showed that methyl-hydrazine derivatives are not only instrumental in inducing specific tolerance in their own right (341) and but that they potentiate the effect of ALS (342), and that the addition of donor lymphoid cells to a limited RO 4–6824/ALS or procarbazine/ALG regimen substantially extends skin (343) and cardiac (344) allograft survival. Because the unresponsive mice possessed anti-donor-reactive lymphocytes, Floersheim postu-lated that the unresponsiveness was mediated by protective antibodies, a hypothesis that was later overtaken by the discovery of cells with suppressor functions and other possible mechanisms.

The use of cell-free tissue extracts

Following the discovery that histocompatibility antigens could be prepared as sub-cellular fractions (345, 346) that possessed antigenic and immunogenic properties, it was only a matter of time before such extracts were used in attempts to induce tolerance to skin grafts in mice, for this held out the hope of tolerance without the risk of GVHD. Billingham and Silvers (347) were the first to attempt this as part of a wider study of the biology of the male-specific Y antigen, which was already known to be one of the weaker non-H-2 histocompatibility antigens (see Chapter 4). Many others soon followed in their footsteps, confirming and improving on the very modest prolongation of graft survival obtained by Billingham and Silvers by the inoculation of cell-free extracts into baby mice, and extending the approach to stronger antigenic disparities, including H-2 (see below). Although Medawar (348) found in 1963 that a single dose of extracted antigen induced a more spectacular unresponsiveness in adult mice in a stronger (but still non-H-2) model when used in combination with sublethal whole body irradiation or A-methopterin (methotrexate), a folic acid antag-onist, it was Abbott, Monaco and Russell who were the first to explore the synergy between extracted antigen and ALS in adult mice (349). Their donors and recipients were H-2 disparate, and repeated injections of cell-free antigen (at weekly intervals) brought about a significant prolongation of skin allograft survival in some recipients when associated with five daily doses of ALS before grafting; the effect was greatly potentiated by previous thymectomy of the young adult mice.

Brent's group (350–352) made a special study of the tolerogenic properties of cell-free extracts when used in conjunction with ALS. Although the ALS was given optimally in the first week after the transplantation of H-2 disparate skin allografts, the best time for administering a single dose of F_1 hybrid spleen cells or liver extract was about two weeks before transplantation. This probably accounts for the fact that this model, which created long-lasting and specific tolerance in a high proportion of recipients, was never applied clinically. The proportion of tolerant mice was further increased by the addition of a single dose of *Bordetella pertussis* vaccine a few days before ALS was given (353), an effect that the authors ascribed to the previously known fact that the vaccine brings about a powerful blood lymphocytosis, thus providing the ALS with a better opportunity of destroying more of the circulating lymphocytes. The addition of a few doses of procarbazine hydrochloride (without *B. pertussis*) led to further potentiation of the tolerance (354), allowing even cocktails of blood (mixed from several donor strains) to be effective tolerogens. Of potential clinical importance, because it greatly simplified the experimental model, was the group's finding that the tissue extract could be replaced very successfully with a single minute quantity of donor strain blood given intravenously (355): depending on the strain combination, 50–90% of the recipients developed long-term (permanent) tolerance.

Apart from offering a possible clinical approach to the induction of specific tolerance in transplant patients, the models analyzed by Brent's group were of interest in that lymphocytes taken from tolerant animals had normal anti-donor reactivity when tested *in vitro* or *in vivo* (356), and because persuasive evidence for the participation of Ts lymphocyte populations came to light. Thus, Kilshaw *et al.* found in 1975 that although the transfer of spleen cells from tolerant animals to normal syngeneic adult mice prolonged skin graft survival by only a few days, transfer into either ALS-treated (357) or sublethally irradiated recipients (358) resulted in long-term survival of a substantial proportion of the grafts. This was confirmed by subsequent studies, regardless of the mouse strains used.

The replacement of cell extracts with minute doses of donor blood in the induction of tolerance likewise led to the generation of suppressor lymphocytes (359). What is more, the cells were clearly T lymphocytes, for treatment with an anti-T cell serum (anti-θ) and complement abolished the suppressive powers of the cells (357) – a finding that received corroboration when it was shown that purified T lymphocytes were on their own capable of transferring unresponsiveness (360). The demonstration of host Ts lymphocytes with specificity for donor histocompatibility antigens was here all the more significant because of the absence of donor cell chimerism (thus eliminating both donor antigen and veto cells as a possible cause) and because skin grafts – immunologically very demanding – were used in the assays. These experiments also showed that the antigenic stimulus from a small skin graft was sufficient to maintain the tolerant state.

Ts lymphocytes had already been described in other immunologic systems (see section on suppressor cells, below), but this was perhaps the clearest indication that they could provide a mechanism for allograft tolerance in adult animals.

That the tolerogenic action of cell-free extracts and ALS was not confined to skin allografts was soon shown by Mybergh's group (361, 362), who obtained promising results for baboon liver allografts, using a soluble glycoprotein extract, and by Judd and Trentin (363), who extended the survival time of murine cardiac allografts. Cerilli and Hattan (364) found later that prolonged survival could be obtained by this method even for skin xenografts (rat to mouse).

The anti-lymphocyte serum story: a summing up

The discovery by Woodruff and Waksman and their colleagues of the immuno-suppressive powers of ALS in the field of tissue transplantation raised great hopes that ALS would become a vital weapon in the clinical armory. Although ALG continues to be used in some transplant centers for the treatment of severe rejection crises (see Chapter 7) these hopes were not realized for several reasons, including the immunogenicity of ALG and the difficulty of producing batches of antisera in horses or rabbits with consistent potency and properties. There have been plenty of impressive experimental models that it might have been profitable to apply clinically, but by the 1970s kidney allograft survival figures, based on azathioprine and pred-nisolone, were already so good that transplant surgeons were understandably unwilling to expose their patients to potentially hazardous and untried new procedures. The 1980s saw the introduction of the powerful immunosuppressive drug cyclosporin A, and there was even less incentive for trying out new treatment regimens, the only direct clinical spin-off being the introduction of donor bone marrow cells into clinical protocols at one or two centers (see Chapter 7).

However, this would be taking too negative a view of the role of ALS in the history of transplantation. ALS was the forerunner for the numerous monoclonal antibodies that have largely replaced ALG in clinical transplantation and in the treat-ment of autoimmune disorders (see below). Those monoclonal antibodies directed against T lymphocytes perform essentially the same function as ALG though they do not always have the same potency as polyspecific antisera. They do, however, have the enormous advantage that they can be mass-produced as a standard product, that they are exquisitely specific and that they can be manipulated to be somewhat less immunogenic (humanized; see below). Clinical aspects apart, ALS/ALG was a powerful immunosuppressive tool that opened new doors for the study of tolerance induction in adult animals and the prevention of GVHD, and which led to a fuller realization of the existence and potential of Ts lymphocytes and other suppressive mechanisms. The full clinical impact of all this has yet to be revealed.

The Introduction of Monoclonal Antibody Technology: Antibody-Mediated Immunoregulation in the 1980s and Beyond

The production of antibodies by the technique of cell fusion was a major innovation introduced in 1975 by Köhler and Milstein, working in Cambridge, United Kingdom (365, 366). It was this discovery that led to the availability of a vast array of highly specific diagnostic and potentially therapeutic antisera which largely came to replace the polyspecific antisera in use up to then. Köhler and Milstein immunized inbred mice with sheep red blood cells (their choice of antigen) and fused antibody-secreting spleen cells with a mouse myeloma cell line in order to confer *in vitro* immortality on the cells. Each cell was expanded into a stable clone secreting an anti-sheep red cell antibody and such clones could be maintained more or less indefinitely. Because each clone was derived from a single cell the antibody response was monospecific; hence the term 'monoclonal antibodies'. It was soon shown that this method could be applied to a wide range of antigens, including major histocompatibility antigens of the rat (367) and the mouse (368). The production of monoclonal antibodies ushered in a new era of immunology and Köhler and Milstein were awarded the Nobel Prize in 1984, jointly with N. Jerne.

So far as transplantation is concerned, monoclonal antibodies had an impact on four fronts.

(1) They made it possible to dissect major histocompatibility complex (MHC) systems, especially human leukocyte antigens (HLA), with much greater precision (see Chapter 4).

(2) Because they made it possible to identify T lymphocyte subpopulations and other cells participating in immune responses it became possible to assess with greater accuracy which cells are primarily involved in graft rejection (see Chapter 2) and in GVHD (see Chapter 8).

(3) They were quickly applied to the suppression of allograft rejection in experimental animals, with specificities against a wide variety of targets – from subpopulations of T lymphocytes and their products such as the interleukins to adhesion molecules and to other molecules involved in graft rejection, and to the induction of tolerance.

(4) They largely replaced ALG or ATG as immunosuppressants in clinical transplantation, certainly prophylactically though not entirely in the treatment of rejection, and provided a tool for the removal of cell populations from human bone marrow before transplantation (see Chapter 8).

(5) Finally, they made it possible to identify cell markers in a wide range of pathologic conditions.

Here I shall confine myself to their use in tolerance induction. The reader is referred to the review by H. Waldmann (369) and I shall discuss only some of the more salient developments.

Anti-T cell antibodies

Anti-CD3 and CAMPATH 1 (pan-T cell)

Since the mid-1950s it has been recognized that T lymphocytes comprise distinct subpopulations with different functions, and the identification of these subpopulations owes much to the development of monoclonal antibodies directed against specific cell surface antigens. Critically important was the production by Reinherz and Schlossman's group in Boston (370) of antibodies called OKT3 and OKT4, the former directed against virtually all human peripheral T lymphocytes. The target is the CD3 molecule of the T cell receptor (TcR); on antigen binding to the Ti molecule, with which it is associated, it acts as a major signal transducer. OKT4 binds to about 55% of T lymphocytes, thus defining a subpopulation that was identified as being associated with T helper (Th) function (371). The OKT4-negative T lymphocytes were subsequently shown to be carrying the CD8 molecule characteristic of the CD8-positive cytotoxic/suppressor (Tc/s) subset (372), cells that appeared to be capable of suppressing Th function.

OKT3 was soon applied to clinical organ transplantation, was found to be effective, and came to replace ALG as the immunosuppressive reagent and also partly prophylactic in rejection crises. Like ALG it operates largely by T cell depletion of CD3-carrying lymphocytes (including the CD4 and CD8 subpopulations), a process that was shown to occur very rapidly (373, 374), although modulation of the Ti/CD3 TcR as the basis of the ensuing unresponsiveness has also been proposed (375, 376). It was Chatenoud et al. (375) who in 1982 first observed modulation after treatment of several human kidney allograft recipients with OKT3 antibody: severe T cell depletion was followed by recovery and the appearance of cells without OKT3, but *in vitro* overnight incubation restored OKT3 expression to the cells. The most recent hypothesis to account for cell depletion is that OKT3 cross-links CD3 on two different cells and thereby induces cell-mediated cytolysis (*377*).

Although anti-T3 antibodies have been mainly studied in patients, thanks to the production of OKT3, mouse models have also been established in which anti-CD3 antibodies have been examined. One of these is that of Hirsch *et al.* (*378*). Again, the rapid peripheral depletion of T lymphocytes was thought not to be the only important factor accounting for the prolonged survival of murine skin allografts; an alteration in TcR expression, and therefore dysfunction of the antigen receptor, was also thought to be involved. It is thus possible that monoclonal antibodies, with their greater specificity for defined molecules on the target cells compared with ALG, owe their immunosuppressive properties to pathways that are at least in part independent of, or secondary to, selective T cell depletion. This is likely to provide a basis for the T cell anergy described in murine (*379*) and human (*380*) T lymphocytes.

Recent work has shown that long-term administration of anti-CD3 antibodies in rats can lead to the permanent survival of cardiac allografts, and that animals carrying healthy heart grafts will also accept skin allografts from the same donor strain, but not from a third-party strain – indicative of true tolerance (*381*). These findings appear to have clinical potential, though the treatment of patients with other immuno-suppressive agents may well complicate the clinical induction of tolerance.

Another pan-T cell monoclonal antibody is CAMPATH 1, prepared and charac-terized by Hale *et al.* in Cambridge (*382*). It is a rat IgM antibody that binds to human T and B lymphocytes as well as to some monocytes, but not to other hemo-poietic cells, and is therefore suitable for the removal of lymphocytes from human bone marrow before transplantation. It is the first anti-lymphocytic monoclonal anti-body shown to fix human complement and this forms the basis of its cell- depleting capacity. It is extraordinarily efficient, killing 99% of peripheral mononuclear cells, and it is therefore hardly surprising that it has been used to great effect in the preven-tion of GVHD after human bone marrow transplantation (*383*) (see Chapter 8). It has also been found to be helpful in clinical renal allotransplantation in the control of rejection crises and as a prophylactic immunosuppressant.

Anti-CD4 and CD8

Once it was realized that T lymphocytes comprise at least two major subpopulations, the Th and the Tc/s subsets (*384, 385*), monoclonal antibodies against them were raised in several species. As the Th subpopulation was incriminated as primarily (though not exclusively) responsible for the rejection of allografts, attention largely focused on the removal of these cells as a means of achieving suppression and tolerance. Although the cell markers of Th were originally designated Leu3/T4 in man, W3/25 in the rat, and Lyt-1 or L3T4 in the mouse, they all belong generically to the CD4 complex, and the antibodies against them are now known as anti-CD4 antibodies (*386*). The discovery of lymphocyte subpopulations and their markers and functional activity is considered in Chapter 1.

Prominent among those who have used such monoclonal antibodies to suppress the immune response, especially to allografts, has been Waldmann's Cambridge group. In 1984 they described the production of several rat-anti-mouse monoclonals and showed that depletion of Th cells in thymectomized mice led not only to reduced antibody responses to sheep red blood cells, but also to the greatly prolonged survival of skin allografts when these differed from their hosts with respect to either minor or major plus minor histocompatibility antigens (387). In contrast, an antibody against Tc/s cells (defined by the Lyt-2 molecule) proved to be ineffective, apparently confirming that Th are the chief mediators of skin allograft rejection. However, because the removal of all T cells was even more effective in bringing about graft prolongation than removal of only the Th subpopulation these authors suggested that there might be some role for Tc/s cells after all, especially in primed mice (388) (see Chapter 2). The same group showed subsequently that two monoclonals (both IgG2b) directed against non-overlapping epitopes of mouse CD4 have a greater suppressive effect than either one used on its own, and that they could be used to block the response to human gammaglobulin, even without elimination of CD4 cells (389) – a finding that was thought to favor the concept of anergy.

This concept was given further support by the demonstration (390) that non-depleting antibodies could likewise induce tolerance to human gammaglobulin as well as to bone marrow and skin allografts, although prolongation of graft survival was dependent on the concomitant use of an anti-CD8 antibody. This tolerance could not be broken by the adoptive transfer of normal spleen cells syngeneic with the hosts, ruling out clonal deletion though not active suppression. The Cambridge group has gone on to demonstrate tolerance of skin allografts with cellular chimerism in mice treated with anti-CD4 and CD8 antibodies and donor strain bone marrow cells in mouse strain combinations differing either for multiple minor antigens only or for minors plus a relatively weak class I locus (391); and likewise for fully mismatched rat heart allo- and xenografts (392). Again, the use of both anti-CD4 and CD8 was obligatory. Among other workers who have found anti-CD4 antibodies to be effective on their own in conferring allograft protection are Jonker et al. in the Netherlands, working with rhesus monkey skin (393) and kidney (394) allografts, and Mottram, Wheelahan and McKenzie in Australia (395), using mouse cardiac grafts, though the latter also found an anti-CD8 (Ly-2) antibody to prolong survival.

It would be wrong to give the impression that the Cambridge group, though highly active and tackling the in vivo induction of tolerance head on, was alone in harnessing monoclonal antibodies for the induction of unresponsiveness. They were, for example, preceded by those who showed with antisera (396, 397) or with monoclonal antibodies (398) against Lyt-2/3 antigens that the cytotoxic activity of effector T lymphocytes could be blocked in vitro, and others have described in vivo unresponsiveness for humoral immunity (399) and cardiac allografts (400, 401). Interestingly, the anti-CD4 antibody used by the latter group (Pearson et al.) to establish tolerance was used in conjunction with donor-specific antigen in the form of whole blood or H-2 transfected L-cells, and it brought about a high level of T cell depletion. Yet, for reasons unknown, the model did not work at all in a second strain combination, thus lessening its appeal for clinical application, even though permanent acceptance of cardiac allografts across the full H-2 disparity was well illustrated in a more recent paper (402).

Finally, Cosimi's group in Boston (403, 404), working with non-human primates, found that although high-dose anti-CD4 antibodies induced donor-specific unresponsiveness to kidney allografts this did not continue on cessation of treatment –

a result rather different from those obtained in murine studies and hardly consonant with true tolerance. One of their findings was that stable graft function correlated well with an absence of interleukin (IL)-2-responsive cells in the allografts.

Monoclonal antibodies to other T cell markers and to other cells involved in allograft recognition

Anti-interleukin-2 receptor antibodies

Because an early step in T cell activation is the secretion of the T cell growth factor IL-2 and the expression of high affinity receptors (R) for IL-2, attempts were made during the 1980s to block the allograft response with anti-IL-2R monoclonal antibodies. A large Boston group was the first to show that IL-2 is required for the reconstitution of the acute rejection response in T cell-depleted rats (405, 406). Another group – again associated with T.B. Strom and N.L. Tilney – demonstrated that treatment with such an antibody substantially prolonged, in many cases long-term, cardiac allograft survival in mice although treatment was discontinued after the tenth day (407). They concluded that "the IL-2 receptor is an important new target for immunosuppression in clinical transplantation", and although experiments with the immunologically more demanding skin allografts proved to be disappointing – it was immunosuppressive only when used in conjunction with X-irradiation (408) – it was later applied clinically. One reason advanced for its inefficacy when used alone was that anti-rat immunoglobulin antibodies were produced, and it was postulated that X-irradiation interfered with this process. Some though not all subsequent publications have upheld a limited measure of immunosuppression by anti-IL-2R antibody, including a study by the Boston group in cynomolgus monkeys, kidney rejection having been significantly delayed (409), although antibodies against the murine monoclonal antibody again clouded the picture. Anti-IL-2R proved to be ineffective for xenogeneic cardiac grafts in cynomolgus monkeys unless coupled to a β radiation emitter (410) but in rats it was shown to act synergistically with low doses of cyclosporin A (411). Even though anti-IL-2R antibody can apparently induce specific tolerance to neural allografts (412) it does not seem to offer a greater clinical potential than antibodies directed against other T cell surface markers; indeed, probably less so.

Anti-adhesion molecule antibodies

Claims have been made for antibodies directed against some of the adhesion molecules that aid in the interactions between cells. LFA-1 (lymphocyte function associated-1) is a molecule present on both T and B lymphocytes, and because it may be involved in adhesions of T lymphocytes to other cells important in the generation of immune responses it has been used in attempts to regulate the allograft reaction. Early data obtained from the transplantation of allogeneic tumors were gently encouraging in that a greater tumor growth rate was observed (413), but regression could not be prevented. Very recently it has been shown that a single dose of anti-LFA-1 is remarkably effective in prolonging the life of thyroid allografts in mice, many grafts surviving for very long periods (414). Although the mechanism remains to be elucidated, it was thought that the antibody brought about anergy by "masking the antigen presentation of the passenger cells in the graft, or by preventing

the migration of dendritic cells to the spleen". There have, however, been less enthusiastic reports, and the case for allografts in general remains to be unproven. Anti-
ICAM-1, an endothelial intracellular adhesion molecule that plays a role in the
contact between the vascular endothelium of grafts and host leukocytes, has also
been put forward as a suitable target for antibody treatment: it evidently promotes
allogeneic bone marrow engraftment (415) and, when used together with anti-LFA-
1, cardiac allograft survival in mice (416).

Anti-major histocompatibility complex antibody

Fabre's laboratory, building on the work showing that class-II positive antigen-
presenting cells such as dendritic cells or macrophages of the host can be important
in triggering the response against allografts (the indirect pathway), have used a single
dose of a mouse-anti-rat class II antibody with anti-host specificity to substantially
prolong the survival of rat kidney allografts (417). The antibody suppressed the MLC
reaction *in vitro* and caused opsonization of class II-positive cells from the circulation.
Graft rejection was suppressed only when the antibody was specific for the recipient
strain's class II molecules, thus distancing itself from conventional enhancement. The
authors proposed that the mechanism of action was largely concerned with the
blocking of antigen presentation of donor antigens displayed on class II-positive host
antigen-presenting cells.

These workers were preceded by Chatterjee, Bernoco and Billing in 1982 (418),
who prolonged the survival of skin allografts in non-human primates with the aid
of monomorphic anti-host class II antibodies, though these were highly toxic; and
by Perry and Williams, who used anti-host class II antibodies in the mouse to prolong
skin allograft survival, though successfully only for class I or minor antigen disparate
combinations (419). The demonstration by T.G. Wegmann's group that engraftment
of parental hemopoietic stem cells in F_1 hybrid mice could be facilitated by the
concomitant intravenous inoculation of anti-host (class I or II) antibody, with long-
term stable and massive chimerism and an absence of GVHD (420), is rather different
as it was concerned with the suppression of GVHD, and the antibodies might
therefore have had an enhancing role.

The use of chimeric or hybrid antibodies

Although the application of monoclonal antibodies directed at lymphocyte subsets
or their cytokine products is rational and clinically promising, their application is
clearly being limited by their immunogenicity, which *in vivo* leads to the formation
of antibodies against them, and consequently to their neutralization. Although a
humanized depleting anti-lymphocyte antibody (CAMPATH-1H) created by the
transplantation of the hypervariable (antigen-binding) regions of a rat antibody into
normal human immunoglobulin genes has been applied with some success to the
treatment of rheumatoid arthritis (421), with no detectable anti-antibody formation
after a course of ten doses, as well as to two non-Hodgkin lymphoma patients (again
without antibody formation) (422), it is too soon to know what clinical impact such
antibodies will eventually have on the rejection of allografts and the induction of
specific tolerance in patients. Even humanized antibodies do not necessarily resolve
the problem of anti-idiotypic and -allotypic antibody formation.

The impact of monoclonal antibodies

What, then, are the conceptual advances that have benefitted the field of tissue transplantation since the introduction of monoclonal antibody therapy, compared with the previous work carried out with the cruder but nonetheless effective ALS/ALG preparations? Perhaps the most important aspect is the far greater precision they have contributed to the dissection of the immunologic events responsible for allograft rejection at both the cellular and molecular level. In the field of immunoregulation, they have led to the realization that T cell depletion is not an essential prerequisite of tolerance induction, a point recently amply confirmed by P.J. Morris' Oxford group (*402*). However, whether non-depleting antibodies act by inducing anergy or suppressor mechanisms must as yet be regarded as an open question. The availability of a vast array of antibodies against cell molecules characterizing lymphocyte subpopulations and their products makes it possible to hit highly specific targets while leaving the remainder of the immune system intact, and the cytotoxicity of the antibodies can be heightened by conjugation to cell toxins such as ricin. This approach is being actively pursued in many laboratories and it is possible that significant clinical developments will eventually accrue.

Finally, quite apart from the reliable production of these antibodies in a pure state, the possibility of making them less or perhaps even wholly non-immunogenic by hybridization and humanization techniques must be regarded as a hopeful possibility. They have on the whole been shown to have a greater potential for therapy than ALG (see Chapter 7). However, only time will tell whether they can be manipulated in clinical transplantation to induce a state of specific and durable tolerance of the kind that has been created in rodent models with relative ease.

Suppressor Cells

Although the discovery of suppression by cells belonging to the CD8-positive subset is referred to in Chapter 5 a brief survey of their historic ups and downs is called for. The reasons for this are two-fold.

(1) Cellular suppression to histocompatibility antigens is a well-documented fact and many examples of tolerance with such a mechanism can be found in the literature, both in experimental animals and in human hyporesponsiveness.

(2) It is of interest that what appears to have been a lack of communication between two groups of immunologists (molecular versus cellular) can lead to the dismissal by one group of phenomena observed, if incompletely understood, by the other.

To quote from the review of immunologic tolerance by R. Schwartz (*1*): "Problems began to emerge in the theoretical constructions, however, when attempts were made to extend the cellular phenomena to the molecular level. Genes could not be isolated, stable T cell clones could not be maintained, and proteins could not be identified. Even the reproducibility of the phenomena was questioned as some of the complex experimental systems could only be performed in a single laboratory. As a result, most molecular immunologists began to question whether Ts cells existed at all". And, in commencing the summary of a recently held workshop on suppression, Green and Webb (423) stated: "There is little doubt that the 'S' word (suppression, as in Ts cells) is the nearest thing to a dirty word we have in cellular immunology. Its use is considered by some (not all) to be synonymous with over interpretation of scanty data and phenomenology (the 'P' word) bordering on the mystical. Many have sought to eliminate its use altogether, substituting terms such as 'down-regulation', 'infectious tolerance' or 'active unresponsiveness'". These authors might well have added the term 'anergy' – a phenomenon frequently described by molecular immunologists working with haptens and other well-defined antigens in which antigen-specific T cells can be shown to be present though in a non-functional state. Yet anergy can only be distinguished from active suppression by the stringent disqualification of possible suppressor mechanisms in the experimental models, a requirement that has often been inadequately met.

First straws in the wind

The pioneering study of Argyris, dating back to 1963 (424), has already been referred to on p. 212 of Chapter 5. Although it was not conclusive it is nonetheless surprising that neither Dröge (425) nor Gershon (426) acknowledged her work in their stimulating reviews of the early work leading to the recognition of active suppression by T lymphocytes. Those readers wishing to study the early investigations leading to the development of the concept of immunoregulation are advised to read these reviews.

Recognition of the immunoregulatory powers of lymphocytes depended on the discovery that the thymus plays a crucial role in the immunologic education of lymphocytes, ushering in the golden age of "thymology" according to J.F.A.P. Miller (427), the realization that there were at least two major (T and B) lymphocyte subpopulations, and that T cells were capable of cooperating with B cells to enable the latter to produce antibody (the second golden age). These crucial discoveries are dealt with in Chapter 1.

The pioneering work on suppressor cells came mainly in the early 1970s and the first few years of that decade witnessed an extraordinary outburst of activity in this area. However, some significant if at first somewhat neglected contributions came from Waksman's laboratory at Yale University when, together with Horiuichi, he extended his laboratory's earlier findings (428) by showing that of all the lymphoid organs into which they inoculated antigen directly, the thymus was by far the best for the rapid induction of systemic tolerance to bovine gammaglobulin (429). They used soluble antigen for tolerance induction (aggregated protein was less effective) and tested for tolerance by challenging the recipient rats with the crude antigen in its most immunogenic form (i.e. in Freund's adjuvant). With the benefit of hindsight these experiments seem to suggest, though did not prove, that appropriately stimu-lated thymocytes can suppress the immune response in the periphery. The authors hinted at this by linking the increase in tolerance over a period of 12 days with the possibility that "time may be required for maturation of thymus lymphocytes which subsequently enter into the peripheral pool". An alternative explanation put forward was that of "recirculation through the thymus (not recognized at the present time)". The authors believed that tolerance induction in the thymus was easy because "the thymus lacks a trapping mechanism which can clear and catabolize the antigen".

and they led the way for more recent investigations concerning the role of the thymus in tolerance induction by direct inoculation of cellular antigens (see below).

Waksman's group was again ahead of the field when in 1965 they showed that the transfer of a tolerant thymus to a mouse that had been thymectomized at birth led to a specific unresponsiveness to bovine gammaglobulin (430), and one year later the same observation was made for skin allografts from the tolerizing strain (431). This transfer of tolerance was again bedeviled by the fact that the tolerant thymuses were chimeric for donor strain cells, as in the experiments of Argyris, but the authors went some way to exclude the possibility that tolerance had been induced by donor cells. It appeared to them "that these animals had adoptive tolerance conveyed by the tolerant thymus cells".

Although Billingham, Brent and Medawar, when publishing their full data on the properties of neonatally induced tolerance, experienced no difficulty in breaking the tolerant state with either normal or presensitized lymphoid cells syngeneic with the tolerant host (432), they were almost certainly aided by the fortuitous choice of donor and host inbred strains of mice, which later proved to be disparate for only class I antigens and for which clonal deletion rather than active suppression provided the main mechanism maintaining tolerance. Others, working either with soluble proteins, sheep red blood cells or histocompatibility differences for class II antigens or right across the H-2 system of the mouse, encountered problems when attempting to break tolerance with normal cells, and this was suggestive of some form of active immunoregulation. Thus, Crowle and Hu (433) succeeded in breaking tolerance induced in adult mice to soluble proteins with presensitized syngeneic cells, but not with normal cells. However, because the tolerance was transferable not only with cells but also with serum, they postulated that antibody rather than lymphocytes played an immunoregulatory role in their model.

Despite the earlier success reported by Weigle and Dixon (434) and by Cohen and Thorbecke (435) in breaking tolerance to soluble proteins, Tong and Boose (436) and later Terman, Minden and Crowle (437), using a bovine gammaglobulin tolerance model, were unable to break tolerance with normal cells, and the former failed even when transferring presensitized cells. Others could not break tolerance in models in which the tolerance was clearly not attributable to antibodies, notably Chase (438), who used chemical allergens, and McCullagh (439), whose rats had been made neo-natally tolerant to sheep red blood cells. Similar observations followed in animals tolerant to histocompatibility antigens, and it became clear that present in the tolerant animals of many, but certainly not all, tolerance models there was an active constraint interfering with the activity of normal lymphocytes. Although in many cases, especially those dealing with immunologic enhancement, the unresponsiveness was thought to be antibody-mediated, there was nonetheless evidence indicative of some synergy between antibody and cells harvested late in the sensitization phase in the transfer of unresponsivenss (see, for example, Batchelor, Boyse and Gorer (440), Cruse, Germany and Dulaney (441) and Hutchin, Amos and Prioleau (442). Further, Asherson, Zembala and Barnes (443), working with a delayed-type hypersensivity model involving tolerance to picryl chloride, found that lymphoid cells transferred unresponsiveness, though in their view the unresponsiveness was "at least in part antibody-mediated". Finally, McGregor, McCullagh and Gowans (444) showed that tolerance could be abrogated by the *in vitro* culture of lymphocytes: they concluded that this indicated that tolerant cells had been present *in vivo*, but not *in vitro*, their data could with the benefit of hindsight, be just as readily explained in terms of the loss of suppressor cells during culture.

Establishment of the phenomenon of suppression

It was against this backcloth of suggestive observations that Gershon, Dröge and McCullagh entered the fray. Gershon and his colleagues had suspected some form of immunoregulation when, in the late 1960s, they found that the concomitant cell-mediated responses detectable in hamsters carrying a transplantable tumor were abrogated by surgical resection of the tumor (see 426). Influenced by the important finding by Claman, Chaperon and Triplett (445) and others who followed them (see Chapter 1) that T lymphocytes cooperate with B cells in the production of anti-sheep red cell antibodies, Gershon's group (426) thought, instinctively it would seem, that these T lymphocytes were the prime candidate for the suppression of cell-mediated responses seen after tumor resection (rather than the removal of the antigenic load). Working at first in the London laboratory of P.C. Koller and A.J.S. Davies, Gershon and Kondo soon came up with evidence that there are indeed T lymphocytes with suppressive properties. Thus, with the aid of some complex experiments in thymectomized, lethally irradiated and bone marrow and thymocyte-reconstituted mice made 'tolerant' to sheep red blood cells (the tolerance was in fact transient and not wholly specific), they concluded in 1970 that the induction of tolerance to sheep red blood cells was T cell-dependent (i.e. that bone marrow-derived cells "seem to require the cooperation of thymus-derived cells" (446) as in the induction of immunity) and that the B cells in their mice were not intrinsically tolerant. The term 'suppression' or 'suppressor cell' was not used in this paper although the implication was clear. One year later and using the same experimental model, these two workers (447) identified thymus-derived lymphocytes in the spleens of the tolerant cellular chimeras that prevented cooperation between normal thymocyte and bone marrow cells when adoptively transferred. Of the three possible explanations considered by them they favored the possibility that tolerance induction was an active process brought about by an immunosuppressive substance released by the transferred T cells. The term 'suppressor cell' was again not used, but they described the transferred unresponsiveness as 'infectious tolerance'. By the time Gershon's team published their 1972 paper (448), in which they elaborated on these experiments, they were sufficiently confident of their data to give it the title of "Suppressor T Cells", and such cells were shown to suppress the responsiveness of other lymphocytes without mediation of B lymphocytes or their products. The concept of T cell suppression had thus been firmly established, and Gershon and his colleagues devoted the next ten years to the study of this phenomenon, including the notion of "contrasuppression", until Gershon's tragically untimely death in 1985. The reader wishing to follow the later literature on suppressor cells – and it is voluminous – may want to consult Gershon's reviews in 1975 (449) and 1980 (450) and his collaborative review of immunoregulatory pathways in 1983 (451).

W. Dröge, whose name has unfortunately been anglicized by British and American journals (causing confusion even to him – see the reference list of reference 452), entered this field from a somewhat different perspective and carried out his work in the young chick rather than in the ubiquitous mouse. When studying the cooperation of thymus cells with bursa-dependent cells in the production of antibodies against *Brucella abortus* and rabbit red cells, he discovered that intravenous inoculation of thymocytes from six-week-old donors into immunologically mature six-week-old recipients that were given the antigens one day later produced a strong suppressive effect. These observations were published in *Nature* late in 1971 (453), but there was no mention of Gershon and Kondo's 1970 paper even though it had been published 18 months earlier. Dröge concluded that "thymus cells thus seem both to amplify and to suppress the production of agglutinating antibody in the chicken". However, whereas amplification was unaffected by neonatal bursectomy of the thymus donor, the suppressive effect proved to be "bursa-dependent". Dröge had no explanation for this, but thought that the suppressive effect "may resemble that found in mice treated with anti-lymphocyte serum". Two years later he confirmed and extended these data, explained the bursa-dependence of the suppressive effect by postulating a bursa-dependent subpopulation of cells in the thymus that may have been directly derived from the bursa, ruled out the possibility that the suppressor cells were typical B cells, and suggested that the suppression was strikingly similar to tolerance induction with antigen in the prenatal or early postnatal period (454). Gershon and Kondo's work was now acknowledged. The cells described by Dröge appeared to be natural suppressor cells found in the thymus of young chicks.

The third line of evidence favoring suppression as a tolerance mechanism came from Australia. Having been involved with work in J.L. Gowans' laboratory in Oxford leading to the realization that the transfer of normal thoracic duct lymphocytes to rats tolerant of sheep red blood cells failed to break the tolerant state (444), P.J. McCullagh embarked on extensive studies of this phenomenon. In 1970 he confirmed that tolerant irradiated hosts were a far less favorable vehicle for the adoptive transfer of antibody-forming capacity than normal irradiated hosts (439). He went on to show that following cell transfer, plaque-forming cell precursors could be recovered in the first three days although no plaque-forming cells could be identified at any stage (455). He concluded that this was due to "some factor in the tolerant host inimical to stimulation of the transferred cells". In the same year, having shown that, by contrast, the transfer of allogeneic lymphocytes led to a break in tolerance, he suggested that "tolerance of sheep erythrocytes in rats represents the repression of a specific reactivity in cells rather than the elimination or irreversible inactivation of reactive cells" (456, 457). A few years later he studied the role of the thymus in suppressing immune responses in the newborn rat. He found that suppression of adoptive responses was achieved in irradiated hosts with thymus cells obtained from rats on their day of birth but not with cells from older donors (458). He concluded that "thymic suppressor cells are responsible for the poor responsiveness of newborn rats to antigenic challenge", with the implication that neonatal tolerance induction involved these suppressor cells. The latter proved to be radiosensitive (459).

These three lines of evidence pointing to the existence of cells capable of suppressing the immune response were established with antigens unconnected with histocompatibility. (Jacobson *et al.* (460), having uncovered prolonged allotypic suppression with mouse spleen cells, probably T lymphocytes, Asherson and Zembala (461) were the first to identify Ts cells in contact sensitivity, having transferred tolerance to lightly irradiated mice, and this was soon confirmed by Phanuphak, Moorhead and Claman

(462).) Among the first to appreciate the fuller significance of suppressive mechanisms were Allison, Denman and Barnes (463) when they outlined a hypothesis according to which "T cells can exert specific feedback control on the synthesis of antibodies by B cells and that relaxation of control – especially in ageing humans and experimental animals – may be an important factor in the development of autoimmunity". Subsequently transplantation immunologists began to look for suppressor lymphocytes in their experimental models, with spectacular results.

T cell suppression in transplantation

Apart from the much earlier papers by Argyris (424) and Toullet and Waksman (431) on the transfer of neonatally induced tolerance, the first really persuasive indication that spleen and lymph node cells could act as specific suppressor cells in the context of allotransplantation came from the study of Elkins in 1972. He showed that mice whose neonatally induced tolerance had been broken by the transfer of normal syngeneic lymphoid cells possessed cells capable of suppressing the ability of normal syngeneic lymphocytes to induce GVHR (464). Among the explanations for this seemingly paradoxical finding (suppressor cells were not demonstrable in the tolerant animals) was the possibility "that suppressor cells produce alloantibody that mediates some form of enhancement phenomenon". Alternatively, he felt that these cells could "react immunologically to the receptor sites present among normal lymphocytes but absent from specifically tolerant chimeras", foreshadowing the concept of anti-idiotypic suppressor cells.

Two years later Jirsch, Kraft and Diener (465) showed that mice made tolerant to fetal heart allografts by whole body irradiation and reconstitution with small numbers of syngeneic bone marrow cells had:

(1) Cells in their spleens that were capable of anti-donor responses *in vitro* (thus arguing against the clonal deletion hypothesis); and
(2) Cells in their lymph nodes that transferred the unresponsiveness to secondary irradiated recipients.

They failed to demonstrate a role for serum-borne factors and concluded that "these data suggest the existence of an active state of repression". Although aware of McCullagh's work they did not connect their results with those workers who had trodden this path before them, albeit with different antigens.

Phillips and Wegmann (466) also found evidence of suppression, this time by spleen cells taken from tetraparental mice, animals that had been chimeric from the eight-cell stage thanks to embryonic fusion. Their spleen cells specifically suppressed *in vitro* responses between the two parental strains, but the effect was not abrogated when the cells were treated with an anti-T cell serum, suggesting that the cells involved were either resistant to the anti-θ antibody or thymus-independent. The interpretation of these workers was, however, complicated by the previous finding that tetraparental mice have 'serum blocking factors' and hence the possibility that the suppressing cells were B cells secreting antibody could not be excluded.

Finally, another early pointer was provided by Weissman (467) when he transferred neonatally induced tolerance to syngeneic neonates: because the transferred tolerance could not be attributed in its entirety to donor cells in the inoculum he postulated that "this active process may involve the generation of specific suppressor T cells or the elaboration of immunospecific suppressor molecules". Proof, however, was lacking.

The nature of the suppressor cells had thus not been clearly established, but a number of other laboratories took up the challenge with a variety of tolerance models and soon it became apparent that the cells responsible for suppression were T lymphocytes. Among the early studies, in the mid-1970s, were those of Dorsch and Roser (468), who collected thoracic duct lymphocytes from DA rats that had been made tolerant at birth to PVG histocompatibility antigens. Such cells, either unfractionated or purified to comprise of T lymphocytes only, were administered to sublethally irradiated DA rats, with the result that tolerance was successfully transferred. The presence of chimeric donor strain cells was eliminated as a factor (but see below). "This phenomenon is not explicable in terms of absence of the clone of antigen sensitive cells but implies that populations of tolerant cells contain cells capable of active, specific suppression of the regenerating immune response in animals recovering from radiation... true transplantation tolerance is a positive immune response mediated by T cells which belong to the recirculating pool of small lymphocytes". Dorsch and Roser confirmed and extended these studies and made a number of other substantial contributions to the literature over the next seven years, not least by the rigorous exclusion of B cells and their products as mediators of tolerance and by the demonstration that the presence of suppressor cells in tolerant animals was not dependent on an intact thymus, at least not up to six months (469); and they concluded that "The target for the suppressor action of these cells is probably the precursor of alloantigen-sensitive lymphocytes, and the effect of suppression may be the deletion or inactivation of the relevant clone of these cells". Although these Australian authors (originally working in Sydney but later in Babraham, United Kingdom) had so far described the suppressor cells as of host origin, their later kinetic studies led them to believe that chimeric (F_1) donor T lymphocytes were primarily responsible (469, 470). Thus, the removal of the chimeric cells abrogated the ability of tolerant inocula to transfer tolerance adoptively, a result that Dorsch and Roser interpreted as suppression "via an anti-idiotypic mechanism, the allo-reactive cells bearing idiotype-positive major histocompatibility complex receptors". Roser reviewed their own work and that of others, both in neonatal and adult tolerance, in 1989 (471).

In the course of a series of studies on the induction of specific tolerance of skin allografts in adult mice using cell-free tissue extracts and a short course of ALS (350, 351), L. Brent's group at St Mary's Hospital Medical School in London described the presence of suppressor cells in the spleens of animals that had been free of immunosuppressive treatment for long periods. Thus, splenic cells and purified T cells from them transferred long-term tolerance to secondary recipients that had received either a short course of ALS treatment (357) or a sublethal dose of whole body irradiation (360). In this model the tolerant animals were patently not chimeric and the suppressor cells were therefore undoubtedly of host origin. The unresponsiveness was rapidly abrogated by *in vivo* treatment with a dose of cyclophosphamide (472) that had previously been shown to enhance contact sensitivity in guinea pigs (473), probably because suppressor cells are especially sensitive to its action (474). An interesting feature of the unresponsiveness studied by Brent's team was that although it could be induced in a number of strain combinations and was frequently complete so far as the test skin allografts were concerned, cells removed from the tolerant milieu and tested *in vitro* could be shown, in several assays, to have anti-donor activity (356, 475) – a finding also made in a variety of other experimental models. Tolerance could be promptly abolished by pre-sensitized syngeneic lymph node cells but not by normal cells (475), and it could be induced equally well if a single minute dose of allogeneic blood took the place of the tissue extract, the unresponsiveness again being mediated by T lymphocytes (355, 476). Although these strategies resulted in a remarkably high level of specific tolerance and clearly established the existence of host T cell suppression, their disadvantage from a clinical point of view lay in the need to give the donor antigen two weeks before transplantation.

Early evidence for the participation of suppressor cells also came from Czechoslovakia, when Rieger and Hilgert (477) showed that neonatally induced tolerance was radiosensitive and that spleen cells from tolerant donors transferred some measure of unresponsiveness to irradiated recipients. However, the possible role of chimeric donor strain cells and the nature of the suppressor cells had not been investigated. According to another Czech group, suppressor activity revealed by an *in vitro* assay resided in a nylon-adherent subpopulation (478). This echoed the earlier work of Folch and Waksman when they described thymus-dependent, glass wool adherent suppressor cells raised *in vitro* in MLC (479) or after incubation with high doses of mitogens (480) (see also Rich and Pierce, 481). Indeed, from a study using endotoxins as antigen Yoshinaga, Yoshinaga and Waksman concluded that in the same system there may be two distinct forms of suppression – one brought about directly by macrophages and the other by macrophage-dependent Ts cells (482). In contrast, Dröge (483) transferred specific suppression of skin allograft rejection with syngeneic thymus cells from young chickens, an effect that was bursa-dependent, as in his earlier experiments.

Overall, a role for suppressor cells, in many cases T cells, had thus been established by the mid-1970s, and this was confirmed in a host of models subsequently developed for the induction of tolerance in adult animals, including that of antibody-induced immunologic enhancement (484, 485), for which Batchelor's group have established an anti-idiotypic mechanism (486). It is, however, clear that T cells are not unique in this respect and that cells such as macrophages, thymus-independent lymphocytes and veto cells can suppress, though not necessarily always in specific fashion. The concept of veto cells has already been discussed (see also the more recent work of Thomas *et al.*, 487) – their mode of action, too, remains controversial, though Kiziroglu and Miller (488) have recently suggested that they might function as deletional antigen-presenting cells.

Active suppression has undoubtedly remained a dominant theme in transplantation immunology up to the present time; recent reviews (489, 491) reveal both the intense interest in suppressor cells and the frustrations encountered in nailing them down. Disappointingly, the mechanism of T cell suppression remains uncertain, largely because it has not been possible to distinguish the Ts cells phenotypically from other CD4-positive or CD8-positive lymphocytes and because the search for factors released from suppressive cells has generally been in vain. Whether they constitute a separate subpopulation remains to be proven and it may well turn out that suppressor cells are simply members of the CD4-positive and CD8-positive subsets that can either be activated or made to enter a suppressive mode depending on factors such as the nature and concentration of the antigen and the absence or presence of co-stimulatory signals.

Anergy Versus Suppression: Peripheral Tolerance

I have already alluded to the fact that immunologists have interpreted many forms of tolerance as anergy (i.e. a down-regulation of the ability of T (or B) lymphocytes to give functional responses to specific antigens despite the presence of cells with appropriate antigen-specific receptors – a form of functional silencing. This differs from the notion of clonal abortion, which Nossal and Pike (492) put forward in 1975 as an explanation for the induction of self-tolerance. Their study was carried out *in vitro* using low concentrations of deaggregated monomeric DNP-conjugated human gammaglobulin (HGG) as antigen, which induced non-responsiveness in B lymphocytes during a relatively short culture period. These workers coined the term "clonal abortion" to distinguish the phenomenon from clonal deletion although, curiously, proof for such a distinction was lacking. Active suppression was ruled out because the unresponsiveness was not transmissible to normal bone marrow cells and the authors concluded that their prediction that it should be possible to switch off permanently (or eliminate) lymphocytes by exposure to antigen at a certain stage of their differentiation (when antigen receptors have already appeared) had been fulfilled. They abandoned the term clonal abortion in favor of anergy when some years later they found that tolerance induction in newborn mice to fluorescein-coupled HGG left the tolerant mice with a normal profile of B lympho-cytes with immunoglobulin receptors, but a clear deficit in responsiveness to HGG (493). Tolerance was thus not due to clonal elimination or modulation of cell surface receptors; "Rather, it is due to the recognition and storage of negative signals amongst cells that continue to display a normal complement of receptors". Nonetheless, active suppression had again not been formally excluded as a possible mechanism.

This set into motion a bandwagon that accelerated throughout the 1980s and that threatened the extinction of the concept of Ts cells, despite the strong evidence in its favor. The bandwagon was helped on its way by the demonstration by Malkovský and Medawar (see 494) that the induction of neonatal tolerance to histocompatibility antigens could be frustrated by the inoculation of the newborn mice with interleukin (IL)-2, and others soon uncovered supporting evidence. For example, Lamb *et al.* (495) described *in vitro* experiments in which human T cell clones specific for defined peptides of influenza A agglutinin became unresponsive after incubation with the antigen. Although clonal deletion was thought to be improbable because the cells continued to respond to T cell growth factor, active suppression was again not formally excluded. Quill and Schwartz (496), again working *in vitro*, induced tolerance to Ia molecules in specific T cell clones by incubation with the antigen, the cells continuing to express normal levels of antigen receptors – a phenomenon that was subverted by the introduction of IL-2. In a paper published in the same year (1987) Jenkins and Schwartz advanced the notion that *in vitro* tolerance induction, this time to pigeon cytochrome C, could be brought about by the chemical modification of antigen-presenting cells (497).

Anergy as an explanation for *in vivo* tolerance to histocompatibility was soon advocated by Waldmann's group in Cambridge when they induced tolerance to skin allografts (multiple minor antigen and H-2D differences) in adult mice following bone marrow transplantation and treatment with non-depleting anti-CD4 and CD8 antibodies; determination of V-β-6 expression indicated that the potentially reactive cells had not been eliminated and the authors concluded that "functional anergy" underpinned the unresponsiveness (391). However, once again this study did not include attempts to exclude suppression as a mechanism, a criticism that is equally applicable to their demonstration of tolerance in MHC-mismatched mice induced with depleting monoclonals followed by non-depleting antibodies (498).

Many other models of anergy can be found in the literature, including for example tolerance for pancreatic islets induced by treatment of mice with a depleting anti-CD4 antibody – the tolerance being at least in part reversible by rIL-2 (recombinant interleukin-2) administration (499) – and tolerance for rat kidney allografts resulting from a single intravenous transfusion of donor blood (500). In this last study by Dallman and her colleagues the tolerant rats displayed a reduced expression of the p55 IL-2 receptor chain on the lymphocytic cell surface as well as fewer high affinity IL-2 receptors, brought about by a dysfunction of IL-2 receptor messenger ribonucleic acid (mRNA) chain transcription. The cells could not synthesize IL-2 in culture and *in vivo* administration of IL-2 abrogated the tolerant state. It was postulated that an altered regulation of the IL-2 pathway was primarily responsible for the tolerance and it remains to be seen whether this will be more generally applicable. The work of Heeg and Wagner is of interest because of the authors' claim that the intravenous inoculation of allogeneic spleen cells led to a state of anergy brought about by donor-specific veto cells (501).

Although clonal deletion can clearly be ruled out as an explanation in systems in which the continued presence of antigen-specific T (or B) lymphocytes can be demonstrated, it is more difficult to distinguish between anergy and suppression unless rigorous experiments are carried out to rule out the latter. This has rarely been done and as a result the literature has been more obfuscating than it need have been. Indeed, in one of their more recent papers Waldmann's group (502) described the tolerance induced by them with non-lytic anti-T cell antibodies as "infectious", for cells from tolerant mice found able to "disable" syngeneic naive T cells that in turn were capable of disabling other naive cells. While the authors were careful to avoid the use of the word 'suppression' these experiments seem to go a long way to suggest that a kind of tolerance previously firmly ascribed to anergy could well be a form of T cell suppression. This impression is further confirmed by a subsequent paper from the Cambridge group (503) in which peripherally induced T cell tolerance could not be broken by normal lymphocytes. This 'resistance' to the transfer of adoptive sensitivity was mediated by T cells; although the authors once again were careful to avoid the use of 'suppression' the two terms are functionally clearly synonymous. That the difference between some forms of suppression and anergy may be non-existent is emphasized by the findings of another previous advocate of anergy, R.I. Lechler. He and his team working at the Royal Postgraduate Medical School in London found that anergic T cell clones could in fact suppress non-anergic T cells *in vitro* (504), an effect ascribed to competition for ligands on the surface of antigen-presenting cells and for locally produced IL-2. If anergic T lymphocytes can indeed suppress the activity of normal cells the difference between anergy and suppression becomes semantic, and it is possible that progress in this area might have been a great deal faster if workers had been more receptive to such a possibility.

It would clearly be quite wrong to suggest that anergy does not occur either in experimental situations or in the physiologic avoidance of anti-self responses. The prevention of autoimmune reactions and disorders is of such crucial importance to the mammalian organism that there is ample room for clonal deletion in the thymus (which must remain the first form of defense) as well as peripheral forms of tolerance comprising active suppression or anergy.

The use of transgenic mice has made it possible in recent years to prove the reality of peripheral tolerance in normal T cell development. Of special interest are the findings of two groups, one in the United States and the other in Australia, published in 1989. Burkly *et al.* (505) and Lo *et al.* (506) – essentially the same group working in the United States – showed that transgenic mice carrying MHC class II I-E molecules on pancreatic β cells but not in the thymus or in peripheral lymphoid organs are tolerant to I-E without deletion of T lymphocytes bearing V-β5 and V-β17a gene segments. Negative selection in the thymus had patently not been possible in these circumstances. Unlike T cells from non-transgenic mice, T cells from the transgenics did not proliferate in response to cross-linkage of their receptors with antibodies against V-β5 and V-β17a, indicating that clonal paralysis had occurred during the course of development. This failed to come about when the mice were irradiated, suggesting that the tolerance was maintained by a peripheral mechanism. Having dismissed Ts cells by *in vitro* and *in vivo* mixing experiments these authors postulated that tolerance was mediated by a "lymphokine sink" brought about by the dilution of non-tolerant T cells by tolerant cells, an explanation that could well be accommodated by the hypothesis of Lechler's group (504). A somewhat similar approach was adopted by Morahan *et al.* (507), using transgenic mice carrying H-2Kb linked to an insulin promoter. In pre-diabetic mice the spleen cells were unresponsive for H-2Kb targets, unlike thymus cells, and the unresponsiveness was reversible by rIL-2. The peripheral induction of tolerance was here dependent on antigen persistence and a lack of IL-2.

Finally, Arnold, Schonrich and Hämmerling (508) have argued persuasively that "depending on the tolerogenic signals, peripheral T cells can reach different levels of tolerance with regard to their reactivation. In addition, it appears that tolerant cells are still susceptible to further tolerogenic signals, driving them into a deeper state of tolerance". This multi-step hypothesis of tolerance induction and maintenance provides a further refinement of a highly complex system of safeguards that have evolved to protect the organism from self-destruction.

A discussion of many of the issues raised above can be found in Nossal's 1989 review (509).

Other Interesting Models for the Induction of Tolerance

A survey of the history of immunoregulation would not be complete without a consideration of several approaches not so far mentioned. Prominent among them are total lymphoid irradiation (TLI) and the inoculation of antigens directly into the thymus. The former was developed in the 1970s and 1980s as a safe method of inducing tolerance with irradiation, and the latter has been one of the major developments of the 1990s. Both have potential clinical application, and TLI has already been used in the treatment of transplant recipients.

Total lymphoid irradiation

The damaging effects of whole body X-irradiation on the tissues of the immune system have been appreciated since the early part of the twentieth century thanks to the pioneering work of Lawen, Hektoen, and Murphy, and much later Craddock and Lawrence, who showed that irradiation of rabbits, rats and dogs could severely interfere with the formation of antibodies to sheep red blood cells or bacterial organisms (see Chapters 2 and 8). They were, likewise, well aware of the potentially lethal effects of this kind of treatment. It was the team of W.J. Dempster (who was responsible for a number of significant contributions to the field of allo-transplantation in the 1950s, but who later unaccountably faded from the picture) who in 1950 was the first to describe the prolongation of skin allograft survival in rabbits brought about by sublethal doses of whole body irradiation (510). Transplant surgeons using whole body irradiation in the 1950s as the chief means of facilitating the survival of human kidney allografts had to balance their radiation doses on a knife-edge, however (see Chapter 7). Because of the hazardous nature of whole body irradiation attempts were made in the 1960s to prevent or delay acute rejection in human kidney recipients by irradiation of the graft soon after transplantation (511, 512) and to prolong the life of kidney allografts in experimental animals by topical irradiation (513, 514). Gleason and Murray (515) analyzed the results from a large number of clinical cases and concluded that there was an improvement overall in the early function of cadaveric kidneys. By giving six doses of 400 rads over a three-week period Gergely and Coles (516) were able to increase the total dose to as much as 2400 rads and found, in these circumstances, that the survival of renal allografts in dogs was substantially prolonged without any other immunosuppression.

This, roughly, was the background against which Slavin, Strober and their colleagues at Stanford University embarked on a series of studies in the mid-1970s in which they applied fractionated, high-dose total lymphoid, as opposed to whole body, irradiation to induce tolerance in adult animals. They were inspired by the fact that this had been used widely in the treatment of malignant lymphomas such as Hodgkin's disease (517) without the disastrous side-effects of whole body irradiation, and their previous work had shown that it was immunosuppressive (518). In applying TLI (totally lymphoid irradiation) to mice (519) they devised an apparatus that ensured irradiation of all lymphoid tissues with the exception of the chest, dorsal spine, hind legs and tail. Thus 200 rads were administered 5 times per week up to a total dose of 2400 rads, and fully allogeneic skin was grafted one day after the last dose. Although a severe leukopenia ensued and blood lymphocytes remained below normal for three months, polymorphonuclear cells had regained normal values by the end of the third week. TLI brought about a five-fold increase in the survival time of the skin grafts but this was reduced to 19 days when the thymus was also shielded. The infusion of 100 million donor strain bone marrow cells led to permanent acceptance of both skin and bone marrow grafts, astonishingly in the total absence of GVHD.

These preliminary data were soon followed up by more extensive studies illustrating not only that the skin graft recipients were specifically tolerant but that the donor chimeric cells were likewise specifically tolerant to host incompatibility antigens (520); and the absence of GVHD was fully confirmed. Patterns of lymphocyte repopulation as well as lymphocyte depletion were tentatively thought to account for the findings, possibly through alterations in the reticular and endothelial structure of the lymphoid tissues (including the thymus), thus leading to perturbation of maturation, homing and cell–cell interactions of T lymphocytes. The authors concluded that "This technique may have relevance for clinical organ transplantation". A year later the same group (521) went on to compare their TLI data with whole body irradiation followed by bone marrow infusions (95% of mice died within two months) and showed that TLI followed by spleen cells resulted in lethal GVHD. Thymic irradiation alone prolonged skin graft survival only marginally and did not facilitate bone marrow engraftment. In this paper, in which they suggested that TLI could be valuable in clinical bone marrow transplantation, they speculated that the protective effect "may be due in part to the lack of development of mature T cells and/or to the development of suppressor cells from immature cells in the bone marrow". Tolerance was found to extend to cardiac allografts, too (522).

The speculation about suppressor cells proved to be near the mark in that Slavin and Strober described the existence of such cells in their tolerant mice in 1979 (523). In the early phase after TLI the action of the cells in suppressing MLR reactions in co-culture experiments were nonspecific (this had also been the experience of Mybergh's laboratory; 524). However, after the first month it became specific for the donor. Because the data were analogous to those obtained with soluble serum proteins as antigen – where Ts lymphocytes had been identified (525) – the authors felt that the same cell type was likely to be involved in their experiments with allografts. However, the mechanism underlying the TLI effect remains controversial and once again we have an impressive experimental protocol for which the precise mechanism remains uncertain despite the fact that it has been successfully applied to large animals (526–530) and even clinically (530–534), albeit with adjunct immunosuppressive agents. The demonstration that TLI-treated patients could in time be taken off all forms of immunosuppression without rejecting their cadaveric kidneys (535) is remarkable and suggests that the immune system of these three patients had indeed become tolerant in the true sense of that word, as judged by graft survival and lack of in vitro anti-donor reactivity.

That TLI has not been applied more widely to clinical transplantation is presumably due to the fact that results with cyclosporine and tacrolimus (FK506) are now so good that clinicians have come to rely on them as a more adaptable form of immunosuppression. The need for TLI treatment to be given before transplantation is another limiting factor, though the recent demonstration by Thomas et al. (536) that TLI together with a short course of antilymphocyte globulin immediately after kidney transplantation in splenectomized rhesus monkeys leads to long-term graft prolongation without further immunosuppression is a hopeful development. The fact that attempts to use TLI and bone marrow grafting in pigs to prolong kidney allograft survival have been disappointing was almost certainly connected with the absence of donor cell chimerism in these animals (537), a finding that was also made by Vaiman *et al.* (538) when using fully allogeneic porcine skin and bone marrow donors. These workers revealed a high level of chimerism as well as skin graft survival, however, when they used MHC matched donors and recipients.

The TLI approach continues to be of considerable interest. Despite great efforts made to establish the mechanism of the tolerance it promotes it remains something of a riddle. There seems to be little doubt that suppressor cells are involved at one stage or another – first nonspecific in nature (523, 524) and later specific (539, 540), but whether they are the sole factor seems unlikely as Slavin's group in Jerusalem has found evidence favoring the elimination or functional inactivation of donor cells with anti-host potential (541, 542). These workers favored the notion that suppressor cells assist in the inductive phase while elimination/inactivation sustains the maintenance phase. The situation is undoubtedly complicated in this system by the fact that TLI-tolerant animals display a two-way tolerance.

The analogy between the tolerance induced neonatally and by TLI has been given some credence by the finding of Strober's group that cloned 'natural suppressor cells' obtained from these two sources have similar *in vitro* immunoregulatory properties (539, 540) and display the same phenotype (CD3-positive, CD4/8-negative) (543). Mice that had undergone TLI showed a long delay in the recovery of Th1 cells – cells that secrete IL-2, interferon (IFN)-γ and lymphotoxin and that mediate delayed-type hypersensitivity reactions – whereas the IL-4, 5 and 6-secreting Th2 cells involved in antibody production recovered rapidly. The role of IL-2 production in TLI tolerance is still a rather grey area. Field and Becker (544) likewise found that TLI produced a shortfall of IL-2-secreting, IL-2 receptor-expressing lymphocytes but in their study it proved to be transient, reactivity being normal by eight weeks. This result does not necessarily conflict with the more recent work of Bass and Strober (545), who described a ten-fold reduction in the strength of the MLR and of IL-2 production after TLI, despite normal levels of IL-2 receptors, but whose study was conducted at 4–6 weeks. Bass and Strober therefore believed that the reducd MLR responsiveness was brought about by a reduction of IL-2-secreting cells. Yet another hypothesis that has been advanced concerns the reduction in cytotoxic precursors and a concomitant increase in suppressor activity (546), but this investigation was carried out with a lower total dose of TLI without bone marrow, and the addition of soluble donor strain histocompatibility antigens. The question of immunosuppressive mechanisms after TLI is far from resolved, and yet again it seems probable that more than one mechanism is, or can be, operative.

Intrathymic inoculation of antigens

The function of the thymus as a site for the education of T lymphocytes became clear when Miller published his seminal paper on the effects of thymectomy in 1961, and others such as Good and Waksman soon followed in his footsteps (see Chapter 1). Waksman and his colleagues in particular were quick to draw attention to the fact that the thymus plays a critical role in the induction of tolerance. In 1965 they published data on this issue (430, 547). Essentially, they showed that when the thymus of rats that had been made tolerant to bovine gammaglobulin was transplanted to adult rats that had been thymectomized and irradiated in adult life, the recipients were found to be tolerant to that antigen for several weeks, as revealed by both delayed-type hypersensitivity reactions and antibody formation. They assumed that the antigen must have penetrated into the thymus and that tolerant cells "are actually produced in the thymus or, if produced in another source organ, pass through the thymus and perhaps mature there". Such cells would then enter the competent small lymphocyte pool. Others before them had shown that thymus grafts can become tolerant of host antigens in thymectomized (548, 549) or non-thymectomized (550) animals. As already mentioned, Toullet and Waksman extended the group's observations likewise to thymuses taken from mice made tolerant neonatally (431). It is of considerable interest that it is now thought that it is the thymic epithelium that is primarily concerned not only with positive selection – shaping the immunologic repertoire of the individual – but also in negative selection, leading to tolerance (551).

Be that as it may, Waksman and his colleagues, working at Yale University, then took matters one vital step further by showing, again in the mid-1960s, that specific tolerance to proteins such as bovine gammaglobulin (BGG) could be induced by the direct inoculation of the antigen into the thymus of rats. Initially this was carried out by using high-dose whole body irradiation with a shielded thymus: such animals recovered their reactivity to BGG unless the antigen was inoculated into the thymus immediately after irradiation (428, 552). Horiuchi and Waksman (553) took this a step further when they succeeded in achieving a similar result in rats that had not been irradiated, though this time monomeric antigen was far more effective than when it was heat-aggregated. Although systemic administration also lowered responsiveness the thymic approach was by far the most effective because "the thymus lacks a trapping mechanism which can clear and metabolize antigen". In none of their papers, which were not given to speculative ruminations, was there any mention of the possible clinical potential of this approach.

Relevant to this story is that years later the degree of donor cell chimerism in the thymus of mice made tolerant neonatally by the inoculation of allogeneic cells was firmly linked to the degree of tolerance induced (554–556).

Enter A.M. Posselt, C.F. Barker and their colleagues in the Department of Surgery, University of Pennsylvania, a quarter of a century later, by which time the investigations by Waksman's laboratory had long been forgotten. In a paper in Science (557) they described the implantation of rat islet allografts into both lobes of the thymus of diabetic adult rats accompanied by the administration of a relatively small dose of ALS, which would be expected to wipe out temporarily the pool of immunocompetent T lymphocytes in the blood. (A modest degree of immunosuppression proved to be necessary and it was used in all subsequent studies by this group.) While the ALS itself led to a moderate but finite prolongation of islets transplanted to the liver or the kidney, the great majority of intrathymic islets survived indefinitely and the hosts became normoglycemic. When some of them received fresh islets under the kidney capsule, having carried their intrathymic islets for more than 200 days, these extrathymic grafts likewise survived; and, because this survival was entirely strain-specific, the authors thought that they had demonstrated that the rats had become systemically tolerant. This tolerance appeared to be uniquely associated with the thymic environment, for other 'immunologically privileged sites' such as the testis proved to be far less satisfactory and certainly not tolerance-inducing.

While FACS analysis and MLC experiments did not reveal any departure from normal, limiting dilution analysis showed that the tolerant animals had a significant and specific shortfall of cytotoxic T lymphocyte precursors, "suggesting that deletion or functional inactivation of class I-restricted RT1 reactive T lymphocytes had occurred". The authors concluded their remarkable article by stating that "This approach offers a novel strategy for successful pancreatic islet transplantation and may be relevant to our understanding of the mechanisms involved in the development of tolerance".

Before describing the avalanche of articles provoked by the paper of Posselt et al. one or two comments are in order. It does seem extraordinary that their approach with alloantigens was not explored many years earlier, once the thymus had been firmly associated with both positive and negative selection of lymphocytes. And yet it was! M. Vojtišková and H. Lengerová, working in Prague, published the results of such an approach in 1965 in a brief communication in Experientia (558), where it was duly buried and forgotten. (I am greatly indebted to Dr C.F. Barker for recently drawing my attention to this thoughtful though far from clearly presented paper.) These workers induced a very prolonged and specific unresponsiveness to skin allografts in mice differing from their donors only at the weak (minor) H-3 locus by giving the recipients sublethal whole body irradiation and a syngeneic thymic implant (either normal or irradiated) that had been inoculated ex vivo with a high dose of donor strain spleen cells. Possibly aided and abetted by the relatively high dose of irradiation, which may have allowed access of some of the cells to the thymic implant, a proportion of mice that had been given the spleen cells subcutaneously near to the implants likewise became tolerant. They concluded that ". . . immunological tolerance can be induced in adult mice by procuring the entry of antigen in thymus (sic) either by its direct inoculation or in an indirect way."

The other question that may be asked is why Posselt et al. were apparently ignorant of the pioneering studies of Waksman's group after they had completed their first exciting series of experiments. While it is easy enough to overlook previous publications among the thousands that are published every year, the computerized literature search Medline goes back to 1966 and would have thrown up some of the papers published by Wakman's group. It was not until late in 1992 that Ohzato and Monaco (559), reporting on their successful induction of tolerance to skin allografts in mice following the inoculation of spleen cells into the thymus, gave credit to the earlier workers. However, Dr C.F. Barker tells me that the genesis of his laboratory's intrathymic approach stemmed from his previous interest (with R.E. Billingham) in immunologically privileged sites, and that it was influenced by his group's speculation that the reason for Billingham, Brent and Medawar's failure to induce tolerance in neonates by intravenous inoculation of non-lymphoid cells was the inability of these cells to reach the thymus.

The paper by Posselt et al. in 1990 was followed by a steady stream of other publications, not least from the same group, who soon showed, quite remarkably, that the diabetes of spontaneously diabetic rats could be reversed by intrathymic implantation of allogeneic islets (regardless of whether they were pre-cultured), and that such animals generally accepted subsequent islet grafts administered by the intraportal route (560). Although they thus confirmed the immunologically privileged status of the thymus, islets transplanted into skin-sensitized rats were destroyed in an accelerated manner, indicating that although resting T cells do not normally penetrate the blood–thymus barrier, activated cells have no such problem – a point that had already been established by others (see Chapter 2). Disappointingly, the intrathymic islets did not induce unresponsiveness to skin grafts from the donor strain, indicating "that the degree of unresponsiveness . . . is not comparable to that which is induced by neonatal inoculation . . . and thus should probably not be referred to as 'tolerance'". It is not impossible, however, that skin was rejected because of skin-specific antigens (see Chapter 2). In this study, as in all others from the Philadelphia group, the experimental design included a single dose of ALS, though it was not an essential requirement in these diabetic hosts, which suffer from a "profound T-cell lymphopenia". Because the transfer of lymphoid cells from islet-bearing hosts into secondary hosts did not bring about unresponsiveness the authors argued that this made the participation of immunoregulatory cells unlikely and that it emphasized the importance of intrathymic deletion or inactivation of T cell clones as the dominant mechanism.

The first independent confirmation of the efficacy of the intrathymic route came from Bergamo in Italy in 1991, when Remuzzi et al. described how the intrathymic implantation of allogeneic rat glomeruli (561) or blood leukocytes (562), using minimal immunosuppression with cyclosporine or none at all, permitted successful transplantation of donor strain kidneys, which then survived indefinitely without further immunosuppression. There followed a string of papers, many published in Transplantation, describing intrathymic induction of specific tolerance to cardiac, skin, liver, and small bowel allografts. An interesting variant of these studies was that of Blakeley et al., who induced tolerance in the donors of allografts of small intestine by injecting the donor thymus with host splenocytes, thus avoiding GVHD (563). Although the first attempt, by M.W. Flye's laboratory, to induce tolerance to xenogeneic skin using a spleen cell inoculum yielded only limited prolongation of survival (656), Barker's Philadelphia team managed to produce indefinite survival of the less immunogenic pancreatic islets, using bone marrow cells as the inoculum (565).

It is noteworthy that tolerance has been induced by intrathymic inoculation of either class II (566) or class I (567) allopeptides and by solubilized antigens comprising both class I and II moieties (568), stressing the role of the indirect pathway of antigen presentation in tolerance induction. In both studies the removal of the thymus five or seven days later led to the prompt rejection of the kidney or cardiac allografts, suggesting that the peptides were held in the thymus and continued to be specifically suppressive for some time.

In the study of Sayegh et al. (566) a marked and specific reduction in the proliferative response (MLR) of host lymphocytes to donor strain antigens was observed. Likewise, ultraviolet light (UV)-B irradiated spleen cells, which cannot replicate, can act as a satisfactory intrathymic tolerogen (569). Of interest, too, is the observation by Knechtle et al. (570) that autologous rat myoblasts and myotubes transfected with only donor class I genes induced specific intrathymic tolerance to both liver and cardiac allografts even though these differed from the host strain right across the histocompatibility spectrum. This recalled the findings of Madsen et al. (571) that recipient cells transfected with a single class I gene were able to induce tolerance for other histocompatibility antigens.

The thymus is thus a remarkably efficient site for inducing specific tolerance, as might have been predicted on theoretic grounds; and there is general agreement that it has opened up a promising way forward for the clinical induction of tolerance. There are, however, some problems that may yet prove to be insuperable.

(1) There have so far not been any reports of success in large animals, with the possible exception of cultured and UVB irradiated islets transplantated to 'minipigs' (*572*).
(2) The human adult thymus may be less amenable to direct inoculation than the thymus of young adult animals, though the approach would presumably be feasible in children and young adults.
(3) J.A. Bradley's group in Glasgow has very recently produced data showing that some rat strain combinations are peculiarly refractory to intrathymic tolerance induction (*573*), though this could turn out to be caused by suboptimal use of ALS.

The bare bones concerning the mechanism of intrathymically induced tolerance are as follows. There is general agreement that the thymus occupies a unique position, for attempts to achieve the same results by inoculating antigen into other sites have consistently met with failure. Although retention of cellular antigen in the thymus has been documented up to three weeks following inoculation of bone marrow, no chimerism was detected in animals that had carried their allografts for 200 days or more (*574*). The fact that intrathymic tolerance is inducible with UVB irradiated cells and with extracted antigens and peptides further suggests that long-term cellular chimerism in the thymus is not a *sine qua non* of tolerance induction, though microchimerism in the periphery could conceivably be established by the transplanted tissue or organ. The tolerance-inducing stimulus must clearly be potentially immunogenic, Campos *et al.* having failed to induce tolerance with islet allografts that had been rendered non-immunogenic by previous culture (*575*). Even the accelerated rejection of cardiac grafts in strongly presensitized rats can be overcome by intrathymic inoculation (*576*), and the same authors have described profound alterations in host humoral alloresponsiveness in the same model (*577*).

It is commonly held that clonal deletion or inactivation (anergy) is the most likely explanation, and this would fit into the general pattern of what is known of the role of the thymus in negative selection. It is therefore hardly surprising that inoculation of bone marrow into only one thymic lobe has yielded inferior results (*578*). Evidence in favor of a deletional/inactivating mechanism includes the following observations.

(1) A reduction in MLR-reactive (*566*) and cytotoxic (*579, 580*) T lymphocytes.
(2) Depletion of V-β6-positive T cells (with reactivity to Mlsa superantigen) in Mlsa-negative recipients of Mlsa-positive cells (*581*).
(3) Failure to identify suppressor cells by the adoptive transfer of lymphoid cells from animals with long-established grafts (*580, 582*).
(4) Abrogation of the tolerogenic effect of allopeptides by the administration of rIL-2 (*583*).

Although the Philadelphia group tends to favor clonal deletion or anergy they have nonetheless provided some evidence for suppressor cell activity, albeit only in animals that had been given intrathymic spleen cells as well as an extrathymic cardiac graft (*584*): without the cardiac allograft, transfer of unresponsiveness to naive animals could not be demonstrated. They concluded that "this finding strongly suggests that an alternate possibility . . . also plays an important role in our results, i.e. induction of regulatory T cell populations in the host". Thus, overall it would seem that both negative selection and the induction of suppressor cells in the periphery play a part in the creative and maintenance of this form of tolerance.

Finally, it is of interest – and yet another demonstration of the extraordinarily potent effect of the intrathymic induction of tolerance – that Posselt *et al.* have succeeded in preventing the occurrence of spontaneous autoimmune diabetes in a rat strain by implanting pancreatic islets from a normal but MHC compatible strain into the neonatal thymus (585). Evidently exposure to normal β cells brought about "a specific modulation of diabetogenic T cells maturing in an islet-bearing thymus".

"Mixed allogeneic chimerism"

An interesting approach adopted by Ilstad and Sachs (586) involves the reconstitution of lethally irradiated mice with a mixture of T cell-depleted syngeneic and allogeneic (congenic) bone marrow cells. This led to the long-term survival of the recipients without GVHD, and the indefinite and specific survival of skin grafts from the allogeneic donor strain. The blood of such animals contained variable proportions of both donor and host lymphoid cells. Similar experiments with xenogeneic (rat) cells led to the prolonged survival of about 25% of skin grafts and there was little evidence of cellular chimerism. The absence of GVHD and the hyporesponsiveness to donor antigens was remarkable. Later studies showed that allogeneic chimeras were equally hyporesponsive *in vitro*, that this was donor-specific, and that such animals are immunocompetent for other kinds of antigens (587), presumably because the presence of syngeneic cells permits cellular interactions that are not possible in fully allogeneic chimeras. However, experiments with a non-congenic strain combination revealed that skin grafts were eventually rejected despite stable and persistent chimerism, "suggesting that skin-specific non-major histocompatibility complex antigens were responsible for rejection of the C3H grafts".

Sharabi and Sachs (588) have gone on to show that the lethal irradiation of the hosts can be replaced by the combined use of anti-CD4 and CD8 antibodies, low sublethal whole body irradiation, and high dose thymic irradiation: this treatment facilitated the establishment of a stable mixed chimerism in a fully mismatched allogeneic mouse strain, again in the absence of GVHD and with specific tolerance for skin grafts of the donor strain. The mechanism underlying these events is, however, not clear. This group has since developed methods of preventing GVHD and inducing tolerance using more conventional means (see Chapter 8).

The curious case of the surviving and tolerogenic livers

It was R.Y. Calne and his colleagues in Cambridge, United Kingdom (589) who first described the prolonged survival of porcine liver allografts in animals that had not been immunosuppressed, which was in marked contrast to the fate of kidney and skin allografts. They were unable to explain this unusual occurrence by chance compatibility and wrote that "We are therefore compelled at present to attribute the long survival of liver transplants in the pig to some quality peculiar to the liver in this species". It clearly was not due to some immunologic quirk of the pig, despite its highly unusual lymphoid system (590), for kidney and skin were rejected promptly, and it later transpired that a similar phenomenon was demonstrable in the rat (see below). Further, Parker, Hickman and Terblanche (591) several years later failed to find compatible pairs of pigs as judged by MLC. Calne's group soon showed that both orthotopic and accessory liver allografts have the power to prolong the life of subsequently transplanted kidney and even skin grafts from the same donor, suggesting that the porcine liver has unique tolerogenic properties (592). These workers also showed that donor liver extracts markedly prolonged kidney graft survival though skin survival only transiently. The tolerogenic properties of liver have remained something of a mystery, but the mechanism has been unraveled to some degree by experimentation in the rat. Interestingly, the phenomenon seems to have a counterpart in urodele amphibians, for Baldwin and Cohen (593) found that the implantation of allogeneic liver fragments into adult urodeles led to a desultory form of rejection and substantially prolonged survival of skin allografts from the same donors. Liver allografts also seem to be partially exempt from the full rigors of rejection clinically (594, 595).

This potentially interesting phenomenon went into limbo until 1980, when two groups began its analysis in the rat. Kamada, Brons and Davies (596), working in Cambridge, showed that in the RT1 mismatched strain combination DA to PVG, allografts survived just as well as isografts, and that subsequently transplanted skin grafts were totally and specifically accepted. The tolerance was associated with an ability of the recipients' serum to block the binding of a monoclonal anti-DA to DA red blood cells, suggesting that DA antigens had been shed into the circulation, but a direct link was not established. The second study by Houssin et al. in Villejuif, France (597) was conducted in a different strain combination in which the tolerogenic effect of liver allografts was determined for skin or kidney grafts from the same donor strain. Again, both the skin and kidney grafts were fully accepted while third party grafts were normally rejected. Among the possible mechanisms suggested were:

(1) Antigenic overload.
(2) Tolerance induction by antigen presentation via hepatic macrophages, the release of humoral factors or the opsonization of alloantigen-reactive T cells.
(3) Intrahepatic activation and/or maturation of Ts lymphocytes.

Clonal deletion was not considered by this French group although evidence for a selective form of deletion directed at T cells with the potential for graft rejection as opposed to GVHR was later proposed as one possibility (598, 599), but the theoretic difficulties of such a proposal were never resolved.

There has been some support for serum blocking factors and Ts lymphocytes. Thus the Cambridge group found a nonspecific serum blocking factor that nonetheless failed to transfer unresponsiveness on passive transfer (600). By contrast Kamada, the leading author of this paper, was later able to bring about the permanent survival of cardiac allografts from the liver donor strain by transferring serum from long-surviving animals (601); this factor involved IgG antibodies, recalling the older 'enhancement' literature. Likewise, factors inhibiting the MLR have been found in the serum of human liver allograft recipients (602), in one case in the form of HLA-A and B antigen (603). As for suppressor cells: although some tentative and limited evidence has been presented favoring splenic (but not blood) suppressor cells – again by Kamada's group – and by Engemann et al. (604), and others have found none at all, the most persuasive evidence for the participation of Ts comes from Grassel *et al.* Thus, Lewis rats that had accepted BN livers possessed splenic Ts cells that transferred the tolerance adoptively to sublethally irradiated recipients syngeneic with the hosts, and this adoptive tolerance extended to the specific survival of skin, hearts and kidneys (*605*). However, these cells, though present in the spleen, were absent from the recirculating lymphocyte pool and this offers an explanation for previous observations, both positive and negative. The concept of "sessile" Ts cells is certainly a novel one and one has to assume that they would likewise have been present in other lymphoid tissues.

Finally, it is possible that the replacement of Kupffer cells by host cells, following initial acceptance of liver grafts, may be a further protecting factor (*606*).

The extraordinary protective powers of rat liver allografts evidently depend on the rat strains used (*607*) and it seems probable that more than one mechanism is responsible.

The liver is, in fact, not unique. In a a brief communication to *Nature* in 1968 J. Salaman described the spontaneous survival of rat kidney allografts between two strains and observed that rats with well established kidney allografts supported the life of skin grafts from the same donor for long periods (*608*). Working with a different strain combination known to have major MHC disparities he later found that renal allografts survived unidirectionally, and that again a successful kidney protected skin grafts from the same donor against rejection (*609*) – reminiscent of the protection afforded to skin allografts by previous transplantation of ovarian grafts in the experiments of Linder (*610*). Dunn and Randall (*611*) observed that in the rat strains they used kidney allografts only occasionally survived for long periods, and in rabbits long-term survival of kidneys was frequently associated with severe early graft damage. This led them to postulate some form of auto-enhancement following early activation of the immune system as a possible mechanism.

The problem was not fully analyzed until P.S. Russell and his colleagues in Boston solved the formidable technical problems of kidney transplantation in mice (*612*). Kidneys from H-2K or D incompatible donors (i.e. class-I disparate) usually survived without immunosuppression and then protected skin grafts from the donor strain from rejection. Although cellular and humoral responses to donor antigens declined during the first few weeks and there was an absence of cytotoxic cells in the spleens, the hosts' lymphoid cells could perform more or less normally in an *in vivo* GVH assay. No suppressor cells could be demonstrated. Yet two years later Russell's laboratory revealed the presence of donor-specific Ts cells in a model involving the spontaneous survival of cardiac allografts in congenic mice (*613*) – an observation that was unfortunately not supported by attempts to transfer the unresponsiveness by adoptive transfer. I will let them have the last word: "Perhaps the Ts cell is not the sole, or even the most important factor mediating specific unresponsiveness to allografts *in vivo* in the systems that we have been studying".

Conclusion

The history of specific immune suppression, which began in the 1930s with some crude and ill-understood studies (the XYZ effect), illustrates that immunologists have succeeded in manipulating the immune system of experimental animals to an astonishing degree during the course of the century. Many mechanisms have been proposed; some hypotheses have been sustained and others have faltered. One of the difficulties has been that experimentalists have overinterpreted their data when relatively modest prolongations of graft survival have been achieved. Often experimental models involved some degree of genetic disparity, organ allografts like the heart that appear to be relatively insensitive to immunologic attack, or animals like the rat in which some measure of tolerance is fairly easily obtained. If it seems disappointing that close to the end of the century, and despite the aid of ever more sophisticated technology, it has not been possible to identify one single overriding mechanism, or to apply the information gleaned from experimental models to the clinic (but see Chapter 7), it must also be seen as a measure of the extraordinary intricacy of the immune system. Vertebrates, and especially mammals, have evolved complex mechanisms that protect individuals against autoimmune manifestations and disorders and, by allowing a battery of protective mechanisms to develop nature seems to have played safe. In our attempts to manipulate the immune system to our advantage we tend to uncover one or other or several of these mechanisms in any one model. Perhaps rather naively the army of investigators in this field have tended to assume that whatever mechanism they happen to have revealed was the all important one, instead of seeing it as merely one band in a complex spectrum. The other comment the historian is in a position to make is that even in the 1990s the collaboration between transplantation/cellular immunologists and molecular biologists has remained fragile. It is only when these two subspecies of immunologists collaborate intimately that a clinically acceptable means of inducing tolerance is likely to become available.

I make no apologies for having allowed this chapter to become the most substantial and kaleidoscopic in the book. Transplantation immunology is, ultimately, an applied science, even though some fundamental phenomena and important theories have emerged from it. I have tried to give the reader an impression of the multiplicity of the experimental approaches used, their limitations, and some of the blind alleys that have been encountered. The biologic and specific control of the rejection process must remain the ultimate objective – the Holy Grail – and when that has been accomplished not only will the transplantation of tissues and organs have been revolutionized but so will the whole of medicine.

The ups and downs of the blood transfusion effect and the controversy concerning the role of donor chimeric cells in the maintenance of tolerance are considered in Chapter 7.

References

1. Schwartz, R. (1993) In *Fundamental Immunology*, ed. W.E. Paul, pp. 677–731, Raven Press, N.Y.
2. Brent, L. (1979) *Transpl. Proc.* **11**, 839.
3. Bulloch, W. (1938) *A History of Medical Bacteriology and Immunology*, pp. 422, Oxford Univ. Press.
4. Parish, H.J. (1965) *A History of Immunization*, E.S. Livingstone Ltd, Edinburgh & London.
5. Topley, W.W.C. & Wilson, G.S. (1990) *Principles of Bacteriology, Virology and Immunity*, 8th edn, eds M.T. Palmer & L.H. Collier, Longman, London.

6. Schöne, G. (1912) *Die Heteroplastische und Homöoplastische Transplantation*, Springer-Verlag, Berlin.
7. Tyzzer, E.E. (1916) *J. Cancer Res.* **1**, 125.
8. Woglom, W. (1919) *Cancer Rev.* **4**, 129.
9. Flexner, S. & Jobling, J.W. (1907) *Proc. Soc. Exp. Biol. Med.* **4**, 156.
10. Bashford, E.F., Murray, J.A. & Haaland, M. (1908) *3rd Sci. Rep. Cancer Res. Fund, Lond.*, 359.
11. Haaland, M. (1910) *Proc. Roy. Soc. B.* **82**, 293.
12. Leitch, A. (1910) *Lancet* **1**, 991.
13. Bisceglie, V. (1926) *Ztschr. f. Krebsforsch.* **23**, 340.
14. Bertolotto, U. (1932) *Tumori* **18**, 601.
15. Favilli, G. *Sper. Arch. di Biol.* **84**, 489.
16. Chambers, H. & Scott, G.M. (1924) *Brit. J. Exp. Path.* **5**, 1.
17. Chambers, H. & Scott, G.M. (1926) *Brit. J. Exp. Path.* **7**, 33.
18. Casey, A.E. (1932) *Proc. Soc. Exp. Biol. Med.* **29**, 816.
19. Casey, A.E. (1934) *Amer. J. Cancer* **21**, 776.
20. Casey, A.E., Ross, G.L. & Langston, R.R. (1949) *Proc. Soc. Exp. Biol. Med.* **72**, 83.
21. Casey, A.E. & Gunn, J. (1952) *Proc. Soc. Exp. Biol. Med.* **80**, 610.
22. Snell, G.D., Cloudman, A.M., Failor, E. *et al* (1946) *J. Nat. Cancer Inst.* **6**, 303.
23. Snell, G.D., Cloudman, A.M. & Woodworth, E. (1948) *Cancer Res.* **8**, 429.
24. Kaliss, N. & Day, E.D. (1954) *Proc. Soc. Exp. Biol. Med.* **87**, 208.
25. Kaliss, N. & Day, E.D. (1954) *Proc. Soc. Exp. Biol. Med.* **87**, 115.
26. Kaliss, N. & Snell, G.D. (1951) *Cancer Res.* **11**, 122.
27. Kaliss, N. (1952) *Science* **116**, 279.
28. Snell, G.D. (1954) *J. Natl. Cancer Inst.* **15**, 665.
29. Kaliss, N. (1955) *Ann. N.Y. Acad. Sci.* **59**, 385.
30. Kandutsch, A.A. & Reinert-Wenck , U. (1957) *J. Exp. Med.* **105**, 125.
31. Kaliss, N. & Molomut, N. (1952) *Cancer Res.* **12**, 110.
32. Kaliss, N., Molomut, N., Harris, L. *et al.* (1953) *J. Natl. Cancer Inst.* **13**, 847.
33. Kaliss, N. (1956) *Proc. Natl. Acad. Sci.* **42**, 269.
34. Kaliss, N. (1956) *Proc. Soc. Exp. Biol. Med.* **91**, 432.
35. Kaliss, N. (1958) *Cancer Res.* **18**, 992.
36. Kaliss, N. (1962) *Ann. N.Y. Acad. Sci.* **101**, 64.
37. Kaliss, N. & Kandutsch, A.A. (1956) *Proc. Soc. Exp. Biol. Med.* **91**, 118.
38. Gorer, P.A. (1947) *Cancer Res.* **7**, 634.
39. Mitchison, N.A. & Dube, O.L. (1955) *J. Exp. Med.* **102**, 179.
40. Billingham, R.E., Brent, L. & Medawar, P.B. (1956) *Phil. Trans. Roy. Soc. B.* **239**, 357.
41. Billingham, R.E., Brent, L. & Medawar, P.B. (1956) *Transpl. Bull.* **3**, 84.
42. Billingham, R.E. & Sparrow, E.M. (1954) *Brit. J. Exp. Biol.* **31**, 16.
43. Möller, G. (1964) *Transplantation* **2**, 281.
44. Voisin, G.A. & Kinsky, R. (1962) In *Transplantation*, eds G.E.W. Wolstenholme & M.P. Cameron, p. 286, Ciba Found. Symp., J. & A. Churchill, London.
45. Voisin, G.A., Kinsky, R.G. & Maillard, J. (1968) In *Advance in Transplantation*, eds J. Dausset, J. Hamburger & G. Mathé, p. 31, Munksgaard, Copenhagen.
46. Voisin, G.A., Kinsky, R.G. & Duc, H.T. (1972) *J. Exp. Med.* **135**, 1185.
47. Voisin, G.A. (1962) In *Mechanisms of Tolerance*, eds M. Hasek, A. Lengerová & M. Vojtisková, p. 435, Czech. Acad, Sci., Prague.
48. Voisin, G.A. (1963) Rev. *Franc. d'Étud. Clin. Biol.* **8**, 927.
49. Medawar, P.B. (1962) In *Transplantation*, eds G.E.W. Wolstenholme & M.P. Cameron, p. 411, Ciba Found. Symp., J. & A. Churchill, London.
50. Brent, L. & Medawar, P.B. (1961) *Proc. Roy. Soc. B.* **155**, 392.
51. Snell, G.D., Winn, H.J., Stimpfling, J.H. *et al.* (1960) *J. Exp. Med.* **112**, 293.
52. Pikovski, M. & Schlesinger, M. (1955) *Cancer Res.* **15**, 285.
53. Mosman, T.R. & Coffman, R.L. (1989) *Annu. Rev. Immunol.* **7**, 145.
54. Kaliss, N. & Bryant, B.F. (1958) *J. Natl. Cancer Inst.* **20**, 691.
55. Kaliss, N. (1958) *Proc. Amer. Assoc. Cancer Res.* **2**, 312.
56. Snell, G.D. (1956) *Transpl. Bull.* **3**, 83.

57. Snell, G.D. (1957) *Ann. Rev. Microbiol.* **11**, 439.
58. Gorer, P.A. (1956) *Adv. Cancer Res.* **4**, 149.
59. Gorer, P.A. (1961) *Adv. Immunol.* **1**, 345.
60. Feldman, M. & Globerson, A. (1960) *J. Natl. Cancer Inst.* **25**, 631.
61. Hellström, I., Evans, C.A. & Hellström, K.E. (1969) *Int. J. Cancer* **4**, 601.
62. Hellström, I. & Hellström, K.E. (1969) *Int. J. Cancer* **4**, 587.
63. Hellström, K.E. & Hellström, I. (1970) *Int. J. Cancer* **5**, 195.
64. Hellström, I., Hellström, K.E. & Sjögren, H.O. (1970) *Cell. Immunol.* **1**, 18.
65. Bansal, S.C., Hargreaves, R. & Sjögren, H.O. (1972) *Int. J. Cancer Res.* **9**, 97.
66. Hellström, I., Hellström, K.E., Pierce, G.E. *et al.* (1968) *Proc. Natl. Acad. Sci. (Wash.)* **60**, 1231.
67. Hellström, I., Hellström, K.E., Pierce, G.E. *et al.* (1968) *Nature* **220**, 1352.
68. Hellström, I., Hellström, K.E. & Allison, A.C. (1971) *Nature* **230**, 49.
69. Bansal, S.C., Hellström, K.E., Hellström, I. *et al.* (1973) *J. Exp. Med.* **137**, 590.
70. Wright, P.W., Bernstein, I.D., Hamilton, B. *et al.* (1974) *Transplantation* **18**, 46.
71. Wegmann, T.G., Hellström, I. & Hellström, K.E. (1973) *J. Exp. Med.* **137**, 291.
72. Hellström, I. & Hellström, K.E. (1973) *Cell. Immunol.* **7**, 73.
73. Quadracci, L.J., Hellström, I., Striker, *et al.* (1971) *Cell. Immunol.* **1**, 561.
74. Sjögren, H.O., Hellström, I., Bansal, S.C. *et al.* (1971) *Proc. Natl. Acad. Sci. (Wash.)* **68**, 1372.
75. Elkins, W.L., Hellström, I. & Hellström, K.E. (1974) *Transplantation* **18**, 38.
76. Batchelor, J.R. (1968) *Cancer Res.* **28**, 1410.
77. Möller, G. (1963) *J. Natl. Cancer Inst.* **30**, 1153.
78. Möller, G. (1963) *J. Natl. Cancer Inst.* **30**, 1177.
79. Möller, G. (1963) *J. Natl. Cancer Inst.* **30**, 1205.
80. Möller, G. (1964) *Transplantation* **2**, 405.
81. Chard, T.C. (1968) *Immunology* **14**, 583.
82. Chard, T., French, M.E. & Batchelor, J.R. (1967) *Transplantation* **5**, 1266.
83. Stuart, F.P., Saitoh T. & Fitch, J.R. (1968) *Science* **160**, 1463.
84. French, M.E. & Batchelor, J.R. (1969) *Lancet* **2**, 1103.
85. Kaliss, N. (1958) *Cancer Res.* **18**, 992.
86. Möller, G. & Möller, E. (1966) In *Antibodies to Biologically Active Molecules*, ed. B. Cinader, p. 349, University Press, Oxford.
87. Batchelor, J.R. (1968) *Cancer Res.* **28**, 1410.
88. Fisher, B. & Lee, S. (1965) *Surgery* **58**, 904.
89. Lee, S. (1967) *Surgery* **61**, 771.
90. Ullmann, E. (1902) *Wien. Klin. Wschr.* **15**, 281.
91. Carrel, A. (1902) *Lyon Méd.* **98**, 859.
92. Woodruff, M.F.A. (1960) *The Transplantation of Tissues and Organs*, pp. 512–16, 550–2, Charles C. Thomas, Springfield, Ill.
93. Moore, F.D. (1964) *Give and Take*, W.B. Saunders Co., Philadelphia & London.
94. Moore, F.D., Smith, L.L., Burnap, T.K. *et al.* (1959) *Transpl. Bull.* **6**, 103.
95. Feldman, J.D., Pick, E., Lee, S. *et al.* (1968) *Amer. J. Path.* **52**, 687.
96. Lee, S. & Edgington, T.S. (1968) *Amer. J. Path.* **52**, 649.
97. Axelrad, M. & Rowley, D.A. (1968) *Science* **160**, 1465.
98. Batchelor, J.R. & Welsh, K.I. (1976) *Brit. Med. Bull.* **32**, 113.
99. Batchelor, J.R. (1978) *Transplantation* **26**, 139.
100. Morris, P.J. (1980) *Immunol. Rev.* **49**, 93.
101. Fabre, J.W. & Morris, P.J. (1972) *Transplantation* **13**, 604.
102. Fabre, J.W. & Morris, P.J. (1974) *Transplantation* **18**, 429.
103. Marquet, R.L., Van Es, A.A., Heystek, G.A. *et al.* (1978) *Transplantation* **25**, 188.
104. Mybergh, J.A. & Smit, J.A. (1972) *Transplantation* **14**, 227.
105. Soulillou, J.P., Keribin, D., Lecoguic, G. *et al.* (1980) *Transplantation* **29**, 314.
106. Wren, S.F.G., Martins, A.C.P., Von Haefen, U. *et al.* (1974) *Surgery* **76**, 112.
107. Fabre, J.W. (1982) *Transplantation* **34**, 223.
108. Hart, D.N.J., Fuggle, S., Williams, K.A. *et al.* (1981) *Transplantation* **31**, 428.
109. Hart, D.N.J. & Fabre, J.W. (1981) *J. Immunol.* **126**, 2109.
110. Hart, D.N.J. & Fabre, J.W. (1981) *Transplantation* **31**, 319.

111. Steinman, R. & Nussenzweig, M.C. (1980) *Immunol. Rev.* **53**, 127.
112. Hart, D.N.J. & Fabre, J.W. (1981) *Transpl. Proc.* **13**, 95.
113. Hirschberg, H., Bergh, O. & Thorsby, E. (1980) *J. Exp. Med.* **152**, 249.
114. Hart, D.N.J. & Fabre, J.W. (1981) *J. Exp. Med.* **154**, 347.
115. Mullen, Y. & Hildemann, W.H. (1971) *Transpl. Proc.* **3**, 669.
116. Mullen, Y., Takasugi, M. & Hildemann, W.H. (1973) *Transplantation* **15**, 238.
117. Hildemann, W.H. & Mullen, Y. (1973) *Transplantation* **15**, 231.
118. Mullen, Y., Raison, R. & Hildemann, W.H. (1977) *Transplantation* **24**, 99.
119. Strom, T.B., Carpenter, C.B., Garovoy, M.R. *et al.* (1975) *Transplantation* **20**, 368.
120. Tokuda, S. & McEntee, P.F. (1967) *Transplantation* **5**, 606.
121. Uhr, J. & Möller, G. (1968) *Adv. Immunol.* **8**, 81.
122. Takasugi, M. & Hildemann, W.H. (1969) *J. Natl. Cancer Inst.* **43**, 843 and 857.
123. Bloom, E.T. & Hildemann, W.H. (1970) *Transplantation* **10**, 321.
124. Voisin, G.A., Kinsky, R.G. & Duc, H.T. (1972) *J. Exp. Med.* **135**, 1185.
125. Takasugi, M. & Klein, E. (1971) *Immunology* **21**, 675.
126. Miller, C.L. & DeWitt, C.W. (1974) *Cell. Immunol.* **13**, 278.
127. Vriesman, P.J.C., Swanen-Sierag, L. & Vlek, L.F.M. (1975) *Transplantation* **20**, 385.
128. Desi, S.B.R. & Ruszkiewicz, M. (1977) *Transplantation* **23**, 230.
129. Fuller, T.C. & Winn, H.J. (1973) *Transpl. Proc.* **5**, 585.
130. Rubinstein, P., Decary, F. & Streun, E.W. (1974) *J. Exp. Med.* **140**, 591.
131. Davies, D.A.L. & Alkins, B.J. (1974) *Nature* **274**, 294.
132. Davies, D.A.L. & Staines, N.A. (1976) *Transpl. Rev.* **30**, 18.
133. Carpenter, B.C., Soulillou, J.P. & d'Aspice, A.F.J. (1976) *Transpl. Proc.* **8**, 199.
134. Jeekel, J., Van Dongen, J., Major, G. *et al.* (1977) *Transpl. Proc.* **9**, 969.
135. Davis, W.C. (1977) *Transpl. Proc.* **9**, 937.
136. Jeekel, J.J., McKenzie, I.F.C. & Winn, H.J. (1972) *J. Immunol.* **108**, 1017.
137. Fabre, J.W. & Morris, P.J. (1974) *Transplantation* **18**, 436.
138. Fabre, J.W. & Batchelor, J.R. (1975) *Transplantation* **20**, 269.
139. Zimmerman, B. & Feldman, J.D. (1973) *J. Immunol.* **103**, 383.
140. McKenzie, J.L., Fabre, W.J. & Morris, P.J. (1980) *Transplantation* **30**, 9.
141. Fabre, J.W. & Morris, P.J. (1973) *Transplantation* **15**, 397.
142. Fine, R.N., Batchelor, J.R., French, M.E. *et al.* (1973) *Transplantation* **16**, 641.
143. Biesecker, J.C., Fitch, F.W., Rowley, D.A. *et al.* (1973) *Transplantation* **16**, 421.
144. Burgos, H., French, M.E. & Batchelor, J.R. (1974) *Transplantation* **18**, 328.
145. Rao, V.S., Bonavida, B., Zhigelboim, J. *et al.* (1974) *Transplantation* **17**, 568.
146. Rao, V.S. & Bonavida, B. (1976) *Transplantation* **21**, 42.
147. Marquet, R.L., Heystek, G.A., Tank, B. *et al.* (1976) *Transplantation* **21**, 454.
148. Debray-Sachs, M., Liegeois, A. & Hamburger, J. (1976) *Transplantation* **22**, 323.
149. Quadracci, L.J., Tremann, J.A., Marchioro, T.L. *et al.* (1974) *Transplantation* **17**, 361.
150. Shoat, B., Cytron, S., Boner, C. *et al.* (1987) *Transplantation* **44**, 34.
151. Clarke, C.A., Donohoe, W.T.A., McConnell, R.B. *et al.* (1963) *Brit. Med. J.* **1**, 979.
152. Freda, V.J., Gorman, J.G. & Pollack, W. (1964) *Transfusion* **4**, 26.
153. Hutchinson, I.V. & Zola, H. (1977) *Transplantation* **23**, 513.
154. Hutchinson, I.V. & Zola, H. (1977) *Transplantation* **23**, 464.
155. Ryder, R. J.W. & Schwartz, R.S. (1969) *J. Immunol.* **103**, 970.
156. Haughton, G. (1971) *Cell. Immunol.* **2**, 567.
157. Ptak, W. & Pryjma, J. (1971) *Eur. J. Immunol.* **1**, 408.
158. Hutchinson, I.V. & Zola, H. (1977) *Transpl. Proc.* **9**, 961.
159. Hutchinson, I.V. & Zola, H. (1978) *Cell. Immunol.* **36**, 161.
160. Hutchinson, I.V., Roman, J. & Bonavida, N. (1979) *Adv. Exp. Med. Biol.* **121B**, 553.
161. Hutchinson, I.V., Rayfield, L.S. & Brent, L. (1982) *Transplantation* **33**, 204.
162. Hutchinson, I.V. & Brent, L. (1982) *Transplantation* **34**, 64.
163. Sinclair, N.R.StC. & Law, F.Y. (1979) *J. Immunol.* **123**, 1439.
164. Hutchinson, I.V. & Brent, L. (1981) *Nature* **292**, 353.
165. Hutchinson, I.V., Barber, W.H. & Brent, L. (1983) *Transplant. Proc.* **15**, 819.
166. Barber, W.H., Hutchinson, I.V. & Morris, P.J. (1983) *Transplantation* **36**, 475.

167. French, M.E. & Batchelor, J.R. (1971) *Transplantation* **20**, 45.
168. Bildsoe, P., Ford, W.L., Pettirossi, D. *et al.* (1971) *Transplantation* **12**, 189.
169. Fabre, W.J. & Morris, P.J. (1972) *Transplantation* **20**, 269.
170. French, M.E. & Batchelor, J.R. (1972) *Transpl. Rev.* **13**, 115.
171. Pearce, N.W., Dorsch, S.E. & Hall, B.M. (1990) *Transplantation* **50**, 1078.
172. Lucas, Z.J., Merkeley, J. & Travis, M. (1970) *Fed. Proc.* **29**, 2041.
173. Salaman, J. (1971) *Transplantation* **11**, 63.
174. Ippolito, R.J., Mahoney, R.J. & Murray, I.M. (1972) *Transplantation* **14**, 183.
175. Hutchinson, I.V. & Brent, L. (1982) *Transplantation* **34**, 305.
176. Tilney, N.L. & Bell, P.R. (1974) *Transplantation* **18**, 31.
177. Fabre, J.W. & Morris, P.J. (1972) *Transplantation* **14**, 634.
178. Ramseier, H. & Lindenmann, J. (1969) *Path. Microbiol.* **34**, 379.
179. Oudin, J. & Michel, M. (1963) *C.R. Acad, Sci. (Paris)* **257**, 805.
180. Ramseier, H. & Lindenmann, J. (1972) *Transpl. Rev.* **10**, 57.
181. McKearn, T.J., Stuart, F.P. & Fitch, F.W. (1974) *J. Immunol.* **113**, 1876.
182. Joller, P.W. (1972) *Nature* **240**, 214.
183. Binz, H., Lindenmann, J. & Wigzell, H. (1973) *Nature* **246**, 146.
184. McKearn, T.J. (1974) *Science* **183**, 94.
185. Kimura, A.K. (1974) *J. Exp. Med.* **139**, 888.
186. Binz, H. & Askonas, B.A. (1975) *Eur. J. Immunol.* **5**, 618.
187. Binz, H. & Wigzell, H. (1976) *Nature* **262**, 294.
188. Binz, H. & Wigzell, H. (1976) *J. Exp. Med.* **144**, 1438.
189. Wigzell, H. & Binz, H. (1977) *Proc. Eur. Dialys. Transpl. Ass.* **14**, 259.
190. Aguet, M., Andersson, L.C., Andersson, R. *et al.* (1978) *J. Exp. Med.* **147**, 50.
191. Fischer Lindahl, K. (1972) *Eur. J. Immunol.* **2**, 501.
192. Brent, L. & Kilshaw, P.J. (1976) *Nature* **262**, 443.
193. Fitch, F.W. & Ramseier, H. (1976) *J. Immunol.* **117**, 504.
194. Binz, H. & Wigzell, H. (1979) *Transpl. Proc.* **11**, 914.
195. Batchelor, J.R. & French, M.E. (1976) *Brit. Med. J.* **32**, 113.
196. Stuart, F.P., McKearn, T.J. & Fitch, F.W. (1976) *Surgery* **80**, 130.
197. Mybergh, J.A. & Smit, J.A. (1978) *Transplantation* **26**, 76.
198. Mybergh, J.A. & Smit, J.A. (1979) *Transpl. Proc.* **11**, 923.
199. Hart, D.A., Wang, A.L., Pawlak, L.L. *et al.* (1972) *J. Exp. Med.* **135**, 1293.
200. Cosenza, H. & Köhler, H. (1972) *Proc. Natl. Acad. Sci. U.S.A.* **69**, 2701.
201. Hart, D.A., Pawlak, L.L. & Nisonoff. A. (1973) *Eur. J. Immunol.* **3**, 44.
202. Eichmann, K. (1974) *Eur. J. Immunol.* **4**, 296.
203. Chew, W.B., Stephens, D.J. & Lawrence, J.S. (1936) *J. Immunol.* **30**, 301.
204. Metchnikoff, E. (1899) *Ann. Inst. Pasteur* **13**, 737.
205. Funck, M. (1900) *Zentralbl. f. Bakt.* **27**, 670.
206. Besredka, A. (1900) *Ann. Inst. Pasteur* **14**, 390.
207. Buchner, H. (1899) *Zentralbl. f. Bakt.* **6**, 561.
208. Flexner, S. (1902) *Univ. Penna. Med. Bull.* **15**, 287.
209. Bunting, C.H. (1903) *Univ. Penna. Med. Bull.* **16**, 200.
210. Christian, H.A. & Leen, J.P. (1905) *Boston Med. Surg. J.* **152**, 397.
211. Pappenheimer, A.M. (1917) *J. Exp. Med.* **26**, 163.
212. Chew, W.B. & Lawrence, J.S. (1937) *J. Immunol.* **33**, 271.
213. Cruickshank, A.H. (1941) *Brit. J. Exp. Path.* **22**, 126.
214. Bogomolets, A.A. (1943–1944) *Amer. Rev. Soviet Med.* **1**, 101. (Adapted by S.H. Fisher from the original.)
215. Linberg, B.E. (1943–1944) *Amer. Rev. Soviet Med.* **1**, 124 (Transl. by A.C. Kling.)
216. Marchuk, P.D. (1943–1944) *Amer. Rev. Soviet Med.* **1**, 113 (Transl. by M.G. Guseva & D.A. Halpern.)
217. Straus, R. (1946) *J. Immunol.* **54**, 151.
218. Straus, R., Runjavac, M., Zaitlin, R. *et al.* (1946) *J. Immunol.* **54**, 155.
219. Straus, R., Horwitz, M., Levinthal, D.H. *et al.* (1946) *J. Immunol.* **54**, 163.
220. Rogoff, B., Freyberg, R.H., Powell, H.M. *et al.* (1947) *Amer. J. Med. Sci.* **214**, 395.

221. Anigstein, L., Whitney, D. & Beninson, J. (1948) *Proc. Soc. Clin. Med.* **69**, 73.

222. Kling, D.H. (1948) *J. Lab. Clin. Med.* **33**, 1289.

223. Rifkinson, N. (1950) *J. Neuropath. Exp. Neurol.* **9**, 198.

224. Keller, J. (1954) *Wien. Med. Wchnschr.* **104**, 593.

225. Doetsch, H. (1956) *Ärztl. Wchnschr.* **11**, 474.

226. Schmidt, S. (1959) *Deutsch. Med. J.* **10**, 59; Schmidt, S. (1959) *Ztschr. Ges. Inn. Med.* **14**, 269.

227. Leger, W. (1956) *Monatsschr. Unfallh.* **59**, 1.

228. Loiseleur, J. (1956) *Ann. Inst Pasteur* **91**, 445.

229. Currey, H.L.F. & Ziff, M. (1966) *Lancet* **2**, 889.

230. Woodruff, M.F.A. & Forman, B. (1951) *Nature* **168**, 36.

231. Inderbitzen, T. (1956) *Int. Arch Allergy* **8**, 150.

232. Waksman, B.H. & Arbouys, S. (1960) In *Mechanisms of Antibody Formation*, p. 165, Czech. Acad. Sci., Prague.

233. Waksman, B.H., Arbouys, S. & Arnason, B.G. (1961) *J. Exp. Med.* **114**, 997.

234. Woodruff, M.F.A. & Anderson, N.F. (1963) *Nature* **200**, 702.

235. Woodruff, M.F.A. & Anderson, N.F. (1964) *Ann. N.Y. Acad. Sci.* **120**, 119.

236. Sacks, J.H., Fillipone, D.R. & Hume, D.M. (1964) *Transplantation* **2**, 60.

237. Gray, J.G., Monaco, A.P. & Russell, P.S. (1964) *Surg. Forum* **15**, 142.

238. Gray, J.G., Monaco, A.P., Wood, M.L. *et al* (1966) *J. Immunol.* **96**, 217.

239. Monaco, A.P., Wood, M.L., Gray, J.G. *et al.* (1966) *J. Immunol.* **96**, 229.

240. Levey, R.H. & Medawar, P.B. (1966) *Ann. N.Y. Acad. Sci.* **129**, 164.

241. Dumonde, D.C.L., Bitensky, G., Cunningham, G.D. *et al.* (1965) *Immunology* **8**, 25.

242. Russe, H.P. & Crowle, A. (1965) *J. Immunol.* **94**, 74.

243. Levey, R.H. & Medawar, P.B. (1966) *Proc. Natl. Acad. Sci.* **56**, 1130.

244. Lance, E.M. (1968) *Nature* **217**, 557.

245. Jeejeebhoy, H.F. (1965) *Immunology* **9**, 417.

246. Monaco, A.P., Abbott, W.M., Othersen, H.B. *et al.*(1966) *Science* **153**, 1264; see also Monaco, A.P., Wood, M.L., Van der Werf, B.A. *et al.* (1967) In *Antilymphocyte Serum*, eds G.E.W. Wolstenholme & M. O'Connor, p. 111, J. & A. Churchill, London.

247. Abaza, H.M., Nolan, B., Watt, J.G. *et al.* (1966) *Transplantation* **4**, 618.

248. Starzl, T.E., Marchioro, T.L., Faris, T.D. *et al.* (1966) *Amer. J. Surg.* **112**, 391.

249. Pichlmayr, R. (1966) *Klin. Wchnschr.* **44**, 594; see also Pichlmayer, R., Brendel, W., Fateh-Moghadam, A. *et al.* (1967) In *Congr. Colloques Univ. Liége*, **43**, 147.

250. Lawson, R.K., Ellis, L.R. & Hodges, C.B. (1966) *Transplantation* **5**, 169.

251. Mitchell, R.M., Sheil, A.G.R., Slafsky, S.F. *et al.* (1966) *Transplantation* **4**, 323.

252. Balner, H. & Dersjant, H. (1967) In *Antilymphocyte Serum*, eds G.E.W. Wolstenholme & M. O'Connor, p. 85, J. & A. Churchill, London.

253. Van Bekkum, D.W., Ledney, G.D., Balner, H. *et al.* (1967) In *Antilymphocyte Serum*, eds G.E.W. Wolstenholme & M. O'Connor, p. 97, J. & A. Churchill, London.

254. Balner, H., Van Bekkum, D.W., De Vries, M.J. *et al.* (1968) In *Advance in Transplantation*, eds J. Dausset, J. Hamburger & G. Mathé, p. 449, Munksgaard, Copenhagen.

255. James, K. & Medawar, P.B. (1967) *Nature* **214**, 1052.

256. Lance, E.M. (1967) In *Cell-bound Immunity with Special Reference to Antilymphocyte Serum and Immunopathology of Cancer*, Congr. Coll. Univ. Liége, **43**, 103.

257. Anderson, N.F., James, K. & Woodruff, M.F.A. (1967) *Lancet* **1**, 1126.

258. Woodruff, M.F.A., Reid, B. & James, K. (1967) *Nature* **215**, 591.

259. Lance, E.M. & Dresser, D. (1967) *Nature* **215**, 488.

260. Dresser, D. (1962) *Immunology* **5**, 378.

261. Clark, J.G., James, K. & Woodruff, M.F.A. (1967) *Nature* **215**, 870.

262. Guttmann, R.D., Carpenter, C.B., Lindquist, J.R. *et al.* (1967) *Transplantation* **5**, 1115.

263. Iwasaki, Y., Porter, K.A., Amend, J.R. *et al.* (1967) *Surg. Gynec. Obstet.* **124**, 1.

264. Lindquist, R.R., Guttmann, R.D., Carpenter, C.B. *et al.* (1969) *Transplantation* **8**, 545.

265. Nehlsen, S.L. (1971) *Clin. Exp. Immunol.* **9**, 63.

266. Simpson, E. & Nehlsen, S.L. (1971) *Clin. Exp. Immunol.* **9**, 79.

267. Lance, E.M. (1968) In *Advance in Transplantation*, eds J. Dausset, J. Hamburger & G. Mathé, p. 107, Munksgaard, Copenhagen.

268. Dalton, R.G., Anderson, N.F. & Sanders, J.H. (1972) *Transplantation* **14**, 65.
269. Denman, A.M. & Frenkel, E.P. (1967) *J. Immunol.* **99**, 498.
270. Howard, R.J., Dougherty, S.F. & Mergenhagen, S.E. (1968) *J. Immunol.* **101**, 301.
271. Hardy, M.A., Quint, J. & Monaco, A.P. (1970) *Transplantation* **9**, 487.
272. Raju, S. & Grogan, J.B. (1969) *Transplantation* **8**, 695.
273. Land, W., Seifert, J., Fateh-Meghadam, A., et al. (1969) *Transplantation* **8**, 748.
274. Pichlmayr, R., Land, W., Wagner, E. et al. (1969) *Klin. Wchnschr.* **47**, 628.
275. Balner, H., Yron, I., Dersjant, H. et al. (1970) *Transplantation* **10**, 416.
276. Svehag, S-E., Haxner, P., Manhem, L. et al. (1972) *Transplantation*, **14**, 21.
277. Golub, E.S. & Weigle, W.O. (1972) *J. Immunol.* **102**, 389.
278. Starzl, T.E., Groth, C.G., Terasaki, P.I. et al. (1968) *Surg. Gynec. Obstet.* **126**, 1023.
279. Bieber, C.P., Griepp, R.B., Oyer, P.E. et al. (1976) *Transplantation* **22**, 478.
280. Taub, R., Brown, S., Kochwa, S. et al. (1969) *Lancet* **2**, 521.
281. Butler, W.T., Leachman, R.D., Rossen, R.D. et al. (1969) *Nature* **224**, 856.
282. Moberg, A.W., Gewurz, H. & Simmons, R.L. (1970) *Transplantation* **10**, 344.
283. Wolf, R.E., Remmers, A.R., Sarles, H.E. et al. (1971) *Transplantation* **11**, 418.
284. Hanto, D.W., Jendrisak, M.D., So, S.K.S. et al. (1994) *Transplantation* **57**, 377.
285. Boak, J.L., Fox, M. & Wilson, R.E. (1967) *Nature* **215**, 1461.
286. Brent, L., Courtenay, T. & Gowland, G. (1967) *Nature* **215**, 1461.
287. Van Bekkum, D.W., Ledney, G.D., Balner, H. et al. (1967) In *Antilymphocyte Serum*, eds G.E.W. Wolstenholme & M. O'Connor, p. 97, J. & A. Churchill, London.
288. James, K. & Jubb, V.S. (1967) *Nature* **215**, 369.
289. James, K. & Anderson, N.F. (1967) *Nature* **213**, 1195.
290. Harris, S. & Harris, T.N. (1966) *J. Immunol.* **96**, 478.
291. James, K., James, V.S. & Pullar, D.M. (1969) *Clin. Exp. Immunol.* **4**, 93.
292. James, K. (1967) *Clin. Exp. Immunol.* **2**, 615.
293. Taub, R.N. (1970) *Progr. Allergy* **14**, 208.
294. Woodruff, M.F.A. (1970) *Symp. Series Immunobiol. Stand.* **16**, 379.
295. Lance, E.M., Medawar, P.B. & Taub, R.N. (1973) *Adv. Immunology* **17**, 1.
296. Levey, R.N. & Medawar, P.B. (1967) In *Antilymphocyte Serum*, eds G.E.W. Wolstenholme & M. O'Connor, p. 72, J. & A. Churchill, London.
297. Martin, W.J. & Miller, J.F.A.P. (1967) *Lancet* **2**, 1285.
298. Leuchars, E., Wallis, V.J. & Davies, A.J.S. (1968) *Nature* **219**, 1325.
299. Lance, E.M. & Batchelor, J.R. (1968) *Transplantation* **6**, 491.
300. Taub, R.N. (1970) *Fed. Proc.* **29**, 142.
301. Martin, W.J. (1969) *J. Immunol.* **103**, 1000.
302. Lance, E.M. (1969) *J. Exp. Med.* **130**, 49.
303. Russell, P.S. & Monaco, A.P. (1967) *Transplantation* **5**, 1086.
304. Levey, R.H. & Medawar, P.B. (1967) *Proc. Natl. Acad. Sci. U.S.A* **58**, 470.
305. Lance, E.M. (1968) Ph.D. Thesis, Univ. London.
306. Nelken, D. & Cohen, M. (1968) *Nature* **218**, 693.
307. Raju, S., Grogan, J.B. & Hardy, J.D. (1969) *J. Surg. Res.* **9**, 327.
308. Guttmann, R.D., Carpenter, C.B., Lindquist, R.R. et al. (1967) *Transplantation* **5**, 1115.
309. Guttmann, R.D., Carpenter, C.B., Lindquist, R.R. et al. (1967) *J. Exp. Med.* **126**, 1099.
310. Inderbitzin, Th. M. (1971) *Int. Arch. Allergy* **41**, 1110.
311. Cohen, M. & Nelken, D. (1970) *Clin. Exp. Immunol.* **6**, 137.
312. Guttmann, R.D., Lindquist, R.R. & Ockner, S.A. (1969) *Transplantation* **8**, 837.
313. Callender, C.O., Simmons, R.L., Toledo-Pereyra, L.H. et al. (1973) *Transplantation* **16**, 377.
314. Denman, A.M., Denman, E.J. & Holborow, E.J. (1968) *Nature* **217**, 177.
315. Rebellato, L.M., Gross, U., Verbanac, K.M. et al. (1994) *Transplantation* **57**, 685.
316. Monaco, A.P., Wood, M.L. & Russell, P.S. (1966) *Ann. N.Y. Acad. Sci.* **129**, 190.
317. Lance, E.M. & Medawar, P.B. (1969) *Proc. Roy. Soc. B.* **173**, 447.
318. Fisher, J.C., Davis, R.C. & Mannick, J.A. (1971) *Immunology* **20**, 901.
319. Nisbet, N.W. (1969) *Transplantation* **8**, 356.
320. Wood, M.L., Monaco, A.P., Gozzo, J.J. et al. (1971) *Transpl. Proc.* **3**, 676.
321. Wood, M.L. & Monaco, A.P. (1978) *Transpl. Proc.* **10**, 379.

322. Wood, M.L., Gottschalk, R. & Monaco, A.P. (1979) *Transplantation* **28**, 387.
323. Wood, M.L. & Monaco, A.P. (1980) *Transplantation* **29**, 196.
324. Simpson, M. & Gozzo, J.J. (1980) *Transplantation* **30**, 64.
325. Maki, T., Simpson, M. & Monaco, A.P. (1982) *Transplantation* **34**, 376.
326. Maki, T., Gottschalk, R. & Wood, M.L. (1981) *J. Immmunol.* **127**, 1433.
327. Muraoka, S. & Miller, R.G. (1980) *J. Exp. Med.* **152**, 54.
328. Rammensee, H., Fink, P. & Bevan, M. (1985) *Transpl. Proc.* **17**, 689.
329. Miller, R.G., Muraoka, S. & Claeson, M.H. (1988) *Ann. N.Y. Acad. Sci.* **532**, 170.
330. Fink, P.J., Shimonkevitz, R.P. & Bevan, M. (1988) *Annu. Rev. Immunol.* **6**, 115.
331. Wood, M.L., Orosz, C.G., Gottschalk, R. *et al.* (1992) *Transplantation* **54**, 665.
332. Thomas, J.M., Carver, F.M., Haisch, C.E. *et al.* (1982) *Transplantation* **34**, 83.
333. Monaco, A.P., Liegeois, A., Wood, M.L. *et al.* (1975) *Adv. Nephrol.* **5**, 135.
334. Thomas, J., Carver, F.M., Foil, M.B. *et al.* (1983) *Transplantation* **36**, 104.
335. Thomas, J., Carver, M., Cunningham, P. *et al.* (1987) *Transplantation* **43**, 332.
336. Mybergh, J.A., Smit, J.A., Mieny, C.J. *et al.* (1971) *Transplantation* **12**, 202.
337. Monaco, A.P., Wood, M.L., Maki, T. *et al.* (1988) *Transpl. Proc.* **20**, 122.
338. Liegeois, A., Charreire, J. & Brennan, J.L. (1974) *Surg. Forum* **25**, 297.
339. Starzl, T.E., Demetris, A.J., Trucco, M. *et al.* (1992) *Lancet* **340**, 876.
340. Starzl, T.E., Demetris, A.J., Murase, N. *et al.* (1992) *Lancet* **340**, 1579.
341. Floersheim, G.L. (1967) *Science* **156**, 951.
342. Floersheim, G.L. (1969) *Transplantation* **8**, 392.
343. Floersheim, G.L. & Brune, K. (1971) *Transpl. Proc.* **3**, 688.
344. Floersheim, G.L. (1973) *Transplantation* **15**, 195.
345. Billingham, R.E., Brent, L. & Medawar, P.B. (1958) *Transpl. Bull.* **5**, 377.
346. Brent, L., Medawar, P.B. & Ruszkiewicz, M. (1961) *Brit. J. Exp. Path.* **42**, 464.
347. Billingham, R.E. & Silvers, W.K. (1960) *J. Immunol.* **85**, 14.
348. Medawar, P.B. (1963) *Transplantation* **1**, 21.
349. Abbott, W.M., Monaco, A.P. & Russell, P.S. (1969) *Transplantation* **7**, 291.
350. Brent, L. & Kilshaw, P.J. (1970) *Nature* **227**, 898.
351. Brent, L., Hansen, J.A. & Kilshaw, P.J. (1971) *Transpl. Proc.* **3**, 684.
352. Brent, L. Hansen, J.A., Kilshaw, P.J. *et al.* (1973) *Transplantation* **15**, 160.
353. Pinto, M., Brent, L. & Thomas, A.V. (1974) *Transplantation* **17**, 477.
354. Brent, L. & Opara, S.C. (1979) *Transplantation* **27**, 120.
355. Wood, P., Horsburgh, T. & Brent, L. (1981) *Transplantation* **31**, 8.
356. Brooks, C.G., Brent, L., Kilshaw, P.J. *et al.* (1975) *Transplantation* **19**, 134.
357. Kilshaw, P.J., Brent, L. & Pinto, M. (1975) *Nature* **255**, 589.
358. Kilshaw, P.J., Brent, L., Brooks, C.G. *et al.* (1975) *Transpl. Proc.* **8**, 637.
359. Horsburgh, T., Wood, P.J. & Brent, L. (1981) *Transpl. Proc.* **7**, 385.
360. Kilshaw, P.J. & Brent, L. (1977) *Transpl. Proc.* **9**, 717.
361. Mybergh, J.A. & Smit, J.A. (1972) *Transplantation* **14**, 191.
362. Smit, J.A. & Mybergh, J.A. (1972) *Transplantation* **14**, 200.
363. Judd, K.P. & Trentin, J.J. (1973) *Transplantation* **16**, 351.
364. Cerilli, J. & Hattan, D. (1972) *Transplantation* **14**, 207.
365. Köhler, G. & Milstein, C. (1975) *Nature* **256**, 495.
366. Köhler, G. & Milstein, C. (1976) *Eur. J. Immunol.* **6**, 511.
367. Galfre, G., Howe, S.C., Milstein, C. *et al.* (1977) *Nature* **266**, 550.
368. Lemke, H., Hämmerling, G.J., Hohmann, C. *et al.* (1978) *Nature* **271**, 249.
369. Waldmann, H. (1989) *Ann. Rev. Immunol.* **7**, 407.
370. Kung, P.C., Goldstein, G., Reinherz, E.L. *et al.* (1979) *Science* **206**, 347.
371. Reinherz, E., Kung, P.C., Goldstein, G. *et al.* (1979) *J. Immunol.* **123**, 2894.
372. Thomas, Y., Sosman, J., Irigoyen, O. *et al.* (1980) *J. Immunol.* **125**, 2402.
373. Cosimi, A.B., Colvin, R.B., Burton, R.C. *et al* (1981) *N. Engl. J. Med.* **305**, 308.
374. Cosimi, A.B., Burton, R.C., Colvin, R.B. *et al.* (1981) *Transplantation* **32**, 535.
375. Chatenoud, L., Baudrihaye, M.F., Kreis, H. *et al.* (1982) *Eur. J. Immunol.* **12**, 979.
376. Russell, P.S., Colvin, R.B. & Cosimi, A.B. (1984) *Ann. Rev. Med.* **35**, 63.
377. Wong, J.T., Eylath, A.A., Ghobrial, I. *et al.* (1990) *Transplantation* **50**, 683.

378. Hirsch, R., Echans, M., Auchincloss, H. *et al.* (1988) *J. Immunol.* **140**, 3766.
379. Jenkins, M.K., Chen, C., Jung, G. *et al.* (1990) *J. Immunol.* **144**, 16.
380. Anasetti, C., Tan, P., Hansen, J.A. *et al* (1990) *J. Exp. Med.* **172**, 1691.
381. Nicolls, M.R., Aversa, G.G., Pearce, N.W. *et al.* (1993) *Transplantation* **55**, 459.
382. Hale, G., Bright, S., Chumbley, G. *et al.* (1983) *Blood* **62**, 873.
383. Waldmann, H., Poliak, A., Hale, G. *et al.* (1984) *Lancet* **2**, 483.
384. Cantor, H. & Boyse, E.A. (1975) *J. Exp. Med.* **141**, 1376.
385. Cantor, H. & Boyse, E.A. (1975) *J. Exp. Med.* **141**, 1390.
386. Jandinski, J., Cantor, H., Tadakuma, T. *et al.* (1976) *J. Exp. Med.* **143**, 1382.
387. Cobbold, S., Jayasuriya, A., Nash, T.D. *et al.* (1984) *Nature* **312**, 548.
388. Cobbold, S. & Waldmann, H. (1986) *Transplantation* **41**, 634.
389. Quin, S., Cobbold, S., Clark, M.R. *et al.* (1987) *Eur. J. Immunol.* **17**, 1159.
390. Quin, S., Wise, M., Cobbold, S. *et al.* (1990) *Eur. J. Immunol.* **20**, 2737.
391. Quin, S., Cobbold, S., Benjamin, R. *et al.* (1989) *J. Exp. Med.* **169**, 779.
392. Chen, Z., Cobbold, S., Metcalfe, S. *et al.* (1992) *Eur. J. Immunol.* **22**, 805.
393. Jonker, M., Goldstein, G. & Balner, H. (1983) *Transplantation* **35**, 521.
394. Jonker, M., Neuhaus, P., Zurcher, C. *et al.* (1985) *Transplantation* **39**, 247.
395. Mottram, P.L., Wheelahan, J. & McKenzie, I.F.C. (1987) *Transpl. Proc.* **19**, 522.
396. Nakayama, E., Shiko, H., Stockert, E. *et al.* (1979) *Proc. Natl. Acad. Sci. U.S.A.* **76**, 1977.
397. Shinohara, N., Hammerling, U. & Sachs, D.H. (1980) *Eur. J. Immunol.* **10**, 589.
398. Wofsky, D., Mayes, D.C., Woodcock, J. *et al.* (1985) *J. Immunol.* **135**, 1698.
399. Goronzy, J., Weyand, C.M. & Fathman, C.G. (1986) *J. Exp. Med.* **164**, 911.
400. Madsen, J.C., Peugh, W.N., Wood, K.J. *et al* (1987) *Transplantation* **44**, 849.
401. Pearson, T.C., Madsen, J.C., Larsen, C.P. *et al.* (1992) *Transplantation* **54**, 475.
402. Darby, C.R., Morris, P.J. & Wood, K.J. (1992) *Transplantation* **54**, 483.
403. Cosimi, A.B., Burton, R.C., Kung, R.C. *et al.* (1981) *Transpl. Proc.* **13**, 499.
404. Wee, S.L., Stroka, D.M., Preffer, F.I. *et al.* (1992) *Transplantation* **53**, 501.
405. Clason, A.E., Duarte, A.J.S., Kupiec-Weglinski, J.W. *et al.* (1982) *J. Immunol.* **129**, 252.
406. Heidecke, C.D., Kupiec-Weglinski, J.W., Lear, P.A. *et al.* (1984) *J. Immunol.* **133**, 582.
407. Kirkman, R.L., Barrett, L.V., Gaulton, G.N. *et al.* (1985) *J. Exp. Med.* **162**, 358.
408. Granstein, R.D., Goulston, C. & Gaulton, G.N. (1986) *J. Immunol.* **136**, 398.
409. Reed, M., Shapiro, M.E., Strom, T.B. *et al* (1989) *Transplantation* **47**, 55.
410. Cooper, M.M., Robbins, R.C., Goldman, C.K. *et al.* (1990) *Transplantation* **50**, 760.
411. Ueda, H., Hancock, W.W., Cheung, Y-C. *et al.* (1990) *Transplantation* **50**, 545.
412. Wood, M.J.A., Sloan, D.J., Dallman, M.J. *et al.* (1990) *J. Exp. Med.* **177**, 597.
413. Heagy, W., Waltenbaugh, C., & Martz, E. (1984) *Transplantation* **37**, 520.
414. Talento, A., Nguyen, M., Blake, T. *et al.* (1993) *Transplantation* **55**, 418.
415. Fischer, A., Griscelli, C., Blanche, S. *et al.* (1986) *Lancet* **2**, 1058.
416. Isobe, M., Yagita, H., Okomura, K. *et al.* (1992) *Science* **255**, 1125.
417. Priestley, C.A., Spencer, S.C., Sawyer, G.J. *et al.* (1992) *Transplantation* **53**, 1024.
418. Chatterjee, S., Bernoco, D. & Billing, R. (1982) *Hybridoma* **1**, 396.
419. Perry, L.L. & Williams, I.R. (1985) *J. Immmunol.* **134**, 2935.
420. Gamble, P., Francescetti, L.H. & Wegmann, T.G. (1984) *Transplantation* **38**, 152.
421. Isaacs, J.D., Watts, R.A., Hazleman, B.L. *et al.* (1992) *Lancet* **340**, 748.
422. Hale, G., Dyer, M.J.S., Clark, M.R. *et al.* (1988) *Lancet* **2**, 1394.
423. Green, D.R. & Webb, D.R. (1993) *Immunol. Today* **14**, 523.
424. Argyris, B.F. (1963) *J. Immunol.* **90**, 14.
425. Droege, W. (1973) *Curr. Titles Immunol. Transpl. Allergy* **1**, 95–7; 131–4.
426. Gershon, R.K. (1974) *Contemp. Topics Immunobiol.* **3**, 1.
427. Miller, J.F.A.P. (1967) *Lancet* **2**, 1299.
428. Staples, P.J., Gery, I. & Waksman, B.H. (1966) *J. Immunol.* **124**, 127.
429. Horiuichi, A. & Waksman, B.H. (1968) *J. Immunol.* **101**, 1322.
430. Işacović, K., Smith, S.B. & Waksman, B.H. (1965) *Science* **148**, 1333.
431. Toullet, F.T. & Waksman, B.H. (1966) *J. Immunol.* **97**, 686.
432. Billingham, R.E., Brent, L. & Medawar, P.B. (1956) *Phil. Trans. Roy. Soc. London, B.* **239**, 357.
433. Crowle, A.J. & Hu, C.C. (1969) *J. Immunol.* **103**, 1242.

434. Weigle, W.O. & Dixon, F.J. (1959) *J. Immunol.* **82**, 516.
435. Cohen, M.W, & Thorbecke, G.J. (1963) *Proc. Soc. Exp. Biol. Med.* **112**, 10.
436. Tong, J.L. & Boose, D. (1970) *J. Immunol.* **105**, 426.
437. Terman, D.S., Minden, P. & Crowle, A.J. (1973) *Cell. Immunol.* **6**, 273.
438. Chase, M.W. (1963) In *La Tolérance Acquise et la Tolérance Naturelle à l'égard des Substances antégeniques définies*, ed. A. Bussard, p. 139. Center National de la Recherche Scientifique, Paris.
439. McCullagh, P.J. (1970) *Aust. J. Exp. Biol. Med. Sci.* **48**, 351.
440. Batchelor, J.R., Boyse, E.A. & Gorer, P.A. (1960) *Transpl. Bull.* **26**, 449.
441. Cruse, J.M., Germany, W.W. & Dulaney, A.D. (1965) *J. Lab. Invest.* **14**, 1554.
442. Hutchin, P., Amos, D.B. & Prioleau, W.H. (1967) *Transplantation* **5**, 68.
443. Asherson, G.A., Zembala, M. & Barnes, R.M.R. (1971) *Clin. Exp. Immunol.* **9**, 111.
444. McGregor, D.D., McCullagh, P.J. & Gowans, J.L. (1967) *Proc. Roy. Soc. B.* **168**, 229.
445. Claman, N.H., Chaperon, E.A. & Triplett, R.F. (1966) *Proc. Soc. Exp. Biol. N.Y.* **122**, 1167.
446. Gershon, R.K. & Kondo, K. (1970) *Immunology* **18**, 723.
447. Gershon, R.K. & Kondo, K. (1971) *Immunology* **21**, 903.
448. Gershon, R.K., Cohen, P., Hencin, R. *et al.* (1972) *J. Immunol.* **108**, 586.
449. Gershon, R.K. (1975) *Transpl. Rev.* **26**, 170.
450. Gershon, R.K. (1980) *J. Allergy Clin. Immunol.* **6**, 18.
451. Greene, D.R., Flood, P.M. & Gershon, R.K. (1983) *Annu. Rev. Immunol.* **1**, 439.
452. Droege, W. (1984) *Immunol. Today* **5**, 161.
453. Droege, W. (1971) *Nature* **234**, 549.
454. Droege, W. (1973) *Eur. J. Immunol.* **3**, 804.
455. McCullagh, P.J. (1970) *Aust. J. Exp. Biol. Med. Sci.* **48**, 369.
456. McCullagh, P.J. (1970) *Aust. J. Exp. Biol. Med. Sci.* **48**, 351.
457. McCullagh, P.J. (1972) *J. Exp. Med.* **132**, 916.
458. McCullagh, P.J. (1975) *Aust. J. Exp. Biol. Med. Sci.* **53**, 413.
459. McCullagh, P.J. (1975) *Aust. J. Exp. Biol. Med. Sci.* **53**, 399.
460. Jacobson, E.N., Herzenberg, L., Riblet, R. *et al.* (1972) *J. Exp. Med.* **135**, 1163.
461. Asherson, G.A. & Zembala, M. (1973) *Nature* **244**, 227.
462. Phanuphak, P., Moorhead, J.W. & Claman, H.N. (1974) *J. Immunol.* **113**, 230.
463. Allison, A.C., Denman, A.M. & Barnes, R.D. (1971) *Lancet* **2**, 125.
464. Elkins, W.L. (1972) *Cell. Immunol.* **4**, 192.
465. Jirsch, D.W., Kraft, N. & Diener, E. (1974) *Transplantation* **18**, 155.
466. Phillips, S.M. & Wegmann, T.G. (1973) *J. Exp. Med.* **137**, 291.
467. Weissman, I.L. (1973) *Transplantation* **15**, 265.
468. Dorsch, S. & Roser, B. (1975) *Nature* **258**, 233.
469. Dorsch, S. & Roser, B. (1977) *J. Exp. Med.* **145**, 1145.
470. Dorsch, S. & Roser, B. (1982) *Transplantation* **33**, 418, 524.
471. Roser, B.J. (1989) *Immunol. Rev.* **107**, 179.
472. Kilshaw, P.J., Brent, L. & Pinto, M. (1975) *Transpl. Proc.* **7**, 225.
473. Turk, J.L., Parker, D. & Poulter, L.W. (1972) *Immunology* **23**, 493.
474. Askenase, P.W., Hayden, B.J. & Gershon, R.K. (1975) *J. Exp. Med.* **141**, 697.
475. Kilshaw, P.J., Brent, L. & Thomas, A.V. (1974) *Transplantation* **17**, 57.
476. Brent, L., Horsburgh, T. & Wood, P.J. (1980) *Transpl. Proc.* **12**, 464.
477. Rieger, M. & Hilgert, I. (1977) *J. Immunogenetics* **4**, 61.
478. Holáň, V., Chutná, J. & Hašek, M. (1978) *Nature* **274**, 895.
479. Folch, H. & Waksman, B.H. (1974) *J. Immunol.* **113**, 140.
480. Folch, H. & Waksman, B.H. (1974) *J. Immunol.* **113**, 127.
481. Rich, R.R. & Pierce, C.W. (1973) *J. Exp. Med.* **137**, 649.
482. Yoshinaga, M., Yoshinaga, A. & Waksman, B.H. (1972) *J. Exp. Med.* **136**, 956.
483. Droege, W. (1975) *Proc. Natl. Acad. Sci. U.S.A.* **214**, 895.
484. Batchelor, J.R., Phillips, B.E. & Greenan, D. (1984) *Transplantation* **37**, 43.
485. Barber, W.H., Hutchinson, I.V. & Morris, P.J. (1984) *Transplantation* **38**, 548.
486. Lancaster, F., Chui, Y.L. & Batchelor, J.R. (1985) *Nature* **315**, 336.
487. Thomas,, J.M., Carver, F.M., Cunningham, P.R.G. *et al.* (1991) *Transplantation* **51**, 198.
488. Kiziroglu, F. & Miller, R.G. (1991) *J. Immunol.* **146**, 1104.

489. Hutchinson, I.V. (1986) *Transplantation* **41**, 547.
490. Bloom, B.R., Salgame, P. & Diamond, B. (1992) *Immunol. Today* **13**, 131.
491. Dorf, M.E., Kuchroo, V.K. & Collins, M. (1992) *Immunol. Today* **13**, 241.
492. Nossal, G.J.V. & Pike, B.L. (1975) *J. Exp. Med.* **141**, 904.
493. Nossal, G.J.V. & Pike, B.L. (1980) *Proc. Natl. Acad. Sci. U.S.A.* **77**, 1602.
494. Malkovský, M. & Medawar, P.B. (1984) *Immunol. Today* **5**, 340.
495. Lamb, J.R., Skidmore, B.J., Green, N. *et al.* (1983) *J. Exp. Med.* **157**, 1434.
496. Quill, H. & Schwartz, R.H. (1987) *J. Immnuol.* **138**, 3704.
497. Jenkins, M. & Schwartz, R.H. (1987) *J. Exp. Med.* **165**, 302.
498. Cobbold, S.P., Martin, G. & Waldmann, H. (1990) *Eur. J. Immunol.* **20**, 2747.
499. Alters, S.E., Shizuru, J.A., Ackerman, J. *et al.* (1991) *J. Exp. Med.* **173**, 491.
500. Dallman, M.J., Shiho, O., Page, T.H. *et al.* (1991) *J. Exp. Med.* **173**, 79.
501. Heeg, K. & Wagner, H. (1990) *J. Exp. Med.* **172**, 719.
502. Quin, S., Cobbold, S.P., Pope, H. *et al.* (1993) *Science* **259**, 974.
503. Scully, R., Quin, S., Cobbold, S. *et al.* (1994) *Eur. J. Immunol.* **24**, 2383.
504. Lombardi, G., Sidhu, S., Batchelor, R. *et al.* (1994) *Science* **264**, 1587.
505. Burkly, L.C., Lo, D., Kanawaga, O. *et al.* (1989) *Nature* **342**, 564.
506. Lo, D., Burkly, L.C., Flavell, R.A. *et al.* (1989) *J. Exp. Med.* **170**, 87.
507. Morahan, G., Allison, J. & Miller, J.F.A.P. (1989) *Nature* **339**, 622.
508. Arnold, B., Schonrich, G. & Hämmerling, G.J. (1993) *Immunol. Today* **14**, 12.
509. Nossal, G.J.V. (1989) *Science* **245**, 147.
510. Dempster, W.J., Lennox, B. & Boag, J.W. (1950) *Brit. J. Exp. Path.* **31**, 670.
511. Starzl, T.E. (1964) *Experiences in Renal Transplantation*, p. 158, Saunders, Philadelphia.
512. Hume, D.M., Lee, H.M., Williams, G.M. *et al.* (1966) *Ann. Surg.* **164**, 352.
513. Kauffman, H.M., Cleveland, R.J., Dwyer, J.J. *et al.* (1965) *Surg. Gynecol. Obstet.* **120**, 49.
514. Ono, K., Lindsey, E.S. & Creech, O. (1969) *Transplantation* **7**, 176.
515. Gleason, R.E. & Murray, J.E. (1967) *Transplantation* **5**, 360.
516. Gergely, N.F. & Coles, J.C. (1970) *Transplantation* **9**, 113.
517. Kaplan, H.S. (1972) *Hodgkin's Disease*, pp. 216–279, Harvard Univ. Press, Cambridge, Mass.
518. Fuks, Z., Strober, S., Bobrove, A.M. *et al.* (1976) *J. Clin. Invest.* **58**, 803.
519. Slavin, S., Strober, S., Fuks, Z. *et al.* (1976) *Science* **193**, 1252.
520. Slavin, S., Strober, S., Fuks, Z. *et al.* (1977) *J. Exp. Med.* **146**, 34.
521. Slavin, S., Fuks, Z., Kaplan, H.S. *et al.* (1978) *J. Exp. Med.* **147**, 963.
522. Slavin, S., Reitz, B., Bieber, C.P. *et al.* (1978) *J. Exp. Med.* **147**, 700.
523. Slavin, S. & Strober, S. (1979) *J. Immunol.* **123**, 943.
524. Stark, J.H., Mybergh, J.A. & Smit, J.A. (1974) *Transpl. Proc.* **19**, 1987.
525. Zan-Bar, I., Slavin, S. & Strober, S. (1978) *J. Immunol.* **121**, 1400.
526. Bieber, C.P., Jamieson, S., Raney, A. *et al.* (1979) *Transplantation* **29**, 347.
527. Gottlieb, M., Strober, S., Hoppe, R.T. *et al.* (1980) *Transplantation* **29**, 487.
528. Mybergh, J.A., Smit, J.A., Browde, S. *et al.* (1980) *Transplantation* **29**, 401.
529. Mybergh, J.A., Smit, J.A., Hill, R.R.H. *et al.* (1980) *Transplantation* **29**, 405.
530. Mybergh, J.A., Meyers, A.M., Thompson, P.D. *et al.* (1989) *Transpl. Proc.* **21**, 826.
531. Waer, M., Vanrenterghem, Y., Ang, K.K. *et al.* (1984) *J. Immunol.* **132**, 1041.
532. Mybergh, J.A., Smit, J.A. & Meyers, A.M. (1986) *World J. Surg.* **10**, 369.
533. Waer, M., Vanrenterghem, Y. & Roels, L. (1987) *Transplantation* **43**, 371.
534. Saper, V., Chow, D., Engleman, E.D. *et al.* (1988) *Transplantation* **45**, 540.
535. Strober, S., Dhillon, M., Schubert, M. *et al.* (1989) *New Engl. J. Med.* **321**, 28.
536. Thomas, J., Alqaisi, M., Cunningham, P. *et al.* (1992) *Transplantation* **53**, 247.
537. Fradelizi, D., Mahooy, G., de Riberolles, C. *et al.* (1981) *Transplantation* **31**, 365.
538. Vaiman, M., Daburon, F., Remy, J. *et al* (1981) *Transplantation* **31**, 358.
539. Okada, S. & Strober, S. (1982) *J. Exp. Med.* **156**, 522.
540. Okada, S. & Strober, S. (1982) *J. Immunol.* **129**, 1892.
541. Morecki, S., Leshem, B., Weigensberg, M. *et al.* (1985) *Transplantation* **40**, 201.
542. Slavin, M., Morecki, S., Weigensberg, M. *et al.* (1986) *Transplantation* **41**, 680.
543. Strober, S., Dejbachsh-Jones, S., Van Vlasselaer, P. *et al.* (1989) *J. Immunol.* **143**, 1118.
544. Field, E.H. & Becker, G.C. (1989) *Transplantation* **48**, 499.

545. Bass, H. & Strober, S. (1990) *Cell. Immunol.* **126**, 129.
546. Florence, L.S., Jiang, G-L., Ang, K.K. *et al.* (1990) *Transplantation* **49**, 436.
547. Isaković, K., Smith, S.B. & Waksman, B.H. (1965) *J. Exp. Med.* **122**, 1103.
548. Miller, J.F.A.P. (1962) *Proc. Roy. Soc. B.* **156**, 415.
549. Dalmasso, A.P., Martinez, C., Sjodin, K. *et al.* (1963) *J. Exp. Med.* **118**, 1089.
550. Dubert, A. & Kaplan, H.S. (1961) *Fed. Proc.* **20**, 40 (abstract).
551. Bonomo, A. & Matzinger, P. (1993) *J. Exp. Med.* **177**, 1153.
552. Horiuchi, A. & Waksman, B.H. (1968) *J. Immunol.* **100**, 974.
553. Horiuchi, A. & Waksman, B.H. (1968) *J. Immunol.* **101**, 1322.
554. Nossal, G.J.V. & Pike, B.L. (1981) *Proc. Natl. Acad, Sci. U.S.A.* **78**, 3844.
555. Wood, P.J. & Streilein, J.W. (1982) *Eur. J. Immunol.* **12**, 188.
556. Morissey, P.J., Sharrow, S.O., Kohno, Y. *et al.* (1985) *Transplantation* **40**, 68.
557. Posselt, A.M., Barker, C.F., Tomaszewski, J.E. *et al.* (1990) *Science* **249**, 1293.
558. Vojtišková, M. & Lengerová, A. (1965) *Experientia* **21**, 661.
559. Ohzato, H. & Monaco, A.P. (1992) *Transplantation* **54**, 1090.
560. Posselt, A.M., Naji, A., Roark, J.H. *et al.* (1991) *Ann. Surg.* **214**, 303.
561. Remuzzi, G., Rossini, M., Imberti, O. *et al.* (1992) *Lancet* **337**, 750.
562. Perico, N., Rossini, M., Imberti, O. *et al.* *Transplantation* **54**, 943.
563. Blakely, M.L., Shaffer, D., Ohzato, H. *et al.* (1995) *Transplantation* **59**, 309.
564. Goss, J.A., Nakafusa, Y., Uchiyama, K. *et al.* (1992) *Transplantation* **54**, 1101.
565. Mayo, G.L., Posselt, A.M., Barker, C.F. *et al.* (1994) *Transplantation* **58**, 107.
566. Sayegh, M.H., Perico, N., Imberti, O. *et al.* (1993) *Transplantation* **56**, 461.
567. Oluwole, S.F., Chowdhury, N.C., Jin, M-X. *et al.* (1993) *Transplantation* **58**, 105.
568. Hamashima, T., Stepkowski, S.M., Smith, S. *et al.* (1994) *Transplantation* **56**, 1523.
569. Oluwole, S.F., Chowdhury, N.C. & Fawwaz, R.A. (1993) *Transplantation* **55**, 1389.
570. Knechtle, S.J., Wang, J., Jiao, S. *et al.* (1994) *Transplantation* **57**, 990.
571. Madsen, J.C., Superina, R.A., Wood, K.J. *et al.* (1988) *Nature* **332**, 161.
572. Une, S., Miyamato, M., Nakawaga, Y. *et al.* (1995) *Transpl. Proc.* **27**, 142.
573. Walker, K.G., Bolton, E.M. & Bradley, J.A. (1996) *Transplant. Internal.* (In press).
574. Odorico, J.S., Barker, C.F., Posselt, A.M. *et al.* (1992) *Surgery* **112**, 370.
575. Campos, L. Posselt, A.M., Deli, B. *et al.* (1994) *Transplantation* **57**, 950.
576. Binder, J., Sayegh, M.H., Watschinger, B. *et al.* (1994) *Transplantation* **58**, 80.
577. Binder, J., Sayegh, M.H., Watschinger, B. *et al.*(1995) *Transplantation* **59**, 590.
578. Odorico, J.S., O'Connor, T., Campos, L. *et al.* (1993) *Ann. Surg.* **218**, 525.
579. Chowdhury, N.C., Fawwaz, R.A. & Oluwole, S.F. (1993) *J. Surg. Res.* **54**, 368.
580. Goss, J.A., Nakafusa, Y., Yu, S. *et al.* (1993) *Transplantation* **56**, 166.
581. Markmann, J.F., Odorico, J.S., Bassiri, H. *et al.* (1993) *Transplantation* **55**, 871.
582. Oluwole, S.F., Chowdhury, N.C. & Fawwaz, R.A. (1993) *Transplantation* **55**, 1389.
583. Sayegh, M.H., Perico, N., Gallon, L. *et al.* (1994) *Transplantation* **58**, 125.
584. Odorico, J.S., Posselt, A.M., Naji, A. *et al.* (1993) *Transplantation,* **55**, 1104.
585. Posselt, A.M., Barker, C.F., Friedman, A.L. *et al.* (1992) *Science* **256**, 1321.
586. Ilstad, S.T. & Sachs, D.H. (1984) *Nature* **307**, 168.
587. Ilstad, S.T., Wren, S.M., Bluestone, J.A. *et al.* (1985) *J. Exp. Med.* **162**, 231.
588. Sharabi, Y. & Sachs, D.H. (1989) *J. Exp. Med.* **169**, 493.
589. Calne, R.Y., White, H.J.O., Yoffa, D.E. *et al.* (1967) *Brit. Med. J.* **4**, 645.
590. Binns, R.M. (1973) *Proc. Roy. Soc. Med.* **66**, 1155.
591. Parker, J.R., Hickman, R. & Terblanche, J. (1975) *Transplantation* **19**, 276.
592. Calne, R.Y., Sells, R.A., Pena, J.R. *et al.* (1969) *Nature* **223**, 472.
593. Baldwin, W.M. & Cohen, N. (1970) *Transplantation* **10**, 530.
594. Starzl, T.E., Porter, K.A., Putnam, C.W. *et al.* (1976) *Surg. Gynecol. Obstet.* **142**, 487.
595. Calne, R.Y. & Williams, R. (1977) *Brit. Med. J.* **2**, 471.
596. Kamada, N., Brons, G. & Davies, H.FF.S. (1980) *Transplantation* **29**, 429.
597. Houssin, D., Gigou, M., Franco, D. *et al.* (1980) *Transplantation* **29**, 418.
598. Kamada, N. & Shinomiya, T. (1985) *Immunology* **55**, 85.
599. Kamada, N. & Teramoto, K. (1988) *Transplantation* **46**, 165.
600. Kamada, N., Davies, H.FF.S., Wight, D. *et al.* (1983) *Transplantation* **35**, 304.

601. Kamada, N., Shinomiya, T., Tamaki, T. *et al.* (1986) *Transplantation* **42**, 581.
602. McDonald, J.C., Landreneau, M.D., Rohr, M.S. *et al.* (1988) *Transplantation* **45**, 474.
603. Davies, H.FF.S., Pollard, S.G. & Calne, R.Y. (1989) *Transplantation* **47**, 524.
604. Engemann, R., Ulrichs, K., Thiede, A. *et al.* (1983) *Transpl. Proc.* **15**, 729.
605. Gassel, H-J., Hutchinson, I.V., Engemann, R. *et al.* (1992) *Transplantation* **54**, 1048.
606. Gassel, H-J., Engemann, R., Thiede, A. *et al.* (1987) *Transpl. Proc.* **19**, 351.
607. Zimmermann, F.A., Davies, H.FF.S., Knoll, P.J. *et al.* (1984) *Transplantation* **37**, 406.
608. Salaman, J.R. (1968) *Nature* **220**, 930.
609. Salaman, J.R. (1968) *Transplantation* **11**, 63.
610. Linder, O.E.A. (1962) *Ann. N.Y. Acad. Sci.* **99**, 680.
611. Dunn, D.C. & Randall, G.K. (1974) *Transplantation* **17**, 406.
612. Russell, P.S., Chase, C.M., Colvin, R.B. *et al.* (1978) *J. Exp. Med.* **147**, 1449.
613. Burton, R.C., Fortin, J.L. & Russell, P.S. (1980) *J. Immunol.* **124**, 2936.

Biographies

**MICHAEL FRANCIS
ADDISON WOODRUFF
(1911–)**

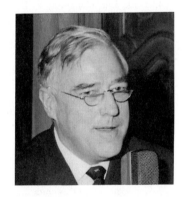

Michael Woodruff was born in London but, his parents having emigrated to Australia when he was young, he received his education first at Wesley College, Melbourne and then at Queen's College, University of Melbourne. His father had become Professor of Veterinarian Science and later Professor of Microbiology, and Michael therefore grew up in an academic environment. As a result he met Macfarlane Burnet after World War II in 1949 and, like many others subsequently, was duly influenced by him. Burnet had just published the Australian edition of his famous monograph with Frank Fenner, and Woodruff was stimulated to make some early attempts to prove experimentally the existence of immunologic tolerance. In the event, and fortunately for Medawar and his colleagues, these were unsuccessful, depending as they did on the transplantation of minute skin allografts to rat fetuses. This did not, however, prevent Woodruff from becoming one of the early pioneers of kidney transplantation – the first kidneys to be transplanted in the United Kingdom were in his unit in Edinburgh in 1962, the first from an identical twin – and his powerful intellect led him and his colleagues to make many crucial experimental observations in the field of tranplantation immunology. Woodruff was a surgeon/scientist *par excellence*.

Woodruff's entry into the field of organ transplantation is quixotically attributed by him (1) to the fact that as an officer in the Australian Medical Corps during World War II he was captured by the Japanese in 1942. He spent the remainder of the war in a prisoner of war camp in Singapore. Conditions were harsh, but he had managed to save a copy of R.H. Maingot's *Postgraduate Surgery*, which he read with interest. He was astonished to be told that human skin grafts transplanted to another person 'took' initially, but then failed to survive. Woodruff wrote in his *Recollections* (1): "I resolved that, if I survived the war, I would investigate the matter". And so he did! After the war he married his wife Hazel (they were to have two sons and one daughter), with whom he still lives happily in his retirement in Scotland and who helped him to carry out an early study of the fate of thyroid allografts transplanted to the anterior chamber of the eye of guinea pigs. It was this work that led him to formulate the concept of graft adaptation, which was to be influential.

His rise in the clinical and scientific communities was astronomic thereafter. His most significant contribution was to resurrect anti-lymphocyte serum, which others had worked on long before but the significance of which had not been appreciated. Woodruff and his colleagues gave it a great boost when they showed for the first time that the life of skin allografts could be prolonged by it. In the mid-1950s, at a time when Woodruff was Professor of Surgery at the University of Otago in New Zealand, P.B. Medawar spent a few months with him, and together they carried out some early tolerance induction experiments in the rat. Woodruff spent most of his working life at the University of Edinburgh, where he became Professor of Surgery and Director of the Nuffield Transplantation Surgery Unit until his retirement in 1976. In 1960 he published a massive and well-researched book *Transplantation of Tissues and Organs* and he has published many clinical and experimental papers. In his later years he developed a keen interest in the immunology of malignant tumors.

Woodruff, who was President of The Transplantation Society 1972–1974, has received many honors, including Fellowship of the Royal Society (1968), a Knighthood (1969), the Lister Medal, and the Gold Medal of the Society of Apothecaries. He was Vice-President of the Royal Society in 1979. He is a keen and expert sailor.

1. Woodruff, M.F.A. (1991) In *History of Transplantation: Thirty-five Recollections*, ed. P.I. Terasaki, p. 185, U.C.L.A. Tissue Typing Laboratory, Los Angeles.

7 Clinical Aspects and Immunosuppression

*"The transplantation of kidneys in medical practice has
already enjoyed greater success than any of us dared to believe
possible as recently as five years ago."*
P.B. Medawar, 1972

*"That chimerism should occur in man is clear proof that the
principle of tolerance applies to human beings as well as to laboratory animals,
and human chimeric twins can accept grafts of each other's skin."*
P.B. Medawar, 1961

Four aspects of clinical transplantation will be covered here.

(1) The early history of kidney allotransplantation. This topic has been chosen because the first successful kidney transplants, carried out against all odds, blazoned the trail for other organs and provided transplantation immunology with a huge impetus.
(2) Although some aspects of immunosuppression have been covered in Chapter 6 (e.g. antilymphocytic serum), I have not so far dwelt on the immunosuppressive drugs, which have made such a great impact on organ transplantation. Clearly, the pioneering attempts at kidney allotransplantation are cosely intertwined with efforts to depress the immune response with, initially, whole body irradiation (WBI) and later with drugs.
(3) The blood transfusion effect is an interesting story worth telling, even though it has not lived up to the high expectations pinned on it.
(4) Thanks to the recent work of T.E. Starzl and his colleagues the question of cellular, donor-specific chimerism – discussed in Chapter 5 in relation to neo-natally induced tolerance – has at last been brought into the clinical realm.

The history of the histocompatibility antigens and tissue typing is fully dealt with in Chapter 4, and transplantation of xenogeneic organs in Chapter 9.

The Dawn of "Modern" Kidney Allotransplantation

The pioneering work of the surgeons working in the early part of the twentieth century is described in Chapter 2. Here I would like to take up the story from the early 1950s. Some of it is covered by M.F.A. Woodruff's (1) book *The Transplantation of Tissues and Organs*, but as that was published in 1960 it is inevitably incomplete. Accounts of the history of organ or kidney transplantation have also been written by F.D. Moore in 1964 (2), J.M. Converse and P.L. Casson (3) in 1968 and by D. Hamilton (4) in 1979. T.E. Starzl's (5) assessment of the development of clinical renal transplantation and the illustrated history of organ transplantation by R. Küss and P. Bourget (6) are among the most recent.

Although much of the early activity took place in the United States and in France, it was in part the experimental work of W.J. Dempster (7, 8) in London and of M. Simonsen (9) in Copenhagen ion renal as well as skin transplantation in dogs that provided an appropriate milieu. Both had mastered the technique of kidney transplantation (pioneered by Carrel and others – see Chapters 3 and 9) (6) and advanced sound evidence for an immunologic basis of kidney allograft rejection. Their studies had in turn been strongly influenced by the incontrovertible proof by Medawar and others (see Chapter 2) from the mid-1940s onward that the fate of skin allografts in experimental animals was determined by the presence in the donor of antigens absent in the recipient inciting a powerful immunologic response. A further factor in encouraging the hope that kidney transplantation might be successful was the demonstration by Billingham, Brent and Medawar (see Chapter 5) in 1953 that mice could be made to accept allogeneic skin grafts permanently by the infusion of the donor's lymphoid cells into neonates – the first time that the rejection barrier to normal tissues had been convincingly and dramatically breached. It provided, according to T.E. Starzl (personal communication) "a blinding beacon of hope".

Sporadic attempts at transplanting human allogeneic kidneys had generally met with failure (10) (see below), and the first impressive successes were kidneys transplanted from monozygotic twin donors. Such grafts do not, of course, involve the recipient's immune system, but their importance lay in showing that transplanted kidneys could function and maintain the recipient in good health for many years, and they helped to make the transplantation of allografts a highly desirable objective.

The first successful monozygotic twin kidney was transplanted in 1954 and recorded in 1956 by Merrill et al. (11), and two years later the same group (12) at the Peter Bent Brigham Hospital in Boston described the results of seven such operations. One of the patients died 4–5 months later, the original disease having devastated the donor kidney, but most survived with well-functioning organs. One had developed the original disease of the patient's own kidneys but was still alive at the time of writing. The Boston team used essentially the operative techniques developed by the French (13–15). Others soon followed in 1960 – Krieg et al. (16), Ginn et al. (17), Woodruff et al. (18) and Dossetor et al. (19). The fact that in some cases the transplanted kidney developed the recipient's glomerular disease was of some concern but did not significantly dampen the euphoria created by these successes.

Some of the attempts made before this development are described by Hume et al. (10). The first 'modern' failure had been described by the Russian surgeon (20) U. Voronoy when he transplanted a cadaveric kidney into the groin of a patient suffering from mercury poisoning. The patient lived for only four days. (Voronoy is not to be confused with S. Voronoff, a Russian endocrinologist working in Paris, who gained notoriety in the 1930s with his attempts to use monkey glands to rejuvenate the elderly and who believed that sooner or later it would be possible to save human lives by transplanting organs from primates; see *21*). Nonetheless, the fact that three of the kidneys described by Hume *et al.* (*10*) survived for more than a month provided some encouragement. Lawler *et al.* (*22*) had a particularly early success, though not wholly conclusive, when they transplanted a cadaveric kidney to a woman with poly-cystic kidney disease. The donor's blood groups were the same as the recipient's and the patient was discharged with a urine output "within normal limits" on the twenty-ninth day. However, the kidney had to be removed on the sixty-third day when it was noted that an incomplete stricture had developed at the point of anastomosis of the two ureters. The appearance of the donor kidney was normal, but no histologic report was presented. The experience of the French, who had begun to transplant kidneys around 1950 (*13–15*), was similar. Michon *et al.* (*23*), for example, trans-planted a maternal kidney into a boy and found it functioned immediately, only to see it rejected abruptly on the twenty-second day. All these attempts, it should be stressed, were made without any form of immunosuppression.

Subsequently, Dammin, Couch and Murray (*24*) noted that uremia of the recipient permitted the prolonged survival of skin allografts, and once Mannick *et al.* (*25*) had demonstrated that renal canine allografts enjoyed substantially prolonged survival in dogs made deliberately uremic it became generally accepted that the transient survival of kidneys in untreated patients was largely brought about by uremia (*26*). Others, whose experience of human renal allografts in the mid-1950s was pretty dispiriting, were the Canadians G. Murray and R. Holden (*27*), regardless of whether they treated the patient with pyribenzamine, whole body irradiation (WBI) or cortisone. In their lengthy article published at about the same time, Hume *et al.* (*10*), having carried out nine transplants despite Dempster's (*8*) statement in 1953 that "It is quite out of the question that kidneys should be homotransplanted in man just in case a permanent survival might be obtained", concluded that "At the present state of our knowledge, renal homotransplants do not appear to be justified in the treatment of human disease". Their paper included a comprehensive review of previous clinical attempts.

Here I would like to add a note about David Hume. He worked for well over a decade at the Peter Bent Brigham Hospital, where he initiated the experimental kidney transplantation program and where he collaborated with Murray and Merrill and others. He subseqently moved to the Medical College of Virginia in Richmond to become Chairman of Surgery. Apart from his early forays into clinical transplantation he carried out experimental studies on renal allotransplantation in dogs and exper-imented with WBI as a means of suppressing the immune response (*28*). In this paper he and his colleagues came to the conclusion that the lymphoid cell infiltrate to be found in kidneys undergoing rejection was of host and not of donor origin, contrary to the speculations of Dempster and Simonsen (see Chapter 8). He was an unusually intelligent, humane and modest man and a bold surgeon and experimentalist, and his death in 1973 in a flying accident at the age of fifty-five was a great loss to the field of transplantation (*29*).

The use of WBI, with or without the replacement of the host's bone marrow with allogeneic bone marrow cells from the donor, was a live subject in the 1950s in a different context and this is described in Chapter 8. Once it was accepted that the poor survival of allogeneic human kidneys was brought about by an immune response of the recipient it was not long before this form of treatment was attempted in kidney transplantation, mainly in Boston and Paris toward the end of the 1950s. The strategy varied between giving sublethal doses of WBI or potentially lethal doses followed by the infusion of donor bone marrow in an attempt to replace that of the patient. The former procedure was followed, for example, by Hamburger *et al.* (30), when they transplanted a kidney from a non-identical twin. Despite an early rejection crisis, treated with a further dose of WBI, renal function became stable and the patient was well four months later and was to remain so for many years.

Meanwhile the Boston group Merrill *et al.* (31) had carried out its first successful transplants between non-identical twins using a potentially lethal dose of WBI and donor bone marrow. In most cases this proved to be an unsatisfactory form of treatment, but in one patient who had received a sublethal dose of WBI their efforts were crowned with the same striking success achieved by Hamburger *et al.* (30). Special features were that before treatment the patient had failed to reject a skin graft from the putative donor (presumed to be due to uremia), that the second recipient kidney, which had become infected, had been removed eleven days after the operation, and that a later rejection crisis had been reversed with cortisone and small doses of irradiation.

Other attempts at manipulating WBI in favor of kidney allograft recipients were made both in the United States and in France. Küss *et al.* (32) were remarkably successful with a sibling kidney, which functioned well (though not perfectly) at three months, but of the six cases described by Murray, Merrill and Dammin (33) in the same year (1960) the only success was that of a kidney from a non-identical twin. Woodruff's team in Edinburgh (34) subsequently reported a patient given a sibling kidney and a low dose of WBI with some additional local irradiation to the spleen; the patient died 30 days later. The results summarized by Küss *et al.* (35) in 1962 were equally discouraging.

Meanwhile Dempster (36) had shown with the greatest clarity in dogs that second kidneys from the same donor, but not from a different donor, underwent "rapid disintegration", thus repeating with kidneys what Medawar had demonstrated with rabbit skin grafts a decade previously (see Chapter 2). The immunologic nature of kidney allograft destruction was therefore no longer in doubt. Dempster removed functioning kidney transplants in the first four days and described the histology in great detail, especially the plasma cell infiltrate, which he wrongly ascribed to a response of the kidneys against their hosts (see Chapter 8). He also showed that a kidney could be successfully retransplanted to the donor after residence in the allogeneic animals for one day, but not after two days. In 1960 an editorial in the *British Medical Journal* (37) expressed the view that "all who have studied the matter" could agree that:

(1) The kidney is a transplantable organ.
(2) "True homografts of the kidney may be expected to fail ... for immunologic reasons."

It was at this stage that azathioprine (or Imuran) became available as an immuno-suppressive drug. The great advantages of using a drug rather than WBI, with its radical and irreversible effects, quickly became apparent. This important innovation and the revolutionary impact it had on renal allotransplantation are discussed in the next section, together with the introduction of the use of corticosteroid hormones.

The Advent of the Immunosuppressive Drugs

Azathioprine (Imuran)

Like many other immunosuppressive agents, the cytotoxic drug 6-mercaptopurine (6-MP) or its imidazole derivative azathioprine (Imuran) was developed as part of the screening process for anti-mitotic agents that might prove useful in the treatment of cancer. Its chemical and biologic properties and its ability to interfere with the use of purines in nucleic acid synthesis had been described by the Americans G.B. Elion and G.H. Hitchings (38) in 1957. Its immunosuppressive potential was revealed a year later by R. Schwartz, J. Stack and W. Damashek (39), working in Boston, when they used it to suppress the antibody response of rabbits to bovine serum albumin (BSA). The drug had to be administered at the same time as the antigen, and it was assumed that it acted only on the primary response. They showed that this was correct a year later (40), and a further paper in 1959 published in *Nature* (41) made it clear that they were not merely suppressing the antibody response but were in fact inducing tolerance to BSA. In other words, the rabbits failed to make the specific antibody after cessation of the drug treatment and being confronted with the antigen.

At this point in the story events became somewhat hectic, with several groups using the drug to prolong the life of skin allografts. Schwartz and Damashek presented a paper at the Seventh European Congress of Haematology in London in September, 1959, but thanks to various delays it was not published until nine months later, in June 1960 (42). They had found that the drug used in a daily dose of 12 mg/kg roughly tripled the survival time of rabbit skin allografts. Schwartz and Damashek illustrated their paper with both macroscopic and microscopic pictures of the grafts and again found that a second-set response (i.e. a secondary response in presensitized animals) could not be suppressed. Although higher doses were more effective they were also toxic, and they wrote that "Its toxicity in man and its limited effects in the rabbit preclude its immediate application to problems of tissue transplantation in humans". In the meantime R.A. Good's group at the University of Minnesota had begun similar studies and their results were published more rapidly; thus their paper appeared in December 1959 in *Proceedings of the Society for Experimental Biology and Medicine* (43). Using somewhat lower doses of 6-MP they too encountered some toxicity but found that the survival of rabbit skin allografts could be significantly prolonged.

Enter R.Y. Calne, the English transplant surgeon working at that time at the Royal Free Hospital in London and the Royal College of Surgeons. He used the drug in dogs in an attempt to bring about the prolonged survival of kidney allografts. His preliminary communication was published in February 1960 in the *Lancet* (44): he too found that the drug was highly toxic, but although most dogs died from toxicity within 10–14 days, the kidneys did not reveal any signs of a host response. On reducing the drug dose, two dogs survived for 21 and 47 days, respectively, with no microscopic signs of an allograft response. They died of pneumonia, presumably due to excessive immunosuppression. Calne wrote: "My observations . . . suggest that this drug can modify the rejection of renal homografts in dogs. It could have advantages over total body irradiation in being less hazardous, and possibly less crippling immunologically, though it seems to increase liability to infection and can cause hepatic biliary stasis. Its use might offer an approach to renal homografting in man, especially in uremic patients in whom homograft rejection is already depressed".

At roughly the same time C.F. Zukoski, a young surgeon working with Hume, had made similar observations in dogs and their data were published with Lee (45) in *Surgical Forum* later in 1960 although the abstract had been submitted for selection as early as mid-February. Their studies were extensive and included a group of dogs in which bilateral nephrectomy had been performed at the time of transplantation of the allogeneic kidneys. The toxicity of 6-MP was confirmed, but histologic signs of rejection were much reduced. Two kidneys functioned beyond twenty-seven days, one with good and the other with indifferent function. Numerous kidneys were examined histologically. These workers noted that the lymph nodes and the spleen of dogs on a regimen of 5 mg/kg for two weeks were "almost totally lacking in lymphocytes and had no follicular structures present", a scenario that they likened to the effects of WBI. They acknowledged Calne's *Lancet* paper, which had appeared while their work was in progress.

It remains a matter of conjecture as to why some articles were published more rapidly than others; the journals chosen by authors were no doubt an important factor. Be that as it may, it is clear that several groups of investigators, working at roughly the same time, established 6-MP as a potentially valuable drug for human application, though pride of place must belong to Schwartz and Damashek for their pioneering studies on the immunologic properties of 6-MP and to Calne for being the first to demonstrate its efficacy in experimental renal transplantation.

Calne then went to Boston to join the group at the Peter Bent Brigham Hospital. There he carried out further studies on the efficacy of 6-MP and other drugs obtained from G.H. Hitchings in suppressing the response to canine kidney allografts, and his extensive data were published in 1961 (46). A variety of doses were tried in an attempt to prevent toxicity without prejudicing graft survival. His most spectacular success was in a dog treated with BW 57–322, an imidazole derivative of 6-MP acting, like 6-MP itself, as an antimetabolite (47): the dog was "alive and well" after 122 days although, like the others, it had been bilaterally nephrectomized at the time of transplantation. Calne found BW 57–322 was as effective as 6-MP, but easier to manage with regard to bone marrow depression, though both drugs decreased the animals' resistance to infection. Unlike Schwartz and Damashek in rabbits he found that rejection occurred ten days after cessation of the treatment in a dog that had up to then carried a very healthy transplant. Tolerance had therefore not been created. Interestingly, Gombos, Tischler and Jacina (48) had reported in the same volume number of *Transplantation Bulletin* the induction of skin graft tolerance by the neonatal exchange transfusion of puppies.

Calne published other experimental papers with Murray (49) and G.P.J. Alexandre (a Belgian visitor to the Brigham Hospital) and Murray (50). In the latter a total of 104 experiments were reported, using several drugs. BW 57–322 in combination with actinomycin C was found to be the most favorable combination, and from the total number of animals used 10% survived for more than three months. The authors felt that the accidental choice of donors with shared histocompatibility antigens might have been responsible for the long survivors. In the same year Good's group (51) reported on their experience with 6-MP in dogs: out of 51 kidney transplants, 15 survived for more than 15 and one beyond 400 days. However, four of the longest-surviving kidneys displayed glomerular, tubular and arteriolar lesions with "round cell" infiltrates.

There now followed a few years of hectic activity, both experimental and clinical. Despite the fact that as late as 1962 the French group Hamburger *et al.* (52) were able to report that three of six patients who had received kidneys from close living relatives and treated with about 450 rad WBI survived for very long periods – the longest more than two-and-a-half years – there was now a growing tendency to abandon WBI in favor of drugs. The drug-orientated activity came mainly from the Peter Bent Brigham Hospital, and Murray, Merrill and their colleagues produced several substantial reports, which left little doubt that drug therapy had come to stay. In their 1962 paper (53) they showed that of 12 patients treated with WBI, only one survived permanently whereas five of six treated with 6-MP or its imidazole derivative Imuran had measurable function, with one surviving beyond four months. Likewise, their large-scale canine experiments pointed in the same direction, the combination of Imuran and actinomycin C having proved to be the best drug combination. They noted a "striking reversibility of the rejection process by the use of the drug in many animals". A year later they reported five cases in which only drug treatment (Imuran with or without azaserine or actinomycin C) was used (54), and they listed the very great advantages of using drugs rather than WBI. Tissue typing was, at this time, "not too highly developed". They concluded that ". . . this report permits a note of cautious optimism in a problem that ten years ago was considered almost insoluble".

The message was strongly reinforced when the same group (55) described a patient whose cadaveric kidney had sustained him for over 15 months, the last five with stable kidney function. He had been treated with azathioprine. Rejection episodes had been countered, not wholly successfully, with actinomycin C, and prednisone treatment was commenced on the 128th day. This brought about stabilization though the procedure had to be repeated some months later. At the time of writing, 15 months after transplantation, the patient was on low doses of azathioprine and prednisone, with relatively poor renal function. In the same year Hume *et al.* (56) reported six patients, mainly with non-twin related donors but one with a cadaveric kidney, who were given a mixed bag of low dose WBI, prednisone and Imuran, which left them to conclude that "Renal homotransplantation is showing signs of coming of age, but it is still a highly experimental procedure . . .". Finally, Murray *et al.* (57), in yet another substantial experimental study in dogs, reported on the mechanism of action of immunosuppressive drugs. More than 1000 animals were used and 24 different drug protocols tested. The combination of azathioprine and azaserine provided the best results, with 90% of kidneys surviving on day 50.

The award of the 1990 Nobel Prize to J.E. Murray for his pioneering role in establishing clinical kidney transplantation raises the question of what contribution others had made. Hume and Merrill, both of whom had been deeply involved, were dead by 1990, but the Frenchmen Küss and Hamburger were not. The pioneering work of the French has, in general, probably been underrated. This came about partly because they tended to publish their data in French journals like *Presse Médicale* and of course in French, a language unfortunately not always mastered by Anglo-Saxon surgeons and scientists. (As I have argued elsewhere (see Chapter 6), G.A. Voisin may have suffered some neglect for the same reason.) However, there is no doubting that the Peter Bent Brigham group, of which Murray was the most prominent leader and F.D. Moore the *'eminence grise'*, was the first to accomplish the first transplant between identical twins and they followed up this seminal demonstration with great energy and singlemindedness in a stream of papers advancing the cause of both experimental and clinical renal allotransplantation. If any one person had to be selected to represent the early kidney transplant pioneers, Murray was the right choice.

The use of corticosteroid hormones

Starzl's group in Denver, Colorado were instrumental in establishing the use of massive doses of prednisolone to reverse rejection crises and to stabilize graft function. Thus, in 1963 Starzl, Marchioro and Waddell concluded (58) in 1963 that rejection crises in human allografts "can be regularly reversed by the addition of actinomycin C and massive doses of prednisone to pre-existing therapy with azathioprine". They believed that "a host–graft non-reactivity followed, lasting for as long as six months", enabling them to return their patients to a pre-crisis maintenance dose. They wondered whether this presaged some sort of host–graft adaptation, an idea first mooted by Woodruff (59, 60). Starzl's group a year later (61) confirmed the benefit of corticosteroids in reversing rejection crises in dogs. All eight dogs that had been given azathioprine routinely developed rejection crises, and the addition of 50–200 mg of prednisolone per day led to rapid improvement in seven out of the eight cases. However, gastrointestinal bleeding proved to be a serious complication. They wrote: "From these experiments it would appear to be a valuable adjunct in reversing established rejection when added in large doses . . . ".

The routine combined use of azathioprine and prednisone soon became established in clinical practice, with additional high doses of prednisone administered in the treatment of rejection crises. This remained the standard immunosuppressive protocol for almost the next two decades until the advent of cyclosporin, despite the many side-effects caused by steroids. Thanks to greater experience with the administration of drugs and better patient management, kidney allotransplantation improved steadily until it reached a plateau towards the mid-1970s. The blood transfusion effect (see below) provided further benefits in increasing the proportion of long-term survivors.

The first Human Kidney Transplant Conference (62, 63) was held in Washington D.C. in 1963, with opening remarks and a summary of data compiled from questionnaires by J.E. Murray – the beginnning of the Kidney Registry, which was to perform a valuable service in monitoring progress over the years. Murray concluded his analysis by stating: "Although the beginnings of clinical success are apparent, strong reservations must be kept in mind regarding the ultimate fate of these patients. Kidney transplantation is still highly experimental and not yet a therapeutic procedure". It was soon to become just that. By 1969 Calne (64) felt able to write: ". . . to see patients with good functioning renal transplants back at work and leading normal lives makes it clear that the effort is worth while and does not differ in principle from the efforts medical men normally make in trying to help their patients". Although some transplant surgeons hoped that the highly prolonged survival of kidney allografts was thanks to the development of tolerance, this generally proved not to be the case though more recently some evidence in favor of this notion has come to light (see later).

The tenth report of the Human Renal Transplant Registry (65) was published in 1972 and illustrated the vast increase in the number of renal transplants of all kinds, from sibling to cadaveric. It was based on reports from as many as 220 centers in the United States, Canada, Europe and Australasia, and it showed graphically that a steady improvement had been maintained until the late 1960s. Thus, 47% of cadaveric kidneys functioned for two years in 1970, compared with only 25% in the period 1951–1966. Somewhat ominously the data for 1969 and 1970 were much the same.

In 1967 The Transplantation Society was formed in Paris under its first elected President, P.B. Medawar, and it took over the function that had up to then been served by a series of international meetings under the aegis of the New York Academy of Sciences and the surgeon J.M. Converse. Both the New York meetings and the biannual conferences of The Transplantation Society, attended as they were by clinicians and experimentalists, provided important focal points in the development of clinical transplantation.

The immunosuppressive potential of corticosteroid hormones in transplantation had in fact been recognized way back in the 1950s and this aspect will now be briefly considered. Two publications in 1951 were seminal. Billingham et al. (66), at that time still in Birmingham, United Kingdom, demonstrated that the daily administration of cortisone acetate to rabbits lengthened the life of skin allografts by a factor of three or four. They argued that this was "partly due to a non-specific reduction of the graft's own ability to incite an immune response, but . . . mainly due to the reduction of the response itself". They added that "It need hardly be said that the response of the rabbit . . . may be very different from that of a human being", but nonetheless stated that "The possible usefulness of this requires no comment". In the same group's second paper (67) they described experiments in which even the local application of cortisone acetate to rabbit skin allografts produced a significant prolongation of survival – an effect that was conspicuously absent if the rabbits had been presensitized. They quoted several publications showing that the conjunctival injection of very small doses of cortisone can be successfully used to treat inflammatory conditions of the eye, and in their first publication they referred to a case study by an American physician, J. Whitelaw (68), who found that the administration of adrenocorticotrophic hormone (ACTH) to a patient with severe burns seemed to facilitate the greatly extended survival of skin allografts. However, in this case it is far from clear whether the graft prolongation was due to stress (i.e. the patient's own hormonal activity) or to the exogenous ACTH.

J.A. Morgan (69) had, quite independently, likewise demonstrated the power of cortisone acetate to prolong the survival of rabbit skin allografts. Medawar's Ph.D. student, E.M. Sparrow (70, 71), carried out similar studies in the guinea pig and found that in this species cortisone alcohol was about twice as effective as cortisone acetate. In inbred mice Medawar and Sparrow (72) investigated several hormones. Cortisone acetate at a dose of 0.4 mg/day prolonged skin allograft survival by about 50%, cortisol was as effective as cortisone, but corticosterone, progesterone, testosterone and estradiol were inactive. They pointed out that cortisone did not counteract a pre-existing immunity and concluded that the action of cortisone was partly explained by the prevention of antigenic matter gaining access to the regional lymph nodes and partly by an effect on the regional lymph nodes themselves.

One of Medawar's colleagues P.L. Krohn, an endocrinologist who had participated in the early studies, made a particularly significant observation in 1954 (73). He set out to study systematically whether the so-called 'second-set' response in rabbits (i.e. the greatly accelerated rejection of grafts in animals that had already rejected grafts from the same donor) could be prevented by cortisone treatment. In keeping with Medawar and Sparrow's results he found that it could not unless cortisone treatment was commenced several weeks before transplantation of the second grafts. In that event the fate of the grafts was more like that expected of first-set grafts. In other words, Krohn had succeeded in abrogating secondary responses by prolonged treatment. Krohn concluded that ". . . these experiments justify the belief that treatment with cortisone, if persisted in, can inhibit even the immune response to a second set of skin homografts". Krohn's study and the earlier observations of Billingham *et al.* (66, 67) were to have a strong influence on Starzl when he decided to use cortisone in renal transplant recipients undergoing dangerous rejection crises. Although it took some time for the significance of these early studies to filter through they nonetheless set the scene for the later introduction of cortisone as an immunosuppressant agent in the treatment of renal allograft recipients.

The cyclosporine era

Because the efficacy of azathioprine and steroid treatment had reached a plateau by the mid-1970s, the advent of another potent immunosuppressive drug with modest side-effects was warmly welcomed by transplant surgeons. During the course of a screening program of fungus extracts Dreyfuss *et al.* (74), working in the Sandoz Laboratories in Basle, discovered in 1976 a new antilymphocytic agent extracted from the fungi *Trichoderma polysporum* (Link ex Pers.) Rifai or *Cylindrocarpon lucidum* Booth. The active ingredient was quickly found to be a cyclic endecapeptide with several known N-methylated amino acids and one new one (75, 76). It was J. Borel *et al.*, also working with Sandoz, who were the first to show that this drug, which was called cyclosporin A (CSA), had remarkable powers of suppressing a variety of immunologic responses. Thus, in their first publication Borel *et al.* (77) showed that oral administration of the drug to mice depressed the appearance of antibody-forming cells and the formation of hemagglutinins, prolonged skin allograft survival, delayed the onset of graft-versus-host disease, and prevented the occurrence of paralysis in rats with allergic encephalomyelitis. Further, it interfered with the development of Freund's adjuvant arthritis in rats and even improved the symptoms of the established condition. The authors pointed out that, in contrast with other immunosuppressive and cytostatic drugs, CSA had a low myelotoxicity, and they concluded that ". . . particularly because of its low degree of myelotoxicity, an appraisal of the present results obtained in animal models should, at a more advanced stage, support its investigation in clinical indications like organ transplantation . . .".

As if these immunologic credentials were not adequate the same group (78), a year later, went on to demonstrate that CSA was effective in several species and that it could interfere with the secondary antibody response and delay the cutaneous hypersensitivity reaction in guinea pigs to a contact allergen as well as to tuberculin. Because the drug failed to suppress antibody formation to lipopolysaccharide antigens in nude mice lacking T lymphocytes the authors felt that this suggested "a selective effect on T cells". Only high doses of the drug proved to be myelotoxic. Although the mode of action was unclear there was evidence suggesting that it acted by triggering immunocompetent lymphocytes, presumed to be T cells. It seemed only a matter of time before this exciting new compound would be tried out in organ transplantation.

Yet there was an element of serendipity about this next step, as Calne (79) explained in his recent recollections. A Greek surgeon, A. Kostakis, had spent two years in the laboratory with Calne's colleague D.J.G. White without having much to show for it and he felt that his Professor would be upset if he returned without useful data. He thought he might like to study immunosuppression, and to this end he acquired the technique of heart transplantation in rats. White had a bottle of CSA sitting on one of his shelves – it had been given to him by Borel some time ago – and he suggested to Kostakis that he might want to try out this new agent. Two months later he told Calne of some very exciting results, which Calne thought so extraordinary that he assumed that Kostakis must have muddled up the rat strains! However, there followed two brief papers, the first (80) describing the prolongation of cardiac allograft survival in rats and the second (81) adding a warning about the drug's toxicity as an alcoholic solution. In their first communication Kostakis et al. had used olive oil as solvent, administered intramuscularly, and rapid communication it prolonged allograft survival five-fold without undue toxicity. A third communication to the same journal by Calne and White (82) showed that oral administration of the drug in olive oil was astonishingly effective in prolonging the life of canine renal allografts, all nine functioning at 20 days (group 1). Among those dogs in which drug treatment had been discontinued between the seventh and fourteenth day was one that was alive seven weeks after transplantation. CSA in alcohol was less effective, and the CSA data were greatly superior to those obtained with azathioprine, which was associated with a high incidence of infection. The authors wrote that ". . . the consistency of the results in group 1 and the lack of toxicity . . . are remarkable when compared with any of the many different agents, including azathioprine . . .". These early experiments of the Cambridge group were the seeds of the cyclosporine era in organ transplantation, and soon many workers – including Calne's group – confirmed the great promise shown by CSA. Indeed, the research floodgates were opened, and looking at the publications in the field of transplantation in the post-1979 years one gains the impression that almost every laboratory in the world was studying various aspects of the drug.

Because the hopes of Sandoz that CSA might prove to be an anti-cancer agent had been disappointed they had decided not to produce the drug for marketing until they were persuaded otherwise by the dramatic results of the Cambridge group and by their advocacy of the drug's potential.

It is not possible or desirable to trace the explosive experimental or clinical development of CSA. I will confine myself to a few publications that confirmed the experimental work of the Cambridge group in the following year and to the first clinical demonstration of the drug's efficacy, leading to the abandonment of azathioprine as the main immunosuppressive agent. C.J. Green and A.C. Allison (83), working in the Medical Research Council's Clinical Research Centre near London, were the first to provide strong confirmation by showing that nephrectomized rabbits treated daily for four weeks not only accepted renal allografts but also sustained them after cessation of treatment for long periods. (This last finding, though confirmed by them (84), was unfortunately not found to apply to human kidney allografts.) Because the authors had evidence suggesting that CSA was toxic for human T and B lymphoblasts, but not for resting lymphocytes they speculated that the drug might be able to elim- inate clones of stimulated lymphocytes thus explaining the survival of grafts after cessation of drug treatment. Their paper was juxtaposed to another by Calne's group (85) showing that the survival of cardiac allografts in major histocompatibility complex (MHC)-mismatched pigs was likewise substantially prolonged.

In the same year (1978) came a cautionary tale from R.L. Powles *et al.* (86) at the Royal Marsden Hospital in Sutton, United Kingdom, who had used CSA in the treatment of patients given allogeneic bone marrow transplants. Although the acute erythematous skin reactions of graft-versus-host disease (GVHD) had resolved within two days, four of five of these patients died within seven weeks with (but not neces- sarily from) liver damage. "We conclude that cyclosporin A is active against acute skin GVHD and is effective within thirty-six hours", they wrote, and they expressed the view that a trial was "now justifiable in man". This was the first time CSA had been used clinically. Two years later the same group (87) reported on a larger trial in allogeneic bone marrow recipients. Although some toxic effects of CSA were observed, mainly in the kidneys, these were reversible. Significantly, only one of 20 patients treated with CSA developed acute GVHD and died, compared with 11 out of 26 who had been treated with methotrexate as a prophylactic agent. "Clearly there is need for caution", they wrote, "but the evidence that cyclosporin can prevent GVHD seems sufficiently strong to encourage further use of the drug".

Calne Cambridge group (88) soon confirmed the data of Green and Allison: rabbit renal allografts could be made to survive for long periods, and the immunosuppressive effect persisted after cessation of treatment, even allowing the survival of a second kidney from a third-party donor. This finding suggested that the long-term action of the drug was nonspecific and argued against tolerance. Of interest, too, were the observations that:

(1) The drug appeared to act only on antigen-stimulated (i.e. proliferating) cells (89).
(2) In the rat, the permanent unresponsiveness induced by a short course of CSA treat- ment did not extend to third-party kidneys transplanted at a later stage (90), although the ability of the rats to produce alloantibody had been grossly impaired.

Of interest, too, was the early observation by Shumway's team in Stanford (91) that CSA was effective in protecting cardiac allografts in cynomolgus monkeys, though infiltration of mononuclear cells was not wholly prevented and there was evidence in some cases of irreversible injury to myocytes. The authors con- cluded that CSA had a powerful immunosuppressive action, "superior to that of azathioprine/corticosteroid regimens", but that continuous administration was required to achieve long-term survival of grafts. In rats, the drug was also effective in ameliorating second-set rejection in presensitized animals (92, 93), and it was confirmed that rejection invariably occurred some time after the drug's withdrawal (93). Of considerable interest was the finding that CSA had a sparing effect on suppressor T lymphocytes (94), providing a pointer to its mode of action.

Calne's team (95) instituted the first pilot study in which the efficacy of CSA in human cadaveric kidney transplantation was assessed. Seven patients received

HLA-mismatched kidneys and were initially given only CSA, though a cyclophosphamide analog was later given additionally to six of them. Five were well with functioning kidneys, and two of these had received no steroids. Both nephro- and hepatotoxicity attributable to CSA clearly worried the team, and they concluded that "Further careful study . . . is necessary before CSA can be recommended in clinical practice". Their full report, involving a total of 34 patients, was published a year later (96). Of 32 cadaveric kidneys 26 were still functioning, three after more than three years, as were two pancreases and two livers transplanted to the same group of patients. It was found that nephrotoxicity could be avoided by hydration and forced diuresis (later it was avoided by reducing the drug dose) and it was concluded that CSA "is effective on its own and is a very immunosuppressive drug. Additional immunosuppressive agents may lead to severe complications", mainly infections and lymphoma.

Despite some further alarms about the nephrotoxicity of CSA and some disappointing early results, thus began the cyclosporine era of organ transplantation. At the 1982 International Congress of The Transplantation Society T. Beveridge (97) of Sandoz, the company that was and still is manufacturing the drug, was able to give a very impressive evaluation of the clinical results, drawing on data from more than a hundred centers. Some 800 patients had received the drug after renal transplantation and 400 after bone marrow grafting. In the latter the drug had been found to be superior to methotrexate in preventing GVHD, and although application of CSA to renal transplant recipients had in general not been carried out in controlled trials (such trials were in progress) the overall picture favored CSA rather than azathioprine. One important new development was the finding that a substantial number of patients on CSA had never received steroids, thus avoiding steroid-induced side-effects. Yet Starzl's team (98, 99) had reported excellent results with CSA and prednisone used in combination, with graft survival of 80% at one year in a consecutive group of 66 patients. The drug had also been used for other organ transplants such as the liver and the pancreas. The main fear had been engendered by its potential toxicity and the development of lymphomas, but the former had generally been reversed by lowering the dose and the latter was within acceptable limits. The provisional conclusion reached by Beveridge was that CSA "is more effective than conventional therapy and that it represents a major advance in clinical immunosuppression". And thus it turned out to be. It did, however, largely vitiate the blood transfusion effect (see below).

CSA became the standard immunosuppressive drug in the 1980s and it gave organ transplantation, including that of the heart, a great boost. In 1985 the indefatigable P.I. Terasaki began his annual series *Clinical Transplants*, with detailed analyses of progress made with various organs and the role played by immunosuppression, tissue typing and other factors (see, for example *100*), and it provides striking testimony for the great clinical advances that had been made. Transplantation not only of the kidney, but also of the heart, liver, pancreas and other organs has become commonplace, largely thanks to better immunosuppression and patient management. It should be added that the advent of CSA also led to a veritable avalanche of experimental models in which the drug was used as a means of inducing specific tolerance in adult animals.

Two reviews dealing with the mechanism of action of CSA are those of S. Britton and R. Palacios (*101*) and, more recently, S.L. Schreiber and G.R. Crabtree (*102*).

A note about antilymphocyte serum or globulin

The experimental genesis of antilymphocyte serum (ALS) and globulin (ALG) has been covered in detail in Chapter 6, as have some clinical aspects. Here I will dwell briefly on the first clinical use of ALG. The critical year was 1967, though K. Gibinski (*103*) retrospectively claimed that ALS, "produced and tested *in vitro*" by Professor I. Lille-Szyszkowicz in the L. Hirszfeld Institute of Immunology, was "first used in man by me in the 3rd medical clinic in Wrozlaw, Poland, as early as 1947" in an attempt to control the leukocytosis of leukemic patients. This letter in the *Lancet* was prompted by the demonstration by R. Schrek and F.W. Preston (*104*) in 1967 that ALS possessed *in vitro* toxicity for human leukemic lymphocytes.

Be that as it may, it became clear from several 1967 publications that ALG, which had been used so successfully in animal models to prolong allograft survival and to facilitate the induction of specific tolerance, was a potent immunosuppressive agent in human allotransplantation. Two groups were primarily involved, T.E. Starzl's (at that time working in Denver, Colorado) and P.S. Russell's in Boston. Starzl's team (Iwasaki *et al.*, 105), which included the British histopathologist K.A. Porter, first described how, basing their approach on that adopted by Monaco, Russell and their colleagues, they prepared ALG from horse sera obtained after immunization of horses with human lymphoid cell sera, and how its activity was tested *in vivo*. In the same year they reported on their first clinical results (*106*). Eight of 11 cadaveric kidney recipients were given ALG from just before the operation in addition to azathioprine and prednisone. All were well 2–4 months later, and it was noted that with ALG it had been possible to reduce the dose of the standard agents. The three patients who had not been given ALG all ran into rejection crises with poor kidney function, but two of them stabilized as a result of ALG therapy, allowing steroid therapy to be reduced. Starzl *et al.* added cautiously that "wider clinical trial is not recommended" until more information has been obtained on the potential toxicity of horse protein, especially the possibility of anaphylactic responses. The same group reported encouraging data in dogs given kidney or liver allografts, and discussed an enlarged group of patients at a Ciba Foundation Study Group meeting in 1967 (*107*). They concluded that "the adjuvant use of heterologous ALG has improved the early course after human renal homotransplantation, and this has been possible without excessive risk from the acute or delayed complications of serum sickness".

At the same meeting, A.P. Monaco, P.S. Russell and their colleagues (*108*) reported on the use of a rabbit antihuman ALS in human volunteers and in patients with chronic uremia (as well as in one with lymphatic leukemia). Although the deep subcutaneous administration of the three doses of ALS produced pain, swelling and transient fever, the normal recipients showed "a profound lymphopenia" that lasted for 2–6 days; in five, the delayed-type skin reactions they had previously produced on testing were either abolished or greatly reduced by the ALG. What is more, skin allografts survived significantly longer than in controls. Three of the 10 individuals developed antibodies to rabbit gammaglobulin, and one of these had transient serum sickness.

ALG gradually became accepted as a legitimate adjunct in organ transplantation, despite the great difficulties of standardizing different batches, even from the same institution. It became a powerful means of overcoming rejection crises. For example, in 1976 J.S. Najarian's team (*109*), in reporting on a seven-year experience with 184 consecutive cadaveric kidney recipients who had been given horse ALG in addition to azathioprine and prednisone, found "significant improvement" in both patient survival and transplant function although they encountered a number of problems. This was before, taking a leaf out of Medawar's book (see Chapter 6), Najarian began to produce a potent ALG in rabbits, 'Minnesota ALG', which was used by him and other centers in the United States to great effect. A decade later Najarian *et al.* (*110*) compared large groups of cadaveric kidney recipients who had been treated either with azathioprine/prednisone/ALG or with cyclosporine/prednisone, and concluded that, mainly because of a lower incidence of rejection crises, "cyclosporine should be used for immunosuppression in most renal allograft recipients". (R.L. Simmons (*111*) has written a brief history of the transplantation program in Minnesota and Najarian's role in it.) The greater efficacy of CSA and the introduction of well-defined and specific monoclonal antibodies to a variety of targets ensured that ALG was gradually phased out, though some centers continue to use it to counter acute rejection.

Enter a new drug, FK 506

The search for new drugs has continued unabated, even though the hope for a potent immunosuppressive drug without adverse side-effects may never be realized. The number of drugs or agents for which immunosuppressive powers have been claimed is legion. They include, in no particular order, the phytomitogen concanavalin A, prostaglandin E, 15-deoxyspergualin, polyunsaturated fatty acids, the imidazole nucleoside mizoribine, low dose heparin, the guanosine analog 8-aminoguanosine, the lymphoblastocidal agent vincristine, the cyclic polypeptide didemnin, 2'deoxy-coformycin (a microbial fermentation product), phytohemagglutinin-P', lentil lectin and rapamycin, a macrolide antibiotic that has been shown to be powerfully immuno-suppressive, both *in vitro* and *in vivo* (*112*). Some of the claims were based on rather unimpressive data in experimental animals. 15-Deoxyspergualin, which was extracted from a bacterial culture filtrate, deserves a special mention because the Japanese group of Suzuki, Kanashiro and Anemiya (*113*) produced substantial prolongation of allogeneic rat hearts with it and because it has been used in a promising clinical trial in renal transplantation in Japan (*114*). The agent appears to have been very effective in reversing rejection crises.

However, a drug that *has* made its mark is FK 506, a drug discovered by the Japanese group of T. Kino (*115*) in 1987 while screening for drugs with antimicro-bial, antineoplastic and immunosuppressive properties. It was isolated from a strain of *Streptomyces tsukubaensis* and was found to be immunosuppressive for rat cardiac allografts. In the same year T. Ochiai *et al.* (*116*) described the action of this powerful drug in beagles. Used on its own in daily doses it produced a highly impressive prolongation of renal allograft survival. Although there were some side-effects these were not severe and the authors concluded that "FK 506 is a powerful immunosuppressant drug in the dog, with tolerable side effects". A stream of publications attesting to the potency of FK 506 followed, foremost among them the demonstration that it sustained skin allografts in rats for as long as it was admin-istered (*117*), and that it reversed acute GVHD in irradiated rats following bone marrow transplantation in all animals, compared with only half of those treated with CSA (118).

The first demonstration of the clinical efficacy of FK 506 came from Starzl's group (119) in 1989. They used it in liver, kidney and pancreas recipients and found it to be impressive, even in rescuing liver transplants in patients who had been treated with CSA and steroids, with or without ALG or azathioprine. FK 506 was used together with low doses of steroids and this combined treatment seemed to avoid rejection crises. Unlike CSA the drug was not nephrotoxic at therapeutic doses. It was concluded that "FK 506 was so potent and free of side-effects that the simplest expedient was to use it alone".

FK 506 (marketed as Prograf) has since been found to cause a form of cardiomyopathy in some patients that is reversible on lowering of the dose or on discontinuing the drug. It is now being used in both renal and liver transplantation, though it has not wholly replaced CSA. Because of an early report by Starzl's group (120) that did not ascribe remarkable results to FK 506 in cadaveric kidney transplantation it was thought that the drug might be particularly favorable for livers. However, in a subsequent direct comparison of the two drugs Starzl's Pittsburgh team (121) found that FK 506 was associated with a somewhat lower incidence of rejection crises, and other multicenter phase III trials of the two agents put them more or less on a par. These trials engendered some controversy, in that Starzl and his colleagues (122) believed his own data had been so convincing that other multicenter trials were unnecessarily "cruel and expensive". R.E. Morris and B.W. Brown begged to disagree (123).

The European Multicenter trial for liver transplants (124) found the two drugs were comparable on grounds of safety, but like Starzl et al., observed a lower incidence of rejection crises for FK 506. To the dispassionate observer it would seem that organ transplanters are fortunate to have two such excellent drugs at their disposal in the 1990s. Although the two drugs are chemically dissimilar their action in inhibiting the production of certain cytokines such as interleukin IL-2 and interferon-gamma (IFN-γ) in T lymphocytes are much the same (125, 126) and they can be used interchangeably, especially if treatment with one or the other fails to be effective. Both inhibit early events in the activation of T cells, and evidently by similar mechanisms (102).

Other patent drugs will no doubt be found, and one such has recently been described, its chief clinical protagonist being H.W. Sollinger of the University of Wisconsin. It is mycophenolate mofetil (MMF), an ester derived from mycophenolic acid (MPA). The latter was shown to be a powerful selective and reversible inhibitor of inosine-5'-monophosphate dehydrogenase by Lee et al. (127) and by Kumagai et al. (128) and its immunologic properties have been studied more recently by Eugui et al. (129), working at Syntex, Palo Alto California. The drug blocks proliferative responses of human, mouse and rat T and B cells in response to mitogens or all antigens and, unlike CSA and FK 506, does not affect IL-2 production or IL-2 receptor expression. One of its features is that it inhibits the mixed lymphocyte reaction (MLR) at a relatively late stage, suggesting that its main action is on deoxyribonucleic acid (DNA) synthesis. It is somewhat specific for lymphocytes. Of considerable interest is the finding (130) that oral administration to mice inhibited antibody to sheep red blood cells and the generation of cytotoxic T lymphocytes. Eugui et al. (129) concluded that "MPA or analogues may have a therapeutic utility in diseases such as rheumatoid arthritis, for prevention of allograft rejection and in lymphocytic or monocytic leukaemias and lymphomas".

A Syntex group improved the bioavailability of MPA by synthesizing the morpho-linoethyl ester (131) and this was soon shown to be strongly immunosuppressive in animal models. In 1992 Sollinger's group set up a phase I clinical trial to test the efficacy of MMF in cadaveric renal transplantation, though it was part of a quadruple regimen also involving CSA, ALG and prednisolone. Patient and graft survival at 18 months were 100% and 95%, respectively, an encouraging interim result (132). Few side-effects were noted. A recent multicenter randomized trial (133) involving only CSA, antithymocyte globulin and MMF (the latter replaced by azathioprine in the controls) revealed a significant reduction in the number of rejection crises and a delay in the appearance of the first crisis, though graft and patient survival at six months was the same. Its inclusion in immunosuppressive regimens for cardiac trans-plant recipients seems to be equally encouraging (134). The mechanism of action of MMF has recently been discussed by Allison, Eugui and Sollinger (135).

A note on the evolution of cardiac and liver transplantation

Pride of place has been given here to the evolution of renal transplantation and the development of immunosuppression to counter rejection, for the kidney led the way for other organs. Unfortunately organs such as the heart and the liver are beyond the scope of this book. So far as the heart is concerned I will confine myself to stating that many years of animal research carried out in several centers preceded the first human allogeneic heart transplant accomplished by C.N. Barnard (136) in 1967. Researchers included J.D. Hardy's group at the University of Mississippi University Medical Center, N.E. Shumway's at Stanford University Medical Center, and M.E. De Bakey's in Houston, Texas. Both Shumway's and De Bakey's teams performed their first human transplants in 1968. It is thanks to the singleminded determination of men like Shumway and their surgical brilliance that cardiac transplantation has become almost as routine as for the kidney and with roughly comparable results.

Much the same can be said of the human liver transplant. F.D. Moore and T.E. Starzl pioneered the technique in dogs well over three decades ago, and some early attempts to provide patients with a new liver were made in the mid-1960s in Denver, Boston and Paris. None were successful. In 1968 Starzl's team (137), which included C.G. Groth and K.A. Porter, reported the first three successful allogeneic transplants in children who were alive at the time of writing from between 49 and 94 days postoperatively. They had been treated with azathioprine, prednisone and ALG. Later that year R.Y. Calne's group (138) described two liver transplants in adult patients, one of which proved to be successful, the patient having returned to work after six weeks.

One may take a less sanguine view of experimental attempts to transplant the brain (139), if only on ethical grounds. But the introduction of CSA and later FK 506 transformed the success rates of a number of transplanted organs other than the kidney – from the heart, heart/lung, liver and pancreas to multiorgan transplants.

One side-effect of immunosuppression has been an increased incidence of malig-nancies. These have been carefully monitored in both the azathioprine and CSA eras by I. Penn (140, 141) and others (142) and, though worrying, seem to be an inescapable price a small number of patients have to pay for the overall benefits of organ transplantation.

The "recollections" of many of the clinical pioneers mentioned here are to be found in Terasaki's book (143), and brief biographic sketches may be found in this book for Carrel (p. 338), Calne, (p. 341), Murray (p. 339) and Starzl (p. 342).

The Blood Transfusion Effect

The genesis of the blood transfusion (BT) effect (i.e. the finding that human kidney allografts show statistically better survival if the patients had previously received BT) is usually attributed to Terasaki's group in Los Angeles. When Opelz et al. (144) first presented their data on this in 1972 to the Fourth International Congress of The Transplantation Society in San Francisco they caused astonishment and some disbelief. Ever since the cause of hyperacute rejection had become understood (see Chapters 2 and 4), prior sensitization to antigens represented in the donor organ, resulting in formation of cytotoxic antibodies was considered to be extremely harmful. Opelz et al., however, acknowledged some antecedents that have since been swept away by the flood of papers generated by their bombshell, and it is worth recalling some of them.

Both Michielsen (145) and Dossetor et al. (146) had observed as early as 1966/7 that multiple blood transfusions associated with long periods of hemodialysis seemed to influence the outcome of renal cadaveric transplantation favorably, even though statistically the data were borderline. Among the possible explanations Dossetor's Montreal group considered was that antibodies with a "non-specific or 'coating' effect might have been responsible;" an alternative was that "each dialyzed uremic patient forms his own allogeneic anti-lymphocyte serum". In view of the much later finding that anti-idiotypic antibodies may be found in many such patients the second hypothesis was perhaps not as wide of the mark as it may have seemed at the time. The paper by Dossetor et al., which analyzed the group's 59 kidney transplants in a variety of ways, did not provide a single reference and this is likely to be unique for the journal *Transplantation* or, for that matter, any other journal!

A year later P.J. Morris and his colleagues (147) published a paper with the title "The paradox of the blood transfusion effect in renal transplantation". Morris was at that time First Assistant in the Department of Surgery at the Royal Melbourne Hospital and his colleagues were A. Ting, then a research assistant, and J. Stocker, listed as a medical student. They duly acknowledged Michielsen and Dossetor et al. before going on to present their own data, which failed to show any correlation between the number of BTs and early graft outcome but certainly did not suggest that a large number of transfusions while on hemodialysis was harmful. Three of 26 patients, who had been treated with azathioprine and prednisone and local irradiation, had developed lymphocytotoxic antibodies: the kidneys of two had to be removed in the first three months and the third had a stormy clinical course. This confirmed the previous observation by Morris et al. (148) (see also 149) that such antibodies are associated with a greater risk of graft failure. As possible explanations for what appeared to be a paradoxical situation Morris et al. suggested:

(1) Some form of immunologic unresponsiveness had been induced, either toler-
    ance or enhancement. They thought that enhancement was unlikely because
    "specific antibody against the graft has not been adequately demonstrated in the
    human recipient of a renal allograft while the graft is exhibiting normal renal
    function".
(2) Uremia might have caused some immunosuppression before transplantation – a
    suggestion that they did not favor because they could not identify a correlation
    between uremia at the time of transplantation and graft outcome.

Morris *et al.* therefore favored the notion of "partial tolerance". They concluded
their prescient discussion by stating: "The practical application of such a hypothesis
would be the treatment of potential recipients with repeated intravenous injections
of purified histocompatibility antigens before grafting. However, the dividing line
between sensitisation and immunological tolerance is ill defined, making such a plan
... rather hazardous in the present state of our knowledge". (In 1974 Morris was
to become Nuffield Professor of Surgery in Oxford, where he has been ever since
and where he has maintained a highly active and productive group of talented transplantation immunologists. He is yet another outstanding example of that band of
transplant surgeons/immunologists who have made their mark in both clinical and
experimental arenas.

The study by Opelz *et al.* (*144*) was specifically designed to explore, retrospectively, the beneficial influence of BT on cadaveric renal transplants in a large group
of patients, for whom the precise BT protocols were known. Most blood used had
been "buffy coat-poor" (i.e. containing relatively few white cells). Patients who had
received more than ten BTs had the best graft survival rate at one year (66%),
whereas that of patients who had received none at all was only 29%. When the
patients were grouped according to the precise number of BTs they had received
before they were found to be negative for cytotoxic antibodies, the results were 80%
and 40%, respectively, with 1–10 BTs showing a survival rate of 48%. "Blood transfusions appear therefore to have preconditioned certain recipients in a way that
improved their graft survival", they wrote. Their further analysis suggested to them
"that graft survival chances for presensitized recipients can be improved by identification of the specificity of cytotoxins prior to transplantation and by selecting suitable (non-specific) mismatches if no HL-A compatible donor can be found". In
another publication (*150*) Opelz, Mickey and Terasaki explained how the failure by
patients on hemodialysis to make cytototoxic antibodies could be used to select
patients more likely to accept HLA-incompatible kidneys subsequently.

A very large number of studies followed these provocative findings and many
centers were able to confirm them. Opelz and Terasaki (*151*) extended their observations in 1974 to a larger number of cadaveric kidneys: in transfused patients the
one-year survival time was 53% compared with 28% in untransfused recipients, and
it was shown that frozen blood did not induce the effect. These data were closely
similar to those previously reported by them. Human cardiac transplants appeared
to be subject to the same effect, for Dong *et al.* (*152*) found that the transplant
patients who had previously received BTs because of open heart surgery fared better.
As Opelz and Terasaki (*151*) pointed out, "The main obstacle to planned transfusion
therapy remains the danger of pre-sensitization". Others among those who confirmed

the effect were Barnes *et al.* (*153*), Van Hooff, Kalff and Van Poelgeest (*154*) and Festenstein *et al.* (*155*).

By 1978 Opelz and Terasaki (*156*) published their analysis of 1360 cadaveric donor kidneys transplanted in a large number of centers in the United States and found "a striking correlation of increased numbers of pretransplant blood transfusions with improved survival", with a p value of less than 0.0001. More than 20 BTs were associated with one- and four-year survivals of 71% and 65%, respectively, compared with 42% and 30% for untransfused patients. They felt that deliberate BTs might be cautiously instituted in some centers – a suggestion they emphasized further two years later (*157*). They listed 18 studies that supported their original findings.

Here I will consider further some particular aspects of the BT effect that aroused both interest and controversy.

(1) Was the magnitude of the effect strictly proportional to the number of BTs?
(2) Did the effect apply to donor-specific BTs?
(3) Was the effect obtainable in animal models?
(4) What was the mechanism responsible for it?
(5) Did a phenomenon that was clearly demonstrable in the azathioprine/prednisone era survive into the CSA era?

How many blood transfusions?

This issue aroused considerable controversy, with the Opelz and Terasaki group tending to find that the larger the number of BTs, the better the survival. For example, in their 1978 survey (*156*) they found a very clear graded correlation, from zero BTs to more than 20. Although the differences were strikingly large in transplant centers that had relatively low baseline levels, they were less pronounced in centers in which a high proportion (70%) of even non-transfused patients sustained functional kidneys at one year; in these the difference between nontransfused patients and those who received more than 20 BTs was a mere 10%. This may well have accounted for the data from some centers that had not found significant BT effects. Four years later Terasaki's group (*158*) confirmed their data concerning the optimal number of BTs, i.e. the more BT the better the outcome.

Others, Feduska *et al.* (*159*) for example, found that 1–5 BTs were as effective as 6–10. The chief protagonists for the notion that a *single* BT was optimal were J.J. Van Rood and his colleagues in Leiden. Thus G.G. Persijn *et al.* (*160*) retrospectively compared a group of 74 cadaveric kidney recipients who had never undergone either a BT or pregnancy with 30 who had received a single BT. One year survival times were 32% and 87%, respectively. They also reported a prospective study, though the comparison was made at only 240 days; the results were much the same. One to three units of leukocyte-free blood were totally ineffective. Further, they found that peroperative BT had no beneficial influence, a point on which conflicting data were obtained in several centers though the majority sided with Persijn *et al.* on this point. Persijn *et al.* argued that a single BT was greatly advantageous in that it would be expected to be associated with a lower rate of sensitization.

The question of whether second cadaveric kidneys transplanted after rejection of a first could benefit from BT produced diametrically opposite results. For example, the British group of Dewar *et al.* from Newcastle (*161*) found that transfused patients had less than half the survival figure at one year – a difference that was only slightly reduced by the beginning of the fourth year. In contrast, the Dutch group Persijn *et al.* (*162*) discovered a significant beneficial influence, their transfused patients having received anything from a few to as many as 100 BTs.

Random versus donor-specific blood transfusion

A number of centers transplanting kidneys to living unrelated (*163*) or related (*164–167*) recipients found that BT from the kidney donor likewise improved the graft survival rate. The patients of Leivestad *et al.* (*167*) included subgroups on azathioprine/prednisolone and on CSA/prednisolone. The kidneys came from one HLA-haplotype-mismatched mixed lymphocyte culture (MLC)-positive donor. The one-year graft survival was extraordinarily high in both groups (about 93%), but it was much the same in a group that had received CSA but no BT. CSA/prednisolone without BT "has therefore become our preferred therapy for haploidentical renal transplants", for it avoided the danger of presensitization.

Animal models: did they throw light on the mechanisms involved?

A large number of animal models were established during the decade following the clinical observations by Opelz *et al.* (*144*) in attempts to imitate the BT effect and to establish the underlying mechanism. However, some interesting data had already been published well before Opelz and Terasaki had made their point in patients. For example, as far back as 1955 Billingham and Sparrow (*168*) had found that the survival time of rabbit skin allografts was prolonged by the intravenous infusion of donor epidermal cells and, less consistently, of donor blood. A decade later Halasz, Orloff and Hirose (*169*) reported a three-fold prolongation of canine renal allografts following two transfusions of very small volumes of donor blood without immunosuppression. This was accompanied by a marked depletion of the recipients' lymph nodes and spleens. Others before them had already pointed the way with skin allografts in rabbits, dogs and rats (*170–173*).

This approach was revived by Marquet, Heystek and Tinbergen (*174*), who demonstrated in rats that allogeneic kidneys and hearts enjoyed greatly extended survival if the recipients had been given a few small aliquots of donor strain blood before transplantation. They excluded specific tolerance as the underlying mechanism because the animals' lymphoid cells were active in an anti-donor graft-versus-host reaction and they therefore favored an enhancement mechanism (see Chapter 6) and some form of graft adaptation. In the same year Jenkins and Woodruff (*175*) prolonged the life of rat cardiac allografts with donor strain blood or thoracic duct cells. The prolongation was specific and depended on blood leukocytes and not other blood elements, and these authors too failed to find enhancing antibodies. Interestingly, third-party blood gave a lesser, but still significant, prolongation. The kinetics of the BT effect in rats was subsequently studied by Fabre and Morris (*176*), who leaned towards an enhancement hypothesis without altogether excluding tolerance (*177*). It was the Oxford group of Morris that many years later described the indefinite survival of cardiac allografts in the rat after both donor-specific (*178*) and random (*179*) BT under cover of a short course of anti-CD4 monoclonal antibody.

A shot across the bows of this approach being applied to bone marrow transplantation was soon fired by R. Storb *et al.* (*180*) in Seattle. Using WBI to condition dogs for allogeneic bone marrow transplants they found to their alarm that when three previous donor BTs had been administered, six out of nine animals rejected their bone marrow grafts acutely, whereas all 12 dogs in the control group showed "prompt and sustained engraftment". BT in bone marrow transplantation was clearly counterproductive, and this was equally true when blood partly depleted of white cells was used (*181*).

That the BT effect was operative in rhesus monkeys was demonstrated by Van Es *et al.* in 1977 (*182*). Animals matched for two or three histocompatibility antigens that had received five non-donor BTs and conventional immunosuppression sustained kidney allografts for considerably longer periods than the untransfused controls. Van Es and Balner (*183*) later found that the BT effect was compromised when the kidney donors and recipients had been matched for DR antigens, a finding confirmed in patients by Thorsby's group (*184*).

Many other experimental BT models have been described. In the next section I will consider the extent to which they, together with two, clinical observations have elucidated the mechanism involved.

What mechanism(s) account for the blood transfusion effect?

No single mechanism emerges as the all-important explanation for the BT effect but a number have been proposed from observations in patients or in experimental animals.

Anti-idiotypic antibodies

It was proposed by Singal and Joseph (*185*) in 1982 that the BT effect could be explained by the appearance of anti-idiotypic antibodies (i.e. antibodies directed against the individual's own T cell idiotypes and therefore suppressive; see Chapter 2). They provided further evidence for this year's later (*186*). Thus, transfused mice developed antibodies that inhibited mixed lymphocyte culture reactions by the lymphocytes of the transfused animals against donor strain targets, a phenomenon that was strictly strain-specific and which was still demonstrable after three weeks. Singal *et al.* (*187*) subsequently provided further evidence favoring the interpretation of their data.

In a study of anti-idiotypic interactions in transfused patients and in kidney allograft recipients, N. Suciu-Foca *et al.* (*188*) showed in 1983 that alloimmune responses were modulated by anti-idiotypic T cells and by anti-idiotypic antibodies, the responses having been developed to T cell receptors for human leukocyte antigen HLA-D/DR gene products. The relevance of this kind of response to HLA antigens was explored by her group in several other publications, among them one by Reed *et al.* (*189*) in which they described the kinetics of the anti-anti-HLA antibody response after donor-specific transfusions and renal transplantation. They confirmed their conclusion that allograft immunity can be downregulated by the development of anti-idiotypic antibodies. They suggested tentatively that kidney transplantation could probably be safely performed in sensitized patients provided that they had such antibodies. In 1987 the same group confirmed that this was indeed the case

(190). Other groups, for example Barkley *et al.* *(191)*, likewise found anti-idiotypic antibodies in transfused patients and this mechanism remains one of the most plausible.

Suppressor cells

Once suppressor T (Ts) cells had been described by R.K. Gershon and K. Kondo *(192)* in 1971 they were soon found in various experimental models of transplantation tolerance (see Chapter 6). Marquet and Heystek *(193)* explored this in rats given a single donor BT seven days before transplantation. This treatment led to the indefinite and specific survival of donor hearts and the unresponsiveness was transferrable to sublethally irradiated secondary recipients by the recipients' splenic T cells. Many others, including A.P. Monaco's group *(194)* in Boston, had similar findings in experimental animals. Smith *et al.* *(195)* studied patients who had been on hemodialysis without ever having been transfused. They were given two units of packed red cells and the incidence of Ts cells and their *in vitro* activity were monitored. Although the number of Ts cells evidently did not change their *in vitro* activity increased, and when the patients were eventually given cadaveric kidneys nine out of 12 were functioning after one year. The presence of cellular suppressor mechanisms in patients who had received donor-specific BT and kidneys was subsequently demonstrated by Burlingham *et al.* *(196)*. Suppressor T cells, like anti-idiotypic antibodies, may therefore play a role in the BT effect.

Clonal deletional tolerance

If antibodies and/or Ts cells are involved it would seem highly improbable that BT induces a form of tolerance brought about by clonal deletion of the recipient's anti-donor lymphocytes. This was indeed confirmed by two groups who set out to prove that deletional tolerance was a factor *(197, 198)*. Even so, Terasaki's group *(199)* found some evidence that was "consistent with the clonal deletion theory although they do not necessarily provide final proof".

Selection of non-responders?

Some workers thought that the action of BT was to select graft recipients for whom kidney allografts were potentially more favorable (i.e. those who failed to make antibodies after BT and who might therefore be considered to be relatively unresponsive to HLA antigens). However, Van Rood *et al.* *(200)* have argued that when only one BT is administered, "This selection phenomenon cannot play a role . . . because then no or only weak antibodies in only a few recipients are formed". Yet they found that a single BT was highly effective, especially when the kidney donors and recipients were mismatched for one DR antigen. More recently Fehrman, Ringden and Moller *(201)* have argued the case for selection on the strength of their data.

Has the blood transfusion effect survived into the cyclosporin A era?

Even at a time when azathioprine was the mainstay of immunosuppression by no means all transplant centers were convinced that they should follow the BT route. The main objection was that some patients would inevitably be sensitized and that this would make it more difficult to find donors for them. It is also true that as the clinical results improved the BT benefit became rather less marked than in the early years when Opelz and Terasaki had been able to demonstrate a doubling of cadaveric kidney graft survival at one year (see above). As CSA was used in more and more centers – and it was not until the mid- to late 1980s that CSA had become the principal drug – the effect diminished even further and the topic excited considerable controversy at meetings of The International Transplantation Society. What is the evidence?

In 1984, Terasaki's group (202) sent a letter to the *New England Journal of Medicine* in which they presented data showing that not only class I and class II matching continued to be of benefit in the CSA era – the difference was of the order of 10% – but that patients drawn from a large number of centers who had received more than five BTs had a 15% better chance of having a functional kidney than those who had not been transfused. Indeed, the CSA data were paradoxically better than those achieved with azathioprine/steroid recipients. The authors urged that "matching and blood transfusion should be pursued even more vigorously in the cyclosporine-treatment era to achieve high transplant-survival rates". Opelz (203) confirmed their matching data a year later, the information having been derived from a huge number of patients from the Collaborative Transplant Study. The difference between zero and four HLA-B and DR mismatches was as high as 20%, but the BT effect was unfortunately not analyzed.

So far as BT is concerned, the 10% difference between transfused and non-transfused patients was also seen in the patients reported to the U.C.L.A. Transplant Registry since 1980 who had been given CSA (204). This effect was supported by Pfaff *et al.* (205) and by Melzer *et al.* (206). In contrast, other centers came to the opposite conclusion. Many of these reports were published in the 1983–1987 *Transplantation Proceedings* – one of them interestingly enough by Opelz (207), who showed that through the use of CSA the survival rates for non-transfused patients had improved so much as to largely obscure the transfusion effect. He wrote: "Our data provide a consistent picture of a decreasing influence of pretransplant transfusion on kidney graft outcome". No wonder that transplant surgeons became transfusion skeptics! His conclusions were fully supported by Lundgren *et al.* (208) and Kerman *et al.* (209), who believed that the need for BT had disappeared.

Although the issue is perhaps not entirely dead there are now relatively few centers in which BT is carried out routinely. Thus ended – more or less – what had appeared to be a most opportune means of significantly improving the results in renal transplantation, one that had been used to good effect for the best part of a decade. The phenomenon has fallen victim to the greatly superior results now obtainable with CSA and FK 506 but it has nonetheless spawned some interesting immunologic findings. It is one of those immunologic phenomena that has never entirely yielded its secret and its mechanism(s) is still under investigation in some laboratories.

Chimerism and Tolerance

Ever since the finding by Medawar's group (210) that cattle dizygotic twins accept each other's skin grafts, preceded by R.D. Owen's (211) remarkable demonstration six years earlier that such twins are nearly always red cell chimeras, it has been assumed that transplantation tolerance and chimerism go hand in hand. Indeed, this became dogma once tolerance had been experimentally established in mice and other species (see Chapter 5): *in vivo* tolerance seemed to go hand in hand with the continued presence of donor cells in the lymphoid tissues of the tolerant animal. This notion was strongly supported when it became apparent in the 1950s that sustained tolerance to soluble protein or other non-replicating antigens required the repeated inoculation of animals with the relevant antigen (see Chapter 5). That the association between tolerance and chimerism was not merely fortuitous was shown by two separate studies by D.M. Lubaroff and W.K. Silvers, who found that removal of the donor cells by various means led to a breakdown of tolerance (see Chapter 5, p. 204). These experiments undoubtedly showed that the maintenance of neonatally induced tolerance depended on the presence of chimeric cells.

Nonetheless, as is seen in Chapter 6, this does not necessarily apply to tolerance induced in adult animals by various stratagems such as the treatment of animals with extracts prepared from donor strain splenic cells and a short course of ALS (see, for example, *212, 213*). Here the question of cellular chimerism did not arise, unless it is supposed that passenger cells from the skin graft migrated into the host tissues – a possibility made unlikely by the finding that removal of the skin graft from an unresponsive mouse for two weeks broke the tolerant state. Evidently the antigens of the graft were sufficient to maintain tolerance. It should, however, be stressed that tolerance in these animals was later found to be mediated by Ts cells. Another example of transplantation tolerance independent of chimerism was described by H. Balner (*214*) in radiation chimeras.

The old literature also provides examples of chimerism persisting after the breakdown of graft tolerance, so-called 'split tolerance.' Billingham and Brent (*215*) were the first to report this in 1959 and the phenomenon was subsequently confirmed (*216*). It is possible for donor cells to persist after rejection of a graft, though this may be exceptional.

Unlike these experimental animals, human transplant recipients continue to receive immunosuppression, usually for as long as the graft remains functional. It is, however, well known that with increasing time the dose of the drugs can be steadily reduced to a maintenance dose, and in some patients a measure of *in vitro* hyporesponsiveness towards the donor's HLA antigens has been shown to develop (*217–220*). That the situation in such patients is far from static has been demonstrated by Starzl's group in Pittsburgh: six of their long-term liver recipients had successfully taken themselves off all drugs (*221*). Equally surprising was the survival of six months to almost three years of liver transplant recipients whose drug intake had to be terminated because of EBV-associated B cell lymphomas (*222*) and the most recent demonstration, again by Starzl's team (*223*), that long-term liver transplant recipients can be weaned off drugs, though this proved not to be successful in about 25% of the group involved. These clinical data support the notion that, with the passing years, the graft recipient develops some measure of tolerance.

The question of whether human transplant recipients become cellular chimeras had not been explored until Starzl *et al.* (*224–226*), using karyotyping and gamma-globulin Gm typing of immunoglobulins, found evidence for the presence of donor cells in long-surviving human liver recipients. Having used cadaveric donors of opposite sex to the recipient they were able to show that the hepatocytes and the vascular endothelium retained donor markers but that the Kupffer cells had been replaced by cells of host origin.

More than two decades later Starzl returned to this issue, techniques for identifying cells in low numbers as well as liver graft survival having meanwhile improved. Thus he and his colleagues (227) in Pittsburgh were able to demonstrate, using *in situ* hybridization and molecular biology techniques as well as karyotyping to identify the Y chromosome of male donors in females, that all the nine female liver transplant recipients examined were chimeras. The subjects had all carried their grafts for 10–19 years. Donor cells were found in the blood, skin and lymph nodes in most of the patients and, of course, in their transplants. The authors concluded: "Although we believe that similar chimerism is the basis for the acceptance of all whole-organ transplants, the disproportionate heavy endowment of hepatic grafts with potentially migratory dendritic cells, macrophages, and other leukocytes of bone marrow origin may help to explain why the liver is more tolerogenic than other organs". The same group (228) in the same year described evidence for the migration of what were thought to be dendritic cells in irradiated mice that had been reconstituted with rat bone marrow, and they published a review article (229) setting down their ideas concerning the importance of this cell migration: rather than prevent it, they argued, everything possible should be done to enhance it. While the migration of dendritic-type (i.e. antigen-presenting) cells would no doubt make the graft less immunogenic, their presence in the recipient's tissues might have been expected to activate an antidonor response. There seems to be something of a paradox here.

In 1993 Starzl *et al.* (230) found evidence for cellular traffic from the graft to the recipient's tissues in all five renal allograft recipients examined by them. These patients had carried kidneys from living related donors for periods of up to 29 years. The blood lymphocytes of the four individuals whose donors were still alive were tested in mixed lymphocyte culture: two gave no antidonor response and the other two relatively low responses compared with third-party stimulator cells. It therefore became clear that cell migration and the resultant chimerism was not unique for the liver.

In 1993 Starzl *et al.* (231) published a lengthy review setting out their thoughts about the significance of the chimeric state and the possible interactions between donor cells and the recipient's immune system, and they argued that "an incipient GVH reaction is a necessary condition for success (this is our fundamental premise). We now know that about 5% of all liver recipients go through a bout of clinical GVHD that in the past usually was attributed to an allergic skin reaction". This then was the basis of what they later called "the two-way paradigm" (232). Certainly, evidence of GVHD in human liver graft recipients had been observed by others (233–235), and Schlitt *et al.* (236) found evidence of microchimerism using polymerase chain reaction amplification specific for donor HLA-DR1 in heart recipients, although the dynamics were complex. Only half of a group of 47 patients could be shown to be chimeric after six months, all were chimeric between six months and two years and only half in the third postoperative year. Yet there was no clinical difference between these groups.

The central question is whether the chimerism is a consequence of the immunosuppressed state of the patient or whether it drives the patient's immune system towards tolerance. There is no clear evidence as yet to answer this, and it is possible that the problem can be resolved only in experimental models. One such attempt has been made by A. Bushell *et al.* (237). Using a model that had been well characterized by them they gave mice a single donor-specific transfusion under cover of a depleting anti-CD4 antibody 28 days before transplanting allogeneic hearts. This protocol always resulted in the indefinite survival of the grafts. The mice were operationally tolerant in that they rejected third-party grafts. It was postulated that the tolerance may have been associated with microchimerism. To discover whether this was the case they irradiated the donor blood before transfusion with 2000 rads, high enough to prevent the cells from replicating and therefore from establishing chimerism. Mice given irradiated cells rejected their cardiac grafts acutely, on the face of it supporting the concept that a chimeric state is a requirement for tolerance. When, however, the dose of irradiated cells was increased by injecting a further three aliquots of blood, indefinite survival was obtained. Bushell *et al.* therefore concluded that in their model "microchimerism is not an absolute requirement for long-term graft survival" although the presence of donor cells was vital for the *induction* of tolerance, and they put forward a working hypothesis to explain their findings.

In both animals (238) and patients (239–241) it has been shown that following the establishment of chimerism by T cell depletion of the allograft recipient, the chimeric cells were likely to have been the cause of an ensuing tolerance that did not depend on further immunosuppression. This point was vividly demonstrated by Sharabi *et al.* (242) when they showed that removal of donor cells led to a breakdown of tolerance. Here donor cell chimerism was clearly an absolute requirement. The role of passenger cells in immunity and tolerance has been discussed in detail in Chapters 2 and 6, respectively.

Another clinical study was that of C. Suberbielle, S. Calliat-Zucman and C. Legrendre (243) in Paris, who found that only about one-third of patients who had carried their kidney allograft for more than 20 years displayed microchimerism. On the other hand, W.J. Burlingham *et al.* (244) identified cells derived from a maternal kidney allograft in the blood and skin of one patient who had good graft function although all immunosuppressive drugs had been discontinued five years previously. This patient seemed to be tolerant in that his *in vitro* antidonor responses were minimal unless IL-2 was added to the cultures, and Burlingham *et al.* speculated that their *in vitro* data were consistent with the action of veto cells. A. Nagler *et al.* (245) have reported some correlation between the presence of donor chimerism and the relative absence of rejection episodes in human liver allograft recipients.

Finally, Streilein's group (246) has recently reported some interesting and relevant observations in mice that had been made neonatally tolerant by the inoculation of F1 hybrid donor cells. Not surprisingly all mice were found to be chimeric according to the polymerase chain reaction assay, but "neither the presence nor the quantity of chimeric cells predicts whether a particular . . . mouse will accept or reject donor-specific skin allografts". Chimerism remained detectable even in mice that had rejected their skin grafts. These workers concluded that "chimerism is essential for the induction of neonatally induced tolerance, and its expansion may play an important role in the maintenance of that tolerance . . .".

In conclusion, the issue of whether cellular chimerism is the cause or the consequence of tolerance is not yet finally settled. Because so many different mechanisms underlying functional tolerance have been uncovered it may well be that chimerism plays a greater or lesser role, or none at all, depending on the mechanism. Certainly in rodent experiments such as those of Streilein's group using donor F_1 hybrid cells, which by definition are incapable of initiating graft-versus-host reactions (see Chapters 5 and 8), Starzl's "two-way paradigm" cannot be operative.

It remains to be seen whether the augmentation of donor-specific cells at the time of clinical transplantation will improve prognosis. W. H. Barber *et al.* (247) made a tentative start in this direction by infusing cryopreserved donor bone marrow cells into patients 17 days after the end of an induction course of ALG. More grafts were lost from rejection in the control group (the mean follow-up period was 16 months for both groups), and Barber *et al.* concluded that there was an overall improvement following bone marrow infusion although they felt that "a more effective induction protocol is needed". Starzl's team (248) have more recently made a similar attempt in kidney, liver and heart recipients, but the bone marrow was administered 1–12 hours after revascularization. All of the first 18 patients have well-functioning organs, with a follow-up period of 4–16 months, and 17 of them were found to have "persistent multilineage leukocyte chimerism in their blood". These data indeed augur well for the future.

References

1. Woodruff, M.F.A. (1960) *The Transplantation of Tissues and Organs*, pp. 1–777, Charles C. Thomas, Springfield, Illinois.
2. Moore, F.D. (1964) *Give and Take. The Development of Tissue Transplantation*, pp. 1–177, W.B. Saunders, Philadelphia, London.
3. Converse, J.M. & Casson, P.R. (1968) In *Human Transplantation*, eds F.T. Rapaport & J. Dausset, p. 3, Grune & Stratton, New York.
4. Hamilton, D. (1988) In *Kidney Transplantation*, 3rd edn, ed. P.J. Morris, p. 1, W.B. Saunders, London.
5. Starzl, T.E. (1990) *Am. J. Kidney Dis.* **16**, 548.
6. Küss, R. & Bourget, P. (1992) *An Illustrated History of Organ Transplantation*, pp. 1–175, Sandoz, Rueil-Malmaison, France (also published in French).
7. Dempster, W.J. (1951) *Brit. Med. J.* **2**, 104.
8. Dempster, W.J. (1953) *Brit. J. Surg.* **40**, 447.
9. Simonsen, M. (1953) *Acta Path. Microbiol. Sc and* **32**, 1, 36.
10. Hume, D.M., Merrill, J.P., Miller, B.J. *et al.* (1955) *J. Clin. Invest.* **34**, 327.
11. Merrill, J.P., Murray, J.E., Harrison, J.H. *et al.* (1956) *J. Am. Med. Ass.* **160**, 277.
12. Murray, J.E., Merrill, J.P. & Harrison, J.H. (1958) *Ann. Surg.* **148**, 343.
13. Dubost, C., Oeconomos, N., Nenna, A. *et al.* (1951) *Bull. Soc. Med. Hop. Paris* **67**, 1372.
14. Servelle, M., Soulie, P. & Rougeulle, J. (1951) *Bull. Soc. Med. Hop. Paris* **67**, 99.
15. Küss, R., Teinturier, J. & Milliez, P. (1951) *Mem. Acad. Chir.* **77**, 755.
16. Krieg, A.F., Bolande, R.P., Holden, W.D. *et al.* (1960) *Am. J. Clin. Path.* **34**, 155.
17. Ginn, H.E., Unger, A.M., Hume, D.M. *et al.* (1960) *J. Lab. Clin. Med.* **56**, 1.
18. Woodruff, M.F.A., Robson, J.S., Ross, J.A. *et al.* (1960) *Lancet* 1, 1245.
19. Dossetor, J.B., Mackinnon, K.J., Luke, J.C. *et al.* (1960) *Lancet* 2, 572.
20. Voronoy, U. (1936) *El Siglo Med.* **97**, 296.
21. Hamilton, D. (1986) *The Monkey Gland Affair*, pp. 1–155, Chatto & Windus, London.
22. Lawler, R.H., West, J.W., McNulty, P.H. *et al.* (1950) *J. Am. Med. Ass.* **144**, 844.
23. Michon, L., Hamburger, J., Oeconomos, N. *et al.* (1953) *Presse Méd.* **61**, 1419.
24. Dammin, G.J., Couch, N.P. & Murray, J.E. (1957) *Ann. N.Y. Acad. Sci.* **64**, 967.
25. Mannick, J.A., Powers, J.H., Mithoeffer, J. *et al.* (1960) *Surgery* **47**, 340.
26. Lawrence, H.S. (1965) *Ann. Int. Med.* **62**, 166.
27. Murray, G. & Holden, R. (1954) *Am. J. Surg.* **87**, 508.
28. Hume, D.M., Jackson, B.T., Zukoski, C.F. *et al.* (1960) *Ann. Surg.* **152**, 354.

29. Pierce, J.C., Lee, H.M., Wolf, J. *et al.* (1975) *Transpl. Proc.* **7** (**suppl. 1**), 915.
30. Hamburger, J., Vaysse, J., Crosnier, J. *et al.* (1960) *Presse Méd.* **67**, 1771.
31. Merrill, J.P., Murray, J.E., Harrison, J.H. *et al.* (1960) *New Engl. J. Med.* **262**, 1251.
32. Küss, R., Legrain, M., Mathé, G. *et al.* (1960) *Presse Méd.* **68**, 755.
33. Murray, J.E., Merrill, J.P. & Dammin, G.J. (1960) *Surgery* **48**, 272.
34. Woodruff, M.F.A., Robson, J.S., Ross, J.A. *et al.* (1962) *Brit. J. Urol.* **34**, 3.
35. Küss, R., Legrain, M., Mathé, G. *et al.* (1962) *Postgrad. Med. J.* **38**, 529.
36. Dempster, W.J. (1955) *Brit. J. Urol.* **27**, 66.
37. Editorial (1960) *Brit. Med. J.* **2**, 1001.
38. Elion, G.B. & Hitchings, G.H. (1957) *The Chemistry and Biology of Purines*, Little, Brown & Co., Boston.
39. Schwartz, R., Stack, J. & Damashek, W. (1958) *Proc. Soc. Exp. Biol. Med.* **99**, 164.
40. Schwartz, R., Eisner, A. & Damashek, W. (1958) *J. Clin Invest.* **38**, 1394.
41. Schwartz, R. & Damashek, W. (1959) *Nature* **183**, 1682.
42. Schwartz, R. & Damashek, W. (1960) *J. Clin. Invest.* **39**, 592.
43. Meeker, W., Condie, R., Varco, R.L. *et al.* (1959) *Proc. Soc. Exp. Biol. Med.* **102**, 459.
44. Calne, R.Y. (1960) *Lancet* **1**, 417.
45. Zukoski, C.F., Lee, H.M. & Hume, D.M. (1960) *Surg. Forum* **11**, 470.
46. Calne, R.Y. (1961) *Transpl. Bull.* **28**, 65.
47. Elion, G.B., Singer, S. & Hitchings, G.H. (1954) *Ann. N.Y. Acad. Sci.* **60**, 200.
48. Gombos, A., Tischler, V. & Jacina, J. (1961) *Transpl. Bull.* **28**, 61.
49. Calne, R.Y. & Murray, J.E. (1961) *Surg. Forum* **12**, 118.
50. Calne, R.Y., Alexandre, G.P.J. & Murray, J.E. (1962) *Ann. N.Y. Acad. Sci.* **99**, 743.
51. Pierce, J.C., Varco, R.L. & Good, R.A. (1961) *Surgery* **50**, 186.
52. Hamburger, J., Vaysse, J., Crosnier, J. *et al.* (1962) *Surgery* **99**, 808.
53. Murray, J.E., Merrill, J.P., Dammin, G.J. *et al.* (1962) *Ann. Surg.* **156**, 337.
54. Murray, J.E., Merrill, J.P. & Harrison, J.H. *et al.* (1963) *New Engl. J. Med.* **268**, 1315.
55. Merrill, J.P., Murray, J.E., Takacs, F.J. *et al.* (1963) *J. Amer. Med. Ass.* **185**, 347.
56. Hume, D.M., Magee, J.H., Kauffman, H.M. *et al.* (1963) *Ann. Surg.* **158**, 608.
57. Murray, J.E., Sheil, A.G., Moseley, R. *et al.* (1964) *Ann. Surg.* **160**, 449.
58. Starzl, T.E., Marchioro, T.L. & Waddell, W.R. (1963) *Surg. Gynec. Obstet.* **117**, 385.
59. Woodruff, M.F.A. (1952) *Ann. Roy. Coll. Surg., Engl.* **11**, 173.
60. Woodruff, M.F.A. (1954) *Transpl. Bull.* **1**, 221.
61. Marchioro, T.L., Axtell, H.K., LaVia, M.F. *et al.* (1964) *Surgery* **55**, 412.
62. Human Kidney Transplant Conference (1964) *Transplantation* **2**, 147.
63. Human Kidney Transplant Conference (1964) *Transplantation* **2**, 581.
64. Calne, R.Y. (1969) *Brit. Med. J.* **2**, 565.
65. Tenth Report of the Human Renal Transplant Registry (1972) *J. Am. Med. Ass.* **221**, 1495.
66. Billingham, R.E., Krohn, P.L. & Medawar, P.B. (1951) *Brit. Med. J.* **1**, 1157.
67. Billingham, R.E., Krohn, P.L. & Medawar, P.B. (1951) *Brit. Med. J.* **2**, 1049.
68. Whitelaw, J. (1951) *J. Am. Med. Ass.* **145**, 85.
69. Morgan, J.A. (1951) *Surgery* **30**, 506.
70. Sparrow, E.M. (1953) *J. Endocrinol.* **9**, 101.
71. Sparrow, E.M. (1954) *J. Endocrinol.* **11**, 57.
72. Medawar, P.B. & Sparrow, E.M. (1956) *J. Endocrinol.* **14**, 240.
73. Krohn, P.L. (1954) *Brit. J. Exp. Path.* **35**, 539.
74. Dreyfuss, M., Haerri, E., Hofmann, H. *et al.* (1976) *Eur. J. Appl. Microbiol.* **3**, 125.
75. Ruegger, A., Kuhn, M., Lichti, A. *et al.* (1976) *Helv. Chim. Acta* **59**, 1075.
76. Petcher, T.J., Weber, H.P. & Ruegger, A. (1976) *Helv. Chim. Acta* **59**, 1480.
77. Borel, J., Feurer, C., Gubler, H. U. *et al.* (1976) *Actions and Agents* **6**, 468.
78. Borel, J., Feurer, C., Magnee, C. *et al.* (1977) *Immunology* **32**, 1017.
79. Calne, R.Y. (1991) In *History of Transplantation. Thirty-five Recollections*, ed. P.I. Terasaki, U.C.L.A. Tissue Typing Laboratory, Los Angeles.
80. Kostakis, A.J., White, D.J.G. & Calne, R.Y. (1977) *IRCS Med. Sci.: Cardiovascular System* **5**, 280.
81. Kostakis, A.J., White, D.J.G. & Calne, R.Y. (1977) *IRCS Med. Sci.: Cardiovascular System* **5**, 243.
82. Calne, R.Y. & White, D.J.G. (1977) *IRCS Med. Sci.: Cardiovascular System* **5**, 595.

83. Green, C.J. & Allison, A.C. (1978) *Lancet* **1**, 1182.
84. Green, C.J., Allison, A.C. & Precious, S. (1979) *Lancet* **2**, 123.
85. Calne, R.Y., White, D.J.G., Rolles, K. *et al.* (1978) *Lancet* **2**, 1183.
86. Powles, R.L., Barrett, A.J., Clink, H. *et al.* (1978) *Lancet* **2**, 1327.
87. Powles, R.L., Clink, H.M., Spence, D. *et al.* (1980) *Lancet* **1**, 327.
88. Dunn, D.C., White, D.J.G., Herbertson, B.M. *et al.* (1979) *Transplantation* **27**, 359.
89. White, D.J.G., Plumb, A.M., Pawelec, G. *et al.* (1979) *Transplantation* **27**, 55.
90. Homan, W.P., Fabre, J.W. & Morris, P.J. (1979) *Transplantation* **28**, 439.
91. Jamieson, S.W., Burton, N.A., Bieber, C.P. *et al.* (1979) *Lancet* **1**, 545.
92. Homan, W.P., Fabre, J.W., Millard, P.R. *et al.* (1980) *Transplantation* **30**, 354.
93. Shulack, J.A., Monson, D., Shelby, J. *et al.* (1983) *Transplantation* **36**, 289.
94. Kupiec-Weglinski, J.W., Filho, M.A., Strom, T.B. *et al.* (1984) *Transplantation* **38**, 97.
95. Calne, R.Y., White, D.J.G., Thiru, S. *et al.* (1978) *Lancet* **2**, 1323.
96. Calne, R.Y., Rolles, K., White, D.J.G. *et al.* (1979) *Lancet* **2**, 329.
97. Beveridge, T. (1983) *Transpl. Proc.* **15**, 433.
98. Starzl, T.E., Weil, R., Iwatsuki, S. *et al.* (1980) *Surg. Gynecol. Obstet.* **151**, 17.
99. Starzl, T.E., Klintmalm, G.B.G., Weil, R. *et al.* (1981) *Surg. Gynecol. Obstet.* **153**, 486.
100. Terasaki, P.I. & Cecka, J.M. (eds) *Clinical Transplants* **1993**, U.C.L.A. Tissue Typing Laboratory, Los Angeles.
101. Britton, S. & Palacios, R. (1982) *Immunol. Rev.* **65**, 5.
102. Schreiber, S.L. & Crabtree, G.R. (1992) *Immunol. Today* **13**, 136.
103. Gibinski, K. (1969) *Lancet* **1**, 183 (letter).
104. Schrek, R. & Preston, F.W. (1967) *Lancet* **2**, 1366.
105. Iwasaki, Y., Porter, K.A., Amend, J.R. *et al.* (1967) *Surg. Gynecol. Obstet.* **124**, 1.
106. Starzl, T.E., Marchioro, T.L., Porter, K.A. *et al.* (1967) *Surg. Gynecol. Obstet.* **124**, 301.
107. Starzl, T.E., Marchioro, T.L., Iwasaki, Y. *et al.* (1967) In *Antilymphocyte Serum*, p. 4, Ciba Found. Study Group, eds G.E.W. Wolstenholme & M. O'Connor, J. & A. Churchill, London.
108. Monaco, A.P., Wood, M.L., Van der Werf, B.A. *et al.* (1967) In *Antilymphocyte Serum*, p. 111, Ciba Found. Study Group, eds G.E.W. Wolstenholme & M. O'Connor, J. & A. Churchill, London.
109. Najarian, J.S., Simmons, R.L., Condie, R.M. *et al.* (1976) *Ann. Surg.* **184**, 352.
110. Najarian, J.S., Fryd, D.S., Strand, M. *et al.* (1985) *Ann. Surg.* **201**, 142.
111. Simmons, R.L. (1992) *The Chimera* **4**, 9.
112. Morris, R.E., Meiser, B.M., Wu, J. *et al.* (1991) *Transpl. Proc.* **23**, 521.
113. Suzuki, S., Kanashiro, M. & Amemiya, H. (1987) *Transplantation* **44**, 483.
114. Amemiya, H., Suzuki, S., Ota, K. *et al.* (1990) *Transplantation* **49**, 337.
115. Kino, T., Hatanaka, H., Miyata, S. *et al.* (1987) *J. Antibiot.* **40**, 1256.
116. Ochiai, T., Nagata, M., Nakajima, K. *et al.* (1987) *Transplantation* **44**, 729.
117. Inamura, N., Nakahara, K., Kino, T. *et al.* (1988) *Transplantation* **45**, 206.
118. Markus, P.M., Cai, X., Ming, W. *et al.* (1991) *Surgery*, **110**, 357.
119. Starzl, T.E., Todo, S., Fung, J. *et al.* (1989) *Lancet* **2**, 1000.
120. Starzl, T.E., Fung, J., McCauley, J. *et al.* (1991) *Transpl. Proc.* **23**, 920.
121. Fung, J., Todo, S., Abu-Elmagd, K. *et al.* (1993) *Transpl. Proc.* **25**, 1130.
122. Starzl, T.E., Donner, A., Eliasziw, M. *et al.* (1995) *Lancet* **346**, 1310.
123. Morris, R.E. & Brown, B.W. (1995) *Lancet* **346**, 1311.
124. European FK 506 Multicentre Liver Study Group (1994) *Lancet* **344**, 423.
125. Johansson, A. & Möller, E. (1990) *Transplantation* **50**, 1001.
126. McCleod, A.M. & Thomson, A.W. (1991) *Lancet* **337**, 25.
127. Lee, H-J., Pawlak, K., Nguyen, B.T. *et al.* (1985) *Cancer Res.* **45**, 5512.
128. Kumagai, N., Benedict, S.H., Mills, G.B. *et al.* (1988) *J. Immunol.* **141**, 3747.
129. Eugui, E.M., Almquist, S.J., Muller, C.D. *et al.* (1991) *Scand. J. Immunol.* **33**, 161.
130. Eugui, E.M., Mirkovich, A. & Allison, A.C. (1991) *Scand. J. Immunol.* **33**, 175.
131. Lee, W.A., Gu, L., Miksztal, A.R. *et al.* (1990) *Pharm. Res.* **7**, 161.
132. Sollinger. H.W., Deierhoi, M.H., Belzer, F.O. *et al.* (1993) *Transplantation* **53**, 428.
133. Sollinger H.W. (1995) (for the U.S. Renal Transplant Mycophenolate Mofetil Study Group) *Transplantation* **60**, 225.
134. Ensley, R.D., Bristow, M.R., Olsen, S.L. *et al.* (1993) *Transplantation* **56**, 75.

135. Allison, A.C., Eugui, E.M. & Sollinger, H. (1993) *Transpl. Rev.* **7**, 129.
136. Barnard, C.N. (1967) *S. Afr. Med. J.* **41**, 1271.
137. Starzl, T.E., Groth, C.G., Brettschneider, L. *et al.* (1968) *Surgery* **63**, 549.
138. Calne, R.Y., Williams, R., Dawson, J.L. *et al.* (1968) *Brit. Med. J.* **4**, 541.
139. White, R.J. (1968) In *Human Transplantation*, eds F.T. Rapaport & J. Dausset, p. 692, Grune & Stratton, New York.
140. Penn, I. & Starzl, T.E. (1972) *Transplantation* **14**, 407.
141. Penn, I. (1987) *Transplantation* **43**, 32.
142. Marshall, V. (1974) *Transplantation* **17**, 272.
143. Terasaki, I. (ed.) (1991) *History of Transplantation. Thirty-five Recollections*, pp. 1–704, U.C.L.A. Tissue Typing Laboratory, Los Angeles.
144. Opelz, G., Sengar, D.P.S., Mickey, M.R. *et al.* (1973) *Transpl. Proc.* **5**, 253.
145. Michielsen, P. (1966) *Eur. Dial. Transpl. Ass. Proc.* **3**, 162.
146. Dossetor, J.B., MacKinnon, K.J., Gault, M.H. *et al.* (1967) *Transplantation* **5**, 844.
147. Morris, P.J., Ting, A. & Stocker, J. (1968) *Med. J. Aust.* **2**, 1088.
148. Morris, P.J., Williams, G.M., Hume, D.M. *et al.* (1968) *Transplantation* **6**, 392.
149. Patel, R., Merrill, J.P. & Briggs, W.A. (1971) *New Engl. J. Med.* **285**, 274.
150. Opelz, G., Mickey, M.R. & Terasaki, P.I. (1972) *Lancet* **1**, 868.
151. Opelz, G. & Terasaki, P.I. (1974) *Lancet* **2**, 696.
152. Dong, E., Griepp, R.B., Stinson, E.B. *et al.* (1972) *Transpl. Proc.* **4**, 787.
153. Barnes, R.M.R., Pegrum, G.D., Williams, G.B. *et al.* (1974) *Lancet* **2**, 1040.
154. Van Hooff, J.P., Kalff, M.W. & Van Poelgeest, A.E. (1976) *Transplantation* **22**, 306.
155. Festenstein, H., Sachs, J.A., Paris, A.M.I. *et al.* (1976) *Lancet* **1**, 157.
156. Opelz, G. & Terasaki, P.I. (1978) *New Engl. J. Med.* **299**, 799.
157. Opelz, G. & Terasaki, P.I. (1980) *Transplantation* **29**, 153.
158. Horimi, T., Terasaki, P.I., Chia, D. *et al.* (1983) *Transplantation* **35**, 320.
159. Feduska, N.J., Vincenti, F., Amend, W.J. *et al.* (1979) *Transplantation* **27**, 35.
160. Persijn, G.G., Cohen, B., Lansbergen, Q. *et al.* (1979) *Transplantation* **28**, 396.
161. Dewar, P.J., Murray, S., Wilkinson R. *et al.* (1980) *Transplantation* **29**, 379.
162. Persijn, G.G., Lansbergen, Q., D'Amaro, J. *et al.* (1981) *Transplantation* **32**, 392.
163. Sollinger, H.W., Kalayoglu, M. & Belzer, F.O. (1986) *Ann. Surg.* **204**, 315.
164. Salvatierra, O., Vincenti, F., Amend, W. *et al.* (1980) *Ann. Surg.* **192**, 543.
165. Solheim, B.G., Flatmark, A., Halvorsen, S. *et al.* (1980) *Transplantation* **30**, 281.
166. Mendez, R., Iwaki, Y., Mendez, R. *et al.* (1982) *Transplantation* **33**, 621.
167. Leivestad, T., Albrechtsen, D., Flatmark, A. *et al.* (1986) *Transplantation* **42**, 35.
168. Billingham, R.E. & Sparrow, E.M. (1955) *J. Embryol.* **3**, 265.
169. Halasz, N.A., Orloff, M.J. & Hirose, F. (1964) *Transplantation* **2**, 453.
170. Monroe, C.W., Andresen, R.J., Hass, G.H. *et al.* (1960) *Plast. Reconstr. Surg.* **26**, 388.
171. Stark, R.B. & Dwyer, E. (1959) *Surgery* **46**, 277.
172. Halasz, N.A. (1963) *J. Surg. Res.* **3**, 503.
173. Marino, H. & Benaim, F. (1958) *Am. J. Surg.* **95**, 267.
174. Marquet, R.L., Heystek, G.A. & Tinbergen, W.J. (1971) *Transpl. Proc.* **3**, 708.
175. Jenkins, A.M. & Woodruff, M.F.A. (1971) *Transplantation* **12**, 57.
176. Fabre, J.W. & Morris, P.J. (1972) *Transplantation* **14**, 608.
177. Fabre, J.W. & Morris, P.J. (1972) *Transplantation* **14**, 634.
178. Pearson, T.C., Madsen, J.C., Larsen, C.P. *et al.* (1992) *Transplantation* **54**, 575.
179. Bushell, A., Morris, P.J. & Wood, K.J. (1994) *Transplantation* **58**, 133.
180. Storb, R., Kolb, H.J., Kane, P.J. *et al.* (1972) *Transplantation* **14**, 248.
181. Storb, R., Kolb, H.J., Erickson, V. *et al.* (1973) *Transplantation* **15**, 129.
182. Van Es, A.A., Marquet, R.L., Van Rood, J.J. *et al.* (1980) *Lancet* **2**, 506.
183. Van Es, A.A. & Balner, H. (1979) *Transplantation* **28**, 135.
184. Moen, T., Albrechtsen, D., Flatmark, A. *et al.* (1980) *New Engl. J. Med.* **303**, 850.
185. Singal, D.P. & Joseph, S. (1982) *Hum. Immunol.* **4**, 93.
186. Nagarkatti, P.S., Joseph, S. & Singal, D.P. (1986) *Transplantation* **36**, 695.
187. Singal, D.P., Ludwin, D., Joseph, S. *et al.* (1986) *Transplantation* **42**, 632.
188. Suciu-Foca, N., Rohowsky, C., Kung, P. *et al.* (1983) *Transpl. Proc.* **15**, 784.

189. Reed, E., Hardy, M., Lattes, C. *et al.* (1985) *Transpl. Proc.* **17**, 735.
190. Reed, E., Hardy, M., Benvenisty, A. *et al.* (1987) *New Engl. J. Med.* **316**, 1450.
191. Barkley, S.C., Sakai, R.S., Ettenger, R.B. *et al.* (1987) *Transplantation* **44**, 30.
192. Gershon, R.K. & Kondo, K. (1971) *Immunology* **21**, 903.
193. Marquet, R.L. & Heystek, G.A. (1981) *Transplantation* **31**, 272.
194. Maki, T., Okazaki, H., Wood, M.L. *et al.* (1981) *Transplantation* **32**, 463.
195. Smith, M.D., Williams, J.D., Coles, G.A. *et al.* (1983) *Transplantation* **36**, 647.
196. Burlingham, W.J., Grailer, A., Sparks-Mackety, E.M.F. *et al.* (1987) *Transplantation* **43**, 41.
197. Burlingham, W.J., Grailer, A., Sondel, P.M. *et al.* (1988) *Transplantation* **45**, 127.
198. Ruiz, P., Coffman, T.M., Howell, D.N. *et al.* (1988) *Transplantation* **45**, 1.
199. Takiff, H., Novak, M., Yin, L. *et al.* (1987) *Transplantation* **43**, 145.
200. Van Rood, J.J., Persijn, G.G., Goulmy, E. *et al.* (1979) *Behring Inst. Mitt.* **63**, 66.
201. Fehrman, I., Ringden, O. & Möller, E. (1983) *Transplantation* **35**, 339.
202. Cats, S., Terasaki, P.I., Perdue, S. *et al.* (1984) *New Engl. J. Med.* **311**, 675 (letter).
203. Opelz, G. (1985) *Transplantation* **40**, 240.
204. Cecka, J.M., Cicciarelli, J., Mickey, M.R. *et al.* (1988) *Transplantation* **45**, 81.
205. Pfaff, W.W., Howard, R.J., Scornik, J.C. *et al.* (1989) *Transplantation* **47**, 130.
206. Melzer, J.S., Husing, R.M., Feduska, N.J. *et al.* (1987) *Transplantation* **43**, 61.
207. Opelz, G. (1987) *Transpl. Proc.* **19**, 149.
208. Lundgren, G., Groth, C.G., Albrechtsen, D. *et al.* (1986) *Lancet* **2**, 66.
209. Kerman, R.H., Van Buren, C.T., Lewis, R.M. *et al.* (1988) *Transplantation* **45**, 37.
210. Anderson, D., Billingham, R.E., Lampkin, G.H. *et al.* (1951) *Heredity* **5**, 379.
211. Owen, R.D. (1945) *Science* **102**, 400.
212. Brent, L. & Kilshaw, P.J. (1970) *Nature* **227**, 898.
213. Brent, L., Hansen, J.A., Kilshaw, P.J. *et al.* (1973) *Transplantation* **15**, 160.
214. Balner, H. (1964) *Transplantation* **2**, 464.
215. Billingham, R.E. & Brent, L. (1959) *Phil. Trans. B* **242**, 439.
216. Brent, L. & Courtenay, T.H. (1962) In *Mechanisms of Tolerance*, eds M. Hašek, A. Lengerová & M. Vojtisková, p. 113, Czech. Acad. Sci., Prague.
217. Ellis, T.M., Mohanakumar, T. & Lee, H.M. (1985) *Transplantation* **39**, 127.
218. Herzog, W.R., Zanker, B., Huber, C. *et al.* (1987) *Transplantation* **43**, 384.
219. Reinsmoen, N.L., Kaufman, D., Matas, A. *et al.* (1990) *Transplantation* **50**, 783.
220. Reinsmoen, N.L. & Matas, A.J. (1993) *Transplantation* **55**, 1017.
221. Starzl, T.E., Demetris, A.J., Trucco, M. *et al.* (1993) *Hepatology* **17**, 1127.
222. Reyes, J., Zeevi, A., Tzakis, A. *et al.* (1993) *Transplant. Proc.* **25**, 3315.
223. Ramos, H.C., Reyes, J., Abu-Elmagd, K. *et al.* (1995) *Transplant. Proc.* **59**, 212.
224. Starzl, T.E., Porter, K.A., Penn, I. *et al.* (1969) *Surg. Forum* **20**, 374.
225. Porter, K.A. (1969) In *Experience in Hepatic Transplantation*, ed. T.E. Starzl, p. 464, W.B. Saunders, Philadelphia.
226. Kashiwagi, N. (1969) In *Experience in Hepatic Transplantation*, ed. T.E. Starzl, p. 394, W.B. Saunders, Philadelphia,.
227. Starzl, T.E., Demetris, A.J., Trucco, M. *et al.* (1992) *Lancet* **340**, 876.
228. Ricordi, C., Ildstad, S.T., Demetris, A.J. *et al.* (1992) *Lancet* **339**, 1610.
229. Starzl, T.E., Demetris, A.J., Murase, N. *et al.* (1992) *Lancet* **339**, 1579.
230. Starzl, T.E., Demetris, A.J., Trucco, M. *et al.* (1993) *Transplantation* **55**, 1272.
231. Starzl, T.E., Demetris, A.J., Murase, N. *et al.* (1993) *Immunol. Today* **14**, 326.
232. Starzl, T.E. & Demetris, A.J. (1995) *J. Am. Med. Ass.* **273**, 876.
233. Burdick, J.F., Vogelsang, G.B., Smith, W.J. *et al.* (1988) *New Engl. J. Med.* **318**, 689.
234. Morubayashi, S., Matsuzaka, C., Takada, A. *et al.* (1990) *Transplantation* **50**, 710.
235. Roberts, J.P., Ascher, N.L., Lake, J. *et al.* (1991) *Hepatology* **199**, 14.
236. Schlitt, H.J., Hundrieser, J., Hisanaga, M. *et al.* (1994) *Lancet* **343**, 1469.
237. Bushell, A., Pearson, T.C., Morris, P.J. *et al.* (1995) *Transplantation* **59**, 1367.
238. Sharabi, Y. & Sachs, D.H. (1989) *J. Exp. Med.* **169**, 493.
239. Sayegh, M., Fine, N., Smith, J. *et al.* (1991) *Ann. Int. Med.* **114**, 954.
240. Jacobsen, N., Taaning, E., Ladefoged, J. *et al.* (1994) *Lancet* **343**, 800.
241. Sorof, J., Koerper, M., Portale, A. *et al.* (1995) *Transplantation* **59**, 1633.

242. Sharabi, Y., Qbraham, V., Sykes, M. *et al.* (1992) *Bone Marrow Transpl.* **9**, 191.
243. Suberbielle, C., Calliat-Zucman, S. & Legrendre, C. (1994) *Lancet* **343**, 1468.
244. Burlingham, W.J., Grailer, A.P., Fechner, J.H. *et al.* (1995) *Transplantation* **59**, 1147.
245. Nagler, A., Ilan, Y., Amiel, A, *et al.* (1994) *Transplantation* **57**, 1458.
246. Alard, P., Matriano, J.A., Socarras, S. *et al.* (1995) *Transplantation* **60**, 1125.
247. Barber, W.H., Mankin, J.A., Laskow, D.A. *et al.* (1991) *Transplantation* **51**, 70.
248. Fontes, P., Rao, A.S., Demetris, A.J. *et al.* (1994) *Lancet* **344**, 151.

Biographies

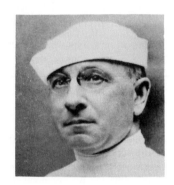

ALEXIS CARREL
(1873–1944)

Alexis Carrel (his real first names were Marie-Joseph-Auguste) was a towering pioneer of vascular surgery, organ transplantation and tissue culture. He studied at the University of Lyon, close to his home in Saint-Foy-les-Lyon, and obtained an L.B. degree in 1890 and an M.D. in 1900. From 1898 he taught anatomy and experimental surgery at the University of Lyon. Among his early scientific papers, published of course in French, were studies on the suturing of blood vessels and the transplantation of organs (1902). Having failed to secure an appointment as a surgeon in Lyon he became disillusioned with the French medical establishment and went to Montreal and from there to Chicago, where the University offered him a post in the Hull Physiology Laboratory. Here began a close collaboration with C.C. Guthrie. It was in Chicago that Carrel pioneered a reproducible technique for suturing severed blood vessels, and this stood him in good stead when he later turned his attention to organ transplantation. In 1906 he accepted a Fellowship in S. Flexner's department in the Rockefeller Institute and thus began an association that continued for more than three decades. Carrel was, however, careful to retain his French nationality. In 1913 he married a French widow, Anne-Marie de la Maire, who came from Brittany, and it was in Brittany that the Carrels later created a permanent home.

In 1910 Carrel published a paper in *The Journal of Experimental Medicine* on the preservation of arterial grafts. He compared a variety of methods such as heating, drying and immersion in formalin or glycerol, but found a vaseline wrapping to be the most effective. In his work on organ transplantation in the period 1907–1912 he distinguished between auto-, homo- and heteroplastic grafts and, having observed that the heteroplastic (xenogeneic) grafts did not survive, he concentrated on auto- and homoplastic (allogeneic) grafts of limbs and kidneys. Although he solved many of the technical problems he was baffled by the relatively short survival of the allogeneic grafts. Because he suspected that the recipients were reacting against their grafts he began to use sibling dogs and cats, with results that were not substantially different. Interestingly, his experimental work soon came to the attention of anti-vivisectionists: he received a death threat and the Institute was forced to impose stringent controls over animal experimentation. However, in 1912 Carrel was awarded the Nobel Prize in Medicine for his "work on vascular suture and the transplantation of organs".

Carrel began his studies on tissue culture before World War I because he believed that the problems of human pathology could only be solved by a close understanding of the "still unknown laws of regeneration, growth and evolution of cells". With M.T. Burrows he soon showed that tissues from a variety of mammals could be grown *in vitro*, that this was equally true for neoplastic cells, and that the addition of embryo extracts to the medium aided survival and growth. This interest preoccupied him for the best part of three decades, almost until the outbreak of World War II. He thus laid the foundations of modern tissue culture, a gigantic achievement. He also carried out large-scale studies on the perfusion of organs with the ambitious aim of establishing organs in culture. In July 1939 Carrel returned to France, knowing that war was imminent. He returned to New York in May 1940, without his wife, and later made his way to Spain and from there to Vichy France, in the hope of being of service to his country. After the war he was accused, probably wrongly, of having been a collaborator, and he died in Paris late in 1944 after a period of ill-health and disillusionment before charges could be brought against him.

I am indebted to T.I. Malinin's *Surgery and Life. The Extraordinary Career of Alexis Carrel* (1979), Harcourt Brace Jovanovich, New York.

JOSEPH EDWARD MURRAY (1919–)

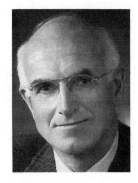

Joe Murray was born in Milford, a small town in Massachusetts, where he spent his childhood. His father was a local judge and his mother a school teacher. Probably influenced by the family's doctor, he knew from an early age that he "was born to be a surgeon", and that is what he became after attending the College of the Holy Cross in Worcester, Massachusetts and studies at Harvard Medical School, which he completed towards the end of World War II. His internship and residency were at the Peter Bent Brigham Hospital, Boston, and his name was to become inextricably linked with that august institution. Apart from his army service (1944–1947), during which he was promoted to the rank of Major, and later a year in The New York Hospital as resident in plastic surgery, he has spent the whole of his professional life at the Brigham. He married Bobby Link in 1945; her father and uncle had developed the Link Trainer, which proved to be useful to the American and British Air Forces during the war. They have had six children, all of whom have pursued successful careers. "We've had a marvelous, blessed family life, now having 14 grandchildren", Murray wrote to me, and his family has clearly been very important to him, despite or perhaps because all the pressures faced by a busy and successful surgeon working at the frontiers of his field.

When Murray returned to the Brigham after his army service he met another ex-army Major and renal physician, John Merrill, and there began a close collaborative partnership that ended only in the premature death of Merrill in 1984 in a yachting accident. Joe Murray likes to stress the complete integration of medical and surgical services at the Brigham, and this also involved G. Dammin's Department of Pathology. The young and highly promising surgeon D.M. Hume joined the team, and F.D. Moore, head of the department, was the *éminence grise* throughout that period. Having devised a more satisfactory surgical technique for kidney transplantation in dogs and having derived some encouragement from kidneys in untreated human recipients, the team performed its first renal transplant between identical twins in 1954. As Murray wrote in *The Chimera* 2, 1, (1990), "The complete, immediate success of this twin transplant was noted worldwide and served as a powerful stimulus to surgeons and basic scientists alike". This led to the transplantation of a number of renal allografts in the late 1950s, using whole body irradiation and bone marrow infusion, but only one of these (between dizygotic twins) was successful. Thanks to the introduction of azathioprine as an immunosuppressive drug by G. Hitchings and T. Elion, and the demonstration in 1960 by R.Y. Calne and D.M. Hume's group of its efficacy in dogs, X-irradiation was soon abandoned in favor of drug treatment, and impressive results were obtained at the Brigham and subsequently elsewhere. Murray played a vital role in this pioneering work and his contribution was recognized when in 1990 he shared the Nobel Prize in Medicine. Typically, he feels that "the greatest satisfaction, the longest lasting, comes from the patients".

Murray has been Professor of Surgery at the Brigham since 1970 and holds a number of other appointments; and he has been widely honored by the award of honorary membership and fellowship of surgical and medical societies in the United States and in many other countries. Prizes, medals and awards, apart from the Nobel Prize, include the Gold Medal of the International Society of Surgeons, the dedication to him (and J.P. Merrill and the Frenchman J. Hamburger) of the 1980 International Congress of The Transplantation Society, honorary fellowship of the Royal College of Surgeons of London, and the Medal for Distinguished Service to Surgery of the American Surgical Society He is an honorary citizen of the City of

Boston. Despite leading an exceptionally busy professional and family life Joe has pursued his hobbies of back-packing, mountain climbing, skiing, and especially tennis, a lifelong passion.

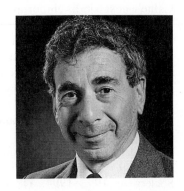

ROY YORKE CALNE
(1930–)

Roy Calne was born in Richmond, Surrey and educated at a well-known English public (i.e. private!) school for boys, Lancing College. He received his medical education at Guy's Hospital Medical School, London and qualified as a surgeon. He spent comparatively short periods in Oxford and at three London teaching hospitals and most of his professional life has been spent in Cambridge, where he became Professor of Surgery in 1965 and where he continues to work. He married Patricia (Patsy) Whelan in 1956 and they have two sons and four daughters.

Calne's interest in transplantation was first aroused when as a medical student he saw patients suffering from fatal diseases that could potentially have been corrected by organ transplantation, but encouragement to enter this embryonic field came only when he met Mr J. Hopewell, a urologic surgeon at the Royal Free Hospital, London. This was the beginning of a distinguished career as a transplant surgeon and although in later years Calne was not averse to berating the professional immunologists for failing to solve some of the clinical problems, he himself sponsored much valuable immunologic research in his department. Through Dr (later Professor) K.A. Porter at St Mary's Hospital he became interested in the (then) recently discovered immunosuppressive properties of 6-mercaptopurine and he proceeded to apply this drug to kidney transplantation in dogs. His 1960 *Lancet* paper describing prolongation of kidney allograft survival was seminal and during a spell at the Peter Bent Brigham Hospital, where he worked as a Research Fellow with F. Moore, J.E. Murray, and P. Merrill, he continued with this work and took part in the first successful clinical transplant using the 6-mercaptopurine analog, azathioprine.

In Cambridge Calne developed a large surgical department which soon became the leading renal transplantation unit in the United Kingdom. Being a man of inexhaustible energy and enthusiasm he fostered a research group that showed, in collaboration with Dr R. Binns at the Agricultural Research Station at Babraham, near Cambridge, that tolerance to kidneys could be induced in the pig by injecting donor cells into the fetus, and that the tolerance applied only partially to skin grafts from the same donor. Their demonstration that liver allografts are often accepted spontaneously by pigs, and that this tolerance also extended to other subsequently transplanted organs from the same donor, remains an intriguing puzzle. Calne's colleagues showed that the same is true for at least some rat strain combinations. Calne's next vitally important contribution, together with Dr D.J.G. White, was the application of cyclosporin A to experimental, and soon after to clinical, kidney transplantation, thus ushering in a new era of clinical immunosuppression. The early application to renal transplantation was carried out with the considerable risk of incurring unacceptable side-effects and reflected Calne's ebullience and his intrepid and sure-footed approach to clinical problems. Other major contributions have been in clinical liver and pancreas transplantation – he pioneered experimental and clinical techniques for the liver – and, with White, in the recent development of xeno-transplantation.

Roy Calne has received honors of all kinds, from Fellowship of the Royal Society in 1973 to a Knighthood in 1986, and he was President of The Transplantation Society in 1993–1994. He has received numerous prizes, medals and honorary degrees, and he shared the prestigious Medawar Prize, awarded for the second time in 1992, with T.E. Starzl and E.D. Thomas. His many publications include several books. He has been a keen and highly competitive sportsman (tennis, squash and skiing) and has developed a considerable talent as a painter, his paintings having been exhibited both in the United Kingdom and abroad. This talent was recognized by the acceptance of one of his paintings for a Summer Exhibition of the Royal Academy of Arts.

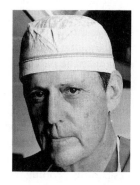

THOMAS EARL STARZL
(1926–)

Tom Starzl was born in LeMars, a small town in western Iowa. His father had been a writer of science fiction stories and owner, publisher and editor of a family newspaper, the *Globe Post*, a man with an "unquenchable . . . instinct to build his own machines". His father's parents had emigrated from central Europe and had an unusually colorful history; Starzl's mother Anna Laura Fitzgerald had, on the other hand, come from Irish stock. Tom's family background and his boyhood years have been lovingly described in his memoirs, *The Puzzle People*, as has much else. Young

Tom learnt to play the cornet and was a talented (American) football player. A few weeks before his mother's death in 1947 he graduated from Westminster College, in Fulton, Mississippi and went on to study medicine at Northwestern Medical School, Chicago, where he completed his Ph.D. and M.D. A powerful influence proved to be the presence of H.W. Magoun, professor of neuroanatomy, who "taught me the true meaning of research", but despite an introduction to the Karolinska Institute to work with Ragner Granit Starzl decided to become a surgeon. In this he was much influenced by the neurosurgeon Loyal Davis, whose daughter Nancy was to marry Ronald Reagan, who later became President of the United States. His internship was spent at The Johns Hopkins Hospital, Baltimore, where he spent "the most formative period of my surgical life". In 1954 Starzl married Barbara June Brothers and they had two sons and a daughter; the marriage came to an end after 22 years. Some years later he married Joy Denise Conger, a black member of his research group.

Starzl became Associate Professor of Surgery at the University of Colorado, Denver in 1961 and stayed there for 17 years. He then moved to Pittsburgh, where he has remained ever since. Once he had entered the field of organ transplantation his steely determination, his capacity for unsparingly hard work, his intelligent and restlessly questioning approach, and his recognition that clinical problems can only be resolved with the aid of laboratory-based research ensured that he made some gigantic contributions to the development of the field. Starzl is a pioneer surgeon–immunologist in the finest tradition. He was among the first to use steroids in conjunction with azathioprine and to apply antilymphocyte globulin to clinical kidney transplantation. Together with his colleagues he pioneered liver transplantation, and he introduced the drug FK 506 at a time when cyclosporine was widely accepted as the standard immunosuppressive agent – an act of considerable faith and courage. He was one of the intrepid surgeons who in the early 1960s transplanted baboon kidneys to patients, and in 1992 he carried out the first clinical transplant of a baboon liver. Thanks to his scientific approach even his failures have yielded worthwhile information. Starzl's latest preoccupation has been his advocacy of cellular donor chimerism as the cause rather than the consequence of graft acceptance, generating lively controversy.

Starzl has been incredibly prolific in his publications, which number 1400, four books and 163 chapters. The honors and awards with which his work has been recognized are far too numerous to list. He was Founding President of the American Association of Transplant Surgeons (1975) and of the Transplant Recipients International Organization (1987), and President of The Transplantation Society in 1990. In 1984 he was elected to honorary membership of the Royal College of Surgeons of England and membre d'honneur étranger de la Societé de Chirurgie de Lyon, A. Carrel's Alma Mater. He has been awarded over a dozen honorary doctorates from universities in the United States and Europe, and among his most cherished prizes are the David M. Hume Memorial Award (1978), the Medallion for Scientific achievement of the American Surgical Association (1990), election as Associé Étranger de L'Academie de Médicine (1991) and the Peter Medawar Prize (1992).

8 Graft-versus-Host Disease and Bone Marrow Transplantation

> *"Many a golden opportunity has been squandered by anti-prophets who do not realise that the grounds for declaring something impossible or inconceivable may be undermined by new ideas which cannot be foreseen."*
>
> P.B. Medawar, 1961

The earliest attempts at clinical bone marrow transplantation were made in the second half of the 1950s, at roughly the same time as kidney transplantation was initiated. They ran into all kinds of difficulties because the recipients had malignant disease, the drugs used to eliminate the malignant cells were still highly experimental, and graft-versus-host disease (GVHD) – at that time not a recognized phenomenon – raised its ugly head whenever allogeneic bone marrow cells did survive in their hosts. This chapter deals with the immunologic consequences of establishing foreign cell populations comprising not only hemopoietic, but also immunologically competent, cells in immunocompromised recipients, and explains how the discovery of GVHD in experimental animals impinged on the development of therapeutic bone marrow transplantation. Two quite distinct experimental avenues led to the recognition of GVHD:

(1) The study of secondary, or homologous, disease in radiation bone marrow chimeras.
(2) The induction of tolerance in immunologically immature animals.

It must be said that the latter had the more decisive impact and that it also threw light on the ill-understood causes of secondary disease.

Secondary (or Homologous) Disease in Lethally Irradiated Mice

The early years

The destructive powers of X-irradiation on lymphoid and myeloid tissue have been appreciated since Heineke's (*1*) observations early in the century and Benjamin and Sluka (*2*) found that X-irradiation diminished the production of precipitating antibodies to 'beef serum' and delayed the disappearance of the antigen from the blood of rabbits. Others, including Hektoen (*3*), studied the effect of irradiation on antibody production. Hektoen found that antibodies to sheep red blood cells were "restrained to a marked degree" if irradiation (dose unknown) was administered repeatedly some days before the sheep blood was injected into rats provided the number of blood leukocytes was greatly reduced. A single large dose of irradiation was eventually lethal, but for about eight days no antibody was formed. He concluded that antibodies must be produced in the spleen, lymphatic tissues and marrow. Craddock and Lawrence (4) returned to this theme and, apart from thoroughly reviewing the literature, confirmed that a known dose (250 rads) of whole body irradiation (WBI) in rabbits resulted in marked lymphopenia and depressed antibody responses provided that the antigen was administered within hours of WBI. Dempster, Lennox and Boag in London were the first to show that not only antibody production, but also the rejection of skin allografts (5) and the development of delayed-type hypersensitivity to tuberculin (6), were inhibited by sublethal irradiation.

The deployment of the atom bomb towards the end of World War II and the impact the effects of radiation had on the world caused a great upsurge of interest in radiation biology and led several countries to establish radiobiologic research institutes. Prominent among them were the Oak Ridge National Laboratory in Tennessee (United States), the Radiobiological Research Unit of the Atomic Energy Research Establishment in Harwell (United Kingdom) and the Radiobiologic Institute in Rijswijk (The Netherlands). The main emphasis was the possible mitigation of radiation-induced damage to the hemopoietic system. Once the lethal dose of irradiation had been established for mice and bone marrow destruction established as the main cause of death, attempts were made to counter the effects of radiation by inoculating foreign bone marrow cells. Cells obtained from genetically different mice – allogeneic in modern terminology – were called homologous in those days, and hence the term homologous disease. This ensued after a delay of at least a few weeks but it was usually lethal despite a transient protection from radiation damage to the recipient's own bone marrow.

American workers of the early 1950s believed that the protective effect was brought about by factors released by the transplanted cells, a notion first proposed by Jacobson et al. (7, 8) on the strength of the observation that shielding of the spleens of lethally irradiated mice enabled some animals to survive. They thought it unlikely that cells would have migrated out of the shielded spleen and proposed that soluble factors were involved. Others showed that bone marrow given to guinea pigs (9) and mice (10, 11) produced similar effects, and that homogenized spleen cells were just as effective as the intact spleen (10, 11), especially when inoculated intravenously. Lorenz et al. (9) suggested that bone marrow cells acted by causing "the generation of new areas of hematopoiesis, contrary to the assumption of Jacobson of a humoral factor". However, as Barnes and Loutit (12) pointed out in an article entitled "What is the recovery factor in spleen?", all these findings were "compatible with either hypothesis – the humoral or the vital", the latter based on the survival of the transferred cells. This was the first time that the cell repopulation hypothesis was given a serious airing, and the evidence presented by Barnes and Loutit indicated that the viability of the transplanted cells was vital for protection to occur – itself not, of course, decisive for the vital hypothesis. It did, however, open the flood gates for new studies incontrovertibly in its favor.

First, Main and Prehn (13) discovered in 1955 that irradiated parental strain mice given F_1 hybrid bone marrow accepted skin allografts from the other parental strain. They concluded that the transferred bone marrow had rescued the recipients from radiation injury and, in establishing 'pseudo-hybrids', had determined the survival of the skin allografts. This strongly suggested that the foreign marrow cells had survived and proliferated in their new hosts. Trentin (14) was soon to confirm these data and to show that CBA–C3H chimeras accepted skin grafts from either parental strain. Second, in the same year Lindsley, Odell and Tausche (15) found that rats irradiated with the LD_{50} dose (at which half the animals died) and inoculated with allogeneic marrow cells had up to 80% of red cells from the donor circulating in their blood within 2–3 weeks, and that these cells persisted for up to five months. They quoted the red cell chimera data of R.D. Owen and the skin graft survival findings of Medawar's group in cattle dizygotic twins (see Chapter 5) and felt that "it is unnecessary to postulate a humoral factor or a transitory activity of the implant as the mechanism responsible for recovery of the erythropoietic and inferentially myelopoietic potential . . .". Together with R.D. Owen they fully confirmed and extended this conclusion two years later (16); while not mentioning GVHD as a possible complication they stated that "the irradiated host marrow cannot compete sucessfully with the implanted marrow". Third, Nowell et al. (17) soon showed that rat granulocytes likewise persisted in irradiated mice given rat bone marrow.

However, definite proof of the survival of implanted hemopoietic tissue came from several quarters in 1956. The Harwell group, with the aid of C.E. Ford, an expert cytogeneticist, demonstrated (18) beyond doubt with the aid of chromosomal markers that allogeneic cells with hemopoietic functions persisted in irradiated mice that had been 'rescued' with spleen cells from infant mice carrying the T6 translocation. All dividing cells in the bone marrow were of donor origin, and the same was true when the inoculated marrow was of rat origin. "These results would seem to establish finally that cellular repopulation is the mechanism by which spleen and other tissues bring about their therapeutic effect", they wrote. Their study was limited to the first few weeks after transplantation and in a subsequent paper (19) they concluded that in the rat–mouse chimeras the rat cells were eventually, "although perhaps never quite completely", replaced by cells of the host. Others came quite independently to much the same conclusion, among them Vos et al. (20), Makinodan (21), Merwin and Congdon (22) and Mitchison (23). The latter used two experimental approaches. First, the histocompatibility antigens of the donor spleen cells were used as markers, in that cells taken from the putative radiation chimera had the power to sensitize normal syngeneic mice against tumor grafts from the donor strain. And second, by using spleen cells from mice that had been immunized by bacterial antigens in the establishment of the chimeras, he was able to show that enhanced titers of specific antibody were present in the irradiated hosts.

"The year 1956 marked a turning point of work on tissue transfusion therapy after irradiation. The cellular hypothesis had been proved substantially correct, but the humoral hypothesis had not been disproved", wrote Koller, Davies and Doak (24) rather cautiously in 1961 in a wide-ranging review of the literature on radiation chimeras. However, a clear understanding of the causes of secondary disease in animals that had been rescued with allogeneic as opposed to syngeneic or F_1 hybrid hemopoietic tissues had to await developments elsewhere, with one important exception. In 1957 D. Uphoff (25) published a study on radiation chimeras in mice in which she observed that F_1 hybrid bone marrow usually 'took' better than parental marrow, and that the latter was associated with many deaths during the second phase of the radiation syndrome. Mice died with extreme diarrhea and emaciation. She found a positive correlation between the H-2 type of the donor strain and the degree of protection, and concluded that "Evidence at present indicates that an immune response of the graft against the host, when the graft and the host have different histocompatibility genotypes at the H-2 locus, is responsible for the secondary phase of the irradiation syndrome". She was clearly unaware of the work published in that year by Simonsen and by Billingham and Brent (see below) and must therefore be credited with the co-discovery of GVHD, in her case in radiation chimeras. She did, however, quote a previous publication by Billingham, Brent and Medawar (26) in which this group discussed the mechanism underlying the termination of tolerance after the adoptive transfer of normal lymph node cells into mice that had been made neonatally tolerant of allogeneic skin grafts. They had written: ". . . it follows that a graft which is immunologically qualified to do so . . . can react against the tissues of the host . . . We particularly urge that the possible reactions of a graft against its host should be kept in mind whenever normal tissues or tumors are transplanted from members of inbred parental lines into their F_1 progeny. The fact that such a graft contains no antigens not also present in the host may cause one to forget that the host contains antigens which are absent from the graft".

The Discovery of Graft-versus-Host Disease (GVHD)

Straws in the wind and a false trail

GVHD was discovered independently by two groups: M. Simonsen in Copenhagen (see biographic sketch, p. 373), and R.E. Billingham (p. 372) and L. Brent in London. It is, however, of considerable historic interest that two Americans, V. Danchakoff (27) and J.B. Murphy (28), having observed the enlargement of the chick embryo spleen after transplantation of adult chicken tissues such as spleen on to the chorioallantoic membrane, had been extraordinarily close to anticipating GVHD. Danchakoff thought that a growth stimulus had come from the adult spleen cells, but she could not decide whether the enlargement of the embryonic spleen was due to local proliferation of the embryonic tissue or to graft cells that "could be transported to the spleen and here under favorable conditions proliferate". A surprisingly acerbic footnote in her lengthy paper indicates that there was some rivalry between her and Murphy concerning precedence of the discovery of splenomegaly. In the event, the time was not ripe for a decisive resolution even though Murphy had got very close to understanding the immunologic function of lymphocytes (see Chapter 2). Not only had Murphy observed splenic enlargement but he had also carefully described and photographed nodules on the chorioallantoic membrane around the site of tissue implantation. Murphy and others after him tended to explain these findings in terms of cellular stimulation by growth factors. It does seem astonishing that Murphy, who in the first three decades of the twentieth century was arguably the most able experimentalist in the field of tumor biology and who managed to get so close to identifying the lymphocyte as the mediator of tumor graft rejection, failed to make that last leap of the imagination with respect to both allograft rejection and GVHD. Simonsen (personal communication) did not know of Murphy and Danchakoff's data when carrying out his splenomegaly studies, though he had become aware of them by the time he wrote his 1957 paper, in which they received a brief mention. In a much later review of graft-versus-host reactions Simonsen (29) discussed the earlier work at some length and speculated as to why Murphy had remained blind to the real causes of the lesions and splenomegaly he had observed so acutely.

There had, however, been some overt suggestions concerning the concept of graft-versus-host reactivity (GVHR), but from a totally different direction. The first came from a London-based transplant surgeon, W.J. Dempster, who was an intelligent and productive experimental surgeon in the 1950s. Dempster not only made some important early observations on the destruction of allogeneic kidneys, skin and adrenals in experimental animals and showed that skin allografts could be prolonged by sublethal WBI (see above), but also wrote some perceptive reviews on allotransplantation. One such review was published in the *British Medical Journal* in 1951 (30). Although primarily devoted to skin transplantation it included a substantial review of current theories and a stout defense of Medawar's 'actively acquired immunity' hypothesis. However, what is of special interest in this context is that his histologic examination of allogeneic kidneys transplanted to non-immunosuppressed dogs led him to speculate about the possibility of an immunologic reaction of the graft against the host. He had noted the "mixed round-cell infiltration around the small blood vessels and glomerular capsule" before tissue destruction set in. He offered two explanations, apart from a cellular reaction interpreted by Loeb "in terms of a purely local interaction between kidney and host in which the lymphocytes and plasma cells react to 'differentials' locally in the kidney substance" (see Chapter 2) – an explanation that clearly did not appeal to Dempster. First, it could be caused by "a proliferation of already existing reticulo-endothelial cells in the kidney", an interpretation that "suggests that the homotransplanted kidney reacts against its host". Second, it was possible that the immune reaction in the kidney was acellular in character but attracted mesenchymal cells of the host. He thought that the former hypothesis was the more likely and he developed it further in a subsequent review of kidney transplantation published in 1953 (31). I shall come back to this presently, but it should be noted that Dempster at that time was thinking primarily of kidney destruction as a result of antibody formation.

The second pointer came from Simonsen (32) in 1953, when he published his data on kidney allograft rejection in dogs. Histologic examination of kidneys undergoing rejection revealed pyronine-positive cells in the cortical interstitium, including some small lymphocytes, particularly around the glomeruli, and he believed that these cells were of local origin (i.e. from the kidney) and engaged in a reaction against the host. While Simonsen's preference was clearly to interpret the occurrence of the infiltrating cells as of graft origin he also left the door open to the possibility that they might have migrated into the kidney tissue from the blood.

As it turned out, the GVHD interpretation of Dempster and Simonsen, though boldly imaginative, was shown to be incorrect when a few years later Hume et al. (33) found that the infiltrate could be suppressed by irradiation of the host and Porter and Calne (34), using radiographic techniques, demonstrated that the infiltrate consisted of host cells. While the GVHR speculations had prepared and inspired Simonsen for his later chicken studies he nonetheless rescinded the interpretation of his histologic observations in his 1962 review (35). Thus he wrote: "It seems at least clear that any claim today of the occurrence of GvH-reactions in the transplanted kidney would have to be established on new evidence".

The discovery of graft-versus-host reactivity (GVHR) in chick embryos – Simonsen's salient contribution

In 1957 Simonsen (36) published his seminal paper describing experiments that "took their origin in a previously formulated concept of transplantation immunity ... claiming that immunization takes place not only in the host against the graft but vice versa as well". He later recounted (37) how he had visited Medawar, Billingham and Brent at University College, London, early in 1954 "where they generously demonstrated their techniques for injection of mouse and chicken embryos. That afternoon changed my career. I never did another kidney transplantation myself, whereas thousands of chicken and newborn mice came to serve my enquiries for many years to come."

In his 1957 paper Simonsen (36) described the inoculation of adult spleen or peripheral blood buffy coat cells into chick embryos, mainly three days before hatching. Most recipients developed severe hemolytic anemia and died within one or two weeks after hatching, usually with a strongly positive Coombs' direct test, and this strongly supported his conclusion that the anemia was caused by immune hemolysis. Because no antibodies formed against the red blood cells of the donor Simonsen assumed that the recipients had become tolerant of the donor's antigens. Post mortem examination revealed splenic enlargement by a factor of two or more and marked changes in the spleen, liver, thymus and bone marrow. "A microscopic study of the development of these changes is fully compatible with the assumption that cell members of the transplant have by host antigens been stimulated to multi-plication and antibody formation. In doing so they largely destroyed and replaced the native population", he wrote. The capacity for inducing splenomegaly could be passaged to new embryos through nine consecutive passages "without significant loss of activity". The recipients had to be young enough to become tolerant and the donors old enough to be able to "form antibodies". Preliminary evidence showed that splenomegaly occurred only when the donors and recipients were genetically different. Simonsen postulated that the use of embryonic rather than adult spleen cells should not cause splenomegaly because tolerance would have been induced in the donor cells, and he provided some preliminary evidence for this. "While these results fit the hypothesis perfectly, they are no formal proof of it. Anyhow, it should be possible to design experiments that would formally prove or disprove the hypothesis." Simonsen went on to interpret 'homologous' disease in radiation chimeras as caused by a GVHR and suggested that diseases such as agammaglobulin-emia and post-irradiation disease in human beings should be treated by fetal rather than by adult cells.

Simonsen, who recently described his discoveries in his Medawar Prize Lecture (37), went on to study GVHD in chicks as well as in newborn mice and made many more contributions, among them the development of the splenomegaly assay as a quantitative test for GVHR (35). He used this assay for identifying immunologically competent cells (38) – as had Terasaki (39) before him – and for characterizing the major histo-compatibility complex (MHC) of the chicken (40). Using inbred lines of chickens he, together with A.G. Cock (41), showed in 1958 that F_1 hybrid cells injected into newly hatched chicks of one of the parental lines caused only a very slight degree of splenomegaly consistent with the known residual diversity in these lines.

Discovery of graft-versus-host disease in the mouse by Billingham and Brent

While Simonsen was engaged in his chicken study, R.E. Billingham and L. Brent had come to the conclusion that the mortality they and P.B. Medawar had encountered when inoculating adult lymphoid tissues into mouse embryos was caused by GVHD and not, as they had originally assumed, by infection or other factors (42). Their tolerance studies had started in 1952 and it is surprising that it was not until 1956, when Billingham and Brent had mastered the art of injecting allogeneic cells into the venous circulation of newborn mice, that GVHD was identified as the cause (43). The circumstances in which this discovery came about have been described by Brent (44) in his Medawar Prize Lecture. The induction of tolerance in newborn mice through the use of the intravenous route, which Billingham and Brent (43) had pioneered, made tolerance induction a predictable event compared with 'blind' inoculation into the embryos, and the delayed mortality encountered – often within 2–3 weeks of inoculation, sometimes much later – demanded an explanation. In their 1957 paper, Billingham and Brent (43) described the following findings.

(1) In some strain combinations, but not in all, the intravenous route was a highly efficient means of inducing specific tolerance to skin allografts.
(2) Tolerant mice were cellular chimeras (i.e. their spleens and lymph nodes possessed significant numbers of donor-derived cells).
(3) Depending on the strain combination used there was a variable mortality, ranging from 100% in some strains to 17% in others.
(4) About half the tolerant mice as shown by donor skin transplantation showed extensive or complete involution of their lymph nodes.
(5) Some of the mice "never developed properly; they were runts and usually died within 40–60 days of birth, their weights not having increased beyond 7–14 gms". (The origin of the term 'runt', familiar to mouse and pig breeders, has been explained by McLaren and Michie (45); it describes a congenital abnormality occurring spontaneously in 1–5% of mouse litters and determining that the affected animal has a natural growth well below that of its littermates.)
(6) Finally, those runts that could be skin-grafted were tolerant, and the runts had virtually no lymph nodes, while their spleens, though outwardly normal, were grossly deficient in Malpighian corpuscles.

Billingham and Brent considered two hypotheses. The first, based on the supposition that the foreign spleen cells might have introduced a pathogen, was more or less dismissed because the subcutaneous administration of allogeneic cells did not produce runts. They favored the alternative hypothesis, that "the abnormalities and deaths may be the outcome of immunological reactions produced by the inoculated adult spleen cells against the tissue antigens in their young hosts". They were struck by the fact that the organs most affected were precisely those to which lymphocytes tended to migrate, and by the finding that there was considerable variability in different strain combinations (i.e. the differences could be "a function of the antigenic disparities between donor and host"). Further, they noted that tolerance induction with cells that did not comprise immunologically competent cells (e.g. kidney, tumors or skin) was not accompanied by runting. They concluded that "If our hypothesis of a graft-versus-host reaction is correct, then it may have important clinical bearings". These included the danger of transfusing immunologically reactive cells into newborn babies, hypogammaglobulinemic patients or heavily irradiated animals given genetically foreign homologous spleen cells. Their paper finished by stating: "We feel that the concept of a graft versus host reaction must be carefully considered before any form of therapy is applied which may not only defeat the surgeon's objective but also cause immeasurable harm to the patient".

While Billingham (46) and Brent (47) enlarged on their findings in 1958, their *magnum opus* on the topic of runt disease, in which their data were collected together and their speculations were more wide-ranging, did not appear until 1959 (48). The reasons for this was Brent's absence for a year in the United States and, just before he returned in 1957, Billingham's departure from University College to join the Wistar Institute in Philadelphia. A further delay in publication came about when they insisted on the inclusion of color photographs; it took almost a year for their paper to appear in print. They showed conclusively that runt disease was caused by a GVHR, quoting the following evidence.

(1) The foreign cells persisted indefinitely.
(2) Inoculation of F_1 hybrid cells into newborn mice was harmless.
(3) Parental strain cells inoculated into F_1 hybrid neonates led to typical runt disease.
(4) The severity and frequency of runt disease were enhanced when presensitized lymphoid cells were used.
(5) Acute runt disease could be avoided by using cells such as bone marrow that had no, or few, immunologically competent cells or by the inclusion of syngeneic adult spleen cells in the inoculum.
(6) The severity and incidence of root disease were affected by antigenic differences between donor and host – when only minor histocompatibility differences were present, runt disease was negligible or non-existent.
(7) Finally, embryonic donor cells, though able to establish tolerance, failed to induce runt disease.

They also showed that if the inoculum comprised spleen cells from two different strains, both of them allogeneic to the neonatal recipient as well to themselves, there was some but not total protection due to a graft-versus-graft effect.

Billingham and Brent also described the circumstances in which they encountered severe splenomegaly in mice that had been given F_1 hybrid cells at birth or later in life after tolerance had been induced and they discussed the possible reasons for this rather bizarre finding. They emphasized the very great similarity between runt disease and homologous disease and thought that their data supported Trentin's (14) hypothesis that homologous disease was brought about by a response of the foreign cells against host antigens. Billingham and Brent pointed out that there was not necessarily any inconsistency in the lethality of allogeneic bone marrow transplants in irradiated adult hosts and the relatively mild effects observed in newborn mice: the irradiated animal might well provide a better opportunity for small numbers of immunologically competent cells to proliferate "and so to reach a fatally high density". In support of this argument they quoted the work of E.O. Owen *et al.* (49), who found that the growth of autologous bone marrow in dogs was greatly facilitated by WBI. Among their speculations as to the clinical significance of their findings was the possibility that some fetal lesions, such as those found in hydrops fetalis, might be brought about by maternal blood leukocytes accidentally entering the fetal circulation and reacting against the antigens of the fetus.

At the time of their GVHD discovery Billingham and Brent were unaware of the far earlier observations on splenomegaly by Murphy and Danchakoff and of Dempster and Simonsen's interpretation of their histologic findings in canine kidney allografts (see above). However, in their 1959 paper these were all duly acknowledged. Attention was also drawn to other workers who had suggested the possibility of GVHD. Thus, Woodruff and Sparrow (50) had encountered some mortality in the course of tolerance induction in newborn rats and, having heard of Billingham and Brent's early data, thought that this might have been caused by the grafted cells reacting against their hosts, a "matter of considerable clinical importance because attempts have already been made by the writer . . . to induce tolerance in human infants", and they quoted Woodruff's publication on this (51). Reactions of grafted cells against their hosts were also observed in 1958 by Egdahl et al. (52) while attempting to induce tolerance in rodents to xenogeneic tissues; and the disease and mortality observed by Nakić and Silobrčić (53) after the parabiosis of adult rats, first encountered by Finerty (54), was interpreted by the Yugoslav workers as probably having been caused by GVHR.

Billingham and Brent (48) believed runt disease to be primarily an "orthodox (i.e. cell-mediated) homograft reaction" but did not rule out the participation of antibodies, as reported by Simonsen (36), for they too had found most runted mice to be anemic. They had noted that some mice arrived at some sort of accommodation with the foreign cells, and vice versa. Simonsen (55) speculated on 'exhaustive sensitization' of the foreign cells as an explanation, supported by his finding that adult parental spleen cells transferred to F_1 hybrids became rapidly and specifically unable to react against host antigens. This hypothesis derived further support from Dineen (56), who was unable to transfer runt disease to secondary recipients despite the presence of donor cells in the inoculum, as well as from Cole and Davis (57), who found that the allogeneic cells in radiation chimeras were specifically unresponsive to host antigens.

Development of the graft-versus-host disease concept

The phenomenon of GVHD was therefore firmly established by 1959 and it was to be described in many experimental species as well as clinically (see below). The early observations led to a major escalation in the number of papers published. Many of these used the two main assays – splenomegaly and runting – as a means of tackling more general immunologic problems, but they were also used to elucidate the mechanisms responsible for GVHD and the cellular mediators involved. Variants of a third type of assay measuring a purely local GVHR were introduced by a number of workers. These included the normal lymphocyte transfer reaction (NLT) described by Brent and Medawar (58, 59) in guinea pigs, in which allogeneic cells inoculated into the skin set up an inflammatory response against host antigens that the authors hoped might be useful as a means of selecting human organ donors. Although this seemed promising (see Chapter 6) it was soon abandoned when serologic tissue typing became possible: by 1965 Nelson, Bridges and McGeown (60), in a direct comparison, found the serologic approach with the antisera available at the time to be at least as discriminating as the NLT test, if not better. The NLT was demonstrated and studied in many species, including for example the hamster (61) and the rat (62), a species in which Ford (63) used thoracic duct lymphocytes to create the skin lesions. Kosunen and Dvorak (64), working with outbred rabbits, estimated that the majority of the cells in the NLT assay were of host origin. Burnet and Boyer (65) used a semi-quantitative test by seeding immunologically competent cells onto the chorioallantoic membrane of chick embryos and counting the number of plaques – a test that led Szenberg and Warner (66) to come to the erroneous conclusion that the main culprit of this GVHD was the large, and not the small, lymphocyte (see the studies of Gowans, Chapter 2).

Perhaps the most valuable of the local GVHR assays were those of Elkins and of Ford *et al.* because they lent themselves to quantitative studies. Elkins (67) inoculated parental strain lymphoid cells under the kidney capsule of F_1 hybrid rats where they incited a GVHR lesion involving the site of injection. In a second study (68) he was able to conclude that the inoculated cells not only instigated the GVHR but also maintained it in a specific manner, although radiosensitive host mononuclear cells migrating to the site also played a role in the pathogenesis of the lesions. A masterly and exhaustive review of the pathogenesis of GVHR was published by Elkins (69) in 1971. Ford, Burr and Simonsen (70) developed the popliteal lymph node weight gain assay, which measured the increase in lymph node weight following inoculation of immunocompetent cells into the footpad. Both these assays have been extensively used. In contrast, P.S. Russell (71) introduced the whole body weight gain assay to measure runt disease quantitatively in newborn mice: by plotting the weight of individual mice he was able to assess the amelioration of runt disease using specific antisera, the immunosuppressive drug amethopterin (methotrexate) and other agents. Mice could be 'rescued' if treatment with methotrexate commenced on the fifth day, suggesting that the irreversible injury to the hosts' organs occurred predominantly thereafter. Russell speculated that the action of the drug lay in its selective elimination of immunologically active cells.

Homologous (or secondary) disease as graft-versus-host disease

Although Uphoff and Trentin (see above) had already thought about the possibility that homologous disease might be caused by a reaction of the transplanted cells against their hosts, 1957 proved to be a turning point in that all workers now interpreted their findings in this way and provided supporting evidence. In the case of Loutit's Harwell group the defining moment came when Medawar and Brent visited them in the autumn of 1957 to put this proposition to them in the light of Billingham and Brent's findings in newborn mice. In a series of papers (72–75) they developed this concept and supplied ample evidence in its favor. For example, the mortality following inoculation of allogeneic embryonic and neonatal spleen cells into irradiated adult mice was greatly reduced (73) compared with adult bone marrow, the hosts' lymphoid organs showed such gross abnormalities as to make them "incapable of normal activity" (74, 75), and F_1 hybrid cells produced better survival than parental cells (74, 75). They also indicated that minor histocompatibility antigens of the host could trigger homologous disease (74) and concluded that "The so-called runt disease of tolerant mice is very similar to 'secondary disease' of radiation chimeras" (74). Schwartz, Upton and Congdon (76) likewise interpreted their findings in terms of the GVHD hypothesis, and Feldman and Jaffe (77) further substantiated it when they showed that donor cells made anti-host antibodies and that fetal liver cells were associated with better survival.

Trentin (78) found that he could induce a lethal disease similar to that of homologous disease in normal (as opposed to irradiated) three-week-old F_1 hybrid mice by inoculating them with a mixture of adult parental spleen and lymph node cells. Further, it was shown that adult blood possessed immunologically competent cells capable of causing homologous disease (79), and Zaalberg and Van Bekkum (80), using rat-anti-mouse antisera, found that after restoration with rat bone marrow, radiation chimeras possessed predominantly rat-type erythrocytes and granulocytes.

Finally, it was shown by several groups that radiation chimeras could be established in monkeys and apes, and Van Bekkum's group in Rijswijk (81) studied the immunologic consequences in rhesus monkeys. While autologous bone marrow was highly successful in protecting the animals, allogeneic marrow produced only a modest prolongation of survival, with an etiology very similar to that observed in the mouse. Using the presence of 'drumsticks' in the polymorphonuclear granulocytes of female bone marrow donors they were able to identify donor cells in most of the recipients, and they concluded that the animals died from severe and early secondary disease. This was to be the forerunner of many other studies in subhuman primates.

The literature on radiation chimeras, as Loutit had named lethally irradiated animals that had been restored with allogeneic bone marrow, became voluminous from the early 1960s on, and it is quite impossible to do justice to it here. Inevitably what had seemed a reasonably straightforward immunologic response directed at histocompatibility antigens (an allograft response in reverse) turned out to be exceedingly complex, involving factors such as the pathogen load of the recipients, the nature of the histocompatibility antigens (class I versus class II versus minor), and the degree of immunodeficiency engendered by the fact that the immune response is MHC-restricted, thus raising problems of cellular cooperation between the lymphoid cells derived from the foreign bone marrow and the host's accessory cells. I am therefore restricting myself to a few selected topics and references. Several excellent reviews are available to the reader who wants more detailed information (35, 69, 82–84).

The nature of the anti-host response

Because it was shown in the 1970s that homologous disease could be significantly mitigated by the use of germ-free animals (85) or animals in which the intestinal flora had been radically altered (86), doubts were cast on the original hypothesis that the disease was essentially caused by a GVHR. This was reinforced by the finding that the removal of immunologically competent cells from bone marrow inocula, though highly successful in preventing homologous disease in semi-allogeneic F_1 hybrids, was not always effective when the recipients were fully allogeneic (87, 88). (Among the first to describe the amelioration of GVHD in irradiated F_1 hybrids were Dicke, Van Hooft and Van Bekkum (89), who removed immunocompetent cells by centrifugation on discontinuous albumin gradients.) However, this remained a controversial subject, some finding that the use of T cell-depleted bone marrow successfully abrogated secondary mortality (90–92) whereas in the hands of others it failed to do so (93, 94). According to Rayfield and Brent (95) neither acute nor delayed GVHR developed in fully allogeneic mouse radiation chimeras following the transfer of T lymphocyte-depleted bone marrow. These workers also provided evidence for the notion that the foreign T lymphocytes could be tolerized through the influence of thymic tissue implanted into the chimeras weeks later. They argued that the late mortality they saw was due to immunoincompetence brought about by defective B cell or accessory cell function "or the way these cells interact with each other and with T lymphocytes". Such a notion – a failure of cooperation between different cell types required to mount an effective immune response – was first proposed by Zinkernagel et al. (93) because allogeneic chimeras in which the bone marrow had been wholly taken over by donor cells could not generate alloreactive or H-2 restricted antiviral cytotoxic T lymphocytes. This whole question has been discussed in detail by Moser, Iwasaki and Shearer (96), who found that spleen cell-induced immunodeficiency brought about by parental T cell recognition of allogeneic F_1 class I plus class II antigens prevented the development of cytotoxic T cell responses "involving both self-X and H-2 alloantigen recognition". In contrast, when parental cell recognition was limited to class I antigens only the self-X cytotoxic response and not the allogeneic response was affected. In their experience the immunodeficiency was associated with deranged cytokine production by the parental cells, in particular an inability to produce IL-2 and IL-2 receptors when stimulated with T cell mitogens.

The cells responsible

From the above it is clear that a consensus of opinion developed in favor of T lymphocytes as the primary cause of GVHD, both in radiation chimeras and in other GVHD models. However, cells of host origin attracted to the inflammatory focus were also involved, contributing nonspecifically to the inflammatory reaction, probably by cytokine production. The coexistence of donor and host cells was established quite early on by Fox (97) in the mouse and by Biggs and Payne (98) in the chick embryo. The many reports in the late 1960s that antilymphocyte serum (ALS) was effective in attenuating or preventing GVHD (99–101) added to the evidence in favor of a T cell mediated reaction, especially when it was shown by Boak and Wilson (102) that the affected cells were in the recirculating lymphocyte pool. ALS was also found to ameliorate GVHD in monkeys (103). (It became clear many years later (104) that the previous exposure of allogeneic bone marrow cells to Fab fragments prepared from a horse anti-mouse thymocyte globulin was sufficient to reduce markedly the capacity of the cells to induce GVHD in irradiated recipients.) Further, in the 1980s various groups, including Waldmann's (105) in Cambridge, confirmed the ALS/anti-lymphocyte globulin (ALG) data with specific anti-T cell monoclonal antibodies. Additional evidence in favor of T lymphocytes as the villains of the piece also accrued from the work of Lonai et al. (106) in Israel when demonstrating that the specific adsorption of normal lymphocytes on allogeneic fibroblast monolayers led to a reduction in GVHR, and from the ingenious experiments by Belldegrün and Cohen (107), who showed that the trapping of specific GVH-reactive T lymphocytes in certain lymph nodes of mice led to a substantial depletion of such cells in the spleen.

Critically important in proving that T lymphocytes were the most important perpetrators of GVHD was the finding by Sprent, Von Boehmer and Nabholz (108), working in Basel, that T lymphocyte-depleted allogeneic bone marrow failed to induce GVHD in irradiated F1 hybrid mice. These mice remained in good health and six months later were shown to have normal numbers of recirculating thoracic duct lymphocytes. Interestingly, their cells were able to respond, if weakly, to host-type histocompatibility antigens in mixed lymphocyte culture (MLC) but failed to generate cytotoxic cells. Sprent, Von Boehmer and Nabholz had used an antiserum directed against the θ antigen of T cells and the earlier study of Tyan (109) had already paved the way. Thierfelder and Rodt (110), through an ingenious stratagem, sensitized mice against a T cell-specific antigen and found that when irradiated and transfused with allogenic spleen and bone marrow cells, the majority of such mice did not succumb to GVHD. Nonetheless, one of the difficulties with the T cell hypothesis was that removal of these cells did not seem to prevent a delayed form of GVHD associated with the presence of minor antigens in the host but absent in the graft (111) (see below). Korngold and Sprent (112), now working in Philadelphia, therefore set out to investigate this question by transplanting H-2 compatible bone marrow that was mismatched for only minor antigens into heavily irradiated recipients. Whereas the untreated marrow caused a high incidence of lethal GVHD, T lymphocyte depletion was very effective in preventing it. Of considerable clinical importance was their finding that the addition of quite small numbers of mature T lymphocytes to the T cell-depleted bone marrow inoculum was sufficient to bring about GVHD "in certain situations", and the authors concluded that "the results imply that mature T cells contaminating marrow inocula are probably the main cause of GVHD seen in the clinical situation".

However, the question remained whether the T cells initiating the GVHR belonged to T helper (CD4-positive) or T cytotoxic (CD8-positive) subpopulations. It was possible to answer this only after the development of specific monoclonal antibodies identifying such subpopulations. Among the earliest attempts to resolve this was that of Vallera, Soderling and Kersey (113). Using monoclonal antibodies directed at the two subpopulations Lyt-1 and Lyt-2, which had originally been defined by Boyse et al. (114, 115), they established that the removal of Lyt-1-positive (helper) cells from allogeneic mouse bone marrow completely prevented the cells from causing lethal GVHD, whereas depletion of Lyt-2-positive (cytotoxic) cells did not. Korngold and Sprent (116) returned to this model but, using mouse strains differing only for class I or class II MHC antigens or both, they were able to take their conclusions one important step further. Thus when GVHD was directed at class I antigens, cytotoxic T cells were primarily responsible for GVHD – the same subset that they had already implicated in the induction of GVHD to minor antigens (117). However, GVHD directed against either class II antigens or the whole MHC spectrum involved predominantly the helper subpopulation, even though the removal of helper lymphocytes did not totally abolish GVHD – a finding that they attributed to the additional presence of minor antigens. These data received strong support from even more sophisticated investigations carried out a few years later by the same group (118), making use of class I or class II mutant mice. Not only did the MHC class determine the cells mediating GVHD but it also affected the induction of splenomegaly in newborn mice and skin allograft rejection. A further refinement in T cell depletion in the prevention of GVHD came from Pietryga et al. (119) when they showed, in 1987, that fully mismatched allogeneic irradiated mice could be protected most effectively if the bone marrow cells were treated with antibodies against both T cell subpopulations. Depletion of T helper cells alone was moderately effective, but removal of only cytotoxic T cells failed to protect, thus confirming the data of Korngold and Sprent (*116*).

Quite recently (1993) the question was re-investigated by a Japanese group using 'nude' mice, which congenitally lack a thymus and therefore possess few T lymphocytes. Thus Uenaka, Kagemasa and Nakayama (*120*) found that in this rather special setting recipients were protected when allogeneic bone marrow was depleted of either helper or cytotoxic subsets. Both seemed to be involved in causing subacute GVHD – the helper T cells acting at an early stage whereas the cytotoxic cells mediated the late onset GVHD, presumably triggered by minor antigens (see below).

One great leap forward in clinical bone marrow transplantation therefore seemed to lie in the depletion of the donor marrow of T lymphocytes combined with full HLA matching. This was a highly attractive idea bearing in mind that the GVHR is not easily suppressed by drugs. (See, for example, early reports on attempts to do this in dogs (*121*) or mice (*122, 123*).) The first human data were published in 1981 by Rodt, Kold and Netzel (*124*): treatment of donor bone marrow with rabbit-anti-human antisera reduced both the incidence and severity of GVHD. Other groups reported similar results following T cell depletion by other means (*125, 126*), but the use of a monoclonal antibody (OKT3) (*127, 128*) when transplanting bone marrow to HLA-matched siblings, though very markedly reducing the incidence of GVHD, did not entirely solve the problem. This prompted the Minneapolis group of Filipovich to attempt to increase the efficiency of T cell depletion by coupling anti-T cell antibodies to the cell poison ricin. In their 1984 report (*129*), which described their experience with only two patients, they concluded that this procedure was effective as well as safe. In the same year Prentice *et al.* (*130*) in London reported excellent results from treating donor marrow with a cocktail of monoclonal antibodies: moderate to severe GVHD was totally prevented. However, promising as these results were, later trials raised an entirely new problem in that T-depleted marrow transplants were often associated with a high leukemia relapse rate, a problem that will be discussed below (p. 364).

The role of minor histocompatibility antigens in graft-versus-host disease

It had therefore become clear by the mid-1980s that acute and chronic GVHD was triggered by MHC antigens and that the cells mediating the reaction belonged to both subsets of T lymphocytes. The role of minor antigens in graft rejection (host-versus-graft, HVG) is discussed in Chapter 2 and it was seen that multiple minor antigens can provoke quite strong HVG reactions. An interesting issue was raised by Wettstein and Bailey (*131*): not *all* the minor antigens possessed by a donor and absent from a recipient were necessarily involved in provoking a cytotoxic T cell response. Thus, in their study of the 40 mouse non-H-2 minor antigens with which the recipients were challenged there was a preferential response to a single immunodominant antigen. This is an interesting phenomenon and the mechanism is not at all clear, though the authors favored the notion that the immune response to other antigens was suppressed by the dominant antigen. Be this as it may, it has already been implied on p. 356 that GVHD can also be triggered by minor antigens of the recipient after bone marrow transplantation and that this GVHD is of late onset.

The evidence incriminating minor antigens in GVHD came from both animal experiments and clinical bone marrow transplantation at roughly the same time. Although it was thought by many in the early 1970s that the minor antigens were relatively unimportant in GVH reactions unless the hosts were neonatal (*132*) or the donor cells had been presensitized against host antigens (*133*), it soon became apparent that provided the conditions were right, mouse minor histocompatibility antigens could incite powerful and destructive responses from transplanted H-2-compatible bone marrow cells. As Billingham and Brent (*48*) had surmised, mouse bone marrow has relatively few immunologically competent cells, but the numbers can increase in appropriate circumstances, as for example in lethally irradiated animals or in neonatal mice. The work of Korngold and Sprent (*112*) has already been referred to in this context. In the same year (1978) O. Halle-Pannenko and her colleagues, working with G. Mathé in Villejuif, France, published the first of a series of papers describing lethal GVHD in adult irradiated mice directed against non-H-2 antigens (*134, 135*). This group went on to show that the GVHD could be reduced by immunization of the bone marrow and spleen donors against the hosts' minor antigens (primarily the Mlsa antigens) or against nonspecific H-2 antigens (*136–138*), and that T suppressor cells were involved in the amelioration of GVHD (*135*). (In contrast, Holda, Maier and Claman (*139*) have described the activity of natural suppressor cells with a phenotype unlike that of T and B lymphocytes in mouse GVH reactions triggered by minor antigens.) Others soon substantiated the power of minor antigens to incite strong and lethal GVH reactions (*140*). Hamilton and Parkman (*141*) concluded that the acute and chronic forms of GVHD observed in their mice showed close clinical and histologic similarities to clinical GVHD after transplantation of bone marrow from HLA-identical and MLC-non-reactive donors. Both forms were initiated by donor T lymphocytes, and acute and chronic GVHD were in their view manifestations of the same disease.

Evidence implicating non-MHC antigens also came from bone marrow grafting in dogs, and they indeed preceded the mouse data. The Seattle group of E.D. Thomas (see biographic sketch, p. 375) and R. Storb, which was to make such major contributions to clinical bone marrow transplantation, published their first observations in 1973. They (*142*) noted that bone marrow transplants in irradiated dogs matched for MHC (DL-A) antigens was followed by the lethal GVHD in more than half the recipients (DL-A is the canine MHC.). The dogs had not been immunosuppressed after transplantation, but when intermittent treatment with methotrexate was given to others a state of "stable graft–host tolerance" ensued. Storb *et al*. pointed out that their results differed from those of Rapaport *et al*. (*143*), who had failed to encounter GVHD in dogs inbred in Cooperstown that had been given serotypically DL-A-identical marrow from littermates or non-littermates. Storb *et al*. thought that their investigation had revealed "that some important antigenic differences are not detected by either serologic canine histocompatibility testing or the MLC test". A few years later Rapaport's group (*144*) did encounter lethal secondary disease in some of their DL-A-identical marrow recipients; whether or not this occurred seemed to depend on differences in the "particular haplotype pedigree combination". Interestingly, they also found that surviving radiation chimeras failed to reject kidney allografts from other DLA- and pedigree-identical donors.

Persuasive evidence for the participation of human minor antigens in the genesis of GVHD came from clinical studies. Whereas HLA-non-identical donors regularly led to the development of GVHD, the use of HLA-identical sibling donors overcame this problem to some extent though by no means completely (145–148): some of the recipients still suffered lethal or non-lethal GVHD. Although in the early 1970s, when these clinical data were first reported, HLA typing was incomplete and the results might well have been due to this, the GVHD was interpreted by most workers, such as Thomas' Seattle group (148), as having been brought about by non-HLA loci. (By choosing sibling donors of opposite sex these workers were able to show cytogenetically that engraftment had taken place.) It is clear from the later literature that this interpretation was correct, for the residual problem of GVHD was not solved by improvements and refinements in HLA matching and the use of HLA-identical, MLC-negative donors (in practice nearly always siblings) continued to offer the best assurance of host survival. Even so, in their 1977 paper Storb, Prentice and Thomas (149) found that 18 of 68 HLA-identical siblings died, the majority with GVHD; but it should be noted that a few of the donors had been positive in MLC, and the CML reactivity of about half was unknown. However, the Copenhagen Study Group in Immunodeficiencies (150) reported one successful transplant from an uncle to an HLA-non-identical, but MLC-negative, infant suffering from severe combined immunodeficiency. The question of major and minor antigens in bone marrow transplantation was discussed at some length by Van Rood and Van Leeuwen (151), who expressed the view that identity for the serologically determined (Class I) HLA antigens was not a prerequisite, but that matching for lymphocyte-defined (Class II) antigens was. The latter were at that time identifiable only by the MLC assay but they were later detected serologically (the DR antigens).

In the 1980s some human minor histocompatibility antigens in addition to the male-specific HY antigen had been identified by the Leiden group and their data were summarized by Goulmy (152) and De Brueger and Goulmy (153). Using MHC-restricted cytotoxic T cell clones, five minor antigens have now been recognized (154); they are the products of single genes segregating in Mendelian fashion (155). While there is no doubt that the sex-linked antigens are a factor to be reckoned with in GVHD – this has been evident since the early clinical analysis of Storb, Prentice and Thomas (149) as well as in mouse experiments by Lengerová and Chutná (156) and Uphoff (157) – it remains to be seen what role these individual antigens play in GVHD. Matching bone marrow recipients for human leukocyte antigens (HLA) as well as minor antigens could be very difficult and, even if practicable, would make the selection of wholly compatible donors a logistically difficult task. Because the human minor antigens appear to be expressed on hematopoietic cells (158) they could certainly incite responses of the host against the graft, and one such example has recently been described (159).

Some Clinical Aspects of Bone Marrow Transplantation

In discussing the development of the concept of GVHD, I have inevitably touched on some of its clinical aspects. It is not the intention here to describe the development of clinical transplantation – the conditioning of the recipients, the selection of donors and the complicated management of the patients. It is perfectly clear from the use of HLA-identical siblings that, short of identical twin donors, they are the most favorable donors. However, recently, with improved strategies for conditioning the recipients and treating them after transplantation to avoid or reduce the danger of GVHD (cyclosporine, FK 506), bone marrow transplantation can now be carried out in unrelated but carefully HLA-matched individuals. However, even in these circumstances GVHD is always a threat. HLA typing therefore remains mandatory and the field of bone marrow transplantation is undoubtedly one in which tissue typing has made its greatest impact.

I have singled out two particular issues for further consideration.

(1) The early history of clinical bone marrow transplantation, mainly because it is an interesting story and the contribution of some European workers, especially the French, has in my view been undervalued.
(2) The effect that T cell depletion has had on the relapse rate in leukemic patients and the question of the 'graft-versus-leukemia effect'.

The pioneering years

Human bone marrow transplantation is strongly associated with the name of E.D. Thomas who, together with his team in Seattle, has played the major role in its development and who has been responsible for a concerted and sustained attack on the many problems that have had to be overcome from the late 1950s to the present day. His outstanding contribution was recognized in 1990 by the award of the Nobel Prize in 1990 and his Nobel Lecture, in which he discussed the past, present and future of bone marrow transplantation, was published in the *Scandinavian Journal of Immunology* (160). The first clinical attempt was reported by his group in 1957 (161). Allogeneic cells were infused intravenously into six patients suffering from various malignancies after the administration of WBI varying from 90 to 600 rad. A temporary 'take' was seen in two of these patients. The authors thought that a higher level of immunosuppression would have been beneficial. In another paper published one year later the same group (162), again including J.W. Ferrebee, who was later to establish an inbred dog colony in Cooperstown with which his team conducted bone marrow and allograft transplantation studies, published a second paper in which they presented five further cases. They concluded that of the total of 12 patients treated by them, only two had shown "significant clinical benefit". By 1959 Thomas, Lochte and Ferrebee (163) had treated two leukemic patients with bone marrow from an identical twin after supralethal irradiation to eliminate the malignant cells. Both recovered hematologically but suffered a recurrence of the leukemia a few months later. This prompted the authors to speculate that in addition to WBI other factors were needed to intervene, one of them being the "unsuitable immunologic environment" provided by allogeneic marrow for the survival of the leukemia (see below).

In 1958 Humble and Newton (164), two consultants from the Westminster Hospital, London, published a preliminary paper describing a technique of bone marrow transplantation and five patients suffering from various malignancies who had received marrow from donors matched for ABO and Rh blood groups. Four of them died, three of them without improvement; the fourth "felt better for the procedure", had an improved white cell count, but died from bronchopneumonia after two months. The health of the fifth patient greatly improved and she was alive five months later, but her leukemic condition was unchanged.

At this point G. Mathé, working in Paris, came on the scene. In 1958 he had begun to work on the antileukemic effects induced by compatible or allogeneic lymphoid or myeloid cells in an attempt to ameliorate GVHD. In that same year six Yugoslav physicists who had been accidentally exposed to high doses (400–700 rad) of WBI were referred to him. Five were treated with bone marrow grafts and the sixth, who had been exposed to the lowest dose, survived without treatment. A transient donor cell chimerism was observed in four patients but the fifth, having received about 700 rad, died. These observations were published by Mathé and his team (165) in 1959 in a French journal. The precise doses of irradiation could, of course, not be established, and it is debatable to what extent the four patients who had been transiently chimeric had been helped by the transplants. In the same year Mathé et al. (166) published their results of bone marrow transplantation in three patients deliberately irradiated with 400 rad: all died from acute GVHD, referred to as "secondary disease".

It is of some interest that Mathé at that time had been in contact with Thomas and Ferrebee in Cooperstown and together they wrote a brief review on the restoration of marrow function in patients after lethal irradiation (167) – Mathé's first foray into the English language. They reviewed Mathé's earlier attempts at marrow transplantation and described the consequences of what appeared to be GVHD; and they went on to draw attention to the finding that unlike the anti-leukemia effect witnessed in mice after irradiation and transplantation of allogeneic marrow (see below), there was no such desirable effect when the human donors had been normal identical twins (163, 168). They concluded by stating that "It will be important, therefore, to see whether foreign marrow reaction (secondary disease) is helpful in eradicating leukemia in man. Certainly radiation alone at the 1000 roentgen level does not appear to do so."

Mathé then became involved with the renal transplantation program in Paris (see Chapter 7) but in 1963 he and his colleages published a paper that is of special interest because it is without doubt the first description of a successful human bone marrow graft (169). A leukemic patient who had been resistant to chemotherapy was given 800 rad WBI, preceded by four days' treatment with methyl-nitro-imidazolyl-mercaptopurine. The patient was then transfused with bone marrow cells from six related donors. "The histocompatibility relations were determined on the basis of the erythrocyte phenotypes (sic), the serum phenotypes, the leukocyte antigens (Dr. J. Dausset) and the histocompatibility test already recommended by us." The latter consisted of an assessment of the intensity of immunization produced by skin from the recipient transplanted to an unrelated individual against skin from the potential donors (170). "After eight months the patient's blood was completely repopulated with red cells which showed the antigenic characteristics of one of the donors", and the patient produced donor-type gammaglobulins and displayed tolerance to that donor's skin. The severe 'secondary syndrome' encountered was controllable and the patient was healthy and in complete remission nine months later.

Thereafter Mathé tried to establish immunotherapy protocols that were less dangerous than the graft-versus-leukemia effect. Among the papers published by his group on bone marrow transplantation was one in 1967 (171), in which they described the fate of 21 patients who had been given 793–950 rad WBI followed by bone marrow from related donors. Engraftment was seen in 15 but all but one died of acute, subacute or chronic 'secondary disease'. (It is strange that they continued to call it secondary disease, although in the discussion they stated that it "seems, as in animals, to be related to graft-versus-host reactivity".) Their donor selection procedure was still extremely primitive – in addition to the tests used in their 1963 study they employed another *in vivo* test in which the reactivity of puta-tive donor and recipient blood leukocytes was ascertained in the skin of irradiated hamsters. Of the 45 references, 21 referred to the group's own work and only one to the work of the Thomas group, confirming the writer's impression that there was a certain lack of generosity in recognizing the work of the Americans.

In 1970, Mathé and his colleagues (*172*) published one other important paper on the use of antilymphocyte globulin (ALG) as the sole immunosuppressive agent in clinical bone marrow transplantation. All 16 patients had related donors who had been matched as far as possible with the then recognized HLA antigens; they were either in the overt phase of leukemia and resistant to chemotherapy or suffering from complete agranulocytosis. In four cases the donors as well as the recipients had received ALG, which was administered to the recipients for 4–12 days. Engraftment occurred in seven. No early acute "secondary disease" was noted in any patient, but the grafts had no anti-leukemic effect and most patients died of leukemia. However, four survived beyond three months, one of them apparently healthy and another showing great clinical improvement. The authors concluded that "these grafts provide the only evidence available at the present time of antilymphocyte serum being a powerful immunosuppressive agent in man for tissue transplantation", all other clinical applications of ALG having been combined with drugs such as azathioprine or prednisone.

Towards the end of the 1960s Mathé moved into the field of active immunotherapy, using live BCG vaccines to destroy human leukemic cells. This is not an appropriate subject for this book, but it may partly explain why Mathé's early contribution has tended to be neglected. A reciprocal lack of generosity, perhaps? The fact that he published his early work in French and in French journals that were not readily available in other countries may have been a contributory factor.

Other successful allogeneic bone marrow transplants were carried out in non-leukemic patients in the late 1960s – by Bach *et al.* (*173*) in a patient with Wiskott–Aldrich syndrome, and in the same year by Good *et al.* (*174*) in a child with lymphopenic agammaglobulinemia. The boy had four female siblings and these, as well as his parents, were examined for HLA compatibility using sera and the MLC assay – a far more stringent selection procedure than previously used. A non-reactive sibling was chosen and her ailing brother was given peripheral leukocytes as well as bone marrow cells. The boy developed a mild GVHD which subsided, and became immunologically responsive. About one-third of his bone marrow cells were demonstrably female. However, two months later he developed bone marrow failure and aplasia, which threatened to be fatal, and he was given a second bone marrow graft from the same donor (*175*). The patient, whose bone marrow became predominantly of donor origin, returned to immunologic normality. The authors wrote: "We contend that these dramatically successful marrow transplants have brought us to the threshold of an era of cellular engineering based on transplantation of bone marrow stem cells or other progenitor cells". A year later (1969) a Dutch group (176) carried out a similar therapeutic protocol using bone marrow and fetal thymus cells for an infant with lymphopenic immunologic deficiency. (Two other groups (177, 178) had, in 1968, restored immunologic reactivity to patients with DiGeorge's syndrome – caused by a congenital absence of the thymus – with allogeneic thymic implants.)

Meanwhile Thomas, Ferrebee and their colleagues in Cooperstown went 'back to the drawing board', and carried out a series of investigations involving bone marrow transplantation in dogs. It was this work, carried out over many years, that enabled them to resume clinical transplantation on a more scientific basis and with some reasonable assurance that GVHD was controllable. This is not the place to summarize their canine studies – a summary may be found in the comprehensive 1975 review of the Thomas team (179). However, it is appropriate to highlight one or two of their findings. For example, dogs given three times the lethal dose of irradiation made a good recovery if preserved autologous marrow was re-introduced (180) – an approach that Rapaport et al. (181) and others returned to 20 years later and that has been attempted clinically, after purging of the patients' bone marrow of leukemic cells (182). Yet after the introduction of cyclosporine (see Chapter 7) in the treatment of bone marrow recipients it was found, disconcertingly, by Hood et al. (183) that some of the patients developed a syndrome that resembled the dermatologic manifestations of GVHD. This was self-limiting and was thought to be caused by autoreactive lymphocytes reacting against class II antigens. Following Uphoff's (184) demonstration that methotrexate given after bone marrow transplantation to irradiated mice could ameliorate GVHD, which was strongly confirmed by Russell (71) in neonatally induced runt disease, Storb et al. showed that the incidence and severity of GVHD in dogs could likewise be significantly reduced with this drug (185). Thus they wrote: "The results show that stable long-term chimerism can be achieved in mismatched recipient dogs when intensive methotrexate is begun immediately after marrow transplantation and continued for a prolonged period of time". Meanwhile Von Bekkum's group (186, 187) had produced good results using cyclophosphamide in monkeys, and thereafter irradiation as a conditioning treatment was supplemented by drugs such as cyclophosphamide.

There now followed a flood of papers from the Seattle group of Thomas as well as from others, with gradually improving results. Thomas et al. (188) now had better clinical results than in their first attempt in 1957 though they were still dogged by non-functioning grafts, GVHD and relapse of the leukemia, even though the patients received HLA-identical sibling grafts. But the patients survived longer, had milder symptoms of GVHD and, in one case out of seven, a cure seemed to have been achieved. More encouraging was their report on four patients with aplastic anemia using sibling donors of opposite sex: out of four patients, two "have excellent-functioning marrow grafts without graft-versus-host disease and are apparently well 138 and 215 days after grafting", the other two having died of graft rejection and GVHD, respectively (148). Two years later (1974) the same group (189) described their experience with 16 leukemic patients who were given marrow from healthy identical twins after cyclophosphamide treatment and supralethal WBI. Eleven had complete remissions for long periods and five relapsed at 3–7 months. It should be added that these patients had been refractory to any other treatment. The authors felt sufficiently encouraged to suggest that "one could even justify using this approach in some patients before they become demonstrably resistant to all other therapy", and proposed that this approach could also be used for other malignancies.

In the same year Storb *et al.* (*190*) published a further paper on 24 patients with aplastic anemia. While some rejected their grafts and others died of GVHD, 11 became stable cell chimeras and were healthy for periods of up to two and a half years. The donors were again HLA-matched siblings. Aplastic anemia, too, proved to be amenable to marrow transplantation from HLA-identical siblings in the 1970s, with a long-term survival rate of about 40% (*190, 191*) although graft rejection and GVHD continued to be the main threats and accounted for most of the mortality. These patients had been conditioned with cyclophosphamide and WBI and treated, after transplantation with methotrexate. It was also shown by Storb, Prentice and Thomas (*192*) that matching for the minor X and Y chromosomes was beneficial.

With these contributions and those of other workers, bone marrow transplantation came of age. Anyone picking up a volume of the journals *Blood* or *Bone Marrow Transplantation* will come across papers grappling with these clinical issues, and while they have not all been resolved there has been a steady improvement in results. The Seattle group, led by E.D. Thomas and with close on 30 years of single-minded endeavor, was largely instrumental in turning the first tentative steps of bone marrow transplantation into clinical reality. It is not surprising that despite the fact that Mathé, Van Bekkum and others in Europe and on the American continent played important roles in these extraordinary developments, Thomas should have been singled out as the recipient of the Nobel Prize in cellular transplantation.

The graft-versus-leukemia (GVL) effect

The modern era of clinical bone marrow transplantation, which has seen the supplementation of WBI with chemotherapy as the conditioning regimen for the patient and the introduction of drugs to prevent GVHD, began around the year 1970. When ALG became available, and later monoclonal antibodies directed against T cell antigens, the obvious way forward seemed to be to deplete the allogeneic bone marrow of T lymphocytes; what could be easier than to avoid GVHD by removing the cells that were known to be intimately involved in the induction of this disagreeable and dangerous – often lethal – disease inflicted on already sick patients? Such a procedure worked extremely well in experimental animals but could lead to a state of immunodeficiency when the donor cells had completely taken over the host's lymphopoietic system (see above). In patients with all kinds of malignancies such as the leukemias one had not taken into account the possibility that allogeneic cells could help to purge the patient of residual malignant cells by what has become known as the "graft-versus-leukemia" effect (see below).

The efficacy of T lymphocyte depletion in animal experiments of the early 1980s has already been referred to, as has the first highly successful clinical application of this procedure by Prentice *et al.* at the Royal Free Hospital, London (*130*). The same group had published a paper in the *Lancet* (*127*) two years earlier (1982) claiming that treatment of human bone marrow cells with the monoclonal anti-T cell antibody OKT3 without the *in vitro* use of complement had substantially reduced the incidence of GVHD from 79% in a previous series to 14%. However, the patients had been observed for only 60 days at the time of writing and it would appear from the follow-up that GVHD had not been totally prevented. The group from Minneapolis, using OKT3 in much the same way, had similar results in that five of ten patients developed acute GVHD requiring the use of steroids (128). In their subsequent study, Prentice *et al.* (130), using two monoclonal antibodies plus rabbit complement were successful, in that only two of 13 patients, none of whom had received any prophylactic post-transplant immunosuppression, had a mild form of skin GVHD and there were no fatal infections. Many other clinical teams subsequently reported a great reduction in GVHD after T cell depletion (193); however, this great gain was frequently offset by a substantially increased leukemia relapse rate.

The graft-versus-leukemia (GVL) concept has quite a colorful history. It was first raised 40 years ago by Barnes *et al.* (194), the group that had made such vital contributions to unlocking the secrets of secondary (or homologous) disease following bone marrow transplantation in irradiated mice. Discussing the problems associated with giving mice a high dose of WBI to cure them of their leukemia, they thought that the 'rescue' of such mice with allogeneic rather than isogeneic bone marrow would be preferable because "the colonizing cells might retain the capacity of the donor to destroy by the reaction of immunity these residual leukaemic cells – and perhaps also the host". Their very preliminary data seemed to give this notion some support.

The idea was taken up by Mathé, who published a 'critical review' in 1960 (195). He concluded that "Most authors admit the rarity of eradicating leukemia by irradiation . . . followed by transfusion of isologous hematopoietic cells. It has been shown that eradication can eventually be obtained when irradiation is followed by transfusion of homologous hematopoietic cells. This, most probably, is due to an immune reaction of those cells against the leukemic cells. Furthermore, even when the leukemia can be eradicated, the animals usually die from the secondary syndrome" (i.e. GVHD). This would appear to be a very clear statement of the problem.

Others studied this problem experimentally in mice. In 1962 Stuart (196) attempted, rather ambitiously, to destroy a mouse ascites tumor *in vivo* by the administration of xenogeneic (rat) lymphoid cells but, after a temporary amelioration the tumors progressed in all animals. In the same year Woodruff and Symes (197), likewise working in Edinburgh, were able to show that the growth of a mammary carcinoma in A strain mice could be "greatly retarded . . . and sometimes completely destroyed, by exposing the recipient to a sublethal dose of irradiation (capable itself of producing only a very slight effect on the tumour) and then injecting allogeneic lymphoid cells from either a normal CBA mouse or a CBA mouse immunized against the A-strain tumour". However, the survival of these mice was not increased because of the intervention of GVHD. The same group (198, 199) had some success with a xenogeneic tumor (Landschutz), again using sublethal irradiation and thoracic duct lymphocytes from rats that were either normal or presensitized. This time the survival of the animals was "markedly prolonged" and three animals appeared to have been cured, but only when presensitized cells were used.

The first clinical attempt to exploit this anti-tumor effect was made in 1964, when Woodruff and Nolan (200) published some preliminary observations. Eight patients with "advanced cancer" were given allogeneic spleen cells after preparatory treatment with a cytotoxic drug or prednisone. ". . . In every case some change occurred in either the patient's symptoms, the physical signs, or the findings on serial biopsy. It is suggested that some of these changes were due to a direct action by the transplanted cells on the tumour". About the same time P. Koldovsky and his colleagues in Czechoslovakia attempted a similar approach in mice, using the sarcoma I and other tumors. The treatment with presensitized spleen cells was effective provided that it was administered either just before or at the same time as the tumor (201, 202) unless it was combined with irradiation, in which case the cells could be given later (201). Woodruff (203) examined the early literature in his more general review on the immunology of cancer, published in 1964.

Woodruff's colleague M.O. Symes went on to study two other mouse tumors. When transplanting an already growing mammary carcinoma survival was prolonged by allogeneic spleen cells in melphalan-treated animals (204), but no benefit was noted when the tumor was a lymphoma, regardless of whether allogeneic or xenogeneic cells were administered (205).

An anti-tumor effect of allogeneic (and indeed xenogeneic) bone marrow in immunocompromised individuals was thus firmly established long before therapy with anti-T cell monoclonal antibodies became possible. It is therefore hardly surprising that many clinical groups ran into difficulties when they used such antibodies in that they succeeded in reducing the danger of GVHD, but found to their dismay an increased relapse rate. For example, Apperley et al. (206), in treating a group of 39 patients with chronic myeloid leukemia, found that T cell depletion of bone marrow from HLA-identical twin donors with the monoclonal anti-T cell antibody Campath-1 significantly reduced the incidence and severity of GVHD, but increased the relapse rate. "We conclude that T-cell depletion used in this manner may be associated with an increased risk of leukaemic relapse", concluded this British group from the Hammersmith and Addenbrookes Hospitals. This has also been the experience of many other groups and their observations have recently been comprehensively reviewed by Giralt and Champlin (207).

Clinicians therefore have to balance on a knife edge, with the dreaded GVHD on the one side and the even more dreaded leukemia relapse on the other. A logical development would be to give the patient a known and carefully selected number of donor lymphocytes after bone marrow transplantation – low enough to avoid the more severe manifestations of GVHD but high enough to induce an effective graft-versus-leukemia effect to wipe out the patient's residual leukemic cells. This is precisely what is being done in the 1990s. For example, Sullivan et al. (208) have used what they called "adoptive immunotherapy" in leukemic patients, who were given either methotrexate or methotrexate combined with the donor's buffy coat cells. The latter increased the incidence of acute (but not chronic) GVHD substantially without affecting the five-year probability of recurrence of the disease. On the other hand, Kolb et al. (209), working in Munich, have treated three patients with a combination of interferon IFN-α and buffy coat cells from the bone marrow donor: all had complete and long-lasting hematologic and cytogenetic remission. Although two developed GVHD this was overcome with the help of immunosuppressive agents. Five years later the same group (210) described their experience with a large group of leukemic patients, again using transfusions of donor lymphocytes. In patients with chronic myeloid leukemia the remission rate was as high as 73%, but the results were less impressive for other kinds of leukemia. However, the incidence of GVHD was as high as 60%.

Mackinnon *et al.* (*211*) have approached the problem rationally by transfusing donor T lymphocytes at various dose levels. Remissions were achieved at 10–500 million kg^{-1} and 15 of 17 evaluable patients were freed of their chronic myeloid leukemia; GVHD was minimal. The authors concluded that "The dose of donor leukocytes or T cells used may be important in determining both the GVL response and the incidence of GVHD. In many patients this potent GVL effect can occur in the absence of clinical GVHD".

Concluding Comments

Perhaps we are close to a resolution of a vexing and vitally important problem that has exercised the minds of immunobiologists and clinicians for the best part of four decades, a resolution that will transform the treatment of those many patients whose lives depend on receiving a bone marrow transplant. There have been other experimental approaches that may yet make an impact, for example the determination of the frequency of cytotoxic T lymphocyte precursor cells in the potential donor's blood as a means of selecting the most suitable donor. This has been carried out with some success for volunteer unrelated (*212*) and HLA-identical sibling (*213*) donors at the Royal Postgraduate Medical School, London, a low frequency having been associated with a low GVHD risk. The fact that this approach has worked with HLA-identical siblings suggests that the assay can detect clinically significant minor histocompatibility differences between donor and host.

It is not inconceivable that in the future it might prove possible to transplant xenogeneic bone marrow for clinical purposes, for it has been argued persuasively by Lafferty and Jones (*214*) that, at least in chick embryos, the introduction of xenogeneic and phylogenetically unrelated lymphoid cells do not initiate GVHRs reactions unless they come from presensitized donors. In this respect the situation is quite unlike that for allografts, and Lafferty and Jones have argued from this that the ability to distinguish between 'self' and 'non-self' operates at two distinct levels.

Finally, it is appropriate to remark that the story of GVHD and bone marrow transplantation has illustrated in a unique way the importance of animal research in the solution of clinical problems.

References

1. Heineke, H. (1905) *Mitt. Grenzgeb. Med. Chir.* **14**, 21.
2. Benjamin, E. & Sluka, E. (1908) *Wien. Klin. Wchnschr.* **21**, 311.
3. Hektoen, L. (1915) *J. Infect. Dis.* **17**, 415.
4. Craddock, C.G. & Lawrence, J.S. (1948) *J. Immunol.* **60**, 241.
5. Dempster, W.J., Lennox, B. & Boag, J.W. (1950) *Brit. J. Path.* **31**, 670.
6. Lennox, B., Dempster, W.J. & Boag, J.W. (1952) *Brit. J. Path.* **33**, 380.
7. Jacobson, L.O., Simmons, E.L., Marks, E.K. *et al.* (1951) *Science* **113**, 510.
8. Jacobson, L.O. (1952) *Cancer Res.* **12**, 315.
9. Lorenz, E., Uphoff, D., Reed, I.R. *et al.* (1951) *J. Natl. Cancer Res.* **12**, 197.
10. Barnes, D.W.H. & Loutit, J.F. (1953) *Proc. Roy. Soc. Med.* **46**, 251.
11. Cole, L.J., Fishler, M.C., Ellis, V.P. *et al.* (1952) *Proc. Soc. Exp. Biol. Med.* **80**, 112.
12. Barnes, D.W.H. & Loutit, J.F. (1954) *Nucleonics* **12**, 68.

13. Main, J.M. & Prehn, R.T. (1955) *J. Natl. Cancer Inst.* **15**, 1023.
14. Trentin, J.J. (1956) *Proc. Soc. Exp. Biol. Med.* **92**, 688.
15. Lindsley, D.L., Odell, T.T. & Tausche, F.G. (1955) *Proc. Soc. Exp. Biol. Med.* **90**, 512.
16. Odell, T.T., Tausche, F.G., Lindsley, D.L. *et al.* (1957) *Ann. N.Y. Acad. Sci.* **64**, 811.
17. Nowell, P.C., Cole, L.S., Habermeyer, J.G. *et al.* (1956) *Cancer Res.* **16**, 258.
18. Ford, C.E., Hamerton, J.L., Barnes, D.W.H. *et al.* (1956) *Nature* **177**, 452.
19. Ford, C.E., Ilbery, P.L.T. & Loutit, J.F. (1957) *J. Cell. Comp. Physiol.* **50** (suppl. 1), 109.
20. Vos, O., Davids, J.A.G., Weyzen, W.W.H. *et al. Acta Physiol. Pharmacol. Neerl.* **4**, 482.
21. Makinodan, T. (1956) *Proc. Soc. Exp. Biol. Med.* **92**, 174.
22. Merwin, R.M. & Congdon, C.C. (1956) *Fed. Proc.* **15**, 129.
23. Mitchison, N.A. (1956) *Brit. J. Exp. Path.* **37**, 239.
24. Koller, P.C., Davies, A.J.S. & Doak, S.M.A. (1961) *Adv. Cancer Res.* **6**, 181.
25. Uphoff, D.E. (1957) *J. Natl. Cancer Inst.* **19**, 123.
26. Billingham, R.E., Brent, L. & Medawar, P.B. (1955) *Ann. N.Y. Acad. Sci.* **59**, 409.
27. Danchakoff, V. (1916) *Am. J. Anat.* **20**, 255.
28. Murphy, J.B. (1916) *J. Exp. Med.* **24**, 1.
29. Simonsen, M. (1985) *Immunol. Rev.* **88**, 5.
30. Dempster, W.J. (1951) *Brit. Med. J.* **2**, 104.
31. Dempster, W.J. (1953) *Brit. J. Surg.* **40**, 447.
32. Simonsen, M. (1953) *Acta Path. Microbiol. Scand.* **32**, 36.
33. Hume, D.M., Jackson, B.T., Zukoski, C.F. *et al.* (1960) *Ann. Surg.* **152**, 354.
34. Porter, K.A. & Calne, R.Y. (1960) *Transpl. Bull.* **26**, 458.
35. Simonsen, M. (1962) *Progr. Allergy* **6**, 349.
36. Simonsen, M. (1957) *Acta Path. Microbiol. Scand.* **40**, 480.
37. Simonsen, M. (1995) *Transpl. Proc.* **27**, 18.
38. Simonsen, M. (1960) In *Cellular Aspects of Immunity*, eds G.E.W. Wolstenholme & M.P. O'Connor, p. 122, Ciba Found. Symp., J. & A. Churchill, London.
39. Terasaki, P.I. (1959) *J. Exp. Embryol. Morph.* **7**, 394.
40. Simonsen, M. (1975) *Acta Path. Microbiol. Scand. C*, **83**, 1.
41. Cock, A.G. & Simonsen, M. (1958) *Immunology* **1**, 103.
42. Billingham, R.E., Brent, L. & Medawar, P.B. (1956) *Phil Trans. B* **239**, 357.
43. Billingham, R.E. & Brent, L. (1957) *Transpl. Bull.* **4**, 67.
44. Brent, L. (1995) *Transpl. Proc.* **27**, 12.
45. McLaren, A. & Michie, D. (1960) In *Congenital Malformations*, p. 178, Ciba Found. Symp., J. & A. Churchill, London.
46. Billingham, R.E. (1958) *Ann. N.Y. Acad. Sci.* **73**, 782.
47. Brent, L. (1958) *Czchsl. Biol.* **7**, 266.
48. Billingham, R.E. & Brent, L. (1959) *Phil. Trans. B* **242**, 439.
49. Owen, E.O., Jacob, S.W., Moloney, W.C. *et al.* (1958) *Transpl. Bull.* **4**, 129.
50. Woodruff, M.F.A. & Sparrow, M. (1957) *Transpl. Bull.* **4**, 157.
51. Woodruff, M.F.A. (1957) *Transpl. Bull.* **4**, 26.
52. Egdahl, R.H., Roller, F.R., Swanson, R.L. *et al.* (1958) *Ann. N.Y. Acad. Sci.* **73**, 842.
53. Nakić, B. & Silobrčić, V. (1958) *Nature* **182**, 264.
54. Finerty, J.C. (1952) *Phys. Rev.* **32**, 277.
55. Simonsen, M. (1960) *Ann. N.Y. Acad. Sci.* **87**, 382.
56. Dineen, M. (1961) *Nature* **189**, 680.
57. Cole, L.J. & Davis, W.E. (1961) *Proc. Natl. Acad, Sci. U.S.A.* **47**, 594.
58. Brent, L. & Medawar, P.B. (1963) *Brit. Med. J.* **2**, 269.
59. Brent, L. & Medawar, P.B. (1966) *Proc. Roy. Soc. B* **165**, 281.
60. Nelson, S.D., Bridges, J.M. & McGeown, M.G. (1965) *Lancet* **1**, 1359.
61. Ramseier, H. & Billingham, R.E. (1964) *Ann. N.Y. Acad. Sci.* **120**, 379.
62. Streilein, J.W. & Billingham, R.E. (1967) *J. Exp. Med.* **126**, 455.
63. Ford, W. L. (1967) *Brit. J. Exp. Path.* **48**, 335.
64. Kosunen, T.V. & Dvorak, H.F. (1963) *Lab. Invest.* **12**, 628.
65. Burnet, F.M. & Boyer, G.S. (1961) *J. Path. Bact.* **81**, 141.
66. Szenberg, A. & Warner, N.L. (1962) *Brit. J. Exp. Path.* **43**, 123.

67. Elkins, W.L. (1964) *J. Exp. Med.* **120**, 329.
68. Elkins, W.L. (1966) *J. Exp. Med.* **123**, 103.
69. Elkins, W.L. (1971) *Progr. Allerg.* **15**, 78.
70. Ford, W.L., Burr, W. & Simonsen, M. (1970) *Transplantation* **10**, 258.
71. Russell, P.S. (1962) In *Transplantation*, p. 350, Ciba Found. Symp., eds G.E.W. Wolstenholme & M.P. Cameron, J. & A. Churchill, London.
72. Barnes, D.W.H., Ford, C.E., Ilbery, P.L.T. *et al.* (1957) *J. Comp. Cell Physiol.* **50** (suppl. 1), 123.
73. Barnes, D.W.H., Ilbery, P.L.T. & Loutit, J.F. (1958) *Nature* **181**, 488.
74. Ilbery, P.L.T., Koller, P.C. & Loutit, J.F. (1958) *J. Natl. Cancer Inst.* **20**, 1051.
75. Barnes, D.W.H. & Loutit, J.F. (1959) *Proc. Roy. Soc. B* **150**, 131.
76. Schwartz, E.E., Upton, A.C. & Congdon, C.C. (1957) *Proc. Soc. Exp. Biol. Med.* **96**, 797.
77. Feldman, M. & Jaffe, D. (1958) *J. Natl.Cancer Inst.* **21**, 297.
78. Trentin, J.J. (1958) *Ann. N.Y. Acad. Sci.* **73**, 799.
79. Cole, L.J., Garver, R.M. & Kunewick, J.P. (1959) *Transpl. Bull.* **6**, 429.
80. Zaalberg, B. & Van Bekkum, D.W. (1959) *Transpl. Bull.* **6**, 91.
81. Crouch, B.G., Van Putten, L.M., Van Bekkum, D.W. *et al.* (1961) *J. Natl. Cancer Inst.* **27**, 53.
82. Billingham, R.E. (1966) *The Harvey Lectures* **62**, 21.
83. Möller, G. (ed.) (1985) *Immunol. Rev.* **88**, 1–238.
84. Wilson, D.B. (1988) *Immunol. Rev.* **107**, 159.
85. Jones, J.M., Wilson, R. & Bealmear, P.M. (1971) *Radiation Res.* **45**, 577.
86. Van Bekkum, D.W., Roodenberg, J., Heidt, P.J. *et al.* (1974) *J. Natl. Cancer Res. Inst.* **52**, 401.
87. Rodt, H., Tierfelder, S. & Eulitz, M. (1974) *Eur. J. Immunol.* **4**, 25.
88. Sprent, J., Von Boehmer, H. & Nabholz, M. (1975) *J. Exp. Med.* **142**, 321.
89. Dicke, K.A., Van Hooft, J.I.M. & Van Bekkum, D.W. (1968) *Transplantation* **6**, 562.
90. Matzinger, P. & Mirkwood, G. (1978) *Transplantation* **148**, 84.
91. Onoe, K., Fernandes, G. & Good, R.A. (1980) *J. Exp. Med.* **151**, 115.
92. Vallera, D.A., Sonderling, C.C.B., Carlson, G.J. *et al.* (1981) *Transplantation* **31**, 218.
93. Zinkernagel, R.M., Althage, A., Callahan, G. *et al.* (1980) *J. Immunol.* **124**, 2356.
94. Norin, A.J., Emeson, E.E. & Veith, F.J. (1981) *J. Immunol.* **126**, 428.
95. Rayfield, L.S. & Brent, L. (1983) *Transplantation* **36**, 183.
96. Moser, M., Iwasaki, T. & Shearer, G.M. (1985) *Immunol. Rev.* **88**, 126.
97. Fox, M. (1962) *Nature* **195**, 1024.
98. Biggs, P.M. & Payne, L.N. (1959) *Nature* **184**, 1594.
99. Boak, J.L., Fox, M. & Wilson, R.E. (1967) *Lancet* **1**, 750.
100. Van der Werf, B.A., Monaco, A.P., Wood, M.L. *et al.* (1968) In *Advances in Transplant*ation, eds J. Dausset, J. Hamburger & G. Mathé, p. 133, Munksgaard, Copenhagen.
101. Brent, L. & Gowland, G. (1968) In *Advances in Transplant*ation, eds J. Dausset, J. Hamburger & G. Mathé, p. 117, Munksgaard, Copenhagen.
102. Boak, J.L. & Wilson, R.E. (1968) *Clin. Exp. Immunol.* **3**, 795.
103. Van Bekkum, D.W., Balner, H., Dicke, K.A. *et al.* (1972) *Transplantation* **13**, 400.
104. Kulkarin, S.S., Kulkarin, A.D., Gallagher, M.T. *et al.* (1981) *Transplantation* **31**, 72.
105. Waldmann, H., Gale, G., Cividalli, G. *et al.* (1984) *Lancet* , **2**, 483.
106. Lonai, P., Eliraz, A., Wekerle, H. *et al.* (1973) *Transplantation* **15**, 368.
107. Belldegrün, A. & Cohen, I.R. (1979) *Transplantation* **28**, 382.
108. Sprent, J., Von Boehmer, H. & Nabholz, M. (1975) *J. Exp. Med.* **142**, 321.
109. Tyan, M.L. (1973) *Transplantation* **15**, 601.
110. Thierfelder, S. & Rodt, H. (1977) *Transplantation* **23**, 87.
111. Van Bekkum, D.W. (1978) In *Natural Resistance Systems Against Foreign Cells, Tumors and Microbes*, eds G. Cudkowicz, M. Landy & G.M. Shearer, p. 69, Academic Press, N.Y.
112. Korngold, R. & Sprent, J. (1978) *J. Exp. Med.* **148**, 1687.
113. Vallera, D.A., Soderling, C.C.B. & Kersey, J.H. (1982) *J. Immunol.* **128**, 871.
114. Boyse, E.A., Mujazawa, M., Aoki, T. *et al.* (1968) *Proc. Roy. Soc. B* **170**, 175.
115. Cantor, H. & Boyse, E.A. (1975) *J. Exp. Med.* **141**, 1376.
116. Korngold, R. & Sprent, J. (1985) *J. Immunol.* **135**, 3004.
117. Korngold, R. & Sprent, J. (1983) *Immunol. Rev.* **71**, 5.
118. Sprent, J., Schaefer, M., Lor, D. *et al.* (1986) *J. Exp. Med.* **163**, 998.

119. Pietryga, D.W., Blazar, B.R., Soderling, C.C.B. *et al.* (1987) *Transplantation* **43**, 442.
120. Uenaka, A., Kagemasa, K. & Nakayama, E. (1993) *Transplant Immunol.* **1**, 132.
121. Schwartz, R.S. & Beldotti, L. (1965) *Transplantation* **3**, 79.
122. Storb, R., Graham, T.C., Shiurba, R. *et al.* (1970) *Transplantation* **10**, 165.
123. Owens, A.H. & Santos, G.W. (1971) *Transplantation* **11**, 378.
124. Rodt, H., Kold, H.J. & Netzel, B. (1981) *Transpl. Proc.* **13**, 257.
125. Reisner, Y., Kapoor, N., Kirkpatrick, P. *et al.* (1983) *Blood* **61**, 341.
126. Filipovich, A.H., Ramsay, N.K.C., McGlave, P.B. *et al.* (1983) In *Recent Advances in Bone Marrow Transplantation*, p. 769, ed. R.P. Gale and A.R. Liss, N.Y.
127. Prentice, H.G., Blacklock, H.A., Janossy, G. *et al.* (1982) *Lancet* **1**, 700.
128. Filipovich, A.H., McGlave, P.B., Ramsay, N.K.C. *et al.* (1982) *Lancet* **2**, 1266.
129. Filipovich, A.H., Vallera, D.A., Youle, R.J. *et al.* (1984) *Lancet* **1**, 469.
130. Prentice, H.G., Janossy, G., Price-Jones, L. *et al.* (1984) *Lancet* **1**, 472.
131. Wettstein, P.J. & Bailey, D.W. (1982) *Immunogenetics* **16**, 47.
132. Cantrell, J.L. & Hildemann, W.H. (1973) *Transpl. Proc.* **5**, 271.
133. Cosgrove, G.E. & Davis, M.L. (1971) *Proc. Soc. Exp. Biol. Med.* **138**, 210.
134. Halle-Pannenko, O., Pritchard, L.L., Motta, R. *et al.* (1978) *Biomed. Express* **29**, 253.
135. Halle-Pannenko, O., Pritchard, L.L., Bruley-Rosset, M. *et al.* (1985) *Immunol. Rev.* **88**, 59.
136. Halle-Pannenko, O., Pritchard, L.L., Motta, R. *et al.* (1979) *Transpl. Proc.* **11**, 652.
137. Halle-Pannenko, O. & Festenstein, H. (1981) *J. Immunogenetics* **8**, 443.
138. Halle-Pannenko, O., Pritchard, L.L. & Rappaport, H. (1983) *Transplantation* **36**, 60.
139. Holda, J.H., Maier, T. & Claman, H.N. (1985) *Immunol. Rev.* **88**, 87.
140. Okunewick, J.P., Meredith, R.F., Raikow, R.B. *et al.* (1982) *Exp. Haematol.* **10**, 277.
141. Hamilton, B.L. & Parkman, R. (1983) *Transplantation* **36**, 150.
142. Storb, R., Rudolph, R.H., Kolb, H.J. *et al.* (1973) *Transplantation* **15**, 92.
143. Rapaport, F.T., Cannon, F.D., Blumenstock, D.A. *et al.* (1972) *Nature New Biol.* **235**, 190.
144. Rapaport, F.T., Bachvaroff, R.J., Watanabe, K. *et al.* (1978) *J. Clin. Invest.* **61**, 790.
145. Van Bekkum, D.W. (1972) *Transpl. Rev.* **9**, 3.
146. Buckley, R.H. (1971) In *Progress in Immunology* **1971**, ed. B.D. Amos, p. 1061, North Holland Publ. Co., N.Y.
147. Thomas, E.D., Rudolph, R.H., Fefer, A. *et al.* (1971) *Exp. Haematol.* **21**, 16.
148. Thomas, E.D., Storb, R., Fefer, A. *et al.* (1972) *Lancet* **1**, 284.
149. Storb, R., Prentice, R.L. & Thomas, E.D. (1977) *J. Clin. Invest.* **59**, 625.
150. Copenhagen Study group in Immunodeficiencies (1973) *Lancet* **1**, 1146.
151. Van Rood, J.J. & Van Leeuwen, A. (1976) *Transpl. Proc.* **8**, 429.
152. Goulmy, E. (1988) *Transpl. Rev.* **2**, 29.
153. De Brueger, M. & Goulmy, E. (1993) *Transpl. Immunol.* **1**, 28.
154. Van Els, C.A., D'Amaro, J., Pool, J. *et al.* (1992) *Immunogenetics* **35**, 161.
155. Schreuder, G.M., Pool, J., Blokland, E. *et al.* (1993) *Immunogenetics* **38**, 98.
156. Lengerová, A. & Chutná, J. (1959) *Folia Biol. (Praha)* **5**, 24.
157. Uphoff, D. (1975) *Transplantation* **20**, 78.
158. Van der Harst, D., Goulmy, E., Falkenburg, J.H.F. *et al.* (1994) *Blood* **83**, 1060.
159. Voogh, P.J., Fibbe, W.E., Marijt, W.A. *et al.* (1990) *Lancet* **335**, 131.
160. Thomas, E.D. (1990) *Scand. J. Immunol.* **39**, 340.
161. Thomas, E.D., Lochte, H.L., Lu, W.C. *et al.* (1957) *New Engl. J. Med* **257**, 491.
162. Ferrebee, J.W. & Thomas, E.D. (1958) *Am. J. Med. Sci.* **235**, 369.
163. Thomas, E.D., Lochte, H.L. & Ferrebee, J.W. (1959) *Blood* **14**, 1.
164. Humble, J.G. & Newton, K.A. (1958) *Lancet* **1**, 142.
165. Mathé, G., Jammet, J., Pendic, L. *et al.* (1959) *Rev. Franc. Étud. Clin. Biol.* **4**, 226.
166. Mathé, G., Bernard, J., de Vries, M.J. *et al.* (1959) *Rev. Franc. Étud. Clin. Biol.* **4**, 675.
167. Mathé, G., Thomas, E.D. & Ferrebee, J.W. (1959) *Transpl. Bull.* **6**, 407.
168. Atkinson, J.B., Mahoney, F.J., Schwartz, I.R. *et al.* (1959) *Blood* **14**, 228.
169. Mathé, G., Amiel, J.L., Schwarzenberg, L. *et al.* (1963) *Brit. Med. J.* **2**, 1633.
170. Matsukura, M., Mery, A.M., Amiel, J.L. *et al.* (1963) *Transplantation* **1**, 61.
171. Mathé, G., Schwarzenberg, L., Amiel, J.L. *et al.* (1967) *Scand. J. Immunol.* **4**, 193.
172. Mathé, G., Amiel, J.L. & Schwarzenberg, L. *et al.* (1970) *Brit. Med. J.* **2**, 131.

173. Bach, F.H., Albertini, R.J., Joo, P. *et al.* (1968) *Lancet* **2**, 1364.
174. Good, R.A., Gatti, R.A., Hong, R. *et al.* (1968) *Lancet* **2**, 1366.
175. Good, R.A., Gatti, R.A., Hong, R. *et al.* (1969) *Exp. Haematol.* **19**, 4.
176. De Koning, J., Dooren, L.J., Van Bekkum, D.W. *et al.* (1969) *Lancet* **1**, 1223.
177. August, C.S., Rosen, F.S., Filler, C.A. *et al.* (1968) *Lancet* **2**, 1210.
178. Cleveland, W.W., Fogel, B.J., Brown, W.T. *et al.* (1968) *Lancet* **2**, 1211.
179. Thomas, E.D., Storb, R., Clift, R.A. *et al.* (1975) *New Engl. J. Med.* **292**, 832, 895.
180. Mannick, J.A., Lochte, H.L., Ashley, C.A. *et al.* (1960) *Blood* **15**, 255.
181. Rapaport, F.T., Bachvaroff, R.J., Akiyama, N. *et al.* (1980) *Transplantation* **30**, 23.
182. Gale, R.P., Horowitz, M.M. & Butturini, A. (1991) *Brit. J. Haematol.* **78**, 135.
183. Hood, A.F., Vogelsang, G.B., Black, L.P. *et al.* (1987) *Arch. Dermatol.* **123**, 745.
184. Uphoff, D. (1958) *Proc. Soc. Exp. Biol. Med.* **99**, 651.
185. Storb, R., Epstein, R.B., Graham, T.C. *et al.* (1970) *Transplantation* **9**, 240.
186. Muller-Bérat. C.N., Van Putten, L.M. & Van Bekkum, D.W. (1966) *Ann. N.Y. Acad. Sci.* **129**, 340.
187. Van Putten, L.M., Balner, H., Muller-Bérat, C.N. *et al.* (1968) *Bibl. Haematol.* **29**, 574, Karger, Basel, N.Y.
188. Thomas, E.D., Buckner, C.D., Rudolph, R.H. *et al.* (1971) *Blood* **38**, 267.
189. Fefer, A., Einstein, A.B., Thomas, E.D. *et al.* (1974) *New Engl. J. Med.* **290**, 1389.
190. Storb, R., Thomas, E.D., Buckner, R.A. *et al.* (1974) *Blood* **43**, 157.
191. Storb, R., Thomas, E.D., Weiden, P.L. *et al.* (1976) *Blood* **48**, 817.
192. Storb, R., Prentice, R.L. & Thomas, E.D. (1977) *New Engl. J. Med.* **59**, 625.
193. Marmont, A.M., Horowitz, M.M., Gale, R.P. *et al.* (1991) *Blood* **78**, 2120.
194. Barnes, D.W.H., Corp, M.J., Loutit, J.F. *et al.* (1956) *Brit. Med. J.* **2**, 626.
195. Mathé, G. (1960) *Blood* **16**, 1073.
196. Stuart, A.E. (1962) *Lancet* **2**, 180.
197. Woodruff, M.F.A. & Symes, M.O. (1962) *Brit. J. Cancer* **16**, 707.
198. Woodruff, M.F.A., Symes, M.O. & Anderson, N.F. (1962) *Brit. J. Cancer* **17**, 482.
199. Woodruff, M.F.A., Symes, M.O. & Stuart, A.E. (1963) *Brit. J. Cancer* **17**, 320.
200. Woodruff, M.F.A. & Nolan, B. (1964) *Lancet* **2**, 426.
201. Koldovsky, P. & Lengerová, A. (1960) *Folia Biol. (Praha)* **6**, 441.
202. Koldovsky, P. (1961) *Folia Biol. (Praha)* **7**, 157.
203. Woodruff, M.F.A. (1964) *Lancet* **2**, 265.
204. Symes, M.O. (1967) *Brit. J. Cancer* **21**, 178.
205. Denton, P.M. & Symes, M.O. (1969) *Brit. J. Cancer* **23**, 100.
206. Apperley, J.F., Jones, L., Hale, G. *et al.* (1986) *Bone Marrow Transplant.* **1**, 53.
207. Giralt, S.A. & Champlin, R.E. (1994) *Blood* **84**, 3603.
208. Sullivan, K.M., Storb, R., Buckner, C.D. *et al.* (1989) *New Engl. J. Med.* **320**, 828.
209. Kolb, H.J., Mittermuller, J., Clemm, Ch. *et al.* (1990) *Blood* **76**, 2462.
210. Kolb, H.J., Schattenberg, A., Goldman, J.M. *et al.* (1995) *Blood* **86**, 2041.
211. Mackinnon, S., Papapodoulos, E.B., Carabasi, M.H. *et al.* (1995) *Blood* **86**, 1261.
212. Spencer, A., Brookes, P.A., Kaminski, E. *et al.* (1995) *Transplantation* **59**, 1302.
213. Schwarer, A.P., Jiang, Y.Z., Brookes, P.A. *et al.* (1993) *Lancet* **341**, 203.
214. Lafferty, K.L. & Jones, M.A.S. (1969) *Aust. J. Exp. Biol. Med. Sci.* **47**, 17.

Biographies

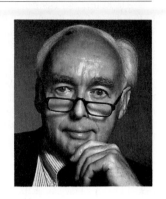

**RUPERT EVERETT BILLINGHAM
(1921–)**

Rupert Billingham – known as "Bill" to all his friends and colleagues – was born in Wiltshire, England, and although he moved to the United States in 1957 with his wife Jean and two children (one more was born in America) he never quite lost his rather endearing Wiltshire burr. Having served as a Lieutenant on Royal Navy anti-submarine escort vessels in Western Approaches Command and on the East Indies Station during World War II, he returned to Oxford to take his D.Phil. under the supervision of P.B. Medawar, with whom he moved to Birmingham in 1947. Thus began a highly creative collaboration, which ended only when he accepted a position on the staff of the Wistar Institute, Philadelphia, ten years later. Although Billingham published a large number of papers in that period and on a variety of topics, the most significant were arguably the collaborative study of skin allografts exchanged between cattle dizygotic twins and the experimental verification of acquired immunologic tolerance, in both of which he played a major role. The other important discovery, made with L. Brent, was of "runt" (or graft-versus-host) disease, made in mice at a time when M. Simonsen was studying splenomegaly in the chick embryo. Billingham was a perfect foil to Medawar's brilliance and intellectual power: always practical with his feet firmly on the ground, immensely inventive in devising techniques and experimental strategies, and with an unquenchable curiosity. He had, and still has, an irrepressible sense of humor, and he was not averse to playing practical jokes. His laboratory at University College was the fulcrum for the tolerance and runt disease studies and Medawar, when engaged in administrative duties, liked to drop in to chat while experimental work was in progress. After Billingham's move to the United States (first to the Wistar Institute and later, in 1965, to the University of Pennsylvania as Professor and Chairman of the Department of Medical Genetics, and in 1971 to the University of Texas as Professor and Chairman of the Department of Cell Biology and Anatomy), his scientific output continued unabated until his retirement in 1986. All who have read his papers will be struck by his experimental ingenuity and his ability to attack difficult problems head-on or from the rear – from the early work with T. Boswell showing that the rabbit cornea is immunogenic when transplanted to the chest of allogeneic rabbits and the demonstration that the cheek pouch of Syrian hamsters is an immunologically privileged site (with W.K. Silvers and others), to the creation of an artificial privileged site lacking lymphatic drainage within pedicle skin flaps, this time with C.F. Barker. While in the United States he also continued to analyze the phenomenon of graft-versus-host disease in mice and rats and he carried out some significant experiments in the field of reproductive immunology.

Billingham attracted outstanding research colleagues, among them W.K. Silvers, D. Steinmuller, J.W. Streilein, P.S. Russell, C.F. Barker, A.E. Beer, and J.R. Head. He was elected to Fellowship of the Royal Society in 1961 and of the American Academy of Arts and Sciences in 1965, and he is an honorary member of many national and professional societies, including the Society for Investigative Dermatology, le Société Française d'Immunologie and the British Transplantation Society. His lectures were always meticulously prepared and well illustrated, and twice he received an award from the University of Texas for excellence in teaching. He was President of The Transplantation Society from 1974 to 1976 and President of the International Society for the Immunology of Pregnancy from 1983 to 1986. Billingham has played an active role on editorial boards and as advisor to research institutions. His great hobby has been photography and he was responsible for providing photographic illustrations for some of the classic scientific papers. He and his wife retired to Martha's Vineyard in 1986, where they continue to live.

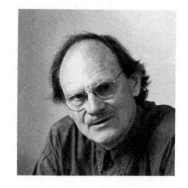

MORTEN SIMONSEN (1921–)

Morten Simonsen was born in Copenhagen, Denmark, where he was brought up and has spent most of his life. He obtained his medical degree from the University of Copenhagen in 1947 and spent his first internship ("by lottery") in a hospital in Aalborg, Jutland, where he was joined by his fellow graduate wife and his young son (now a nephrologist). He tells of the primitive conditions in which he had to establish a suitable operating room for his research and how he taught himself the appropriate techniques. Experimental animals including dogs had to he bought from his own salary "and the noisy dogs had to be installed in the yard of a nearby municipal workhouse, and the inmates were not supposed to mind" (*Scandia-transplant*, 1985). The dogs were "doped with morphine and carried across in a laundry basket at night, as the operations were usually performed on evenings or

Sundays". This was pioneering work with a vengeance! In 1948 Simonsen returned to Copenhagen to work in the General Pathology Department of the University, where the sympathetic head was able to provide him with animals as well as with encouragement. His thesis entitled "*Biological Incompatibility in Kidney Transplantation in Dogs*" was published in 1953 and it comprised not only a comprehensive review of the field but careful clinical, morphologic and histologic observations on the fate of kidney allografts in non-immunosuppressed recipients. The finding that mononuclear leukocytes were to be found around the kidney blood vessels and glomeruli was original, and he interpreted their presence as primarily a reaction on the part of interstitial cells of the graft against the recipient's histocompatibility antigens, an interpretation that he later withdrew. It did, however, prepare his mind for his subsequent studies on graft-versus-host disease in chick embryos which, together with Billingham and Brent's mouse investigations, made him a co-discoverer of graft-versus-host disease, a phenomenon that was to preoccupy him for much of his scientific life.

Simonsen has a lively and questing mind and he made many other contributions to the development of transplantation immunology and immunologic theory. In the mid-1950s he spent some time at the Institut Pasteur, Paris and at the Chester Beatty Research Institute, London. Having been a Senior Research Fellow at the University of Copenhagen from 1955 to 1961 he became Director of Research at the McIndoe Memorial Research Unit in England and Honorary Professor at the Royal College of Surgeons. There he continued his investigations in transplantation immunology and in graft-versus-host disease in particular. He returned to Copenhagen in 1967 to become Professor of Experimental Immunology, where he remained until his retirement in 1991. Simonsen's effort was very much part of the great upsurge in the field of experimental transplantation in the postwar years and he was a regular contributor to international conferences, including the small symposia organized by Milan Hašek in Czechoslovakia. As an idealistic communist in those years – not the most popular political stance to maintain in western Europe in the 1950s – Simonsen seemed more at ease than other western scientists in such an environment, and he and Hašek developed a close friendship that was founded on shared scientific interests, mutual respect, and shared political beliefs.

Simonsen wrote numerous papers and reviews and among the honors bestowed on him were the Paul Ehrlich Prize (1975), the Anders Jahre Prize (1986) and the NOVO-Nordisk Prize (1990). In 1994 he shared the Peter Medawar Prize of The Transplantation Society with R.E. Billingham and L. Brent in recognition of his co-discovery of graft-versus-host-disease. He has been elected to honorary membership of several national and international professional organizations and he continues to work in his retirement at the Statens Seruminstitut, Copenhagen.

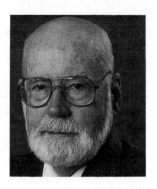

EDWARD DONNAL THOMAS
(1920–)

Don Thomas recounts in his Nobel Lecture (1991, Les Prix Nobel 1990, The Nobel Foundation, p. 219) that his father's family moved to Texas in a covered wagon in 1874 when his father was a young boy. His father gained an M.D. without any formal schooling and became a general practioner in a small Texas village. Thomas himself had graduated from the University of Texas with a B.A. in 1941 and an M.A. two years later, when he began his medical studies at Harvard. By then he had married Dorothy (Dottie) Martin, whom he had encountered accidentally in a snowball fight! They still live happily together and have three children and eight grandchildren, and Dottie worked in his laboratory for many years. It was during his medical residency at the Peter Bent Brigham that Thomas first met Joseph Murray, then a surgical resident, and thus began a lifelong friendship. He became interested in bone marrow and leukemia while still a student, and when allocated his first laboratory by Dr Sydney Farber he began to work on bone marrow-stimulating factors. In 1955 he was invited to join J.W. Ferrebee in Cooperstown, where he began to work on bone marrow transplantation in dogs and humans. "Except for an occasional patient with an identical twin, we quickly learnt that allogeneic marrow transplants in man were going to be very difficult." He remembers the Cooperstown years as being highly formative for his career.

Thomas moved to Seattle in 1963, where he became Professor of Medicine and Head of the Division of Oncology at the University of Washington School of Medicine; he has remained in Seattle ever since. R. Storb, his principal collaborator, joined him in 1965, and he recalls that the laboratory was 'tiny' and the staff consisted of "three physicians, one secretary, two animal technicians and one lab technician. All our work was done on animals, and the clinical applications seemed to be way in the distant future". From these inauspicious beginnings Thomas developed a large and thriving laboratory and the world's leading clinical bone marrow transplantation program, the success of which owes everything to the wide-ranging and sustained experimental studies carried out in dogs. As these became more and more successful Thomas raised the funds to convert an abandoned maternity ward at the Public Health Hospital into accommodation suitable for bone marrow transplantation, and the clinical program commenced in 1969. More than 4000 human bone marrow transplants have been performed. His clinical services, expertise and advice are much sought after: he is Attending Physician at six hospitals in Seattle and, through his appointments as Director of Medical Oncology and Associate Director of Clinical Research Programs, he has been intimately involved with the Fred Hutchinson Cancer Research Center, to which he transplanted his team in 1975. Throughout his tenure as head of the Division of Oncology, Storb recalls "he participated as any other member of the now growing group of investigators in attending duties and night calls and . . . carried the same clinical load as the most junior attending".

The honors that have been bestowed on Thomas, apart from the Nobel Prize, are far too numerous to list; they include the Philip Levine Award of the American Society of Pathologists, The Robert Roesler de Villiers Award of the Leukemia Society of America, and the Karl Landsteiner Award of the American Association of Blood Banks. Thomas was President of the American Society of Hematology from 1977 to 1978 and he has received Honorary Doctorates from several Italian and Spanish universities. In 1990 he became Professor Emeritus of Medicine at the University School of Medicine, Washington. His abiding passion – apart from bone marrow transplantation and his family – is fishing for salmon and steelhead and hunting, hobbies he was happy to share with his chief animal technician. He has remained notably modest despite a hugely successful life.

9 Xenotransplantation

"We shall solve the problem of using heterografts if we try hard enough, and maybe in less than fifteen years."

P.B. Medawar, 1968

Xenotransplantation – the grafting of tissues and organs from animals of one species to recipients belonging to another species – has a history virtually as old as allotransplantation. Its mythologic roots in the shape of the Lamassu, Chimera, Griffon, Hippocamp and Cockatrice have been touched on by Cooper (1) in an amusing foreword to the book *Xenotransplantation*, explaining that the editors chose the Lamassu, which is part human and part lion and with wings "to represent spiritual elevation", to put on their book's cover because "it appears to have been endowed with a much more benign and desirable character than many of its mythological associates". Nonetheless it is the Chimera (lion, goat and serpent) that immunobiologists chose as their symbol when describing the induction of tolerance in animals and humans when there was evidence of the continued survival of donor cells in the tolerant host.

Although moderately well-documented experiments involving xenotransplantation were conducted in the nineteenth century, most of the earlier attempts are anecdotal and unreliable. There was a great upsurge of interest when it became possible to transplant whole kidneys and certain other organs at the turn of the century, thanks to the pioneering work of Carrel in the anastomosis of blood vessels. Because the notion of using human organs from living volunteers or even cadavers was too exotic at a time when surgical techniques and asepsia still left a lot to be desired, some surgeons of that era turned to animals as organ donors even though the experimental evidence generally indicated that success was not to be expected. These early attempts were, of course, made entirely without immunosuppression, a vital weapon that the second great wave of surgeons in the 1960s had at their disposal. Even so, the clinical attempts in the "middle period" by men like Reemtsma and Starzl were doomed to failure, as will be shown below. Though much criticized at the time for "jumping the gun", before there was solid scientific evidence of how precisely xenografts were rejected, these surgeons nonetheless prevented clinical xenotransplantation from being consigned to the dustbin of history. The headlong advances made in understanding the mechanisms of allograft rejection and the development of powerful immunosuppressive agents were important factors leading to a renewal of interest in xenotransplantation, and since the mid-1980s there has been a veritable explosion in the number of experimental investigations. New journals catering entirely for this new (yet old) science were set up, conferences were organized, and two international congresses have been entirely devoted to the subject in the last five years. At a guess, well over 95% of all papers ever published on xenotransplantation have appeared in the last 15 years, making the writing of its history exceedingly hazardous.

However, the main drive for the renewed interest in xenotransplanation stems from the fact that, as allotransplantation of organs has become more and more routine, a great shortage of donors has been experienced. As Cooper (2) has recently argued, despite an increase in the sharing of organs in the United States through the setting up of UNOS (United Network for Organ Sharing) and the transplantation of a greater number of organs, the wait list has lengthened substantially in the period 1988–1991. The organ shortage therefore jeopardizes life, Cooper claims, and raises acute ethical dilemmas concerning the selection of organ recipients. According to Cohen and Wright (3), the gap is even greater in Europe. The formidable ethical dilemmas involved have recently been discussed by Sells (4). At their most extreme they include the use of organs from executed criminals, but also the problem of an "entrepreneurial profit-led market" in living unrelated kidneys, and the fact that the use of cadaveric organs is unacceptable in some societies. The use of animal organs, though raising other pressing biologic as well as ethical problems, could conceivably resolve the shortage, and Cooper (5) is optimistic that the solution of the problem of hyperacute rejection "will enable the pig or other mammal to be used as an unlimited supply of organs for man". Non-human primates, despite their phylogenetic closeness to the human, are unlikely contenders, not only because of their scarcity but also because, unlike the pig, they carry viruses and other transmissible infections that could pose grave dangers for human organ recipients, as Michaels and Simmons (6) have pointed out.

A number of historic reviews on xenotransplantation have been published, from sections dispersed in Woodruff's (7) 1960 tome to reviews by Saunders (8), Reemtsma (9, 10) and Auchincloss (11, 12). The latter's overview in *Transplantation* (11) is particularly well documented, although it does not cover the older literature and a huge amount of work has been done since. Another very recent review is that by Kaufman, Gaines and Ildstad (13), which has a historic introduction and reviews the literature right up to the present time. Not infrequently references to the older literature, which have often been derived from secondary sources, have been found to be misleading. An account by S.W. Lambert (14) of a highly disreputable transaction between a woman patient and a pig, resurrected by Saunders (8), strikes one as wholly frivolous as well as worthless, if indeed it ever occurred. In this chapter a bird's eye view of the early history will be presented and an attempt will be made to explain some of the very recent and current lines of investigations that are most likely to lead to a clinical solution.

An Ancient Dream of the Pioneer Surgeons

Transplantation of skin

In Chapter 2 I referred to the work of the outstanding sixteenth-century Italian plastic surgeon G. Tagliacozzi, who has been credited with the transplantation of allogeneic noses. He himself seemed to be well aware of the difficulties of allotransplantation, if only because of the practical difficulties. Although he believed that allotransplantation might be possible, he thought that for a number of reasons xenotransplantation was not in the realm of the probable. The work of the great Scottish experimental surgeon, J. Hunter, working in the eighteenth century, has likewise been described in Chapter 2. Most of his transplantation studies were carried out with allografts, but among his not at all well substantiated claims was one involving the transplantation of a human tooth into the comb of a cockrel (15). In the nineteenth century many surgeons claimed that human skin allografts had been successfully transplanted (Chapter 2) and these claims, based on poor observation, wishful thinking and the well-known ability of host epidermis to overgrow a graft undergoing rejection, were also extended to xenografts from a variety of species. For example, in 1895 A. Miles, another Scottish surgeon, claimed to have healed ulcers by transplanting skin from young dogs, rabbits, kittens and frogs, though on the strength of a single frog graft he concluded that "undoubtedly the frog's skin was least satisfactory". (16) Others likewise claimed success (see Chapter 2). Despite the warnings of men like Lexer and Schöne in the first decade of the twentieth century that allotransplantation, let alone xenotransplantation, was beset with the utmost difficulties, an American surgeon, C.S. Venable (17), claimed as late as 1914 that porcine Ollier–Thiersch grafts had a success rate of 85–100% when transplanted to patients. In the same year E. Lexer (18) came to a very different conclusion: even the value of epidermal or skin allografts was extremely limited, his own data making him doubt the successes of others, and he believed that xenotransplantation was doomed to failure.

Blood transfusion

Following W. Harvey's elucidation of the circulation of blood many attempts were made to cure patients of a variety of conditions by the transfusion of blood (see Chapter 2). For example, in a paper by R. Lower (19) a physician from Oxford, and communicated by Robert Boyle in the first volume of the prestigious *Philosophical Transactions of the Royal Society*, the possibility of tranfusing blood from one animal to another was discussed at some length and, in particular, whether it could be carried out safely when the recipient belonged to another species. Also considered was the question of whether the biologic nature of an animal could be altered as a result of repeated transfusions from donors of another species. "The prescriptions . . . have hitherto been attended with good success, and that not only upon Animals of the same species (as two Dogs first, and then two Sheep) but also upon some of very differing species (as a Sheep and a Dog); the former emitting, the other receiving." Some of these speculations were soon put to the test. According to Samuel Pepys (20), who claimed to have watched the proceedings, R. Lower and E. King in the same year (1666) transfused the blood of a lamb into a man, Arthur Coga. Pepys felt that the result was a matter of dispute, as some members of the Royal College thought that the patient had become "less frantic" whereas others thought not. Hot on the heels of Lower was the Frenchman J. Denis. After having successfully carried out transfusions in dogs this "Professor of Philosophy and Mathematicks", as he was described in *Philosophical Transactions of the Royal Society* in which he published his lengthy letter in 1667 (21), wrote that "we were strongly perswaded (*sic*) that the transfusion would have no such dangerous consequences, as some people endeavor'd to presage". Accordingly, we thought good to try it in some form of different species, and accordingly we took a Calfe and a Dog." This operation successfully accomplished, and repeated more than once, "whence we became confirm'd in the opinion, that there was more ground to hope effects rather advantageous than hurtful to mankind, from this discovery of Transfusion of Blood".

Denis answered the criticisms of the skeptics, and evidently there were plenty of those, and argued that the transfusion of blood into patients could be made "more boldly, and with greater success by employing Brutes", and he stated that the "dangers and inconveniences which would occur in opening the Arteries of a man are not inconsiderable". Accordingly, having first removed some blood he injected three times as much from a lamb into the circulation of a young man who was suffering from a "contumacious and violent fever" that had failed to improve after 20 blood lettings, and his condition was thought to have been improved. This case was published in *Philosophical Transactions of the Royal Society* (21), as was a second case of a healthy (!) man in his fourty-fifth year. Denis was evidently keen to try a larger transfusion, but because the vessels were "very low and not well fill'd" he withdrew only about 10 ounces and transfused about twice as much blood from a lamb. Advised to rest in a prone condition, the man leapt up full of energy and proceeded to engage in vigorous exercise, starting with the slaughtering and "fleaing" (fleecing?) of the "poor Lamb". When Denis met him the following day he found him well, without pain and with more strength than before.

In the same year Denis (22) published yet another long letter, citing the case of a madman whose wife had implored him and his assistant M. Emmerez to treat her husband with a blood transfusion. I will spare the reader the sordid details, but they removed about 10 ounces of blood from the patient and replaced it with 5–6 ounces of blood from a calf. The transfusion had to be terminated when the patient began to faint. The beneficial effects did not last long and it was repeated, this time with a larger quantity of calf blood. The effects were quicker (*sic*!) and "more considerable": the pulse became very variable and the patient perspired and complained of kidney and stomach pains and was on the verge of choking. The transfusion was terminated and after vomiting (ascribed to eating too much bacon) the patient slept and thereafter felt very much better. What urine he produced in the next two days was black as if "mix't with the soot of Chimneys". However, the story had a happy outcome in that after praying and confessing the patient was "in a very calm spirit, performs all his functions very well" and slept all night. Denis concluded: "I shall here suspend judgement ... till I have made many experiments more". Finally, in yet another letter published in the same journal a year later Denis (23), after complaining that false rumors had been circulated to the effect that the Magistrates of London had prohibited all transfusions, described in great detail the sequel to the case mentioned above. After the two transfusions there was a relapse in the patient's condition and his wife implored Denis and Emmerez to administer a third transfusion. Despite severe misgivings they relented, but at an early stage the patient had a violent fit and died. The widow charged both physicians with manslaughter, but after a full investigation it was discovered that she had poisoned her husband with arsenic! It did, however, "cause the enemies of the Experiment" to triumph and considerably set back the cause of blood transfusion. Transfusion in France was "not absolutely prohibited", but the French Court decided that it should be carried out only by "prescript of Physicians of Paris". It was later (1678) banned by the French Parliament as well as by the Royal Society of London and, after the Pope had likewise raised objections, interest in transfusion fell away and was not rekindled until a century later (24). Transfusion of xenogeneic blood was never to make a comeback.

The early kidney transplanters

One of the earliest scientific workers of the nineteenth century to study tissue transplantation scientifically was P. Bert (25), a French biologist, and reference to his work has been made in Chapter 2, p. 57. Although he believed that he had been partially successful in an attempt to parabiose a rat and a cat, he nonetheless realized that implanted xenogeneic tissues were invariably resorbed while allogeneic tissues seemed to survive for quite long periods. However, his experimental model involved ten-day-old rats of an ill-defined "white" breed that could have been partially inbred. Tolerance might therefore have intervened.

Although it is easily possible to delude oneself into thinking that a skin graft has happily survived when in fact the dermal pad has been overgrown by native epithelium, it is not possible to misinterpret the results of kidney transplantation provided the recipient has undergone bilateral nephrectomy. Once A. Carrel had so brilliantly solved the purely surgical problems of whole kidney transplantation, especially those connected with the anastomosis of blood vessels (see Chapter 7 and reference 8, in which Saunders also discusses the less than happy relationship between Carrel and his collaborator C.C. Guthrie), the kidney was widely used as an experimental tool in the first decade of the twentieth century. Most attempts used allografts, but despite the warnings of Bert, which may not have been known to the surgical fraternity, a number of attempts at xenotransplantation were made. The intrepid surgeons involved were mainly German and French.

Although E. Ullman (26) has been credited by Reemtsma (9) with the first kidney xenotransplant (dog to goat) I have been unable to find any reference to this in his 1902 paper. There he demonstrated the successful reimplantation of an *autologous* canine kidney, with immediate urine production, and he stated that further experiments will show whether transplantation into another dog or even from one species into another is possible, and whether a nephrectomized recipient can be kept alive. In fact, Ullmann had a wholly realistic view of the problems posed by xenotransplantation. Thus, by 1914 he was able to express the view (27) that "The hopes which we entertained 15 years ago regarding tissue and autotransplantation have been partially fulfilled; in heteroplastic transplantation it appears that the obstacle to success lies in anaphylaxis, while in homoplasty inherent chemical characteristics interfere with healing". He came to other farsighted conclusions. "The cell protoplasm, specific for each organism, varies with the individual. There are as many protoplasms as there are individuals." Had he used the term 'histocompatibility antigen' instead of protoplasm he would have been well ahead of his time! And again: "Then in homotransplantation the appearance in the body of a foreign protoplasm calls forth ferments into the circulation which destroy the transplanted tissue". Finally, he thought that "Whether it is possible or not to artificially alter the bloods of two individuals so that homotransplantation will be successful, is questionable". (28).

A surgeon who vigorously pursued the crock of the xenogeneic rainbow was E. Unger, another German. In his 1909 paper (29), having praised Carrel and Guthrie for having been "systematic and genial" in their approach to kidney transplantation, especially their study in which they bilaterally nephrectomized a dog and success-fully reimplanted one of the kidneys, he described one experiment with an allogeneic canine kidney in a bilaterally nephrectomized recipient. Although the two dogs were of different breeds the kidney functioned well for eight days, but the dog became ill and died on the eighteenth day. Urine secretion continued until the end. Histology showed hemorrhages and necrotic areas, with some glomeruli appearing fairly normal. They went on to carry out 50 experiments in cats and 20 in dogs, but none of the kidneys lasted for more than a few days. The causes of death were mostly unknown. Slightly better success with three allogeneic transplants (survival for about five days) showed to Unger's satisfaction that "the transplanted kidneys can function, adequate to sustain the recipient". He seemed happy to contemplate the first human allograft and more or less indicated (in German of course) to the reader to 'watch this space', as it were. And low and behold, his paper a year later (30), in the same journal, was entirely concerned with xenotransplantation and described the first xeno-geneic kidney in a patient.

Once again Unger (30) began his paper by singing the praises of Carrel and Guthrie as the originators of the "daring idea" of removing the recipient's own kidneys. Having explained that all four xenografts transplanted by him (piglet to dog, dog to goat, and cat to dog) were "as expected" all destroyed within ten hours, prob-ably because of thromboses, he described putting a child's kidney into a monkey, which died within 18 hours. Unger dismissed the notion of removing a kidney from a healthy human donor and, finding the logistics of obtaining an organ from a fresh cadaver too problematic, Unger turned to the question of whether it might be justifiable to transplant a monkey kidney into a patient. He knew that Uhlenhuth had shown that the apes were most closely related to the human and that even cynomolgus monkeys bore some similarities. Thus, when a young woman in "desperate condition" presented herself, Unger obtained a ten-year-old Macaque male from the local zoo and transplanted both kidneys without previous perfusion. Blood flow was established in just over an hour, but after a minimal production of bloody urine, the patient became sick and collapsed and died after three days. The kidneys looked white and they were swollen, and microscopic examination showed hemorrhages, pus in the mesenteric nodes, but no infiltration with "small cells". There was no certainty that the kidneys had ever functioned and the result having been considered inconclusive (!), Unger suggested that the problem needed to be pursued "with great care".

Two other clinical attempts in the first decade of the twentieth century will be briefly mentioned, if only to show that these intrepid surgeons, like Unger, were disastrously ahead of the basic sciences; both were French. First, Princeteau (31) treated a child suffering from renal insufficiency with slices of rabbit kidney inserted into a nephrostomy. The postoperative course was encouraging but the child died on the sixteenth day of pulmonary congestion. Second, in 1906 Jaboulay (32) implanted a goat and a pig kidney in the antecubital space of two patients; the early failure was attributed to thromboses in both cases though there was some function. It was left to Carrel (33) to emphasize that the results from xenotransplantation had so far proved to be negative, including his newly reported experiment involving one rabbit kidney transplanted to a cat. In contrast, his canine renal allografts sometimes remained functional for some time, in one case for several months.

It is hardly surprising that interest in allotransplantation of organs, let alone xenotransplantation, waned despite a few scattered and equally unsuccessful attempts in the 1920s. Further developments had to await the second half of the century, by which time the immunologic mechanisms bringing about the rejection of allografts (and to a lesser extent xenografts) were at least partly understood (see Chapter 2), powerful immunosuppressive drugs (see Chapter 7) raised the hope that even xenografts could be sustained, and some degree of immunologic tolerance had been induced for some xenografts, albeit mainly in the special environment of the neonatal rodent (see Chapter 5).

The Middle Era: The Dream Revived

The contribution of cancer research workers

Among the factors that led to a renewed interest in xenogeneic organ transplantation in the 1960s – and three of these have been alluded to above – there were also the studies by those who hoped to be able to elucidate the biologic and physiologic characteristics of human tumors by growing them *in vivo* in animals. An early worker in this field was H.S.N. Greene who, in a series of publications commencing in 1938 (34), transplanted fragments of human and animal tumors into the anterior chamber of the guinea pig eye, this being one of the 'immunologically privileged sites' (see Chapter 2, p. 100). In his 1952 paper (35), in which he described experiments with 123 different human tumors, he concluded that the transplantable tumors were usually associated with a fatal course for the patient whereas patients whose tumors failed to grow generally lived "for a considerable time". H. Toolan (36) managed to establish human tumors in mice treated with cortisone, and Handler *et al.* (37) found the hamster cheek pouch to be a hospitable site, with cortisone or X-irradiation providing useful adjuncts. This approach was widely adopted, especially in the 1970s when antilymphocyte or thymocyte serum became available for suppressing the immune response of experimental animals. Some used such antisera on their own (38, 39) whereas others combined it with adult thymectomy and whole body irradiation with (40) or without (41) bone marrow replacement. It thus became possible to grow some human tumors in mice and to study their susceptibility to anticancer drugs.

A further development of some importance was the discovery of the athymic ("nude") mouse, which proved to have a great shortfall of T lymphocytes. The nude hairless gene was first discovered by Isaacson and Cattanach (42) in 1962. Four years later Flanagan (43) described its pleiotropic effects, but overlooked the fact that nude mice were athymic – a discovery that we owe to E.M. Pantalouris (44). The latter linked the congenital athymia of homozygous nude mice to their striking susceptibility to intercurrent viral infections, especially hepatitis, and assumed that this was caused by the absence of T lymphocytes. Rygaard and Povlsen(45) were the first to demonstrate that a human adenocarcinoma of the colon grew in these mice, and the nude mouse became a much favored vehicle for the study of xenogeneic tumors (46–50).

Although these developments were unquestionably important it is doubtful that they influenced subsequent events in organ xenotransplantation, for the surgeons at 'the sharp end' of those experiments seem to have been unaware of this corpus of work. Nor did the tumor transplantation studies throw any light on the prime problem encountered in the transplantation of vascularized organs – hyperacute rejection (HAR).

The fact that in the 1950s xenogeneic tissues were made partially acceptable in animals that had been tolerized before or immediately after birth (51, 52), though again not a direct influence, may have helped to form the climate of opinion that allowed a second wave of xenotransplants to patients to be attempted in the 1960s. But the most important factor was no doubt the fact that kidney allotransplantation had begun to take off early in that decade (see Chapter 7).

Re-enter the surgeons

Although very little basic research had been carried out on the immunology of the xenograft response, R.Y. Calne (53) reported in 1961 a single attempt to transplant a goat's kidney into the iliac fossa of a dog without immunosuppression. Despite good initial blood flow the kidney became pale and then blue and within 90 minutes the renal artery had thrombosed. The kidney was removed and showed acute vascular disintegration with hemorrhages in the juxtamedullary region. A piece of goat's skin transplanted subsequently under daily 6-mercaptopurine immunosuppression was rejected in 12 days, compared with 6 days for a control. This information was included in a paper on experimental allotransplantation and did not receive any further comment.

1964 proved to be an extraordinary and controversial year in that it saw the publication of several accounts of clinical xenogeneic kidney and heart transplantation. Looking back at this year it seems as if some sort of collective madness had taken over in the United States, where the attempts were made, for despite the introduction of azathioprine and steroids in the treatment of patients who had been given renal allografts the omens cannot have been good. Nonetheless, Reemtsma and his surgical team (54) in New Orleans, when describing their first two cases, felt that "New exploration of this field now seems warranted because of success with immunosuppressive measures in homografts". These patients were heavily immunosuppressed with a combination of azathioprine, steroids, actinomycin C and azarine, and the donors were a rhesus monkey and a chimpanzee. Both donor kidneys were transplanted in each case. The rhesus kidney recipient died on the twelfth day – the kidneys revealing "a sprinkling of inflammatory cells" and relatively normal-looking glomeruli – but the chimpanzee recipient survived for as long as nine weeks, the cause of death having been diagnosed as bronchopneumonia. No cellular infiltrate was present. This case was presented together with several others in greater detail a few months later (55), when the authors concluded that "the early graft-rejection phase following renal heterotransplantation in man may be reversed". Indeed, one of the chimpanzee kidney recipients survived, remarkably, for more than six months. When Reemtsma (56) presented his team's findings at the spring meeting of the

American Surgical Society J.E. Murray, the human kidney allograft pioneer, commented that "although as yet not of clinical usefulness, (he) has opened up this phase of transplantation biology for further experimental investigation. None of us one year ago would have guessed that any primate graft would have survived for 12 weeks".

After performing a number of cardiac allografts in calves, though without long-term survival, J.D. Hardy and his team at the University of Mississippi Medical Center (57) embarked on the transplantation of a chimpanzee heart into a comatose patient with 90% occlusion of the coronary vessels. They had been impressed with the relative success of Reemtsma *et al.* (56) and went ahead after a vote among members of the surgical team, though they were aware that the operation "was even more likely to arouse controversy" than transplantation of a human heart. They felt that in the particular circumstances their decision "was well within ethical and moral boundaries". In the event, within an hour it became clear that the chimpanzee heart could not cope with the large venous return and no further support was given. The azathioprine that had been intended for intravenous inoculation was not adminis-tered. The authors listed among the positive features of their attempt that "it is clear that the heart can be transplanted in man, and that with further refinements in physiology and drug therapy this operation may some day add years of life to many patients". The news of this operation caused a sensation and generated extensive public debate on the ethics of using animal organs.

Two further reports were published in the same year, both involving renal xenografts from baboons. Hitchcock *et al.* (58) from Minneapolis carried out a trans-plant in a 65-year-old woman after a three-day-old allograft had run into trouble with poor function and imminent gangrene of the ureter. The patient was receiving azathioprine and an analog of leucine. The baboon kidney functioned immediately and secreted three liters of urine in the first 24 hours, but four days later the patient developed a severe gastrointestinal hemorrhage. Urine output suddenly ceased and exploration revealed thrombosis of the renal artery. The baboon kidney was removed and the patient died eight days later. A "minimal cellular infiltrate" was found and the authors were sufficiently encouraged to proceed to further trials. The donor had not been typed for red cell antigens. The authors concluded by stating that "Immunologic studies of the baboon, in addition to such studies in humans who receive kidneys from baboons, are of paramount importance".

The second study, by Starzl *et al.* (59) working in Denver, was more substantial. It involved six cases and, thanks to the collaboration of K.A. Porter, the histopathol-ogist from St Mary's Hospital, London, it included a careful histologic appraisal of the baboon kidneys. Allografts had been unsuccessfully sought "in one case for as long as 2 months". Immunosuppression with azathioprine and actinomycin C was given before and after transplantation and the kidneys were irradiated locally after transplantation. Although rejection episodes could be reversed "relatively easily" they recurred frequently and vigorously, so that the immunosuppressive treatment had to be maximal. This led to infections and these proved to be the cause of death in most cases. However, the patients lived for 19–98 days, but these survival times included two patients whose still functioning kidneys were removed at 60 and 49 days, to be replaced by allografts that had become available. (Both died within 5–6 weeks because of "septic complications" following the insertion of the allografts.) The other four baboon kidneys were still in place 19–49 days later when the patients died. "Complete cessation of heterograft urine excretion appeared only in two cases, although renal function was failing in the remainder prior to death or the removal of the heterografts."

All grafts were found to be heavily infiltrated with plasma cells and large pyroninophilic lymphoid cells. The pathologic changes were varied and more severe than those observed by Reemtsma's group. Both donors and recipients had been typed for red blood cell antigens and some of the blood samples were tested for anti-baboon heteroagglutinin activity; all patients started with anti-baboon antibodies, the levels of which fell immediately after transplantation and then rose again. Chromium^{51}-labeled donor cells were cleared from the bloodstream very rapidly, again indicative of the presence of antibodies soon after transplantation. It was found that patients with blood types that were compatible with their donor's has "more sustained function than those which did not". Starzl et al. concluded that "the primary cause of failure in all but one case was inability to control rejection", and they speculated that the reasons for the absence of immediate rejection by preformed antibodies may have been that the antibody had not saturated the antigenic sites of the kidney. "It is impossible to be certain from present evidence if there is any fundamental difference in the mechanism of rejection in these heterografts as opposed to homografts", they wrote somewhat surprisingly. In this they were influenced by some evidence suggesting that humoral factors as well as cell-mediated immunity might be involved in the rejection of allografts. They advised that red cell mismatched donors should be avoided in future attempts.

It should be added that in addition to the factors already mentioned that encouraged surgeons to attempt xenotransplantation in the mid-1960s, there was one other referred to by Starzl (60) in his fascinating book, *The Puzzle People Memoirs of a Transplant Surgeon*. At that time dialysis facilities were still in their infancy and it was rarely possible to maintain a uremic patient by dialysis. According to Starzl (personal communication) there were only "six slots for chronic dialysis in the entire United States". The lives of uremic patients were therefore at incomparably greater risk than is the case at the present time.

There now followed a lull in clinical xenotransplantation while immunologists were beginning to study the mechanisms of rejection in animals, though in 1978 the South African team of C.N. Barnard (61) reported an unsuccessful attempt to get a baboon and a chimpanzee heart to assist the patient's left heart. The lull developed into a storm in 1985 when Bailey et al. (62) published their 'heroic' attempt to save a human neonate suffering from congenital and life-threatening heart disease by the transplantation of a baboon heart. Though technically satisfactory it was not successful despite immunosuppression with cyclosporine, surviving for only 20 days. The donor had been selected from a panel of six baboons because in a xenogeneic mixed lymphocyte culture assay the neonate's response had been the weakest. Despite the presence of low titers of heteroagglutinins hyperacute rejection did not occur. Although anti-baboon cytotoxic antibodies were absent before transplantation they were identified throughout the postoperative period. The parents of baby Fae, as the neonate became known, had given their consent in preference to interventional surgery and the consent process was subsequently reviewed by the National Institutes of Health (N.I.H.) Office of Protection from Research Risks (63). The surgical team was criticized for having overstated the possible benefits and for not having included in their protocol a clear indication that "a search for a human heart suitable for transplant into the infant would be made". The case created a furore, causing the journal in which Bailey's paper had been published to include an editorial by O. Jonasson and M.A. Hardy (64). They concluded as follows: "Until the lesions caused by preformed antibodies can be prevented by immunologic or pharmacologic manipulation of the recipient or of the donor organ, successful xenografting for the long term will be impossible. What Dr. Bailey has demonstrated, however, in this remarkable experiment with Baby Fae is that orthotopic heart transplantation is technically feasible in the newborn . . .".

In the same year the Council for Scientific Affairs (65) published a review of the literature and the current status of xenografts and concluded, rather lamely that "the process of xenograft rejection qualitatively resembles allograft rejection, involving both cellular and humoral immune mechanisms, but differs quantitatively depending on the genetic disparity between donor and recipient". The Baby Fae case also prompted Caplan (66) to publish a major critique of the ethical problems raised by research involving xenografts, concluding: "Only when it is clear to the medical community, regulatory bodies . . . and the general public that both researchers and their subjects or surrogates fully understand that clinical trials involving xenografts have as their primary goal the acquisition of generalizable knowledge should further research be undertaken".

These clinical attempts, unsuccessful as they proved to be, have become very much part of the history of xenotransplantation. Despite the criticism they engendered from those who felt that the attempts had been made prematurely I believe that they re-kindled interest in xenotransplantation and encouraged immunologists to turn to the very complex mechanisms involved. They also drew attention to fact that the use of non-human primate organs was beset with both ethical and logistic difficulties, and they encouraged surgeons as well as immunologists to investigate other species as potential organ donors even though they were more distantly related.

The Modern Era

Developments came about within a few years of the ill-fated clinical attempts in 1964. By 1966 it had become clear that human kidney allografts underwent hyper-acute rejection (HAR) – a cessation of function within minutes or hours – if kidneys were transplanted to patients who had preformed antibodies against the donor's HLA antigens (see Chapter 2). Calne et al. (67) did not encounter this in its more acute form when they transplanted pig kidneys into baboons, but four of seven recipients died in 6–30 hours from uncontrollable hemorrhages. Four animals had been immunosuppressed with azathioprine and/or hydrocortisone and the longest survivor in this group died of bronchopneumonia on the fourth day, with "well preserved hepatic parenchyma". However, there was no information on the presence of anti-pig antibodies.

Preceding this paper by two years (1966) two groups identified the involvement of antibodies and complement in the destruction of renal xenografts from widely divergent donor species. First, Perper and Najarian (68) showed that pig kidneys transplanted to dogs became non-functional within 20 minutes and dog kidneys in pigs within four hours, that the shut-down was accompanied by congestion, endothelial destruction and hemorrhage, and that complement was consumed during the rejection process. They were certain that preformed antibody had mediated rejection and various strategies, including the use of immunosuppressive agents, did not affect the outcome. They pointed out that Algire, Weaver and Prehn (69) had demonstrated the formation of antibodies after xenotransplantation in 1957, but that there had been conflicting reports in the clinical studies. A year later (1967) Perper and Najarian (70) strongly confirmed their data by showing that even in relatively closely related species such as the goat and the sheep the passive transfer of antibody could lead to a very rapid form of rejection. Polymorphonuclear cells were found in the glomeruli and arterioles within 20 minutes and gammaglobulin was found in the walls of arterioles and venules.

Another contribution of note came from R.A. Good's group (71) in Minneapolis. In the course of a wide-ranging investigation of the involvement of complement (C') in the rejection of allo- and xenografts they concluded that a variety of renal xenografts transplanted to dogs were rejected with remarkable rapidity (4–60 minutes, depending on the donor species) and that this was a very "pure" form of humoral rejection. They showed that C' components and complement-fixing antibodies were associated with the pathologic changes in the endothelium and vessels of the grafts, and demonstrated the importance of C' and antibodies by the use of C' inhibitors and passive antibody transfer. They concluded that "C', activated and directed by C'-fixing antibodies, *can* be an effector mechanism of graft rejection, and indeed *is* such an effector in renal xenografts in the dog". This much neglected, but prescient paper, is well worth reading.

The story was taken a step further by another American group, this time from Detroit. Rosenberg *et al.* (72), from studies involving transplantation of pig kidneys into dogs, were able to state that "the pathophysiological basis of hyperacute rejection . . . is the induction of platelet aggregation, leading to the formation of platelet plugs and activation of the clotting and fibrinolytic system. The end result is progressive intrarenal intravascular coagulation of the cortical vessels and cortical necrosis". The basis for more recent studies had therefore been laid by 1969: preformed antibodies, complement, platelets and the vascular endothelium of the graft were conclusively incriminated in HAR of xenogeneic kidneys, and a host of subsequent papers confirmed and embroidered these conclusions. As Perper and Najarian had found before them, numerous investigators were relatively unsuccessful in preventing HAR using a wide range of strategies (11) (see below). The majority of experiments have been carried out with renal grafts, but it would seem that xenogeneic cardiac and even skin grafts can be susceptible to destruction by humoral antibodies. The literature is extensive and the reader is referred to the review by Auchincloss (11). However, a few points should be highlighted.

Having described the gross appearance of human skin allografts and the vascular changes they undergo (73), Converse and Rapaport found that in very strongly sensitized individuals a freshly transplanted allograft never becomes vascularized and remains a "white graft" (74). Similar observations have been made in other experimental animals such as the mouse and the rat. It would therefore appear that high titers of pre-existing alloantibodies can interfere with the healing-in process, leading to a failure of vascularization. The same has been found to be true for xeno-geneic skin, which is clearly vulnerable in the face of xenogeneic antibodies, as Ben-hur, Solowey and Rapaport (75) and Steinmuller (76) have shown. The vulnerability of skin xenografts to antibodies was later carefully studied by the Boston groups of Winn and Russell (77, 78), who encountered antibody-mediated rejection even in closely related species such as the rat and the mouse. Jooste et al. (79, 80) revealed in the early 1980s that antibody action was directed at the vascular endothelium, for grafts that had been in place for some time in immunosuppressed hosts lost their sensitivity to antibody. Such a dispensation did not, however, apply to cardiac xenografts (81), and it was assumed that this was due to endothelial host cell replacement in the heart "occurring less readily" than in the blood vessels of the skin. Certainly the xenogeneic heart has in many cases proved to be susceptible to HAR (11).

Workers who helped to keep the cause of xenotransplantation alive during the 1970s before it became fashionable, at a time when most research focused on allo-grafts and how to make them acceptable, included W. Brendel's group in Munich. They transplanted kidneys in many xenogeneic combinations, generally using large animals, and were particularly interested in the action of preformed antibodies and their phylogenetic significance. For example, Messmer et al. (82) found that the rejec-tion of pig kidneys by dogs could be delayed from survival for a few minutes in the controls to more than ten hours when the kidneys were perfused and the recipients subjected to hemodilution, and the delay was directly related to depletion of preformed antibodies, complement, platelets and blood leukocytes. In 1973 Hammer et al. (83) studied natural antibodies in a large number of species, including the human, and concluded in the light of their own experience (84) that xenogeneic kidneys invariably underwent HAR. Humans were shown to have natural antibodies against a wide range of species, with the exception of a few very closely related primate species, and they concluded that until such antibodies could be excluded the transplantation of xenogeneic tissues to humans was "not advisable". Pretreatment of dogs for six weeks with a soluble porcine liver extract administered intravenously in increasing doses prolonged survival 16-fold, but this amounted only to around eight hours compared with the controls (85). Rather better were the results with more closely related species, such as fox kidneys transplant to dogs when antilym-phocyte globulin (ALG) and prednisolone were used (86). These and other investi-gations by the Munich group did not bring forth solutions, but they drew attention to the many problems encountered in xenogeneic organ transplantation. Even in their fairly recent review of evolutionary and immunologic aspects of xenotransplantation Hammer, Suckfüll and Saumweber (87) felt pessimistic with regard to a solution to the problems posed by natural antibodies and rather gloomily (and unjustifiably?) concluded that "total depletion of preformed natural antibodies is not compatible with normal life".

Two faintly encouraging contributions came from Calne's and Medawar's groups. Back in 1970 Calne et al. (88), including workers from the Netherlands, found that a rhesus monkey liver graft survived for as long as three weeks in an ALS-treated cynomolgus recipient, the liver showing cellular infiltration and focal necrosis not unlike that found in allografts. Two other recipients died in the early postoperative period. However, once again more distantly related liver xenografts (pig to rhesus monkey) could not be rescued from the dire action of what were assumed to be preformed antibodies, despite ALS treatment. The work of Medawar's group on the use of ALS in prolonging xenogeneic skin graft survival was summarized by Lance (89) in the same year (1970). ALS worked remarkably well, but the species were the rat and the mouse (i.e. extremely closely related phylogenetically) and some degree of tolerance induction was achieved. Lance found it necessary to remark "that the barrier to survival is purely immunological", and concluded that so far as skin was concerned the reaction was viewed by them as "an allograft response of special intensity, depending principally on cell mediated rejection but reserving the possibility that the participation of humoral antibodies may be more important than . . . for allografts".

Calne (90) rendered a great service in 1970 by introducing the terms 'concordant' and 'discordant'. He proposed that "organ transplants between widely differing species that are rejected violently should be termed 'discordant' grafts as opposed to 'concordant' grafts between closely related species". The former subsequently proved to be those destroyed rapidly by preformed antibodies. This new terminology was promptly and universally adopted, and it added some clarity to a complex and amorphous field. Concordant grafts were those described by Lance as subject to allograft responses of special intensity (see above), but because of the logistic and ethical difficulties of using non-human primate organs in clinical transplantation much of the more recent work has been carried out with the objective of making discordant grafts acceptable, despite the far greater problems posed by them.

The concept of "accommodation"

The term was first coined by J.L. Platt and F.H. Bach and their colleagues (91, 92) in Minneapolis although evidence for its existence was already available from clinical experience with kidney allografts transplanted into ABO-incompatible recipients. 'Accommodation' describes the acceptance of discordant organ grafts that have escaped HAR by the removal or inactivation of preformed antibodies and/or complement and which continue to survive despite the subsequent recovery in anti-donor antibody levels. Some form of accommodation between transplant and host has evidently taken place once the graft has been in residence for some time, and many recent investigations have been directed at uncovering the mechanism underpinning this phenomenon.

It was G.P.J. Alexandre's team in Brussels (93) who reported in 1985 the successful transplantation of living-related ABO-incompatible kidney allografts after the removal of preformed antibodies by plasmapheresis. This procedure was coupled with immunosuppression with azathioprine, splenectomy, the administration of soluble A or B blood group antigens to mop up residual antibody and infusion of donor platelets. Of 14 transplants, ten were successful; one underwent chronic rejection, and three (all in patients who had not been splenectomized) were rejected by HAR. ABO antibody levels after transplantation varied from lower than pre-treatment levels to very high, and this was equally true for immunoglobulin IgM and IgG antibodies. Theirs was a remarkable achievement in view of the fact that, with few exceptions, ABO-incompatibility is a recipe for disaster (94, 95). Two years later Alexandre et al. (96) confirmed these findings in another 16 cases: 15 of 16 patients had functioning grafts, though one of these patients lost his graft from chronic rejection and was given a second graft from another relative. Only one graft was lost from acute rejection on the seventh day. Although the authors did not offer any explanation for their findings they stated that their success "warrants further and renewed interest for experimentation in the field of xenotransplantation. . . It is hoped that similar manipulation of the recipient could constitute a key by which xenografting would become a reality". Their hope shortly became reality, up to a point, when the same group (97) showed that more or less the same strategy could be used to overcome HAR of pig kidneys in the baboon, the kidneys having survived for up to 23 days in heavily immunosuppressed recipients. Gianello, Latinne and Alexandre (98) have recently reviewed these data more fully. Although results such as these do not compare with allotransplantation they nevertheless hold out the hope that, with further manipulations and perhaps different kinds of immunosuppression, discordant xenografts will become a realistic option. Another study of this Belgian group (98) has shown that the preformed natural IgM antibodies of baboons, which play such a vital role in HAR, are very efficiently removed by splenectomy and plasmapheresis, together with coagulation and complement factors, and that splenectomy inhibits the rebound of antibody production seen with plasmapheresis alone.

Platt (99), in a recent review of the problems of xenotransplantation and the notion of accommodation, stated that "Regardless of the biological nature of accommodation, further understanding of this process will be very useful, if not critical, in the clinical application of xenotransplantation".

Meanwhile many other groups have worked towards similar objectives. One such is that of Bach and Platt and their colleagues (91, 92, 100), who have developed the hypothesis that HAR occurs by a sequence that begins with the binding of natural antibodies to the vascular endothelium (VE) and goes on to the activation of complement, changes in the anticoagulant environment of the VE, the binding of polymorphonuclear cells and platelets to the activated cells of the VE and, as the end result, thrombosis. Their ideas and those of others have recently been reviewed (101) and it is impossible as well as inappropriate to give but the barest outline here of what the most promising lines of enquiry have been so far. They fall into four main categories: the removal of natural antibodies by various devices, the *in vivo* or *ex vivo* use of soluble xenoantigens, the introduction into the pig genome of human genes that inactivate human complement, and the induction of tolerance.

Removal of antibodies

The effects of plasmapheresis have been discussed above and this method continues to hold considerable promise. A daring experiment involving a patient awaiting a cadaver kidney allograft was carried out in the mid-1980s by Welsh *et al.* (102) although it was not formally published until 1991, or repeated, "because worldwide press coverage led to several threats made by animal rights campaigners against the hospital and the members of the medical team". The patient had been one of a group whose anti-HLA antibodies had been depleted by immunoadsorption for clinical reasons; the patients were under immunosuppression to prevent antibody resynthesis. It was found that this procedure (plasma exchange) "effectively removed human anti-pig IgM" although there was a return to pretreatment levels within 6–8 weeks. Having shown that sera from these patients prepared at a time when anti-pig antibodies were at a low ebb did not cause HAR of *ex vivo* pig kidneys, the team pumped blood from one patient through an *ex vivo* pig kidney. There was no HAR and the kidney secreted urine immediately and continued to do so until termination of the experiment six hours later. The patient suffered no significant side-effects and histology of the kidney confirmed the absence of HAR and IgM deposition. The patient's anti-pig antibodies gradually returned at the normal rate. This experiment demonstrated rather dramatically that removal of natural antibodies can be a very effective way of avoiding HAR, thus eliminating the immediate threat to xenogeneic organ transplants. (It is of passing interest that the animal rights campaigners seemed to be less interested in the fate of the patient than in the use of the pig as the organ donor, an unbalanced and extreme approach that has frequently marked their activities in Britain.) The Guy's Hospital team published their data on the extracorporeal immunoadsorption of anti-HLA antibodies in 1989 (*103*).

A group that has attempted to make pig hearts acceptable to baboons is that of Cooper (*104*), at that time working in Capetown. Using antibody adsorption by perfusing the baboon blood through one of the donor's kidneys, as well as immunosuppression, they surmounted the HAR hurdle, three of four hearts surviving for more than 24 hours. It may therefore be concluded that natural preformed antibodies play a critical role in the induction of HAR and that HAR can be successfully avoided by previous removal of anti-donor antibodies.

The use of soluble xenogeneic antigens

One very important development in the last few years has been the identification of the antigens that are responsible for HAR of organ xenografts. The notion that the antigens might be carbohydrates, inciting the formation of heterophile antibodies, was first put forward by Laus, Ulrichs and Müller-Ruchholtz (*105*) working in Kiel, Germany, in 1988. This hypothesis was taken up and developed with remarkable speed by D.K.C. Cooper, who had meanwhile moved from Capetown to Oklahoma, and his colleagues. Their work has been described in detail by Cooper, Koren and Oriol (*106*) and only the most salient findings will be alluded to here.

By infusing human plasma through pig hearts or kidneys Koren *et al.* (*107*) found that human preformed antibodies against the pig included IgG, IgA and IgM subclasses, and that all three bound most consistently to a molecule of 206 kD present on vascular endothelial as well as on other pig cells. Although other antigens, all of low molecular weight, were identified in some tissues, they thought that the 206 kD molecule was likely to be the one triggering HAR. The purified antibodies against this molecule were then tested against a variety of synthetic carbohydrates. The strongest binding was obtained with an α-galactosyl(αGal) terminal residue, which included certain di- and trisaccharides (*108, 109*). *In vitro* experiments revealed that the cytotoxicity of human serum, regardless of ABO group, could be markedly reduced against various pig cells by passage through an immunoaffinity column containing any of three αGal-1–3Gal oligosaccharides (*108*). This antibody depletion also protected sheep and bovine red blood cells against lysis. These findings have been confirmed by other groups. Cooper, Koren and Oriol (*106*) believe that the antibodies identified by them "belong to the anti-αGal antibodies first described in 1984 by Galili and his colleagues (*110*) and which, like anti-ABH natural antibodies, are thought to develop in the neonate as a result of stimulation by micro-organisms (*111*). The antigens identified by Cooper's group were subsequently shown to be present on vascular endothelial cells (*112*) – a vital demonstration in view of the fact that these cells are intimately involved in HAR.

Attempts to apply this knowledge to *in vivo* transplantation have been hampered by the scarcity of the relevant αGal di- and trisaccharides. Instead of using extracorporeal immunoadsorption or infusion of the pure materials into baboons, Cooper's group had to be satisfied with the infusion of melibiose (αGal-1–6Glc) and arabinogalactan (an impure plant polysaccharide with an αGal terminal residue) into baboons at high concentration, having first shown that both these molecules reduce the cytotoxicity of both human and baboon sera. The cytotoxicity of 4 of 15 baboon sera was completely abrogated and that of the remainder reduced (*106*). However, continued administration for more than a few days led to toxicity. Their only attempt at extracorporeal adsorption of these antibodies by passing baboon plasma through a melibiose affinity column on four consecutive days led to a reduction of cytotoxicity to less than 20%.

This group is presently collaborating with D. Taube's Transplant Unit at St Mary's Hospital, London in applying affinity columns with the purified disaccharide and an analog of the trisaccharide to the transplantation of pig hearts to baboons, with promising preliminary results (D. Taube, personal communication). It would appear to be a worthwhile approach.

The transgenic approach

Several groups (*113–116*) suggested in 1993 that the most elegant solution to the problem of HAR would be to breed pigs that do not express αGal epitopes on their vascular endothelium or have them masked by increased expression of another carbohydrate molecule (*115*). The deletion of the gene coding for α-galactosyl epitopes is far from easy and, as Galili (*114*) has pointed out, it might prove not to be feasible if these epitopes are found to play an important role in the development of mammals. However, Tearle et al. (*115*) have very recently managed to generate mice in which the α(1,3)-galactosyltransferase gene has been deleted, causing the relevant epitope to be absent ('knockout' mice). The tissues of such mice bound "substantially less" xenoantibody from human serum and human complement was less efficiently activated. Although the mice were viable they developed cataracts. An even more sophisticated approach would be to inhibit expression of the epitope selectively (i.e. on the cells of the vascular epithelium). This has been suggested by Gustafsson, Strahan and Preece (*117*) at the Institute of Child Health, London, using anti-sense- or ribozyme-constructs that will inhibit expression of the α1,3GT gene in *ex vivo* pig organs with the aid of adenoviral- or liposome-vector systems. Again, it remains to be seen whether this is possible.

A potentially easier option would be to insert genes into the pig genome that code for inhibitors of the human complement cascade. There can be little doubt that activation of complement through the binding of natural antibodies to the vascular endothelium plays an important role in HAR. For example, by inactivating complement with cobra venom factor Kemp et al. (*118*) found in 1982 that the survival of rabbit kidneys transplanted to cats could be prolonged from 5–15 minutes to up to four days, though this result was achieved with the additional use of cyclosporine as well as a drug inhibiting platelet aggregation. However, complement inactivation was found to be of prime importance, one graft surviving for one week with cobra venom factor alone. The efficacy of cobra venom factor has been strongly confirmed by Leventhal *et al.* (*119*) in rats given guinea pig hearts and a single baboon which received a porcine heart. Other approaches such as the use of complement-deficient guinea pigs by Braidley *et al.* (*120*) or the inoculation of soluble recombinant complement receptor type 1 by Pruitt *et al.* (*121*) have overcome the HAR barrier with discordant xenogeneic organs to some degree. Of interest is the observation by Johnston *et al.* (*122*) that newborn pigs that have not been allowed to acquire maternal antibodies from the colostrum and therefore lack antibodies can reject rabbit hearts by HAR, and that this can be overcome by treatment with cobra venom factor. These workers believe that the alternative pathway of complement activation not requiring antibody was responsible for HAR in the antibody-free piglets. This could, however, be exceptional, and natural antibodies are more likely to be the usual trigger. Certainly, Platt *et al.* (*123*) have made a strong case for the importance of IgM in the HAR seen in cynomolgus monkeys against porcine cardiac and renal grafts, as have Gambiez *et al.* (*124*) in a guinea pig to rat model.

The evidence for the assumption that the prevention of complement activation would help to solve the problem of HAR is therefore strong, even though it is unlikely to be the whole story. Several inhibitors of complement have been identified (*125, 126*) and they include molecules with decay-accelerating activity (DAF or CD55), membrane cofactor protein (MCP or CD46), and CD59, which is a membrane inhibitor of reactive lysis. These regulatory proteins are present on human cells and protect those cells against the effects of self-destruction by the accidental activation of complement. (Microbes do not possess them.) Successful attempts have been made to transfect the genes for some of these molecules into foreign cells. Thus DAF (though not MCP) protected foreign cell lines against lysis with antibody and human complement, as shown by Atkinson *et al.* (*126*); and Dalmasso *et al.* (*127*) have demonstrated convincingly that human DAF transfected into porcine endothelial cells protected them against complement-mediated lysis. "Our eventual objective is to engineer a transgenic donor animal, such as the pig, with human membrane-associated C inhibitor genes to achieve a high level of expression of the corresponding proteins in the endothelial cells of the xenograft", they wrote in 1991. "When a human is transplanted with such an organ the critical role of C in hyperacute rejection would be largely, or perhaps fully, compromised." In the same year Walsh, Tone and Waldmann (*128*) found that CD59 likewise protected cells of a rat line from human complement-dependent lysis. Notwithstanding the negative results obtained by Atkinson *et al.* (*126*), both Oglesby *et al.* (*129*) and Lublin and Coyne (*130*) have succeeded in showing that MCP, like DAF, has protective powers. It is of interest that Charreau *et al.* (*131*) succeeded in abolishing the protective effect with antibodies against the regulatory molecules.

Although complement may not itself directly cause tissue injury, as Dalmasso *et al.* (*132*) have pointed out, the incorporation of regulatory genes into potential donors such as the pig could nonetheless help to overcome the danger of HAR. Cozzi and White (*133*) have recently reviewed the prospects for this, the technology involved, and the difficulties still to be overcome. This approach is being followed by numerous groups, including White's in Cambridge, which has succeeded in producing 46 transgenic pigs into which the human DAF gene has been incorporated. In presenting the histologic analysis of these transgenic animals, Rosengard *et al.* (*134*) found DAF expression to be somewhat variable and they stressed the need to select 'founder' animals with high expression in the endothelial and smooth muscle cells that transmitted this expression to their offspring. DAF expression was without deleterious effects and the animals developed and grew normally and were capable of reproduction (*133*). *Ex vivo* hearts from transgenic animals were found to be resistant to HAR (*133*) but full publication of these data and the results of *in vivo* transplantation studies are eagerly awaited. Fodor *et al.* (*135*) have likewise achieved a high level of human CD59 in transgenic mice and pigs on a variety of tissues, including the vascular endothelium, and found such cells to be resistant to lysis by high titer antiporcine antibody and human complement.

Finally, McCurry *et al.* (*136*) were the first to report on the successful use of hearts transplanted from transgenic pigs carrying the genes and gene products for human DAF and CD59 into baboons. Control hearts were rejected within 60–90 minutes whereas the transgenic organs survived for 4–30 hours. While this increase in survival time is highly significant and the transgenic approach had carried the grafts through the period in which HAR would be expected, this can be regarded as only a beginning. Histology of an organ one hour after transplantation revealed "markedly reduced injury", including a "remarkable absence of haemorrhage, microthrombi and myocyte injury". The rejected hearts showed signs of injury, but this was focal rather than widespread. Both IgM antibody and the third and fourth components of C' were identified "along endothelium . . . indicating activation of the classical complement pathway". There seemed to be little difference in the measurable levels of C' complexes compared with non-transgenic hearts. The authors expressed the view that possibly higher levels of the regulatory proteins needed to be achieved. It should be stressed that the recipient baboons had not been immunosuppressed.

Induction of tolerance to xenogeneic antigens

Partial tolerance to xenogeneic skin induced in embryonic or neonatal mice or chicks was described in the 1950s (see Chapter 5) and the construction of stable xenogeneic chimeras after whole body irradiation was reported during the same period (see Chapter 8). These successes were almost without exception with concordant transplants, mainly rat to mouse or vice versa, or with avian species such as the turkey to the chicken. Auchincloss (*11*), in his comprehensive review of xenotransplantation, lists 44 references to papers in which some degree of tolerance to xenogeneic antigens had been established. He concluded that it was usually more difficult to induce tolerance to xenogeneic tissues than to allografts, larger cell doses having been required to establish stable chimeras in adult irradiated recipients (*137–139*) compared to comparable allogeneic chimeras.

An interesting model is that of Ildstad and Sachs (*140*). They overcame the problem of graft-versus-host disease (GVHD) in radiation chimeras by reconstituting the recipient with T lymphocyte-depleted bone marrow from both host and donor. This procedure led to the long-term survival of the recipients in the absence of GVHD and such animals later accepted skin grafts of the donor type for substantially prolonged periods, regardless of whether the model was allo- or xenogeneic. The tolerance was specific in that the animals were normally responsive to third-party skin grafts. The xenogeneic donors in this case were rats, so that the question of

HAR did not arise. Ildstad *et al. (141)* went on to show that these animals exhibited specific hyporesponsiveness in mixed lymphocyte culture and cell-mediated lysis assays, and that the lymphoid tissues had low levels of detectable donor cells, if any. The precise mechanism remained unclear. Sharabi and Sachs *(142)* then showed that engraftment of unmanipulated allogeneic mouse bone marrow could be obtained in mice by substituting lethal doses of radiation with anti-CD4 and anti-CD8 antibodies combined with sublethal irradiation and thymic irradiation. When applying this kind of regimen to xenogeneic (rat) marrow Sharabi *et al. (143)* found that, in addition to the antilymphocyte antibodies, they had to treat the mice additionally with antibodies against natural killer (NK) cells. These animals became chimeras, including the T cell compartment, and accepted donor-type rat skin grafts after about four months. The skin graft tolerance was donor strain-specific and the rat cell chimerism was gradually lost. There was no correlation between loss of tolerance and chimerism. The authors postulated that non-tolerized NK cells had been responsible for the loss of chimerism.

Finally, Cosimi's Boston group *(144)* applied their model to renal allograft tolerance in the cynomolgus monkey, but using a complex mix of antithymocyte globulin, sublethal whole body irradiation, thymic irradiation, and donor bone marrow infusion. Both monkeys rejected their kidneys by day 15. When the irradiation was fractionated and cyclosporine was administered additionally for one month, cellular chimerism was established and the survival of the renal allografts was substantially prolonged in the absence of further immunosuppression.

From these and other experiments the authors concluded that at least transient engraftment of donor bone marrow was essential to induce tolerance to the kidneys. When this kind of model was applied to concordant kidney xenografts (baboon to cynomolgus monkey) one recipient accepted his graft for more than 120 days *(145)*. It is difficult to assess whether this approach will have a clinical future.

Various approaches to the induction of xenotolerance have recently been discussed at length by Sykes, Lee and Sachs *(146)*.

A clinical xenogeneic liver transplant in the FK 506 era

The irrepressible T.E. Starzl and his team *(147)* described in 1993 a single case of a baboon liver transplanted to a patient with B virus-associated chronic active hepatitis and human immunodeficiency virus (HIV) infection. Because their own work had revealed that "the humoral component of xenograft rejection could be diminished by a short course of antimetabolite therapy, such as cyclophosphamide, which targeted the B-cell proliferative response", the patient's liver was thought to be resistant to hepatitis B infection. Because of the patient's "urgent clinical status" the decision was taken to transplant a liver from a 15-year-old baboon, on the assumption that a baboon liver would not be susceptible to HIV infection. FK 506, prednisone and prostaglandin were given postoperatively, and non-myelotoxic doses of cyclophosphamide were administered on the second day and continued for 55 days. The patient was eating and walking within five days, was released from intensive care after one month, and then developed several infections that had to be treated with nephrotoxic antibiotics. Complications included renal failure and dialysis was initiated on the twenty-first day. The patient had to be readmitted into intensive care with jaundice on day 55, was plasmapheresed five times between days 65 and 70, and suddenly lost higher nervous system function to be declared brain dead some hours later. On necropsy baboon DNA was found in his heart, lung, kidney, and lymph nodes, and blood samples collected earlier also proved to be positive. The liver revealed a number of pathologic changes including small platelet aggregates in the sinusoids and portal and hepatic veins, but no hepatocyte necrosis or necrotizing vasculitis. Death proved to have been caused by a subarachnoid hemorrhage and brainstem herniation secondary to invasive aspergillosis in multiple sites in the left brain. The authors stated that "the liver is thought to have immunologic advantages compared with other potentially transplantable organs, including greater resistance to humoral rejection". The presence of baboon DNA "is construed as the first step toward chronic acceptance and ultimately donor-specific tolerance". The case raised several important questions that could not be answered because of the relatively brief survival of the organ.

Starzl *et al.* (*148*) have recently reviewed the biologic basis and strategies for clinical xenotransplantation.

Conclusion

It will be apparent to the reader that the field of xenotransplantation has come a long way from its humble beginnings. In the last ten years in particular there has been an explosion of interest, engendered partly by the acute shortage of allogeneic donors and partly by the remarkable success in preventing the rejection of organ allografts with ever more powerful drugs. As a result, understanding of the mechanisms of xenograft rejection has increased sharply. In this context it is of interest that both xenogeneic graft-versus-host reactivity (*149*) and mixed lymphocyte reactivity (*150, 151*) have long been known to be weaker than comparable allogeneic reactions. Recent work has confirmed the hypothesis of Lafferty and Jones (*149*) that the reason for this is that xenogeneic cells do not produce an adequate level of costimulatory signals to facilitate the proliferation of cells. This has been demonstrated by Benfield *et al.* (*152*), who found that exogenous human interleukin IL-1 added to human lymphocytes at an early stage in culture with mouse cells brought about maximal proliferation.

In his summation of the 1966 Seventh Transplantation Conference in New York, L. Brent (*153*) stated: ". . . we have heard little of the xenograft, or heterograft to the diehards. At the last conference this was raised and discussed at some length from a clinical point of view, and I remember vividly that I was assailed for stating my view (which I still hold) that to think of using xenografts in clinical transplantation was premature". A great deal has happened in the intervening three decades, in which the basis for an understanding of the immunobiology of xenotransplantation has been laid. Once HAR has been mastered, as surely it will, it is possible that the cellular response to xenoantigens can be controlled by the available drugs or by new agents. But even this statement needs to be qualified, for Bach *et al.* (*154*) have drawn attention to the finding that after the immediate endothelial activation by antibody in HAR (called stage 1 activation by them) there follows a second stage, lasting several days, which is characterized by the influx of inflammatory mediators and NK cells. The latter have been shown to be injurious to the vascular endothelium

(*155*) and they are not as amenable as T lymphocytes to suppression with conventional immunosuppressive agents.

Nonetheless, it would not be too surprising if a cautious start were made in the clinical application of organ xenografts by the beginning of the new millennium. Yet it is clear from this historic account that it is vital that no such attempts are made before success can be fully assured, and before virologists are satisfied that organs from potential donors such as the pig will not infect patients with potentially harmful organisms such as retroviruses.

References

1. Cooper, D.K.C. (1991) In *Xenotransplantation*, eds D.K.C. Cooper, E. Kemp, K. Reemtsma, & D.J.G. White, p. vii, Springer-Verlag, Berlin.
2. Cooper, D.K.C. (1993) *Xeno* **1**, 25.
3. Cohen, B. & Wright, C. (1993) *Xeno* **1**, 21.
4. Sells, R.A. (1992) *Transpl. Proc.* **24**, 2401.
5. Cooper, D.K.C. (1992) *Transpl. Proc.* **24**, 2393.
6. Michaels, M.G. & Simmons, R.L. (1994) *Transplantation* **57**, 1.
7. Woodruff, M.F.A. (1960) *The Transplantation of Tissues and Organs*, pp. 1–777, C. Thomas, Springfield, Ill.
8. Saunders, J.B. (1972) In *Transplantation*, eds J.S. Najarian & R.L. Simmons, p. 3, Urban & Schwarzenberg, Munchen-Berlin-Wien.
9. Reemtsma, K. (1968) In *Human Transplantation*, eds F.T. Rapaport & J. Dausset, p. 357, Grune & Stratton, New York.
10. Reemtsma, K. (1991) In *Xenotransplantation*, eds D.K.C. Cooper, E. Kemp, K. Reemtsma & D.J.G. White, p. 9, Springer-Verlag, Berlin.
11. Auchincloss, H. (1988) *Transplantation* **46**, 1.
12. Auchincloss, H. (1991) In *Xenotransplantation*, eds D.K.C. Cooper, E. Kemp, K. Reemtsma & D.J.G. White, p. 23, Springer-Verlag, Berlin.
13. Kaufman, C.L., Gaines, B.A. & Ildstad, S.T. (1993) *Annu. Rev. Immunol.* **13**, 339.
14. Lambert, S.W. (1938) *Proc. Caharaka Club* **9**, 38, (R.R.Smith, New York).
15. Hunter, J. (1771) *Treatise on the Natural History and Diseases of Human Teeth*, J. Johnson, London.
16. Miles, A. (1895) *Edinb. Hosp. Rep. p.* 647.
17. Venable, C.S. (1914) *Southwest. J. Med. Surg.* **22**, 341.
18. Lexer, E. (1914) *Wien. Klin. Wchschr.* **27i**, 875.
19. Lower, R. (1666) *Phil. Trans., Lond.* **1**, 353. (Communicated by Robert Boyle.)
20. Wheatley, H. (ed.) (1896) *The Diary of Samuel Pepys*, vol. 7, p. 28, Bell & Sons, London.
21. Denis, J. (1667) *Phil. Trans., Lond.* **2**, 489.
22. Denis, J. (1667) *Phil. Trans., Lond.* **2**, 617.
23. Denis, J. (1668) *Phil. Trans., Lond.* **3**, 710.
24. Hoff, H.E. & Guillemin, R. (1967) *Cardiovasc. Res. Center Bull.* **6**, 47.
25. Bert, P. (1864) *J. Anat. Physiol.* **1**, 85.
26. Ullmann, E. (1902) *Wien. Klin. Wchschr.* **15**, 281.
27. Ullmann, E. (1914) *Ann. Surg.* **60**, 195.
28. Ullmann, E. (1914) *Wien. Klin. Wchschr.* **27i**, 875.
29. Unger, E. (1909) *Berl. Klin. Wchschr.* **46i**, 1057.
30. Unger, E. (1910) *Berl. Klin. Wchschr.* **47i**, 573.
31. Princeteau, M. (1905) *J. Med. Bordeaux* **26**, 549.
32. Jaboulay, M. (1906) *Lyon Med.* **107**, 575.
33. Carrel, A. (1908) *Arch. Klin. Chir.* **88**, 379.
34. Greene, H.S.N. (1938) *Science* **88**, 357.
35. Greene, H.S.N. (1952) *Cancer* **5**, 24.
36. Toolan, H. (1953) *Cancer Res.* **14**, 660.

37. Handler, A.H., Davis, S. & Sommers, S.C. (1956) *Cancer Res.* **16**, 32.
38. Phillips, B. & Gazet, J.C. (1970) *Brit. J. Cancer* **24**, 92.
39. Tibbetts, L.M., Chu, M.Y., Hager, J.C. *et al.* (1977) *Cancer* **40**, 2651.
40. Cobb, L.M. & Mitchley, B.C.V.C. (1974) *Eur. J. Cancer* **10**, 473.
41. Berenbaum, M.C., Sheard, C.E., Hager, J.C. *et al.* (1974) *Brit. J. Cancer* **30**, 13.
42. Isaacson, A.B. & Cattanach, C.D. (1962) *Mouse Newsletter* **2**, 31.
43. Flanagan, S.P. (1966) *Genet. Res.* **8**, 295.
44. Pantalouris, E.M. (1968) *Nature* **217**, 730.
45. Rygaard, J. & Povlsen, C.O. (1971) *Acta Path. Microbiol. Scand.* Sect. 1, **79**, 159.
46. Giovanella, B.C., Stehlin, J.S. & Williams, L.J. (1974) *J. Natl. Cancer Inst.* **52**, 921.
47. Kuga, N., Yoshida, K., Seido, T. *et al.* (1975) *Gann* **66**, 547.
48. Shimosato, Y., Kameya, T., Nagai, K. *et al.* (1976) *J. Natl. Cancer Inst.* **56**, 1251.
49. Osieka, R., Honchens, D.P., Goldin, A. *et al.* (1977) *Cancer* **40**, 2640.
50. Azar, H.A., Fernandez, S.B., Bros, L-A. *et al.* (1984) *Pathol. Annu.* **19**, 245.
51. Hašek, M. (1957) *Proc. Roy. Soc. B.* **146**, 67.
52. Billingham, R.E. & Brent, L. (1957) *Proc. Roy. Soc. B.* **146**, 78.
53. Calne R.Y. (1961) *Brit. J. Surg.* **48**, 384.
54. Reemtsma, K., McCracken, B.H., Schlegel, J.W. *et al.* (1964) *Science* **143**, 700.
55. Reemtsma, K., McCracken, B.H., Schlegel, J.W. *et al.* (1964) *J. Amer. Med. Ass.* **187**, 691.
56. Reemtsma, K., McCracken, B.H., Schlegel, J.W. *et al.* (1964) *Ann. Surg.* **160**, 384.
57. Hardy, J.D., Chavez, C.M., Kurrus, F.D. *et al.* (1964) *Ann. Surg.* **188**, 114.
58. Hitchcock, C.R., Kiser, J.C., Telander, R.L. *et al.* (1964) *Ann. Surg.* **189**, 934.
59. Starzl, T.E., Marchioro, T.L., Peters, G.N. *et al.* (1964) *Transplantation* **2**, 752.
60. Starzl, T.E. (1992) *The Puzzle People. Memoirs of a Transplant Surgeon*, pp. 92–93, University of Pittsburgh Press, Pittsburgh & London.
61. Barnard, C.N., Wolpowitz, A., Losman, J.G. *et al.* (1978) *S. Afr. Med. J.* **52**, 1035.
62. Bailey, L.L., Nehlsen-Cannarella, S.L., Concepcion, W. *et al.* (1985) *J. Amer. Med. Ass.* **254**, 3321.
63. Knoll, E. & Lundberg, G.D. (1985) *J. Amer. Med. Ass.* **254**, 3359.
64. Jonasson, O. & Hardy, M.A. (1985) *J. Amer. Med. Ass.* **254**, 3358.
65. Council for Scientific Affairs (1985) *J. Amer. Med. Ass.* **254**, 3353.
66. Caplan, A.L. (1985) *J. Amer. Med. Ass.* **254**, 3339.
67. Calne, R.Y., White, H.J.G., Herbertson, B.M. *et al.* (1968) *Lancet* **1**, 1176.
68. Perper, R.J. & Najarian, J.S. (1966) *Transplantation* **4**, 377.
69. Algire, G.H., Weaver, J.M. & Prehn, R.T. (1957) *Ann. N.Y. Acad. Sci.* **64**, 1009.
70. Perper, R.J. & Najarian, J.S. (1967) *Transplantation* **5**, 514.
71. Gewurz, H., Clark, D.S., Finstad, J. *et al.* (1966) *Ann. N.Y. Acad. Sci.* **129**, 673.
72. Rosenberg, J.C., Broersma, R.J., Bullemer, G. *et al.* (1969) *Transplantation* **8**, 152.
73. Converse, J.M. & Rapaport, F.T. (191956) *Ann. Surg.* **143**, 306.
74. Converse, J.M. & Rapaport, F.T. (1958) *Ann. Surg.* **144**, 273.
75. Ben-hur, N., Solowey, A.C. & Rapaport, F.T. (1969) *Israel J. Med. Sci.* **5**, 322.
76. Steinmuller, D. (1970) *Transpl. Proc.* **2**, 438.
77. Baldamus, C.A., McKenzie, I.F.C., Winn, H.J. *et al.* (1973) *J. Immunol.* **110**, 1532.
78. Winn, H.J., Baldamus, C.A., Jooste, S.V. *et al.* (1973) *J. Exp. Med.* **137**, 893.
79. Jooste, S.V., Colvin, R.B., Soper, W.D. *et al.* (1981) *J. Exp. Med.* **154**, 1319.
80. Jooste, S.V., Colvin, R.B. & Winn, H.J. (1981) *J. Exp. Med.* **154**, 1332.
81. Burdick, J.F., Russell, P.S. & Winn, H.J. (1979) *J. Immunol.* **123**, 1723.
82. Messmer, K., Hammer, C., Land, W. *et al.* (1971) *Transpl. Proc.* **3**, 542.
83. Hammer, C., Chaussy, Ch. & Brendel, W. (1973) *Eur. J. Surg. Res.* **5**, 162.
84. Chaussy, Ch., Hammer, C., Eisenberger, F. *et al.* (1972) *Eur. J. Surg. Res.* **4**, 262.
85. Land, W., Hammer, C., Fiedler, L. *et al.* (1972) *Res. Exp. Med.* **158**, 1.
86. Brendel, W., Duswald, K.H., Von Scheel, J. *et al.* (1977) *Transpl. Proc.* **9**, 349.
87. Hammer, C., Suckfüll, M. & Saumweber, D. (1992) *Transpl. Proc.* **24**, 2397.
88. Calne, R.Y., Davis, D.R., Pena, J.R. *et al.* (1970) *Lancet* **1**, 103.
89. Lance, E.M. (1970) *Transpl. Proc.* **2**, 497.
90. Calne, R.Y. (1970) *Transpl. Proc.* **2**, 550.
91. Platt, J.L., Vercelotti, G.M., Dalmasso, A.P. *et al.* (1990) *Immunol. Today* **11**, 450.

92. Bach, F.H., Turman, M.A., Vercelotti, G.M. *et al.* (1991) *Transpl. Proc.* **23**, 205.
93. Alexandre, G.P.J., Squifflet, J.P., De Bryère, M. *et al.* (1985) *Transpl. Proc.* **17**, 138.
94. Wilbrandt, R., Tung, K.S.K., Deodhar, S.D. *et al.* (1969) *Am. J. Clin. Path.* **51**, 15.
95. Paul, L.C., Van Es, L.A., de la Rieviere, G.B. *et al.* (1978) *Transplantation* **26**, 268.
96. Alexandre, G.P.J., Gianello, P., Latinne, D. *et al.* (1989) In *Xenograft 25*, ed. M.A. Hardy, p. 259, Elsevier, Amsterdam, New York, Oxford.
97. Besse, T., Duck, L., Latinne, D. *et al.* (1994) *Transpl. Proc.* **26**, 1042.
98. Gianello, P.R., Latinne, D. & Alexandre, G.P.J. (1995) *Xeno* **3**, 26.
99. Platt, J.L. (1994) *Immunol. Rev.* **141**, 128.
100. Winkler, H., Ferran, C. & Bach, F.H. (1995) *Xenotransplantation* **2**, 53.
101. (1994) *Immunol. Rev.* **141**, 1–276.
102. Welsh, K.I., Taube, D., Thick, M. *et al.* (1991) In *Xenotransplantation*, p. 501, eds D.K.C. Cooper, E. Kemp, K. Reemtsma & D.J.G. White, Springer-Verlag, Berlin.
103. Palmer, A., Taube, D., Welsh, K.I. *et al.* (1989) *Lancet* **1**, 10.
104. Cooper, D.K.C., Lexer G., Rose, A.G. *et al.* (1988) *J. Heart Transplant.* **7**, 238.
105. Laus, R., Ulrichs, K. & Müller-Ruchholtz, W. (1988) *Arch. Allergy Appl. Immunol.* **85**, 201.
106. Cooper, D.K.C., Koren, E. & Oriol, R. (1994) *Immunol. Rev.* **141**, 31.
107. Koren, E., Neething, F.A., Ye, Y. *et al.* (1992) *Transpl. Proc.* **24**, 595.
108. Good, A.H., Cooper, D.K.C., Malcolm, A.J. *et al.* (1992) *Transpl. Proc.* **24**, 559.
109. Cooper, D.K.C., Good, A.H., Koren, E. *et al.* (1993) *Transpl. Immunol.* **1**, 198.
110. Galili, U., Rachmilewitz, E.A., Peleg, A. *et al.* (1984) *J. Exp. Med.* **260**, 1519.
111. Galili, U., Mandrell, R., Hamadeh, R.M. *et al.* (1988) *Infect. Immunol.* **57**, 1730.
112. Oriol, R., Ye, Y. & Cooper, D.K.C. (1993) *Transplantation* **56**, 1433.
113. Sandrin, M.S., Vaughan, H.A., Dabkowski, P.L. *et al.* (1993) *Proc. Nat. Acad. Sci. U.S.A.* **90**, 11391.
114. Galili, U. (1993) *Immunol. Today* **14**, 480.
115. Tearle, R.G., Tange, M.J., Zannettino, Z.L. *et al.* (1996) *Transplantation* **61**, 13.
116. Cooper, D.K.C., Koren, E. & Oriol, R. (1993) *Lancet* **342**, 682.
117. Gustafsson, K., Strahan, K. & Preece, A. (1994) *Immunol. Rev.* **141**, 59.
118. Kemp, E., Kemp, G., Starklint, H. *et al.* (1982) *Transpl. Proc.* **24**, 116.
119. Leventhal, J.R., Dalmasso, A.P., Cromwell, J.W. *et al.* (1993) *Transplantation* **55**, 857.
120. Braidley, P.C., Dunning, J.J., Wallwork, J. *et al.* (1994) *Transpl. Proc.* **26**, 1259.
121. Pruitt, S.K., Kirk, A.D., Bollinger, R.R. *et al.* (1994) *Transplantation* **57**, 363.
122. Johnston, P.S., Wang, M-W., Lim, S.M. *et al.* (1992) *Transplantation* **54**, 573.
123. Platt, J.L., Fischel, R.J., Matas, A.J. *et al.* (1991) *Transplantation* **52**, 214.
124. Gambiez, L., Salame, E., Chereau, C. *et al.* (1992) *Transplantation* **54**, 577.
125. Lachmann, P.J. (1991) *Immunol. Today* **12**, 312.
126. Atkinson, J.P., Oglesby, T.J., Adams, E.A. *et al.* (1991) *Clin. Exp. Immunol.* (suppl.) **86**, 27.
127. Dalmasso, A.P., Vercellotti, G.M., Platt, J.L. *et al.* (1991) *Transplantation* **52**, 530.
128. Walsh, L.A., Tone, M. & Waldmann, H. (1991) *Eur. J. Immunol.* **21**, 847.
129. Oglesby, T.J., White, D., Tedja, I. *et al.* (1991) *Trans. Ass. Am. Physiol.* **104**, 164.
130. Lublin, D.M. & Coyne, K.E. (1991) *J. Exp. Med.* **174**, 35.
131. Charreau, B., Casssard, A., Tesson, L. *et al.* (1994) *Transplantation* **58**, 1222.
132. Dalmasso, A.P., Vercellotti, G.M., Fischel, R.J. *et al.* (1992) *Am. J. Pathol.* **140**, 1157.
133. Cozzi, E. & White, D.J.G. (1995) *Nature Med.* **1**, 964.
134. Rosengard, A.M., Cary, N.R.B., Langford, G.A. *et al.* (1995) *Transplantation* **59**, 1325.
135. Fodor, W.L., Williams, B.L., Matis, L.A. *et al.* (1994) *Proc. Nat. Acad. Sci. U.S.A.* **91**, 11153.
136. McCurry, K.R., Kooyman, D.L., Alvarado, C.G. *et al.* (1995) *Nature Med.* **1**, 423.
137. Zaalberg, O.B., Vos, O, & Van Bekkum, D.W. (1957) *Nature* **180**, 328.
138. Santos, G.W., Garber, R.M. & Cole, L.J. (1960) *J. Natl. Cancer Inst.* **24**, 1367.
139. Van Bekkum, D.W. (1964) *Nature* **202**, 1311.
140. Ildstad, S.T. & Sachs, D.H. (1984) *Nature* **307**, 168.
141. Ildstad, S.T., Wren, S.M., Sharrow, S.O. *et al.* (1984) *J. Exp. Med.* **160**, 1820.
142. Sharabi, Y. & Sachs, D.H. (1989) *J. Exp. Med.* **169**, 493.
143. Sharabi, Y., Aksentijevich, I., Sundt, T.M. *et al.* (1990) *J. Exp. Med.* **172**, 195.
144. Kawai, T., Cosimi, B., Colvin, R.B. *et al.* (1995) *Transplantation* **59**, 256.

145. Sachs, D.H., Sykes, M., Greenstein, J.L. *et al.* (1995) *Nature Med.* **1**, 969.
146. Sykes, M., Lee, L.A. & Sachs, D.H. (1994) *Immunol. Rev.* **141**, 245.
147. Starzl, T.E., Fung, J., Tzakis, A. *et al.* (1993) *Lancet* **341**, 65.
148. Starzl, T.E., Valdivia, A., Murase, N. *et al.* (1994) *Immunol. Rev.* **141**, 213.
149. Lafferty, K.J. & Jones, M.A.S. (1969) *Aust. J. Exp. Biol. Med. Sci.* **47**, 1754.
150. Wilson, D.B. & Nowell, P.C. (1970) *J. Exp. Med.* **131**, 391.
151. Widner, M.B. & Bach, F.H. (1972) *J. Exp. Med.* **135**, 1204.
152. Benfield, M.R., Witson, J.C., Alter, B.J. *et al.* (1993) *Scand. J. Immunol.* **38**, 130.
153. Brent, L. (1966) *Ann. N.Y. Acad. Sci.* **129**, 876.
154. Bach, F.H., Robson, S.C., Winkler, H. *et al.* (1995) *Nature Med.* **1**, 869.
155. Inverardi, L., Samaja, M., Motterlini, R. *et al.* (1992) *J. Immunol.* **149**, 1416.

Biographies

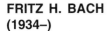

**FRITZ H. BACH
(1934–)**

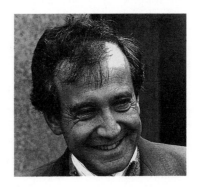

Fritz Bach was born in Vienna into a Jewish family. His father was a musician and sound engineer and his mother "just that, and wonderfully so". His family, including his brother, escaped from Austria in 1939 and Fritz spent the next nine years in England. In 1948 the family went on to the United States where he gained a B.A. from Harvard College. Before qualifying as a doctor at Harvard Medical School in 1960 he had already married Marilyn Brenner, who at the time was working for her Ph.D. at the Massachusetts Institute of Technology. They had one daughter and two sons, the latter destined to become physicians. Marilyn and Fritz were close scientific collaborators for some years but they parted in 1979. He became a professor in the Departments of Medical Genetics and Surgery at the University of Wisconsin, Madison in 1973 and subsequently Director of the Immunobiology Research Center. Later he filled the same positions at the University of Minnesota, Minneapolis. Apart from remarrying – he and Jeanne Gose, a pediatric allergist, have three daughters – another significant development in Bach's life was his appointment as Director of the Laboratory of Transplantation Immunology in Vienna, established by Sandoz. Life had therefore come full circle for a man who had to flee from Nazi Austria before the war. He is now Director of the Sandoz Center for Immunobiology at the New England Deaconess Hospital, Boston and the Lewis Thomas Professor at Harvard Medical School.

Bach regards Lewis Thomas as a major formative influence in his scientific development when he became a resident in internal medicine at New York University, and it was Thomas who persuaded him to attend a lecture P.B. Medawar gave in New York in 1961 in which Medawar discussed the antigens important in graft rejection and the mechanisms thought to be involved. Bach likes to recall how after the lecture he had asked Medawar whether he really believed that one could analyze it all *in vivo*; should one not try to do it *in vitro*? Apparently the reply was: "I think you should do just that, young man". Not many years later Bach and his colleagues had developed the mixed lymphocyte culture (MLC) assay, which provided an *in vitro* analog of allograft reactivity and the basis for the cell-mediated lympholysis assay. Both became indispensable tools in the analysis of allograft effector mechanisms, and Bach and his colleagues used them to great effect in the study of histocompatibility antigens. It was Bach's group that first put forward the notion that there are two kinds of histocompatibility antigens – the serologically identifiable (later class I) and those defined by mixed lymphocyte cultures (later class II). Bach played an important role in the study of these molecules and it is no accident that R. Ceppellini, J.J. Van Rood and D.B. Amos became close friends of his. Together with R.A. Good, Bach was involved in the first bone marrow transplants to patients suffering from immunodeficiency diseases, using his skills at human leukocyte antigen (HLA) matching. The donors for both proved to be MLC-negative and both patients are still alive and chimeric for donor cells. In recent years Bach has returned to the problem of xenotransplantation and together with his colleagues, prominent among them J.L. Platt and A.P. Dalmasso, he has made major contributions to the elucidation of the mechanism of hyperacute rejection.

Bach is a member of numerous professional bodies and editorial boards and among a number of awards are the Distinguished Scientist Award of the American Red Cross (1983), the Medal of the Collège de France (1984), foreign membership of the Royal Dutch Academy of Sciences (1987), The Emilio Trabucchi Foundation Award (1989), and honorary membership of the American Society of Transplant Surgeons (1991). Fritz Bach is well known for the clarity of his well-prepared scientific talks and lectures. His passionate interest is music, and as a regular participant of the W. Brendel Symposia in Austria he has become a competent and keen skier.

10 The Mammalian Fetus: Nature's (Almost) Perfect Allograft

". . . certain trends in the evolution of viviparity raise special immunological difficulties for the foetus."

P.B. Medawar, 1953

Full recognition that the survival of the mammalian fetus – a natural allograft thanks to the inheritance of histocompatibility and red blood cell antigens from the father – is remarkable came in 1953 with a landmark paper by P.B. Medawar (1) on "Some immunological and endocrinological problems raised by the evolution of viviparity in vertebrates". It was based on a lecture he had delivered to the Society of Experimental Biology soon after he had become Professor of Zoology at University College, London, and at a time when he still thought of himself primarily as a zoologist rather than an immunologist. It was written with the clarity, analytical sharpness and speculative brilliance that characterized so much of Medawar's later writings.

The paper began with an outline of the evolution of viviparity, stated the immunologic problems it raised, reviewed the endocrinologic features of pregnancy, discussed the implications of hemolytic disease of the newborn in terms of maternal immunization by fetal rhesus (Rh)-positive red blood cells, and set out the three most probable factors that could account for the undeniable fact that the mammalian fetus normally survives in a potentially hostile environment. The three factors he discussed were:

(1) The anatomic separation of fetus from its mother.
(2) The antigenic immaturity of the fetus.
(3) The immunologic inertness of the mother.

Much of the research that this paper generated fell into these three categories although one or two mechanisms that were later put forward were on rather different lines, such as the generation by the mother of blocking antibodies or antigen–antibody complexes or the uterus as an immunologically privileged site. Medawar concluded that "There can be little doubt that the first of these is by far the most important".

In discussing the question of anatomic separation, he stressed that the barrier separating maternal and fetal circulations "is normally impermeable to cells". Medawar's lecture was given before the adoptive transfer of sensitized lymphoid cells had revealed that the rejection of allogeneic grafts was largely brought about by lymphoid cells rather than by antibodies (see Chapter 2), and this prompted him to make the following statement: ". . . although it is generally agreed that purely cellular responses of the type envisaged by Loeb (1945) do not provide a sufficient explanation of transplantation immunity (*sic*), it may yet be found that cells of the immunized animal must participate in the reaction if immunity is to be given effect. If this proves to be the case, the vascular quarantine of the mammalian foetus clearly provides both for preventing the immunization of the mother by foetal tissue cells and, should the occasion arise, for withholding the consequences of immunization from the foetus". Although the relative impermeability of the placental barrier has since been a subject of controversy it has, nonetheless, remained the prime candidate in the search for the causes of protection.

Medawar pointed out that very little was known about the time of development in embryonic and fetal life of the "ordinary tissue antigens", but that "there are general reasons for thinking that the antigens of tissue cells develop much earlier than the antigens of highly differentiated end-cells like erythrocytes". The time of origin of the isoantigens of ordinary tissue was "on the agenda of our future research".

So far as the immunologic inertness of the pregnant mother is concerned, Medawar asked why it was that Rh "immunization occurs in practice very much less often than it might be expected to do on purely immunologic grounds": antigenic incompatibility between mother and fetus clearly was a necessary, but not a sufficient condition for the occurrence of hemolytic disease. He quoted some speculations by Mitchison (2) in a paper in which he had shown in mice that immunization of the prospective mother against paternal antigens did not affect the survival or litter size of the offspring. Mitchison had put forward "a theoretically and ingenious" hypothesis explaining why about 50% of Rh-negative individuals do not make antibodies when transfused with Rh-positive blood: having been exposed to the Rh antigen *in utero*, they had become "partially desensitized". Medawar added that if this were the case, "there should be a relative excess of Rh-negative grandmothers of children with haemolytic disease", but he ruled this out because "I understand that inspection of the available records has failed to bear this out".

Medawar asked: "Is pregnancy accompanied by any physiological change which may to some degree prevent the foetus, qua tissue homograft, from immunizing the mother against itself?". He immediately answered this question by stating that "The gist of the answer is simply that certain secretions of the adrenal cortex manifestly subdue the immunity reaction provoked by grafting tissue from one animal to another; these hormones are probably secreted in relative excess during pregnancy, with the effect that the female should become specially tolerant (*sic*) to the residence in it of genetically foreign cells." In support of this statement he quoted the work of his own group (3) and of Morgan (4), according to which the life of rabbit skin allografts was prolonged three- or four-fold by the daily administration of 10 mg cortisone acetate, and of his Ph.D. student E.M. Sparrow (5), who found much the same effect in guinea pigs although larger doses were required. He felt that there was a special significance in the finding by Billingham, Krohn and Medawar (6) that cortisone acetate could be made to act locally by painting the allografts every third day with a watery emulsion, suggesting that locally secreted hormones (in the ovary, for example) could affect the survival of the fetus. There followed a lengthy discussion of the secretion of hormones by cells of the adrenal cortex during the course of pregnancy.

Having established a link between the enhanced secretions of hormones during pregnancy, the protective effect of cortisone-like steroids administered to non-pregnant animals, and the protection of the embryo, 'qua tissue homograft', from the danger of maternal immunization, Medawar considered the immunologic reactivity of pregnant animals. He thought that "only a beginning has been made" in ascertaining whether the survival of foreign tissue was prolonged in pregnancy. However, he quoted the work of Heslop, Krohn and Sparrow (7) showing that skin allografts transplanted to rabbits on the 22nd day of pregnancy had significantly prolonged survival. Medawar concluded: "A prima facie case has been made out for the hypothesis that the enhanced secretion of cortisone-like steroids in pregnancy . . . has the effect of protecting the foetus from the dangers of immunizing its mother; but the hearing is still in progress, and a verdict has yet to be returned."

Medawar's perspicacious discussion has formed the theoretic framework for a great deal of later research and it therefore proved to be highly influential. However, as is the case so often when examining the roots of a scientific topic, Medawar was not the first to have regarded the mammalian fetus as an allograft. For example, C.C. Little (8), in his 1924 review of the genetics of tissue transplantation in mammals, raised this issue, though more or less *en passant*. He was concerned with the question of whether an implant needs to be genetically identical with its host to survive. He thought not, "provided it has no factors recognized by the host as foreign". In support of this argument he cited "the growth of the embryo of mammals as an implant in the uterus". He believed that "the mother has a well developed system of protective mechanisms, but it seems likely that most of the structures developed for the care of the embryo have, in evolution, a morphogenetic or mechanical function rather than any attempt to keep the physiological nature of the embryo apart from that of the mother". This is a far more opaque statement of the problem than Medawar's, and Little went on to assume that embryonic tissue has "distinctly fewer individually characteristic differences than has the tissue of the same individual when adult", an assumption that was not borne out by later research.

Having made his mark, Medawar did not pursue the topic of "the foetus qua homograft" any further, but his former colleague R.E. Billingham and his team, including A.E. Beer and J.R. Head, greatly helped to unravel some (though not all!) of its mysteries, as did M.F.A. Woodruff and a host of others. Most hypotheses – and there were many – had their proponents; some have stood the test of time and others have fallen by the wayside. The protection of the mammalian fetus from maternal attack is such a fundamentally important biologic feature that no single factor can be implicated on its own; it is far more likely that evolution has seen to it that multiple defenses are involved, leaving little to chance. Interest in reproductive immunology, which goes well beyond the narrower problem of the fetus as an allograft, has escalated to such a degree that an International Society of the Immunology of Reproduction was founded in 1975, and two specialist journals have been established: the *Journal of Reproductive Immunology* (1979) and the *American Journal of Reproductive Immunology* (1980).

A brief historic account of the evolution of thought on how the fetus usually manages to survive and flourish is given below.

Does the Fetus Lack Antigens?

It has become clear since the late 1950s that fetal tissues do not lack histocompatibility antigens, in that the implantation of allogeneic fetal tissues into extrauterine sites of adult animals provokes normal responses. This was first shown by Woodruff (9) in 1957 and soon confirmed by others, including Hašková (10) and Terasaki (11). In

Woodruff's study female rats were given skin grafts from males with which they were mated some weeks later. On the 15th day of pregnancy one embryo was removed and the hind limbs transplanted subcutaneously to the pregnant mother. These limbs were removed for histologic examination at 6 and 14 days after implantation. The grafts were rejected very briskly, unlike similar grafts transplanted to non-sensitized control animals, which showed reasonable survival even at 14 days though with some round cell infiltration. Similar results were obtained with rabbits. In both species the females became pregnant normally, preimmunization not having affected their fertility and capacity to sustain the embryos. Woodruff concluded that rat and rabbit fetuses possessed tissue antigens, though he thought that the moderately good survival in normal animals was suggestive of some degree of antigenic immaturity in the fetuses or, alternatively, some degree of immunologic inertness on the part of the mothers. He concluded that "these factors are . . . not necessary and that the decisive factor – which is both necessary and sufficient – is the anatomical separation of mother and fetus".

G. Möller (12) in Stockholm demonstrated that 13–14-day-old mouse embryos possessed major histocompatibility antigens (H-2) although his assays – sensitization to skin grafts and the production of anti-H-2 antibodies – left some doubt as to the precise time of appearance of the antigens. He had previously (13) failed to reveal such antigens on 15-day-old fetal cells using the indirect fluorescent antibody technique, but thought that these differences were caused by differences in the sensitivity of different assays. Shortly afterwards M. Edidin (14), an American working in Medawar's laboratory and using a cytotoxic antibody test, showed that fetal H-2 antigens were present in nine-day-old mouse fetuses, though he encountered some strain variability. This was confirmed by several other workers, using antibody absorption assays or direct visualization of antigenic sites with the aid of fluorescein-conjugated alloantibodies (see 15). Billington, Jenkinson and Searle (16) a decade or so later, and using more sophisticated methods, had no difficulty in revealing both H-2 and non-H-2 (i.e. minor) antigens on 4–8 cell embryos of the mouse, on the morula as well as on the cells making up the blastocyst (all before implantation). They likewise found both kinds of histocompatibility antigen on the inner cell mass and the embryonic sac after implantation (i.e. in the 7–8-day-old conceptus).

In the human fetus, major histocompatibility antigens (HLA) have been found in the early stages of pregnancy. For example, class I antigens have been detected in mesenchymal cells of the chorionic villi at 2–3 weeks by Sutton, Mason and Redman (17), though they were weakly and sporadically expressed, and Haynes et al. (18) found both class I and II antigens in the thymic epithelial cells of seven-week-old fetuses.

As fetal tissues appeared to possess antigens, a lack of paternal antigens was sought in the trophoblast – the fetal component of the placenta that is at the critical interface between the maternal blood and the fetus. Before considering the trophoblast it is, however, necessary to explore the question of how impermeable the mammalian placenta is to maternal cells and, conversely, to fetal cells.

Is the Placenta a Cell-impermeable Barrier?

Medawar (see above) clearly felt that, no matter what other mechanisms nature had to offer for the protection of the fetus, the separation of the maternal and fetal bloodstreams was by far the most important, and others thought likewise, for example, Beer and Billingham (19). Were it not so it is doubtful that mammals would have survived and evolved, for the ready migration of maternal lymphocytes into the fetus would have opened up the possibility of widespread destruction of fetuses by an immunologic response against paternally inherited antigens. Clearly this did not and does not happen. What is more there would have been a corollary, in that even if some other mechanisms had prevented the destruction of the fetus, the latter would have developed immunologic tolerance to maternal histocompatibility antigens – a possibility that has been looked for, but not found (see Chapter 5). The vascular anastomosis that is the rule between cattle dizygotic twins and that happens rarely between human fraternal twins is, by contrast, harmless because the fetal lymphocytes of each twin develop tolerance to the histocompatibility antigens of its partner, so that tolerance and cellular chimerism result (see Chapter 5).

Nonetheless, the accidental and local breakdown of the tissue barrier between the two circulations, however transient, could cause the mother to become sensitized to paternally inherited antigens, but even this need not be fatal to the fetus provided that the activated lymphocytes are unable to make their way across the placental membranes into the fetal circulation. This would appear to be the case, for first Mitchison (2) and after him many others have failed to prejudice the survival of fetal animal litters by previous sensitization of the mother with tissues of the paternal strain. Especially informative was a study by Lanman, Dinerstein and Fikrig (20) in 1962, in which they failed to impair the normal development of blastocysts transferred to the uteri of pseudopregnant rabbits powerfully presensitized by skin allografts obtained from both parents of the embryos. It must be concluded that the placenta does act as a fairly efficient barrier to lymphocytes and that it is not as porous as some have claimed.

Leaks of maternal blood into the human fetal circulation have, however, been recorded, both for radiolabeled red blood corpuscles (21) and leukocytes (22). What is more, Beer and Billingham (23) have shown that it is possible to bring about a condition indistinguishable from runt disease (graft-versus-host disease (GVHD), see Chapter 8) in the offspring of female rats sensitized either adoptively or actively against paternal antigens. This observation would seem to be a paradoxical in view of the failure of others to prejudice the survival of litters by similar means, but Beer and Billingham argued that previous data might have suffered from the fact that litters were not followed up for long enough and that the cell donors had usually been hyperimmunized, thus raising the possibility that protective (enhancing) antibodies had been induced. In their own experiments, in which about 50% of the offspring developed fatal GVHD within 45 days of birth, the cell donors in the adoptive transfer experiments had been given a skin graft from the paternal strain, followed by a single intraperitoneal dose of spleen cells. The effect depended upon the number of cells transferred, was antigen-specific, was markedly less when normal cells were transferred, and could be mimicked by active sensitization. Although it might be argued that sensitization of these rats was artificially powerful Beer and Billingham pointed out that "Careful clinical examination of infants failing to thrive has produced some excellent examples of runt disease" (24). Evidently the placental barrier, though generally effective, needs to be supplemented by other protective mechanisms.

Placental permeability to immunoglobulin G antibodies in many species is well known (25), and it is therefore just as well that humoral antibodies do not usually act as the principal mediators of allograft rejection (see Chapter 2).

Does Fetal Trophoblast Lack Paternal Antigens, or are they Masked?

The trophoblast is a more or less uninterrupted layer of fetal origin and it is the ultimate 'frontier' between the maternal and fetal blood circulation in many mammalian species. Much attention has therefore been focused on it, for a lack of paternally inherited histocompatibility antigens would at least partly explain the failure of maternal blood cells to be activated against the fetus. It was E. Witebsky and his colleagues (26, 27) who drew attention to the fact that human placental villi lack blood group antigens and who suggested the notion that if the trophoblast was non-antigenic the placenta might act as an effective barrier. This suggestion predated Medawar's 1953 paper by more than two decades and as it was not mentioned by him it must be assumed that he was unaware of it. Another suggestion came from Bardawil and Toy (28): the existence of a layer of fibrinoid material separating the maternal and fetal tissues where the invading trophoblast comes up against the maternal decidual tissue could form "an immunological no man's land, walling the fetus off from the chemical interaction with its host". In other words, the fibrinoid layer might mask the presence of antigens were they present on the trophoblast. Both these hypotheses were to derive experimental support but the latter was eventually abandoned.

Early studies

In 1962 Simmons and Russell (29) carried out an elegant study designed to answer the question of whether the trophoblast is non-immunogenic to the mother. Working with inbred strains of mice they separated early placental tissue at various stages of development from pregnant animals carrying F_1 hybrid fetuses. Small pieces of this tissue were then implanted under the kidney capsule of adult mice of the maternal strain to ascertain whether this provoked an immunologic response against the paternally derived antigens. They found that mid-gestational placenta, which contained fetal cells in addition to trophoblastic tissue, strongly sensitized the recipients and the paternal skin grafts were rejected in an accelerated fashion. When a similar experiment was conducted with tissue obtained from embryos seven days after implantation, when the fetal tissue could be cleanly separated from the ectoplacental cone (the trophoblastic rudiment), two quite distinct results were obtained. Fetal tissue was strongly destroyed in the presence of a mononuclear cell infiltrate, indicative of the presence of histocompatibility antigens, but the ectoplacental cones "survived well for their expected normal inherent life span". When fertilized eggs were similarly transplanted they found that the pure growth of trophoblast giant cells failed to incite a reaction even though the hosts had been presensitized against paternal antigens. Finally, they noted that the accidental inclusion of trophoblast cells in embryonic grafts transplanted to presensitized recipients left these cells unaffected, but their non-trophoblastic neighbors were destroyed. Simmons and Russell concluded "that histocompatibility antigens are either absent from trophoblastic giant cells or that they are not expressed in a manner which is appreciated on grafting . . .", and they argued that the trophoblast may therefore act as "an immunologic buffer zone between the mother and the fetus".

Later studies considerably muddied this attractively simple explanation. Many investigations on the antigenicity of the mouse trophoblast had been carried out with mice differing at multiple histocompatibility loci and with polyspecific antisera. They were therefore far from reliable, as Billington and Bell (30) pointed out in their 1983 review. Techniques involving the short-term culture of early mouse embryos and autoradiographic localization of binding sites for radiolabeled monoclonal antibodies have changed the picture substantially. It would seem that non-H-2 antigens are indeed expressed on trophoblast from an early stage (16, 31), that class II major MHC antigens are not expressed at all (32, 33) and that class I antigens, although present on diploid trophoblast cells of the early post-implantation embryo, are expressed only on certain trophoblast cells of the mature placenta (31, 34). According to Billington (35) in a fairly recent review of the role of the trophoblast, the giant cells of this tissue "have no expression of class I, nor probably class II, MHC antigens". He concluded that ". . . trophoblast nonantigenicity is no longer an acceptable hypothesis to explain the lack of immunologic rejection of the murine allogeneic conceptus and that there must be some other mechanism(s) to counteract any potentially deleterious maternal immune response". Nonetheless, the absence of class II antigens would presumably make the trophoblast a less immunogenic fetal tissue at the critical interface between maternal and fetal circulations.

Very similar conclusions have been drawn for the trophoblast of the rat. In the human placenta, in which maternal blood comes into direct contact with the syncytiotrophoblast, the situation appears to be different. Although work in the 1970s by Seigler and Metzgar (36), Goodfellow et al. (37), Faulk and Temple (38) and Faulk, Sanderson and Temple (39) strongly suggested that the syncytiotrophoblast of human chorionic villi lacked MHC antigens, this was disputed by Loke, Joysey and Borland (40) and others. The more sophisticated studies of the 1980s, making use of the monoclonal antibody technology, threw an entirely new light on the situation.

Modern investigations: human leukocyte antigen-G (HLA-G)

The more recent studies on what has proved to be a complex and controversial subject have recently been well reviewed by Sargent (41). The absence of HLA class II antigens has been wholly confirmed (42,43), trophoblast cells failing to stimulate maternal T lymphocytes. However, the question of class I antigen expression has proved to be more complex. Thus, Sunderland et al. (44), working in Oxford, found that HLA class I-specific antibodies reactive with HLA-A, B and C were not bound by syncytiotrophoblast and the underlying villous cytotrophoblast, but reacted strongly with the invasive extravillous cytotrophoblast in the placental bed and in the amniochorion (45). However, the possibility that these class I antigens might sensitize maternal lymphocytes through the indirect pathway of antigen presentation (see Chapter 2) was made unlikely by the observation that they lacked specificity for HLA-A, B or C, suggesting that they were structurally and immunologically different from the class I antigens found in other embryonic and adult cells. This has proved to be the case. The trophoblast class I antigen was found to differ biochemically (46, 47) and molecularly (48), in that it is non-polymorphic and has a lower molecular weight. It has been designated HLA-G (49), and it has recently been confirmed by Loke's group (50) that it is restricted to the extravillous cytotro-phoblast – that part of the fetal placenta in direct contact with maternal blood. As HLA-G appears to be unable to activate maternal T lymphocytes *in vitro* (51, 52) it could be a prime candidate for the "immunologic buffer zone" envisaged by Simmons and Russell (29) and others in the 1960s (but see footnote, p. 418.)

The latest research suggests that HLA-G may even have an immunoregulatory function, for it has been shown by Sanders, Giblin and Kavathas (53) that it can interact with CD8, the lymphocyte differentiation molecule that acts with the T cell receptor in peptide presentation by MHC class I molecules. These researchers have therefore proposed that it could serve as a recognition element by CD8-positive suppressor T lymphocytes and thus interfere with putative antifetal responses by the mother, especially if it were shed from the cell membrane in a soluble form. Regardless of whether this can be substantiated, Sargent's (41) conclusion that "The trophoblast forms the barrier between maternal and fetal cells and therefore plays a major role in preventing maternal immune rejection of the fetus" seems very persuasive. If some class I antigens are indeed expressed on the trophoblast, Wegmann's suggestion (54) that this layer acts as an immunosorbent barrier for potentially harmful cytotoxic antibodies would not seem in the least far-fetched.

The "masking" concept

This concept has been overtaken by modern developments and is of purely historic interest. It was first proposed by Bardawil and Toy (28, see above) in 1959 and was developed by another group working in Oxford led by D.R.S. Kirby (55), who provided detailed experimental evidence for the existence of a fibrinoid layer in the mouse placenta. They claimed that the majority of trophoblast cells were surrounded by a layer of amorphous electron-dense material, 0.1 to 2 µm in thickness, which was especially conspicuous around the trophoblastic giant cells. Schiebler and Knoop (56) had made a similar observation for the rat placenta a few years earlier. Kirby *et al.* stated that "the morphological evidence that this material overlies the free surface of the labyrinthine trophoblast bordering on the maternal lacunae is not so convincing. High resolution electon-micrographs, however, show a very thin, ill-defined, filamentous layer in this position". The material was mucoprotein in nature, "probably rich in hyaluronic and sialic acids" and resembled fibrinoid material found in other physiologic situations. There was more of it in F_1 hybrid placentae than in those of inbred strains, and Kirby *et al.* suggested that its existence might explain the survival and development of mouse blastocysts in extrauterine sites, where they produce a highly invasive trophoblast. Histochemically the fibrinoid seemed to bear a close resemblance to the material found in the cheek pouch of the hamster where it accounted, according to Billingham and Silvers (57), for the behavior of the sub-cutaneous layers of the cheek pouch as an immunologically privileged site. Kirby *et al.* thought that the fibrinoid "prevents the escape of foetal antigens into the maternal system" and suggested that its enzymatic removal might well reveal histocompati-bility antigens.

Two other British workers, G.A. Curry and K.D. Bagshawe, were attracted to the notion of masked antigens because of their interest in the immunogenicity of tumors, and in 1967 they proposed (58) that the sialomucin layer on trophoblast cells and on certain cancer cells acted in much the same way, affording protection through a high electronegative cell surface charge, and that removal of the layer should make cancer cells more vulnerable to immunologic attack. Their demonstration that this was the case (59) aroused much interest, but others were unable to substantiate their claims and the whole concept soon met with oblivion. This came about despite the demonstration by Curry (60) that pure mouse trophoblast treated with neuraminidase sensitized adult recipients against subsequently transplanted skin grafts, whereas untreated tissue did not. I was unable to find a single reference to the masking hypothesis in more than half a dozen reviews written since 1978, including one that was written by W.D. Billington (35), one of the co-authors of the 1964 *Nature* paper by Kirby *et al.* There is no convincing explanation for the remarkable rise and fall of what was undoubtedly an interesting and experimentally supported hypothesis.

And yet . . . ! It would appear that human trophoblast is relatively resistant to both antibody- and cell-mediated destruction unless it has been pretreated with neuraminidase or, alternatively, interferon-boosted natural killer cells are used (61, 62). Likewise, the trophoblast of the early ectoplacental cone of the mouse is relatively resistant to immune lysis, according to Jenkinson and Billington (63), though the same is not true once the trophoblast cells have developed histocompatibility antigens (64). Thus, as Billington (35) has pointed out, at least in the mouse the trophoblast is a potential target for immunologic attack in the later stages of pregnancy.

The Uterus as an Immunologically Privileged Site

In their extensive 1971 review on the immunobiology of reproduction, Beer and Billingham (15) stated that "despite considerable evidence that the success of fetuses qua homografts is dependent upon an ineffective expression of transplantation antigens by the trophoblast, whether any special immunologic dispensations apply to the uterus, at least at the site of implantation of conceptuses, is still equivocal". Nonetheless, even at that time there was some evidence against such "dispensations". For example, the Israeli immunobiologist M. Schlesinger (65) had transplanted small allogeneic tumor grafts into the uterine horns of rats and mice and found that they had short life-spans and that they were rejected in an accelerated fashion in presensitized female mice regardless of their pregnancy status. As Beer and Billingham pointed out (15), these results would have been invalidated if the allogeneic tumors had penetrated the myometrium. However, the same results were obtained when P.S. Russell's group (66) transplanted parathyroid tissue into the uterus, a finding that was criticized by Kirby (67) because of the inability of such grafts to provoke a decidual reaction.

The question was further examined by Beer, Billingham and Hoerr (68), who transplanted small allogeneic skin grafts to the uteri of estrogen-treated virgin female rats. Such grafts were rejected at the normal speed unless they were implanted into females during the preimplantation stage of pregnancy involving males of their own inbred strain, when they had a significantly prolonged survival. Although this did not apply to skin grafts transplanted to the chest, these experiments are somewhat difficult to interpret because local hormonal and quite nonspecific changes may have been operative. However, Beer, Billingham and Hoerr found that a decidual reaction did not prevent the accelerated rejection of skin allografts implanted into the uteri of presensitized animals and that they could be destroyed promptly by the adoptive transfer of sensitized lymphoid cells. "Thus, at best in rats", they concluded, "decidual tissue can only play a minor role in insuring the success of mammalian fetuses as homografts".

Physiologic and Immunologic Changes in the Pregnant Female

It has been suggested at various times that as a consequence of some interaction between the fetus and its mother, the latter generates protective mechanisms. These have included the production of blocking antibodies or antigen–antibody complexes (see Chapter 6), suppressor cells (see Chapter 6) and corticosteroid hormones and plasma proteins, either local or systemic. The trophoblast, too, has been implicated in the production of hormones that might have a protective effect in the extraordinarily complex placental tissues. The merits of such proposals will now be briefly discussed.

It appears to be reasonably well established that some elements of sensitization to paternal antigens can be found in at least some pregnant animals and women. This has been studied by Billington's group (see 35), who concluded that in mice antipaternal antibodies may be demonstrated in some but not all hybrid matings, that they tend to occur only in second or after multiple pregnancies, and that the antibodies react with a strictly limited number of MHC specificities and do not inhibit cellular *in vitro* responses.

In human pregnancy Jonker, Van Leeuwen and Van Rood (69) found that only a small fraction of primiparous women develop anti-HLA antibodies, and about half overall (i.e. regardless of parity). The evidence for antipaternal cell-mediated responses in pregnant mice (70) and women (71) is weak and that is undoubtedly good news for the mammalian fetus. In this context, it is of interest to note some studies carried out by Breyere and Barrett in the early 1960s, when they found that the survival of paternal skin (72) or tumor (73) grafts was markedly prolonged in multiparous mice, though the mechanism was not clarified (see below).

Are maternal immune responses weakened during pregnancy?

The work in the early 1950s showing that skin allografts enjoy a longer survival time in pregnant rabbits and guinea pigs (3–5) has already been alluded to. The responsiveness of pregnant animals and women has been much studied since, but the data that have emerged have conflicted and there is no consensus for the notion that a nonspecific weakening of the maternal immune system can account to any great extent for the survival of the fetus. Nonetheless, a number of immunosuppressive factors have been identified in the serum of pregnant women, from α-2-globulins and β-1-globulins to α-fetoprotein. The literature is voluminous and the claims often conflicting, and the reader is referred to Gill and Repetti's detailed and scholarly 1979 review (74). These molecules do appear to be able to block many *in vitro* reactions but their *in vivo* role, if any, is less certain. Much the same is true for corticosteroids, estrogens, progesterone and androgens, the latter being precursors of estrogens. To quote Gill and Repetti: "Thus, corticosteroids exert an inhibitory effect on mitogenic stimulation of human lymphoid cells *in vitro* at physiologic concentrations. However, it remains unclear whether this *in vitro* sensitivity suggests a possible modulatory role for corticosteroids *in vivo* ... The evidence is not supportive of the concept that estrogens are effective inhibitors of the immune response ... A variety of studies are not wholly compatible with the implication that progestational agents possess immunosuppressive properties," and they noted that these hormones can stimulate as well as depress some immunologic functions". As for androgens: "Although it appears unlikely that the major androgens exert an immunosuppressive effect at physiologic concentrations, it remains possible that other derivatives or metabolites may possess immunoregulatory properties".

As Staples and Heap (75) concluded after a careful survey of the role of steroids and proteins during pregnancy in sheep: "The evidence for an indispensable role of hormones in immunoprotection of the conceptus must still be regarded as circumstantial ...".

Possibly of greater relevance are hormones secreted in the placental tissue itself or in the uterus, where they can potentially act locally and achieve higher concentrations. Among such protein hormones are human chorionic gonadotrophin (HCG) and human placental lactogen (HLP), both secreted by cells of the trophoblast, and the prostaglandins (74). The levels of all these tend to increase as pregnancy proceeds. They can all be detected in the maternal serum and have been found to be immunosuppressive *in vitro*. Their natural biologic *in vivo* role has been difficult to ascertain. Although far more has become known about pregnancy hormones since 1953, Medawar's (1) conclusion that "the hearing is still in progress, and the verdict has yet to be returned" seems as valid now as it was then. Indeed, the failure to pin down hormonal influences as a prime protective influence would suggest that they do not play a highly significant role. However, any level of nonspecific immunosuppression at the placental interface must be regarded as helpful.

Specific Immunoregulation

The notion that specific (i.e. antipaternal) antibodies demonstrable in the serum of pregnant mice might contribute to the protection of fetuses was first developed by Hellström, Hellström and Brawn (76), when they showed that maternal sera blocked *in vitro* reactivity to paternal antigens. Blocking antibodies or antigen–antibody complexes have been discussed in Chapters 5 and 6; they were very fashionable in the 1970s as mediators of hyporesponsiveness before they were displaced by suppressor T lymphocytes as one of the key mechanisms capable of ensuring specific non- or hyporeactivity.

The observation that antipaternal antibodies can result from pregnancy was far from new, for in 1958 Van Rood, Eernisse and Van Leeuwen (77) (see also Chapter 4) had used the sera of multiparous women to demonstrate antileukocyte antibodies with specificity for paternal HLA. Human pregnancy sera with specific inhibitory effects on the mixed lymphocyte culture reaction were later described by Greenberg, Reinsmoen and Yunis (78), Robert, Betuel and Revillard (79) and Brochier, Roitt and Festenstein (80). Antibodies with similar specificity have been eluted from human placentae (81), and Wegmann, Singh and Carlson (82) and others after them have shown experimentally that alloantibodies can be selectively absorbed by antigens in the placenta. Relevant is the finding by Rocklin *et al.* (83) that some women who had experienced chronic abortions lacked blocking factors in their serum. The implication was that such blocking factors or antibodies were akin to the antibodies that are known to bring about a state of specific hyporeactivity known as enhancement (see Chapter 6). Such antibodies were demonstrated in pregnant mice by many workers, including Voisin and Chaouat (84), who also showed that maternal antibodies are normally absorbed by the trophoblast cells of the placenta. The eluted antibodies had the power to bring about the specific enhancement of tumor allografts of the paternal strain.

Head and Billingham (85) compared the effects of multiple syngeneic and allogeneic pregnancies in rats: the latter weakened the capacity of the mothers to produce antipaternal alloantibodies and to reject paternal skin allografts. This weakening appeared to be largely mediated by the draining para-aortic lymph nodes and the source of the antigenic stimulus was shown to be the trophoblast. However, despite so much evidence in favor of blocking antibodies, Redman, Sargent and Sutton (86) concluded that "The major problem is that if blocking antibodies are defined by their action on maternal–fetal/panertal mixed lymphocyte reaction then they are found in only half the sera of parous women" (68) and they are present in only a small fraction of women undergoing their first pregnancy. "Consequently it cannot be argued that they are essential for normal pregnancy. This is the key issue."

Among other pregnancy-induced antibodies with immunoregulatory properties are anti-idiotypic antibodies as described by Suciu-Foca *et al.* (87), and antibodies to antigens restricted to the placental trophoblast have also been described. The existence of trophoblast-specific antigens was first mooted by Hulka, Hsu and Beiser (88). Following the subsequent identification of such antigens by Searle and Jenkinson (89), Davies and Browne (90, 91) have been able to study the kinetics of antibodies formed against them during the course of first and second human pregnancies. The titers were lower in second pregnancies, and reduced titers during the second and third trimesters appeared to be due to the formation of antigen–antibody complexes from which five trophoblastic proteins of differing molecular weight could be isolated (92).

It was thought that antitrophoblast antibodies might play a role in protecting the fetus, a hypothesis first put forward by Faulk *et al.* (93) on the strength of a non-MHC antigen system that, being cross-reactive between trophoblast and lymphocytes, they termed TLX. Taylor and Faulk (94) and Faulk and McIntyre (95) have developed from this and other observations the concept that maternal recognition of non-MHC trophoblast antigens followed by antibody formation holds the key to successful pregnancy, and that an absence of such recognition explains the occurrence of recurrent spontaneous abortions (see below). A similar approach was followed by Beer *et al.* (96) in the same year (1981). Possible immunologic mechanisms for recurrent abortions are discussed briefly below. It is, however, first necessary to mention yet another possible immunoregulatory mechanism of pregnancy – suppressor T lymphocytes. These have been discussed in the context of allotransplantation and tolerance in Chapters 5 and 6.

Fetal mouse liver and splenic T lymphocytes have been shown to be capable of suppressing immune responses, an activity that has been reviewed by Gill and Repetti (74). The Israelis Umiel and Trainin (97) found that fetal or neonatal liver cells prevented subsequently inoculated adult spleen cells from mounting an *in vivo* graft-versus-host reaction when transferred into lethally irradiated F_1 hybrid adult mice. This was further elucidated by Globerson, Zinkernagel and Umiel (98). Fetal and neonatal liver cells suppressed both *in vitro* MLRs and CML assays, regardless of whether the liver cells were syngeneic or unrelated to the stimulator cells. Commencing in 1983, D.A. Clark and his colleagues (99, 100) in Canada systematically studied the question of active, antigen-specific suppression by T lymphocytes in the uterus, and they concluded that such cells play an important role in making the trophoblast resistant to immune attack *in vivo*. Their studies were carried out in the mouse but they believed that similar events occur in the human uterus. Although conclusive evidence may be hard to come by, it would seem that suppressor cells provide yet another safeguard against the destruction of the mammalian fetus.

Tolerance in Pregnancy?

Some of the evidence quoted (3–5) suggested that pregnant animals are hyporesponsive but that this is not specific to the paternal antigens. The work mentioned in the preceding section suggests that highly specific events can likewise take place, such as the induction of suppressor T lymphocytes. According to a very recent paper by Tafuri *et al.* (101) from Heidelberg, Germany, maternal mouse T cells acquire a transient tolerance for the paternal alloantigens. This was revealed through the use of mice transgenic for a T cell receptor to the MHC H-2Kb histocompatibility antigen, allowing the authors to follow the fate of T cells reactive to the paternal antigens. Thus, mice bearing a Kb-positive conceptus had reduced numbers of Kb-reactive T cells and accepted Kb-positive tumor grafts, but this was not the case with syngeneic or third-party allogeneic pregnancies. Normal T cell profiles and responsiveness returned after delivery of the litters. This transient tolerance, which in terms of mechanisms seems to be akin to partial clonal deletion, may prove to be another safety device provided by evolutionary processes, and Tafuri *et al.* make the interesting suggestion that it could also "in part explain why certain autoimmune diseases, such as multiple sclerosis and rheumatoid arthritis, undergo remission during pregnancy, apparently in the absence of general immunosuppression". It is possible that the significant changes recorded by A.G. Clarke (102) during the course of pregnancy in the mouse bear on the development of tolerance.

As G.M. Stirratt (103) stated, "there is little firm evidence that pregnant women are more susceptible to infectious diseases" (see 104) and specific immunoregulatory mechanisms such as antigen–antibody complexes, suppressor cells or the development of tolerance would not be in conflict with such clinical observations.

Recurrent Spontaneous Abortions: Do they have an Immunologic Cause?

A surprisingly high proportion of human pregnancies – 15% – end spontaneously in abortion, an estimate made by Roth (*105*) more than three decades ago but which seems to have been, if anything, an underestimate. The more recent estimate by Edmonds (*106*) puts the figure as high as 60%, the conceptuses being lost before the fourth week of gestation and therefore freqently unrecognized. Until fairly recently the causes of abortion were unknown although various possibilities, from infection to endocrine disturbances, were put forward. There were, however, some interesting straws in the wind resulting from experimental rodent studies in the 1960s and 1970s, mainly in the United Kingdom. For example, Billington (*107*), quickly confirmed by James (*108*), found that dissimilarity between the MHC antigens of mouse mothers and fetuses affected the size of the placenta. Michie and Anderson (*109*) showed that in the rat there are intense intrauterine selective pressures against fetuses that are homozygous with their mothers, and Palm (*110*) in the United States a decade or so later described the selective elimination of rat MHC homozygotes either prenatally or soon after birth as a result of maternal–fetal MHC compatibility. She also noted abnormalities in lymphoid development in affected individuals and thought that her observations had an immunologic basis. Beer, Scott and Billingham (*111*) made a careful study of this phenomenon. They confirmed that "allogeneic placentae" were heavier than syngeneic ones, presensitization of mothers against paternal antigens led to heavier placentae compared with those of normal females, and mothers that had been made specifically tolerant to paternal antigens had smaller placentae. They undermined the "classic notion" that the observed effects were brought about by hybrid vigor by means of experiments involving the transfer of parental or hybrid blastocysts into genetically tolerant hybrid females, the placentae being of the same size. "Maternal immunologic reactivity against the fetus qua allograft may make a significant contribution here", they wrote. Among their other findings was that genetic disparity between conceptus and mother significantly improved its chances of implantation and survival.

The work of Faulk's group (*94, 95*) from 1981 made it even more plausible that for a pregnancy to continue normally, positive recognition by the maternal immune system of trophoblast antigens is a necessary prerequisite, although they had non-MHC antigens in mind. It was postulated that if the trophoblast–lymphocyte cross-reacting (TLX) antigens were shared by the father and the mother, such recognition could not occur and abortion would follow. The clinical attempts to rectify this by active immunization were founded on a somewhat flimsy theoretic foundation, but it was subsequently established that HLA (not TLX!) compatibility is higher in couples with a history of recurrent abortions than in couples who face no such problems (*112*). Furthermore, the analysis by Thomas et al. (*113*) indicated that couples with a history of abortion have a greater incidence of HLA-B and DR antigen sharing. This observation could provide the basis for a genetic interpretation involving homozygosity for recesssive MHC-linked genes; alternatively, it could lend further support to the immunologic hypothesis.

It is against this conceptual background that some tentative clinical attempts to overcome the problem of recurrent abortions by active immunization of mothers commenced in 1981. Two groups were involved – Taylor and Faulk (*94*) in the United kingdom and Beer et al. (*96*) in the United States – but the strategy adopted by them was different. Taylor and Faulk chose three women with three previous abortions who shared some, but by no means all, HLA antigens with their husbands. On the assumption that an immune response against the "trophoblast/lymphocyte cross-reactive (TLX) antigens" needed to be induced, the women were repeatedly transfused with leukocyte-enriched plasma from "at least 16 different erythrocyte-compatible donors". Each woman produced a healthy baby. The discussion concerning the possible involvement of HLA and TLX antigens was sufficiently opaque as to leave the interpretation open although the authors seemed to favor a role for the putative TLX antigens. This small-scale clinical trial was not in any way controlled, and it was not possible to rule out that the 'tender loving care' bestowed on the women may have been a contributory, or even the sole, factor.

The trial by Beer et al. (96) was part of a more general study of HLA compatibility between husband and wife and the effect this had on the mixed lymphocyte culture reaction, using the woman's lymphocyte as responders and the husband's as stimulators or vice versa. All had a history of recurrent chronic abortions. The subjects were divided into two groups – those with no known causes for the abortions and those "in whom an etiology had been demonstrated". The former shared more HLA-A, B, and D/DR antigens than the latter and were specifically less responsive to their husbands' cells, though there was great variability. Three couples sharing A, B and D/DR antigens and hyporesponsive in MLR were selected for therapy. This time blood leukocytes from the husband were injected intradermally into the wife, and six months later the MLR tests were repeated. The reactivity of two remained unchanged, whereas one had a stronger response. Two of the women, including the one whose MLR response had been enhanced, became pregnant, and at the time of publication one healthy baby had been born and the other was in a normal mid-term pregnancy. The authors of this study, which again was small and uncontrolled, concluded that "genetic homozygosity with regard to MHC antigens . . . is associated with reproductive inefficiency. At the present time we are not able to link this inefficiency comfortably with alterations in immune responses on the part of the woman during pregnancy . . .".

Having published some encouraging preliminary findings (114), which did not, however, confirm HLA sharing and hyporesponsiveness as prerequisites of recurrent spontaneous abortions, Mowbray et al. (115) in London presented their data from a large controlled double-blind trial. Successful pregnancy was significantly more common in women injected intravenously and intradermally with purified lymphocytes from their husbands (77%) compared with women who, unknown to themselves, had received their own lymphocytes (37%). An absence of cytotoxic antibodies was one of the criteria for entry into the trial but the majority of women in the experimental group made antibodies following sensitization. Although this would seem to be a very remarkable result it needs to be seen in the context of an earlier study in which women who had had recurrent spontaneous abortions and received counseling and psychologic support had a pregnancy success rate of 86% compared with 33% in women who had not been given this treatment (116). The results are astonishingly similar. Nonetheless, success rates for ten leukocyte immunization trials reported between 1981 and 1991 showed a very impressive consistency, according to Sargent's summary (117).

Psychologic factors can certainly be discounted in the treatment of spontaneous abortion in two mouse models described by Clark, McDermott and Szewczuk (118) and Chaouat and Clark (119), for in both strain combinations immunization against paternal antigens lowered the abortion rate (120, 121). Here the induction of suppressor cells seems to have been an important factor.

The mechanisms of recurrent spontaneous abortion and its prevention by immunization of the mother have yet to be fully unraveled, and non-immunologic mechanisms have been postulated by some. The story is further complicated by the data of Sargent, Wilkins and Redman (122), who found no evidence for either maternal cell-mediated or humoral antibody activity in normal pregnancy or in recurrent aborters, and no correlation between the production of cytotoxic antibodies and serum blocking activity. And there are some (117) who continue to harbor doubts as to the justification and safety of immunization procedures.

Conclusion

The study of the survival of the mammalian fetus in the face of a potentially hostile immunologic environment has yielded an immense amount of information and a plethora of hypotheses since Medawar's analysis in 1953. Because of the profundity and complexity of the problems posed it is perhaps not surprising that no definitive resolution has been achieved. What has become evident is that evolutionary processes have established a number of safeguards, the most important of which are the separation of maternal and fetal bloodstreams and the unique characteristics of the fetal trophoblast – the layer that is at the cutting edge of whatever interactions take place between the mother and fetus.

It is a matter of some interest that a quite disproportionate number of British workers have been drawn into the field of developmental immunobiology since Medawar's seminal paper in 1953 (1) – from Billingham, who has himself made so many salient contributions and who has been instrumental in establishing the American school of developmental immunobiology, right down to the present day, when a number of active groups together with their colleagues in other countries are continuing the quest for the solution of nature's highly successful if puzzling experiment.

When this chapter had been completed my attention was drawn to a newly published review by P. Parham (123) in which he expressed some doubt about the role of HLA-G in fetal protection. His skepticism was based mainly on the finding that this monomorphic molecule has not yet been identified in non-primate species, "suggesting that HLA-G is not an essential part of what it is to be a mammal. Instead it seems possible ... that recognizable HLA-G-like genes arose after divergence of the lineages leading to rodents and humans... Let us now play devil's advocate and contend that HLA-G is not a protector of fetuses but a retired classical antigen-presenting molecule that by chance has been exiled to the trophoblast". Parham's reservations do not, however, exclude the possibility that HLA-G nonetheless plays a protective role in primates with their long gestation periods and small number of offspring.

References

1. Medawar, P.B. (1953) *Symp. Soc. Exp. Biol.* **7**, 320.
2. Mitchison, N.A. (1953) *J. Genet.* **51**, 406.
3. Billingham, R.E., Krohn, P.L. & Medawar, P.B. (1951) *Brit. Med. J.* **1**, 1157.
4. Morgan, J.A. (1951) *Surgery* **30**, 506.
5. Sparrow, E.M. (1953) *J. Endocrinol.* **9**, 101.
6. Billingham, R.E., Krohn, P.L. & Medawar, P.B. (1951) *Brit. Med. J,* **2**, 1049.
7. Heslop, R.W., Krohn, P.L. & Sparrow, E.M. (1954) *J. Endocrinol.* **10**, 325.
8. Little, C.C. (1924) *J. Cancer Res.* **8**, 75.
9. Woodruff, M.F.A. (1957) *Proc. Roy. Soc. B* **148**, 68.
10. Hašková, V. (1959) *Folia Biol. (Praha)* **6**, 54.
11. Terasaki, P.I. (1959) *J. Embryol. Exp. Morph.* **7**, 409.
12. Möller, G. (1963) *J. Immunol.* **90**, 271.
13. Möller, G. (1961) *J. Immunol.* **86**, 56.
14. Edidin, M. (1964) *Transplantation* **2**, 627.
15. Beer, A.E. & Billingham, R.E. (1971) *Adv. Immunol.* **14**, 1.
16. Billington, W.D., Jenkinson, E.J. & Searle, R.F. (1977) *Transpl. Proc.* **9**, 1371.
17. Sutton, L. Mason, D.Y. & Redman, C.W. (1983) *Immunology* **49**, 103.
18. Haynes, B.F., Scearce, R.M., Lobach, D.M. *et al.* (1984) *J. Exp. Med.* **159**, 1149.
19. Beer, A.E. & Billingham, R.E. (1976) *The Immunobiology of Mammalian Reproduction*, Prentice-Hall Inc., Englewood Cliffs, N.J.
20. Lanman, J.T., Dinerstein, J. & Fikrig, S. (1962) *Ann. N.Y. Acad. Sci.* **99**, 706.
21. Zarou, D.M., Lichtman, H.C. & Hellman, L.M. (1964) *Am. J. Obstet. Gynec.* **88**, 565.
22. Desai, R.G. & Creger, W.P. (1963) *Blood* **21**, 665.
23. Beer, A.E. & Billingham, R.E. (1973) *Science* **179**, 240.
24. Kadowaki, J-I., Zuelzer, W.W., Brough, A.S. *et al.* (1965) *Lancet* **2**, 1152.
25. von Brambell, F.W.R. (1966) *Lancet* **2**, 1087.
26. Oettingen, Kj. & Witebsky, E. (1928) *München. Med. Wchschr.* **75**, 385.
27. Witebsky, E. & Reich, H. (1932) *Klin. Wchschr.* **11**, 1960.
28. Bardawil, W.A. & Toy, B.L. (1959) *Ann. N.Y. Acad. Sci.* **80**, 197.
29. Simmons, R.L. & Russell, P.S. (1962) *Ann. N.Y. Acad. Sci.* **99**, 717.
30. Billington, W.D. & Bell, S.C. (1983) In *Biology of the Trophoblast*, eds Y.W. Loke & A. Whyte, p. 571, Elsevier, Amsterdam.
31. Sellens, M.H., Jenkinson, E.J. & Billington, D. (1978) *Transplantation* **25**, 173.
32. Jenkinson, E.J. & Searle, R.F. (1979) *J. Reprod. Immunol.* **1**, 3.
33. Chatterjee-Hasrouni, S. & Lala, P.K. (1981) *J. Immunol.* **127**, 2070.
34. Jenkins, E.J. & Owen, V. (1980) *J. Reprod. Immunol.* **2**, 173.
35. Billington, W.D. (1987) *Curr. Top. Develop. Biol.* **23**, 209.
36. Seigler, H.F. & Metzgar, R.S. (1970) *Transplantation* **9**, 478.
37. Goodfellow, P.N., Barnstable, C.J., Bodmer, W.F. *et al.* (1976) *Transplantation* **22**, 595.
38. Faulk, W.P. & Temple, A. (1976) *Nature* **262**, 799.
39. Faulk, W.P., Sanderson, A.R. & Temple, A. (1977) *Transpl. Proc.* **9**, 1379.
40. Loke, Y.W., Joysey, V.C. & Borland, R. (1971) *Nature* **232**, 403.
41. Sargent, I.L. (1996) In *Clinical Immunology*, ed. P.C. Sen Gupta, Oxford Univ. Press, Oxford.
42. Starkey, P.M. (1987) *J. Reprod. Immunol.* **11**, 63.
43. Giacomini, P., Tosi, S., Murgia, C. *et al.* (1994) *Hum. Immunol.* **39**, 281.
44. Sunderland, C.A., Naiem, M., Mason, D.Y. *et al.* (1981) *J. Reprod. Immunol.* **3**, 323.
45. Redman, C.W., McMichael, A.J., Stirrat, G.M. *et al.* (1984) *Immunology* **52**, 457.
46. Ellis, S.A., Sargent, I.L. & Redman, C.W. (1986) *Immunology* **59**, 595.
47. Kovats, S., Librach, C., Fisch, P. *et al.* (1991) In *Cellular and Molecular Biology of the Materno-Fetal Relationship*, eds G. Chaouat & J. Mowbray, p. 21, John Libbey, Paris.
48. Ellis, S.A., Palmer, M.S. & McMichael, A.J. (1990) *J. Immunol.* **144**, 731.
49. Kovats, S., Main, E.K., Librach, C. *et al.* (1990) *Science* **248**, 220.
50. Chumbley, G., King, A., Gardner, L. *et al.* (1994) *J. Reprod. Immunol.* **27**, 173.
51. Hunt, J.S., King, C.R. & Wood, G.W. (1984) *J. Reprod. Immunol.* **6**, 377.

52. Burt, D., Johnston, D., Rinke de Wit, T. *et al.* (1981) *Int. J. Cancer* (suppl.) **6**, 117.
53. Sanders, S.K., Giblin, P.A. & Kavathas, P. (1991) *J. Exp. Med.* **174**, 737.
54. Wegmann, T.G. (1981) *J. Reprod. Immunol.* **3**, 267.
55. Kirby, D.R.S., Billington, W.D., Bradbury, S. *et al.* (1964) *Nature* **204**, 548.
56. Schiebler, T.H. & Knoop, A. (1959) *Z. Zellforsch.* **50**, 494.
57. Billingham, R.E. & Silvers, W.K. (1962) In *Transplantation*, eds G.E.W. Wolstenholme & M.P. Cameron, p. 90, Ciba Found. Symp., J. & A. Churchill, London.
58. Curry, G.A. & Bagshawe, K.D. (1967) *Lancet* **1**, 708.
59. Curry, G.A. & Bagshawe, K.D. (1968) *Brit. J. Cancer* **22**, 843.
60. Curry, G.A. (1968) *Proc. Roy. Soc. Med.* **61**, 1206.
61. Paul, S. & Jailkhani, B. (1982) *Am. J. Reprod. Immunol.* **2**, 204.
62. Pross, H., Mitchell, H. & Werkmeister, J. (1985) *Am. J. Reprod. Immunol.* **8**, 1.
63. Jenkinson, E.J. & Billington, W.D. (1974) *J. Reprod. Fertil.* **41**, 403.
64. Smith, G. (1983) *J. Reprod. Immunol.* **5**, 39.
65. Schlesinger, M. (1962) *J. Nat. Cancer Inst.* **28**, 927.
66. Poppa, G., Simmons, R.L., David, D.S. *et al.* (1964) *Transplantation* **2**, 496.
67. Kirby, D.R.S. (1968) *Transplantation* **6**, 1005.
68. Beer, A.E., Billingham, R.E. & Hoerr, R.A. (1971) *Transpl. Proc.* **3**, 609.
69. Jonker, M., Van Leeuwen, A. & Van Rood, J.J. (1977) *Tissue Antigens* **9**, 246.
70. Smith, G. & Chappell, F. (1984) *Immunology* **52**, 49.
71. Sargent, I.L. & Redman, C.W.G. (1985) *J. Reprod. Immunol.* **7**, 95.
72. Breyere, E.J. & Barrett, M.K. (1960) *J. Nat. Cancer Inst.* **25**, 1405.
73. Breyere, E.J. & Barrett, M.K. (1961) *J. Nat. Cancer Inst.* **27**, 411.
74. Gill, T.J. & Repetti, C.F. (1979) *Am. J. Path.* **95**, 465.
75. Staples, L.D. & Heap, R.B. (1984) In *Immunological Aspects of Reproduction in Mammals*, ed. D.B. Crighton, p. 195, Butterworth, London.
76. Hellström, K.E., Hellström, I. & Brawn, J. (1969) *Nature* **224**, 914.
77. Van Rood, J.J., Eernisse, J.G. & Van Leeuwen, A. (1958) *Nature* **187**, 1735.
78. Greenberg, L.J., Reinsmoen, N. & Yunis, E.J. (1973) *Transplantation* **16**, 520.
79. Robert, M., Betuel, H. & Revillard, J.P. (1973) *Tissue Antigens* **3**, 39.
80. Brochier, J., Roitt, I.M. & Festenstein, H. (1974) *Eur. J. Immunol.* **4**, 709.
81. Doughty, R.W. & Gelsthorpe, K. (1976) *Tissue Antigens* **8**, 43.
82. Wegmann, T.G., Singh, B. & Carlson, G.A. (1979) *J. Immunol.* **122**, 270.
83. Rocklin, R.E., Kitzmiller, J.L., Carpenter, C.B. *et al.* (1976) *J. Exp. Med.* **295**, 1209.
84. Voisin, G.A. & Chaouat, G.J. (1974) *J. Reprod. Fertil.* (suppl.) **21**, 89.
85. Head, J.R. & Billingham, R.E. (76) *Transpl. Proc.* **8**, 267.
86. Redman, C.W.G., Sargent, I.L. & Sutton, L. (1987) In *Immunological Aspects of Reproduction in Mammals*, ed. D.B. Crighton, p. 219, Butterworths, London.
87. Suciu-Foca, N., Reed, E., Kung, P. *et al.* (1983) *Proc. Nat. Acad. Sci. U.S.A.* **80**, 830.
88. Hulka, J.F., Hsu, K.C. & Beiser, S.M. (1961) *Nature* **191**, 510.
89. Searle, R.F. & Jenkinson, E.J. (1978) *J. Embryol. Exp. Morph.* **43**, 147.
90. Davies, M. & Browne, C.M. (1985) *J. Reprod. Immunol.* **7**, 285.
91. Davies, M. & Browne, C.M. (1985) *J. Dev. Physiol.* **7**, 269.
92. Davies, M. (1985) *Clin. Exp. Immunol.* **61**, 406.
93. Faulk, W.P., Temple, A., Lovins, R.E. *et al.* (1978) *Proc. Nat. Acad. Sci. U.S.A.* **75**, 1947.
94. Taylor, C. & Faulk, W.P. (1981) *Lancet* **2**, 68.
95. Faulk, W.P. & McIntyre, J.A. (1983) *Immunol. Rev.* **75**, 139.
96. Beer, A.E., Quebbeman, J.F., Ayers, J.W. *et al.* (1981) *Am. J. Obstet. Gynec.* **141**, 987.
97. Umiel, T. & Trainin, N. (1975) *Eur. J. Immunol.* **5**, 85.
98. Globerson, A., Zinkernagel, R.M. & Umiel, T. (1975) *Transplantation* **20**, 480.
99. Clark, D.A., Slapsys, R., Croy, B. *et al.* (1983) In *Immunology of Reproduction*, eds T.G. Wegmann & T.J. Gill, p. 342, Oxford Univ. Press.
100. Clark, D.A., Chaput, A., Slapsys, R.M. *et al.* (1987) In *Immunoregulation and Fetal Survival*, eds T.J. Gill & T.G. Wegmann, p. 63, Oxford Univ. Press.
101. Tafuri, A., Alferink, J., Möller, P. *et al.* (1995) *Science* **270**, 630.

102. Clarke, A.G. (1984) In *Immunologic Aspects of Reproduction in Mammals*, ed. D.B. Crighton, p. 153, Butterworths, London.
103. Stirratt, G.M. (1994) *Brit. Med. J.* **308**, 1385.
104. Hart, C.A. (1988) *Clin. Immunol. Aller.* **2**, 735.
105. Roth, D.B. (1963) *Int. J. Fertil.* **8**, 431.
106. Edmonds, D.K. (1982) *Fertil. Steril.* **38**, 447.
107. Billington, W.D. (1964) *Nature* **202**, 317.
108. James, D.A. (1965) *Nature* **205**, 613.
109. Michie, D. & Anderson, N.F. (1966) *Ann. N.Y. Acad. Sci.* **129**, 88.
110. Palm, J. (1974) *Cancer Res.* **34**, 2061.
111. Beer, A.E., Scott, J.R. & Billingham, R.E. (1975) *J. Exp. Med.* **142**, 180.
112. Gill, T.J. (1983) *Transplantation* **35**, 1.
113. Thomas, M.L., Harger, J.H., Wagener, D.K. *et al.* (1985) *Am. J. Obstet. Gynec.* **151**, 1053.
114. Mowbray, J.F., Gibbings, C.R., Sidgwick, A.S. *et al.* (1983) *Transpl. Proc.* **15**, 896.
115. Mowbray, J.F., Gibbings, C., Liddell, H. *et al.* (1985) *Lancet* **1**, 942.
116. Stray-Pedersen, B. & Stray-Pedersen, S. (1984) *Am. J. Obstet. Gynec.* **148**, 140.
117. Sargent, I.L. (1992) In *The Human Placenta: a Guide for Clinicians and Scientists*, eds C.W.G. Redman, I.L. Sargent & P.M. Starkey, p. 414, Blackwell, Oxford.
118. Clark, D.A., McDermott, M. & Szewczuk, M.R. (1980) *Cell. Immunol.* **52**, 106.
119. Chaouat, G. & Clark, D.A. (1986) *J. Reprod. Immunol.* (suppl.) **1**, 135.
120. Chaouat, G., Kiger, N. & Wegmann, T.G. (1983) *J. Reprod. Immunol.* **5**, 389.
121. Clark, D.A., Chaput, A. & Tutton, D. (1986) *J. Immunol.* **136**, 166.
122. Sargent, I.L., Wilkins, T. & Redman, C.W.G. (1988) *Lancet* **2**, 109.
123. Parham, P. (1995) *Am. J. Reprod. Immunol.* **34**, 10.

11 The Interaction between Immunology and Transplant Surgery (and Other Matters)

"To deride the hope of progress is the ultimate fatuity, the last word in poverty of spirit and meanness of mind. There is no need to be dismayed by the fact that we cannot yet envisage a definitive solution of our problems, a resting-place beyond which we need not try to go."

P.B. Medawar, 1969

This quotation is taken from Peter Medawar's Presidential Address to the British Association, a body embracing the whole of science and whose role is to make scientific knowledge accessible to the general public in the United Kingdom. Medawar was therefore speaking as much to the layperson as to scientists themselves. The latter – and immunologists not least among them – would certainly subscribe to this statement. Indeed, its sentiments brilliantly summarize the intellectual and humane approach adopted by those in the field of transplantation, from the very early pioneers trying to understand and influence malignant tumor growth to workers such as Carrel and the many surgeons after him who had the dream of overcoming human disease by the transplantation of kidneys and other organs – not to mention immunologists probing the very frontiers of knowledge. The audacity of the early workers in making fundamental discoveries – vaccines, antibodies, complement, phagocytosis – and putting forward theories (*pace* Ehrlich's receptor hypothesis) is quite breathtaking, and those who have followed them have been equally imaginative and inventive. The progress made in both immunology and transplantation since the beginning of the century is by far their best testimonial.

Although it would be absurd to attempt to draw up a balance sheet as to which field influenced the other most profoundly, it is nonetheless worth discussing, in the light of the preceding ten chapters, how basic immunology, transplantation immunology and transplantation have related to each other. This is especially worthwhile because it has occasionally been asserted that immunologists have failed rather dismally in solving the problems of organ transplantation, meaning I think that the manifold models of transplantation tolerance in adult animals in particular, some of them highly impressive, have in the main not proved to be applicable to the clinic. In 1977, on the tenth anniversary of the foundation of The Transplantation Society, I (*1*) drew attention to the implied criticism by R.Y. Calne (*2*) when he wrote, in the same year: "Better immunosuppressive drugs with less toxicity may well be developed, and I would speculate that it is more than likely that clinical grafting will advance in this way rather than by the application of immunological research". In many respects it was a prophetic statement, except that he seemed to have overlooked the fact that the assessment of the putative immunosuppressive drugs' immunologic potential depended very much on input from immunologists! While at the time I conceded that there was a case to answer, my defense was that "... we may have to accept a time scale of progress that is greater than self-interest and our natural urge for human advance demand".

As will have been seen in Chapter 7, clinicians are beginning to realize that sometimes long-term organ graft recipients do become tolerant in that their grafts continue to survive even without immunosuppression. The wonder of it is that this is not a far more regular occurrence, bearing in mind the animal models (see Chapter 6). Furthermore, a beginning is being made to speed the process of tolerance induction by giving the patient, in addition to the organ, viable bone marrow cells to boost the level of donor chimeric cells in the patient's immune system. It is fair to say that this approach has its roots in the old observations of the Medawar group and of Monaco and his colleagues and many others (see Chapters 5 and 6) and has recently been revived by Starzl's enthusiastic advocacy (see Chapter 7 p. 330).

Transplantation immunologists are immunologists who have made it their business to study the immunologic basis of tissue and organ graft rejection and how to overcome it – simple enough stated baldly like this but in fact encapsulating one of the most fundamental problems in immunology. Although it is half a century since Billingham Brent and Medawar established acquired tolerance in fetal or neonatal mice and birds by the simple expedient of confronting them with viable allogeneic cells (see Chapter 5, p. 189), clinical tolerance remains something to strive for. Yet, the induction of a true specific tolerance in human beings would completely revolutionize not only organ and tissue transplantation, but the whole of medicine; it is therefore well worth waiting for! Transplantation immunologists are sometimes looked down upon by "pure" immunologists working with well-defined soluble antigens because of the applied nature of their art and because they have to grapple with problems that until very recently often could not be defined with precision. They are the workers at the coal face, so to speak, and often get blackened and bruised for their pains. For them cells that have the power to transfer tolerance to animals that have never seen the relevant histocompatibility antigens are, by definition, suppressor cells. Some purists would have it that such cells do not exist because a unique phenotype, different from that of helper or cytotoxic T lymphocytes, has not been found for them and no T cell gene rearrangement has been uncovered. However, agreement is now being reached that some T cells are immunoregulatory and it is the precise mechanism by which they operate that is still unresolved.

The early tumor and transplantation researchers did not consider themselves to be immunologists at all. How could they, when the immunologic basis of tumor and normal tissue rejection was not fully appreciated until the 1930s and 1940s? They were biologists or pathologists and sometimes geneticists by training, and even the fathers of immunology before and soon after the turn of the twentieth century thought of themselves as chemists or pathologists rather than immunologists. A.M. Silverstein (3) drew attention to the fact that Medawar and his immediate colleagues in the 1950s were all trained as zoologists, and although they clearly grappled with immunologic problems they did not regard themselves as professional immunologists until round about the mid-1950s, by which time tolerance had taken center place in immunologic theory. Earlier their main forum for the discussion of their discoveries had been provided by surgeons and physicians who hoped, sooner or later, to be able to transplant organs.

The Contribution of Transplantation Immunology to Basic Immunology

The debt owed by the transplantation immunologists to basic immunology is too well known to discuss here (see Chapter 1). The other side of this coin will now be briefly considered.

The first major input was Medawar's proof of the immunologic nature of skin allograft rejection in rabbits (see Chapter 2, p. 71), followed by the discovery of immunologic tolerance (see Chapter 5, p. 188). Tolerance was quickly incorporated into the latest theories of antibody formation and it became a central plank of Burnet's clonal selection hypothesis (see Chapter 1, p. 29). This development gave immunology a new direction in that it turned away from its preoccupation with the physical chemistry of antibodies and redirected towards events at the cellular level. Together with the earlier work of Chase and Landsteiner, Mitchison and the Medawar team were instrumental in establishing the cellular school of immunology when they showed that immunity to tumor and skin allografts could be adoptively transferred to animals that had never "seen" the relevant histocompatibility antigens before. Cellular immunology became a dominant field of study in the 1950s and 1960s and it was to lead to the full appreciation of the importance of lymphocytes and their subpopulations. At the same time the work with skin grafts provided immunology with yet another clinical focus and objective and it added a certain glamor to its somewhat staid image.

With the revival of antilymphocyte serum (see Chapter 6, p. 252) immunologists were provided with a powerful biologic immunosuppressive agent that allowed them to study responsiveness in T lymphocyte-depleted animals and to examine lymphocyte kinetics in a new way. Perhaps it would be pursuing the argument too far by claiming that Miller's discovery of the function of the thymus was carried out with the aid of skin allografts! But arguably the most profound contribution transplantation immunology has made to basic immunology was through the discovery of the histocompatibility antigens. This exciting story has been described in detail in Chapter 4. It was knowledge of the existence and complexity of these molecules, known at first as transplantation antigens, that the phenomenon of major histocompatibility complex (MHC)-restriction became recognized (Chapters 1 and 4), the precise interactions between cells of the immune system became understood and the physical basis of peptide presentation became clear (see Chapters 1 and 4). The study of histocompatibility antigens in patients with a variety of diseases also led to the realization that there are a large number of associations between human leukocyte antigens (HLA) and infectious or autoimmune diseases.

There are, I expect, other hidden benefits. For example Festenstein's Mls antigens were later recognized to be powerful 'superantigens' (see Chapter 4, p. 146), the minor histocompatibility antigens contributed to an understanding of the role of other minor antigens such as those of viruses, and the proliferation of monoclonal antibodies derived a considerable impetus from transplantation immunologists anxious to study the impact of such antibodies on cells and molecules (such as cytokines) involved in the rejection process.

The Impact of the Surgeons

It is seen in Chapter 7 that the first surgeons to attempt renal transplantation in the modern era, that is in the 1950s, did so in a climate of opinion that was on the whole ranged against such a daring venture. The immunologic basis of allograft rejection had by then been firmly established in a wide range of experimental animals; and it had likewise been demonstrated with human skin grafts by Conway *et al.* (4) and Converse, Rapaport and their colleagues (5, 6) (see also Chapter 2). The immunologic barrier to the clinical transplantation of allografts was therefore seen as formidable and even awesome: here was a fundamental barrier that only the induction of tolerance in immunologically immature rodents had succeeded in breaching. Attempts to transplant allogeneic kidneys into patients without recourse to immunosuppression had all failed even though the patient's uremia could be immunosuppressive and sometimes result in surprisingly long survival times. No wonder the Peter Bent Brigham group decided to conduct their first serious attempt in identical twins (see Chapter 7, p. 307), mainly to establish the technique and to demonstrate that a patient can live happily with a transplanted kidney.

Although neonatally induced tolerance was an important influence, those involved in its discoveries suffered from no illusions as to its clinical applicability. Thus Calne (7) likes to tell the story of how a medical student asked Medawar after a lecture in Oxford on the subject of tolerance whether he thought that it had any application, and how Medawar replied "Absolutely none!". The only guidance to surgeons in the mid-1950s came from the field of radiobiology, which had succeeded in creating allogeneic and even xenogeneic cellular chimeras with the aid of lethal doses of X-irradiation and bone marrow transplantation. The use of whole body irradiation in sublethal doses, or in lethal doses accompanied by bone marrow infusions, was therefore a great act of faith and courage on the part of the Paris and Boston surgeons. The fact that some patients survived the treatment and sustained a functional kidney for varying periods provided the spur for further attempts when azathioprine became available in the early 1960s, and the modest successes undoubtedly encouraged transplantation immunologists and immunogeneticists to redouble their efforts.

The Contribution of Transplantation Immunology to Clinical Transplantation

Although it is true that the three drugs that have had a major impact on organ transplantation and that have been mainly responsible for the steady improvement in clinical results in the last three decades – azathioprine, cyclosporine and FK 506 – have been discovered in the context of screening programs for cytostatic drugs, their immunologic potential was discovered by immunologists. Generally it was only when these drugs had been shown to be powerfully immunosuppressive in suppressing antibody production, delayed-type hypersensitivity reactions, graft-versus-host responses and/or skin allograft rejection in rodents that they were applied to organ grafts in dogs and in patients. It would therefore be wrong to exclude immnunologists from the triumphs of immunosuppression, though this does not in the least detract from the ingenuity of the chemists who isolated and/or synthesized the drugs, and the astonishing courage of the surgeons (and their early patients!) in applying them.

Although the modern era of antilymphocyte serum was initiated by a surgeon, M.F.A. Woodruff, the extensive animal work that led to its use in clinical transplantation was largely the work of immunologists (see Chapter 6). The monoclonal antibodies that are used not only in research but also diagnostically and therapeutically (see Chapter 7, p. 33) were developed thanks to the work of Kohler (immunologist) and Milstein (biochemist).

Although there had been great hopes in the 1960s that tissue typing would make a major contribution to the solution of the clinical problem it is true that these hopes have not been realized. At the same time it must be said that in arguing the case against tissue typing, it would be foolish to throw out the baby with the bathwater! Thus there is no doubt at all that tissue matching is a great bonus when transplanting kidneys from living related donors (see Chapter 4), that it is of some importance in corneal transplantation and that it is an indispensable prerequisite in bone marrow transplantation (see Chapter 8). It also encouraged the establishment of large organ-sharing pools on both sides of the Atlantic and these have made a considerable impact on the supply of organs. Even now, most centers will choose an organ that is reasonably compatible with the putative recipient, especially if there is a positive cross-match as in presensitized patients, unless the clinical condition of the patient demands immediate transplantation.

The blood transfusion effect, first discovered by Opelz and Terasaki (see Chapter 7, p. 323), improved the renal transplantation results in many centers during the azathioprine era, though it seems to be true that the effect has diminished almost to a point of no return in the cyclosporine and FK 506 eras. Immunosuppression has become so effective that the blood transfusion effect has been almost squeezed out, so to speak. Nonetheless, not a few patients owe the good functioning of their kidneys to this effect, the basic mechanisms of which are still under active consideration.

There are three other ways in which immunology has benefitted clinical transplantation.

(1) The discovery of graft-versus-host disease (see Chapter 8, p. 347) by immunobiologists provided the all-important warning against clinical therapy involving the transplantation of tissues rich in lymphoid cells, such as allogeneic bone marrow, until such time as this life-threatening phenomenon could be overcome by one means or another.

(2) The proof of the immunologic basis of graft rejection and its detailed study is one of the success stories of transplantation immunology and it is doubtful that without that knowledge modern organ transplantation would have been carried out, even though this knowledge pointed to the difficulties that lay ahead.

(3) And finally, the recent attempts to augment the microchimerism described in organ recipients has its roots in experiments in rodents, in which functional tolerance is frequently accompanied by persistent cellular chimerism (see Chapter 7, p. 329).

Other Matters

There are two issues that I have not aired in these pages, except in passing. First, the many ethical problems facing transplant surgeons. These include the criteria of brain death in the use of cadaveric donors, the risks to the donor – however small – when transplanting living related kidneys, the future use of xenogeneic organs, the indefensible removal of organs from executed prisoners in at least one country, and the trade in organs in some Asian countries that encourages unrelated donors to offer a kidney for payment. So far as the last of these is concerned, the Indian Parliament is to be applauded for passing a bill recently outlawing trade in human organs (8) and it is to be hoped that other countries will follow suit.

The other issue is the extent to which so-called animal rights campaigners have disrupted experimental work with animals in many developed countries and the impact this has had on research. Unfortunately both these problems are beyond the scope of this book.

I hope that those who have read this book will agree that astonishing advances have been made during the course of the twentieth century in our understanding of the complex events following allo- and xeno-transplantation. The participants and their allies in basic immunology have every right to feel proud of what has been achieved. It is to be hoped that the rate of progress will not be slowed down by the regrettable modern tendency to patent discoveries and to form limited companies.

References

1. Brent, L. (1977) (Presidential address) *Transpl. Proc.* **9**, 1343.
2. Calne, R.Y. (1977) *Brit. Med. Bull.* **32**, 107.
3. Silverstein, A.M. (1989) *A History of Immunology*, p. 290, Academic Press, New York.
4. Conway, H., Joslin, D., Rees, T.D. *et al.* (1952) *J. Plast. Reconstr. Surg.* **9**, 557.
5. Converse, J.M. & Rapaport, F.T. (1956) *Ann. Surg.* **143**, 306.
6. Rapaport, F.T., Thomas, L., Converse, J.M. *et al.* (1960) *Ann. N.Y. Acad. Sci.* **87**, 217.
7. Calne, R.Y. (1991) In *History of Transplantation. Thirty-five Recollections*, ed. P.I. Terasaki, p. 229, U.C.L.A. Tissue Typing Laboratory, Los Angeles.
8. Editorial article (1994) *Brit. Med. J.* **308**, 1657.

Subject Index

Author Index

Page numbers in **bold** type indicate biographies; pages on which references appear in full are in *italic* type